PHYSIOLOGY OF EXERCISE AND SPORT

PHYSIOLOGY OF EXERCISE AND SPORT

BRUCE J. NOBLE, Ph.D.

Professor
School of Physical and Health Education
University of Wyoming
Laramie, Wyoming

With 165 illustrations

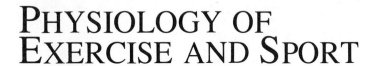

Times Mirror/Mosby College Publishing
St. Louis • Toronto • Santa Clara   1986

MOSBY

A TRADITION OF PUBLISHING EXCELLENCE

Editor: Nancy K. Roberson
Developmental editor: Michelle A. Turenne, Kathy Sedovic
Editing supervisor: Elaine Steinborn
Manuscript editor: Mike Molloy
Book design: Nancy Steinmeyer
Cover design: Christine Leonard Raquepaw
Production: Jeanne A. Gulledge, Ginny Douglas

Library of Congress Cataloging in Publication Data

Noble, Bruce J.
  Physiology of exercise and sport.

  Includes index.
   1. Sports—Physiological aspects. 2. Exercise—
Physiological aspects. I. Title.
RC1235.N63   612'.044   85-29702
ISBN 0-8016-3711-2

A/VH/VH   9 8 7 6 5 4 3 2 1   03/D/316

To
SALLY, BRUCE, MARJORIE, AND JOHN

For providing, over the past thirty years,
the purpose and sustenance of life

PREFACE

As I began this book, my mind ran back 25 years to the first course I took in the "science" of physical education. I was a political science major who had for 3 years in college resisted following in my father's footsteps as a physical educator and coach. My resistance had been partially based on my belief that the field lacked a scientific base or mechanisms to achieve such a base. Thanks to the enthusiasm, intelligence, and guidance of Wayne Van Huss, my beliefs were changed, and my career was vaulted into an orbit that persists to this day. My personal goals continue to center on a desire to discover and teach about this scientific base of physical education.

The audience

This book has been written with undergraduate physical education majors as the primary target audience. Most students do not have extensive training in science and mathematics. Therefore this book assumes that the reader is without this extensive previous scientific training and needs to address the question of "How is exercise physiology of practical importance to the teacher, coach, and exercise specialist?"

The importance of exercise physiology

Answers to the question of why the study of exercise physiology is important will be a continuing theme throughout the text. At the outset, however, it should be recognized that this question needs to be addressed by all the subspecialties within physical education. Sports, dance, and exercise are not just physiological entities. Biomechanics, motor learning, sports psychology, sports sociology, and other specialties all contribute to the explanation of human performance. Physiological explanations will always come up short in attempts to answer more global performance questions. Exercise physiology can answer questions such as "Why does inactivity lower physical fitness scores?" or "How can I train my cross-country team?" Students will have to look elsewhere to answer questions such as "How do I get my basketball team 'up' for the tournament?" or "How can I motivate children to be more active?" In other words, human performance explanations are complex and often require many disciplines for complete answers.

For those like myself, devoted to a career of studying physiological response to exercise, the importance of exercise physiology is obvious. On the other hand, I realize that the future teacher, coach, or exercise specialist may not recognize the importance so readily. For the teacher or exercise specialist, part of the importance lies in the selection of knowledge for inclusion within the physical education curriculum or program. Exercise physiology is *one* of the sources of knowledge. What we teach people about sport and exercise should reflect what has been scientifically verified and appears in the scientific literature. Do we build programs based on what we *know,* or what we think might be fun to do? Fun is important, but it should not be the primary criterion for curriculum development.

The coach, who has limited time and resources to bring a team to peak performance levels, requires knowledge of physiological response and understanding of the principles of applying physical stress most effectively. Too often we have relied on past practices of a winning coach, instead of individually prescribing new programs that are directly related to the scientific basis of coaching. No two teams or individuals behave exactly alike. Coaches must wear many hats. One hat should be that of the clinical exercise physiologist —solving the problems of athletes in the field laboratory.

Exercise physiology will help future teachers, coaches, and exercise specialists to better understand the role that exercise can play in the development of a healthy life-style. The general public has become very conscious of preventive health practices in recent years. Recognition of the positive benefits of a life-style that includes physical activity, diet, and stress management has reached peak proportions. Hardly a month goes by that a new "prescription" for health and longevity does not appear on the newsstands or in the bookstores. Physical educators, whether in schools, YMCAs, or corporate fitness programs, serve not only as disseminators of health knowledge, but also as interpreters of the many "get fit quick" programs on the market. Exercise physiology can provide you with a basis for making sound life-style recommendations and detecting programs that have a legitimate scientific base.

By studying exercise physiology you can gain an appreciation for how the body functions under conditions of exercise stress. However, perhaps of greater importance is the role this knowledge plays in decision making—both personal and as a practitioner.

Following are a few examples of the areas in which knowledge can be used in making decisions relative to subjects that I have stressed in this book:

1. The diagnosis of exercise- and sport-related problems
2. The prescription of exercise
3. The development of training programs
4. The choice of curricular content
5. Consumer protection, that is, providing correct information to the lay public
6. The determination of when it is *safe* to exercise, that is, in heat, cold, altitude, and underwater environments
7. The effects of exercise one can expect, and the role of these effects on general health, growth, and aging

The theme of this book—physical fitness

The predominant theme in this book is physical fitness. Most teachers have it as a goal, and all coaches know that athletes who are physically fit perform better. Physical fitness can be a goal in and of itself but, for the most part, motives for obtaining physical fitness arise from two somewhat independent sources. First, average people, who make up the majority of the population, seek physical fitness to achieve functional health, that is *health-related fitness*. Second, athletes wish to become physically fit to improve physical performance in some sport, that is, *performance fitness*. A major difference between the two lies in the specificity required. A great many exercise modes can lead to health-related fitness. For instance, running, swimming, and cycling, applied properly, can lead to many physiological changes related to improved body efficiency. Physical fitness for improved sport performance, however, involves exercise modes and physiological changes very specific to the sport in question. Cross-country running, for example, requires very specific fitness characteristics. It is important to recognize that some overlap may exist between physical fitness achieved for functional health and that achieved for improved physical performance. The recreational jogger will gain some of the characteristics of the competitive runner, for example. However, the weight lifter will probably not demonstrate characteristics that resemble either the recreational jogger or competitive runner.

Thanks to media publicity, physical education professionals are faced with great opportunities and many problems as well. The opportunities come from increased public expectations of what exercise and sport programs should provide. People want up-to-date facilities and trained professionals. Problems are created from information and misinformation. We can no longer pass off questions by the media-educated public like we used to, with answers such as ''That's just the way the body works!'' or ''Do it because it's good for you.'' Attitudes like this cannot be tolerated in the private sector, and they meet with great resistance in the public sector. On the other hand, the brevity of media exposure sometimes creates gaps in knowledge that need to be corrected. A well-trained exercise specialist should be able to easily counteract misinformation, but it is a constant source of aggravation. Another related problem involves the lag between the growth of the "exercise business" and the ability of institutions to prepare qualified professionals. However, great opportunities do await those who have absorbed the knowledge available in exercise physiology and can translate that knowledge into effective programs.

Organization

As an instructor, I have found the organization of topics presented in *Physiology of Exercise and Sport* to be optimal. In addition to serving an integral role in the text as a whole, most chapters are independent entities as well. Therefore the instructor can easily select topical coverage based on time, student interest, and personal teaching style.

Chapters 1 to 9 are devoted to basic physiological mechanisms stressing muscular contraction and systems that support this process. This sets the stage for practitioners' understanding of training theory and human response to physical activity. Chapters 1 to 5 are logically sequenced from the specific (details of muscle structure) to the general (aerobic and anaerobic power). Chapters 6 to 9 also develop similarly, from the specific to the general. The student is presented with the progression of oxygen intake and transport from the environment, to the lung, to the blood, to tissue, and is finally shown how this process is facilitated by the movement of blood by the heart.

Chapters 10 to 21 are sequenced by compatibility, addressing those factors that may beneficially or adversely affect muscular contraction during exercise and sport.

Content features

In the study of exercise physiology, there are several topics that may be of particular interest to both student and instructor. These topics are addressed in *Physiology of Exercise and Sport* and are worth noting. Unique to this text, I have integrated the female response throughout, rather than relegating it to a single chapter, thus recognizing that every chapter is relevant to females. In Chapter 4, dietary intake is specifically related to muscle function, rather than being presented simply as information for "good nutrition." Given the important role that the kidney plays in acid-base balance and water balance, both relevant to muscle fatigue, I have devoted Chapter 8 to this topic. Because increased numbers of students are interested in receiving certification as fitness instructors, exercise technologists, and exercise specialists, Chapters 10 and 11 have been included to address graded exercise testing and exercise prescription. Comprehensive coverage of a topic that is of special interest to many students today, body composition and weight control, is provided in Chapter 13. Given the growing numbers of athletes and recreational exercisers participating in the heat, cold, underwater, and at varying altitudes, an entire section (Chapters 15 to 18) is devoted to these environmental influences on performance. Chapter 20 addresses current topics related to drug use by athletes, including blood doping and the use of steroids, because knowledge of these topics is essential for the future exercise specialist. Exercise sensations, a topic that is not presented in other exercise physiology texts, is covered in Chapter 21. This chapter recognizes the body as a wholistic entity that operates during exercise and sport. It is not merely a physiological entity, but a psycho-biological entity.

Pedagogical aids

To facilitate the use of this text by students and instructors, many unique pedagogical and design features are included:

Chapter Objectives and Applications. The major learning objective of each chapter is clearly defined, and a sport-related application of each is provided for the student.

Key Terms. Key terms are highlighted in italics as they appear, and the list of terms is defined at the end of each chapter. For additional accessibility to the student, a comprehensive glossary is included at the end of the text.

Summary. Each chapter contains a summary that outlines the major points discussed.

Review questions. To test the student's comprehension of the material presented, thought-provoking questions for further review and analysis are included in each chapter.

Case Studies and Laboratory Applications. Each chapter includes one or more case studies that aid the student in applying the principles learned. When additional application as a laboratory experience is appropriate, these have also been provided at the end of the chapter.

References and Suggested Readings. Up-to-date references and suggested readings are provided in each chapter to direct the student to sources for additional reading or study.

Color Illustrations. Numerous illustrations and the extensive use of color accentuate and help teach important concepts to the student.

Acknowledgments

As the publisher's reviewers provided significant contributions which helped to enhance the quality and utility of this text, I would like to express my sincere gratitude to:

Michael Buono, Ph.D.
San Diego State University

Russell Pate, Ph.D.
University of South Carolina-Columbia

S. Kay Burrus, Ph.D.
Indiana University-Bloomington

Guy Penny, Ed.D.
Middle Tennessee State University

David Cundiff, Ph.D.
University of Southern Mississippi

J. Douglas Seelbach, Ph.D.
University of Oregon

Gary Sforzo, Ph.D.
Ithaca College

William Thorland, Ph.D.
formerly of University of Nebraska

William Stone, Ed.D.
Arizona State University

Anthony Wilcox, Ph.D.
Kansas State University

Nancy Stubbs, Ed.D.
Wichita State University

The completion of this book has been measurably assisted by several colleagues, graduate students, and institutions. Principal among institutions is the University of Wyoming. The flexibility of this institution and particularly my chairperson, Ward Gates, contributed significantly. St. Luke's Medical Center in Kansas City offered considerable aid and comfort during my sabbatical leave as Beyer's Medical Lecturer. Carl Maresh, then the Director of the Health Institute at St. Luke's and now at the University of Connecticut, provided me with time and personal support for my writing. Many thanks, Carl. Also, part of the manuscript was written while I was serving as Visiting Research Professor at the University of Liverpool. Grateful appreciation is extended to David Brodie, the Director of Sport Science at UL.

During most of the years I was writing this book, Bill Kraemer was pursuing a doctorate in exercise physiology under my supervision. Bill, currently conducting research at the U.S. Army Institute of Environmental Medicine, endured my monastic behavior with quintessential patience and support of every kind. His assistance was most consistent and I am significantly in his debt. Several graduate students served as masterful ''gophers'' without whom my job would have been greatly aggravated. Significant contributions were made by Jema Allen, Paula Garbarino, and Tish Woodard. I would like to single out Claire Karwacki who joined me on a number of chores during the final revision stage and did so with great skill, motivation, and friendship. Special thanks, Claire. Many people were involved as typists. I would be seriously remiss if I didn't give special recognition to Christine McKim and Patricia Rivera.

Many times my endurance waned, but my friend Jamie provided me with the spiritual energy to wax again. Her alchemy was indeed golden.

The editorial staff of Times Mirror/Mosby clearly met their lifetime challenge of incorrigibility with this author. When the final page of this book was set in print, a wave of expiration from St. Louis was felt throughout the country. Thanks to Nancy Roberson, Kathy Sedovic, and especially Michelle Turenne for their thoroughly professional efforts. Both their hardships and mine were secondary to a product that escorts the next generation down a dark road with the lamp of learning in the lead. We have all chosen a difficult road but reached the end with a sincere feeling of fulfillment and pleasure.

A final word

This text will never replace the spark that a competent teacher can bring to the student. Hopefully, however, a text will not detract from the teacher's effort. My wish, in this case, is that the teaching process will be facilitated. You are embarking on a journey that will not always be easy, but that reaches into the heart of your profession. It is my hope that this text will help to make your trip an enjoyable and successful one. Good luck!

Bruce J. Noble

CONTENTS

PART TWO Cardiorespiratory function

PART THREE   Exercise prescription, training techniques, and physiological effects

PART FIVE   Special considerations

PHYSIOLOGY OF
EXERCISE AND SPORT

PART ONE

MUSCLE FUNCTION

chapter 1

SKELETAL MUSCLE STRUCTURE

MAJOR LEARNING OBJECTIVE

The basic unit of muscle concerning contraction is the fiber. Fibers are of three basic types. Although the number and percentage of each type are genetically determined, there is considerable variability between individuals and between muscle groups.

APPLICATIONS

Certain sports demand a high percentage of certain fiber types. Identification of the type *may* help determine those persons with potential for athletic success.

■ A simple test involving repeated maximal contractions of a particular muscle group can roughly determine those persons with predominantly slow-twitch (red) or fast-twitch (white) fibers.

THE objective of this first chapter is to help you understand how muscles function to produce movement. Many types of movement take place in the body. For example, the tongue moves to produce speech and the intestines engage in peristalsis to move metabolic waste. In exercise physiology, we are concerned with the gross movement of body segments resulting from the contraction of skeletal muscles. When you hit a baseball, many muscle fibers from several fiber bundles contract to bring about the swinging motion. For the sake of simplicity, we can examine just the forearm extension movement of the swing. The goal is to cause rotary motion at the elbow joint by contracting the triceps muscle, at the point where the tendon crosses the joint and attaches to the ulna. Contraction causes the triceps to shorten, which pulls the forearm through an arc to approximately 180 degrees. This shortening is caused by many fibers receiving stimulation from the

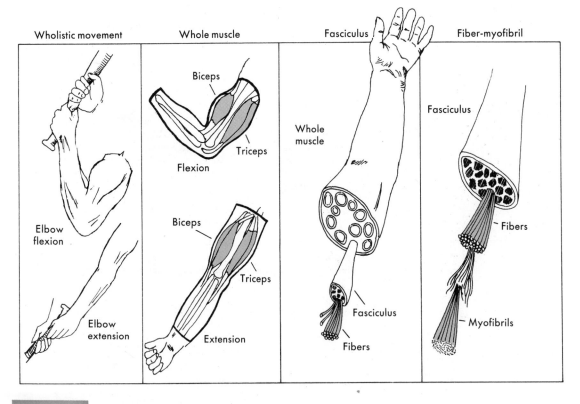

Wholistic movement   Whole muscle   Fasciculus   Fiber-myofibril

Biceps

Triceps

Flexion

Elbow flexion

Biceps

Triceps

Elbow extension

Extension

Whole muscle

Fasciculus

Fibers

Fasciculus

Fibers

Myofibrils

FIG. 1-1   Forearm extension in the baseball swing: from wholistic movement to the myofibril.

nervous system. The key to understanding the process is comprehending how a single fiber shortens to cause movement. Figure 1-1 illustrates the progressive reduction of muscle activity from skilled movement to the single fiber. In the respective insets in this figure, the triceps muscle is depicted as a whole muscle, a series of bundles, and a series of muscle fibers.

MUSCLE STRUCTURE AND FUNCTION
The fiber

Skeletal muscle consists of bundles of fibers. A single bundle is called a *fasciculus*. The fiber is basically cylindrical with a length of a few millimeters to many centimeters. Fiber diameter ranges from 10 to 100 micrometers. A sheath or membrane called the *sarcolemma* surrounds the fiber. The sarcolemma separates the muscle fiber from the interstitial fluid. The muscle fiber contains one or more nuclei, generally distributed beneath the sarcolemma. Nuclei are arranged along the fiber axis. As seen in Figure 1-1, the fiber is composed of a number of smaller units called *myofibrils*. The average myofibril diameter is 1 micrometer. Myofibrils have no membrane sheath and are immersed in the fluid portion of the cell called *sarcoplasm*. The sarcoplasm comprises the cellular structures that produce energy *(mitochondria)* and interchange material between the fiber and the interstitial spaces *(sarcoplasmic reticulum [SR])*. In the mitochondria, oxygen chemically interacts with food fuels to form energy for muscular contraction (see Chapter

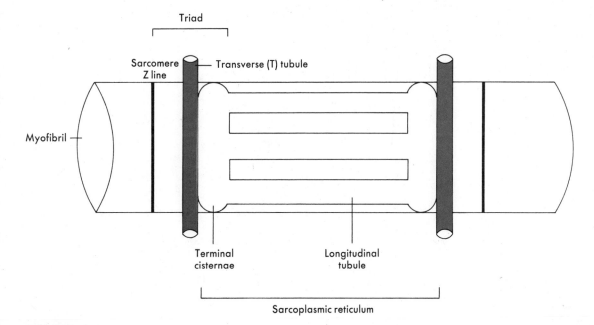

FIG. 1-2   The sarcoplasmic reticulum (SR). The point where the Z line of the sarcomere, T tubule, and SR come together is referred to as the triad.

3). Each mitochondrion has a smooth outer membrane with a folded inner membrane; these two membranes form compartments called *cristae*. Generally, the oxidative requirements of the cell are correlated with the number, size, and enzymatic content of the mitochondria. *Adenosinetriphosphate (ATP),* the source of energy for muscular contraction, is formed in the mitochondria by oxidative phosphorylation. Molecules of the respiratory chain are located in the cristae.

The SR surrounds the myofibrils with both longitudinal and transverse structures

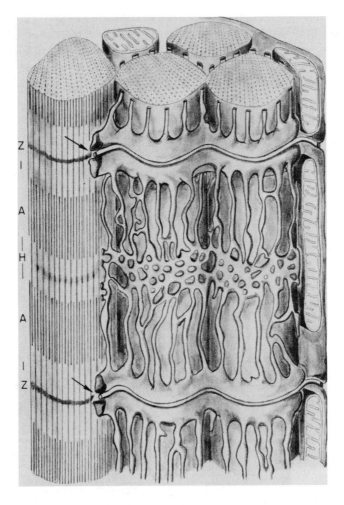

FIG. 1-3   **Anatomical proximity of various muscle fiber structures. (From Dowben, R.M.: Contractility, with special reference to skeletal muscle. In Mountcastle, V.B., editor: Medical physiology, ed. 14, vol. 1, St. Louis, 1980, The C.V. Mosby Co.)**

(Figure 1-2). Calcium stored in the SR, as we see later in this chapter, plays an important role in the contraction of muscle. The *longitudinal tubules* run parallel to the myofibrils and perpendicular to the *transverse tubules (T tubules)*. At the end of the longitudinal tubules, and adjacent to the T tubules, are calcium-containing sacs called *terminal cisternae*. The T tubule and terminal cisternae located on either side are called the triad. T tubules, although technically not a part of the SR, are functionally related by providing a direct link between the interior of the muscle fiber and the fiber membrane.

The SR and T tubules were first identified in 1902.[2] This discovery answered the question of how ionic changes on the surface of the muscle cell can spread throughout the fiber so rapidly. The function of the T tubule is to conduct signals from the nervous system into the fiber. Presumably, the arrival of electrical signals to the area of the terminal cisternae is related to the release of calcium, necessary for muscle contraction.

Figure 1-3 illustrates the anatomical location of the various structures discussed above. To further illustrate the relative orientation of these structures, Figure 1-4 shows an electron micrograph of a transverse section of skeletal muscle. This figure also shows the proximity of these structures to a capillary.

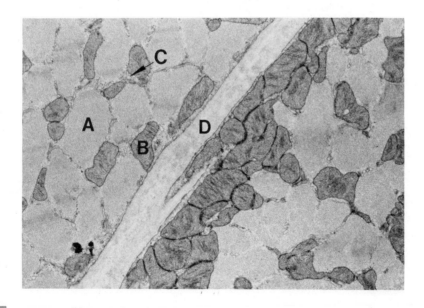

FIG. 1-4   Electron micrograph of a transverse section of skeletal muscle: *(A)* muscle fiber, *(B)* mitochondrion, *(C)* sarcoplasmic reticulum and T tubule system, *(D)* capillary.

The sarcomere

Skeletal muscle appears striated under microscopic inspection. This ''striped'' appearance is caused by the variable density of the contractile proteins that make up the myofibrils. The principal contractile proteins are *actin* and *myosin*. Muscle contraction is the result of chemical energy from the food we eat being transformed into mechanical energy mediated by the movement of actin and myosin.

Scientists have identified the basic components that make up the complex of striations that repeats itself along the myofibril, the *sarcomere*. Figure 1-5 shows a graphic representation of the designations that identify each of the sarcomere components. An actual micrograph of the striated muscle is shown in Figure 1-6. In a two-dimensional sense, each fiber can be thought of as an alternating dark- and light-banded cord. Each sarcomere

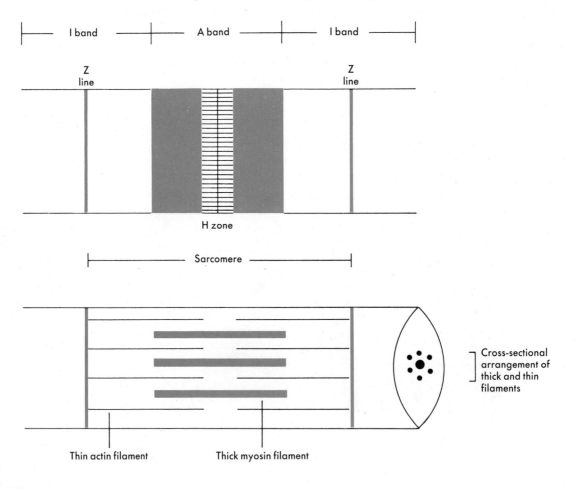

FIG. 1-5   The sarcomere.

extends between Z lines. The I bands grow out of the Z lines and are composed of thin filaments (actin) that give a lighter appearance. The darkest appearing band is composed of both thin and thick filaments (myosin) and is called the A band. The H zone, moderate in color, is formed by thick filaments only. In cross section, a pattern of dispersion of actin and myosin filaments can be seen in which one myosin filament is surrounded by six actin filaments.

It is important to remember that the protrusions called *cross-bridges* extend from the thick filaments. These cross-bridges attach to thin filaments, causing them to move inward; thus shortening has occurred. Cross-bridges are arranged in six rows around the myosin filament. They are spaced about 400 Å (10^{-10} m) along each row. Since the rows are staggered, cross-bridges appear every 60 to 70 Å. Cross-bridges are movable and represent sites where ATP is split to provide energy for muscle contraction. Myosin is composed of a light component (L-meromyosin) and a heavy component (H-meromyosin). The stem of the cross-bridge is made up of L-meromyosin, and the bilobed head consists of H-meromyosin. The H-meromyosin contains the enzyme ATPase, which is involved in filament sliding.

The sliding filament hypothesis

When a muscle contracts dynamically (concentrically), it shortens, as indicated earlier. How is shortening possible? Before 1950, it was thought that muscle shortening occurred by length changes in the muscle fiber as a whole. However, in 1954 Huxley and Hanson refuted this theory with results from their study of skeletal muscle using electron microscopy.[15] This study provided evidence of filament sliding as a mechanism for muscle shortening; that is, the whole fiber does shorten, but without a change in length of the component parts.

In a figurative sense, the muscle fibers in use will telescope inward. The distance between the Z lines shortens without actually shortening either thin or thick filaments. In

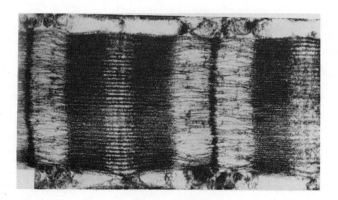

FIG. 1-6   **Electron micrograph of skeletal muscle sarcomere. (From Anthony, C.P., and Thibodeau, G.A.: Textbook of anatomy and physiology, ed. 11, St. Louis, 1983, The C.V. Mosby Co.)**

fact, the filaments slide past one another, retaining their individual lengths but reducing the length of the sarcomere. This description gives rise to the sliding filament hypothesis, which is concerned with how muscles shorten.

The inquisitive student should then wonder what makes the filaments slide past one another. Keep in mind that we are dealing only with a hypothesis based on certain established anatomical characteristics. In simple terms, the hypothesis states that the cross-bridges of the thick filaments bind with selected sites on the thin filaments. After binding, the head of the cross-bridge rotates, causing the thin filament to slide toward the center of the sarcomere. This sliding action requires the splitting of ATP. This high-energy compound consists of the nucleotide, adenosine, and three phosphates. When the latter (terminal) phosphate is split off, forming *adenosine diphosphate (ADP),* energy is liberated. ATP must be formed again on the cross-bridge head for actin and myosin to

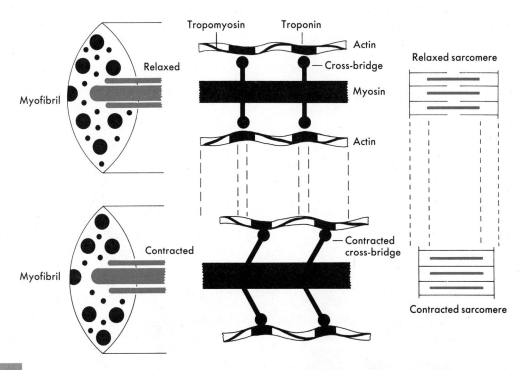

FIG. 1-7   The action of the cross-bridges as predicted by the sliding filament hypothesis. On the left, a cross-sectional view of the myofibril illustrates the larger myosin filament surrounded by smaller actin filaments. The top center shows the unconnected cross-bridges. The bottom center illustrates both connected cross-bridges and the "ratcheting" (lateral movement) of cross-bridges during the contracted state. Note the lateral movement of the actin filament while the myosin filament remains stationary. The right side shows how actin and myosin position is manifested in the sarcomere; the sarcomere shortens in reaction to the movement of actin filaments toward the center while myosin filaments remain stationary.

become unbound and for the action to be able to be repeated. Figure 1-7 demonstrates the interaction between the cross-bridge action and the shifting of position of sarcomere components. The cross-bridges are essentially perpendicular extensions with jointed heads. The heads attach to the actin filament and pull it toward the middle with ratchetlike action. This process may occur very many times during one contraction.

The role of calcium

The presence of ATP alone will not produce muscle contraction. An electrical impulse of the proper magnitude must stimulate the muscle, which in turn stimulates the release of calcium (see Chapter 2). It has been known for some time that the calcium concentration within the muscle cell must increase for contraction to occur. How is calcium released, and what role does it play in the contractile process?

First, we should mention the presence of two more proteins in the muscle cell and briefly discuss their role. These proteins are *tropomyosin* and *troponin*. They are located along the actin protein. The actin molecule is sphere shaped and arranged in a helical formation—it is shaped like a twisted cord. Tropomyosin binds with actin in the grooves formed by the twisting. The protein troponin, in turn, binds only to selected sites on tropomyosin. These troponin sites are where the cross-bridges must connect.

As mentioned earlier, during rest ATP is present on the cross-bridge head. It will take the action of the enzyme *myosin ATPase* to split ATP to ADP + P_i, and provide the energy for pulling the actin filament toward the center. As long as ATP remains unsplit, no contraction takes place. Troponin has an inhibiting effect on myosin during rest so that ATP splitting cannot occur. The following is one hypothesis concerning this inhibition process. When the calcium concentration is low in the muscle (relaxation), tropomyosin takes a position in which the troponin binding sites are blocked; therefore, the cross-bridges cannot bind. However, when calcium concentration increases (contraction), the binding site changes position, exposing it to binding with the cross-bridge. In other words, as long as troponin is allowed to play its role, no contraction can take place.

We now look at the action and role of calcium. The T tubules, as mentioned earlier, have a direct link with the cell membrane. Nervous stimulation travels along the fiber membrane and through the T tubules to the sarcoplasm, causing an influx of calcium from its storage place in the SR. (Depolarization of cell membranes is discussed in Chapter 2.) Calcium, when it increases beyond a certain threshold concentration, binds with troponin, thus releasing actin binding sites. That is, it activates myosin. Calcium does not increase as such but is redistributed from the SR to the actin filaments. Myosin ATPase is then free to split the ATP located on the cross-bridge, which, in turn, attaches and pulls the actin filament along. The more cross-bridge attachments that are made throughout the whole muscle, the stronger is the contraction. During the process of relaxation, this procedure reverses. When nervous stimulation to the muscle ceases, calcium is pumped back into the SR. Lowering the calcium concentration below threshold allows troponin to again inactivate myosin by not allowing ATP to be split. Therefore production of energy for shortening is not possible until the muscle is stimulated again.

We will briefly review the sliding filament hypothesis to make sure that the steps are understood:

1. During rest, troponin inhibits myosin from binding to actin.
2. When muscle is stimulated, the nervous impulse releases calcium from the SR, which activates myosin; that is, actin and myosin combine. This binding process allows myosin ATPase to break down ATP to ADP + P_i. The energy released from this reaction causes the sarcomere to shorten.
3. During relaxation, the process reverses.

Smooth and cardiac muscle structure

For the sake of clarity, it will be helpful for you to know a few characteristics of two other types of muscle tissue: smooth and cardiac. Smooth muscle, found in the vascular system for example, is not striated and shows small invaginations along its surface membrane. All muscle proteins that are found in skeletal muscle are also found in smooth muscle, except for troponin, which has not been identified as yet. Smooth muscle is not under voluntary control and contracts more slowly than skeletal muscle. Contraction is more rhythmical and sustained.

Cardiac muscle, found only in the heart, like skeletal muscle is striated, containing sarcomeres. However, cardiac fibers are shorter and show branching. Mitochondria are larger and more abundant. Fibers are interwoven with *intercalated disks* located at fiber junctions. The heart muscle responds as a *functional syncytium*—that is, the heart contracts and relaxes as a total synchronous unit. Wherever the heart is stimulated, the contraction spreads throughout. In contrast, in skeletal muscle only those fibers that are stimulated contract. Thus, the heart is capable of only one force production (excluding chemical influences), whereas in skeletal muscle force production can be graded. Basically, however, the contractile process is the same in cardiac and skeletal muscle.

Fiber type characteristics

Although the general structural characteristics of muscle fibers are similar, differences can be noted in their functions. Functional differences exhibited by fibers have been characterized according to speed of contraction, aerobic capacity, anaerobic capacity, number of mitochondria present, number of capillaries present, strength of contraction, ATPase activity, and fatigability.

Scientists have known for some time that muscle fibers could be classified into at least two broad categories. For example, the concentration of *myoglobin* in fibers enables classification by color—red and white. Red fibers were associated with endurance capacity (distance running) because they were high in mitochondria and capillaries and low in fatigability. In contrast, white fibers were associated with sprinting capacity (100 meter dash) because they were high in speed, strength of contraction, and fatigability.

How were these characteristics identified? Early classification was done mostly on animals. Fiber samples were taken, and the tissue was stained for certain characteristics, for example, ATPase activity. Fiber type is identified by its reaction to an alkaline pH. In the sampling area an intermixing of types has been seen, like an arrangement of small mosaic tiles. Figure 1-8 contrasts identification of fiber type using two different pH incubations. In one case, an acid incubation, pH 4.3, results in white fibers staining white and red fibers staining dark. In the other case, with alkaline incubation, pH 10.6, the ATPase of the white fiber stains dark and the red fiber stains light.

Over the years many staining techniques have been developed, and researchers still argue over the number of distinct types of fibers. Some scientists believe that it is unwise to assign to fibers names that imply dominant functions. Therefore, designations like *type I* (red) and *type II* (white) are common. Others prefer functional classifications, such as *slow twitch* (ST) or *fast twitch* (FT) to refer to red and white muscle, respectively. Three predominate types have been identified based on staining procedures:

SO—Slow, oxidative (type I)

FOG—Fast, oxidative, glycolytic (type IIa)

FG—Fast, glycolytic (type IIb)

These types show up as dark (FG), gray (FOG), and white (S) in the right panel of Figure 1-8. Slow and fast refer to contractile velocity, while oxidative and glycolytic focus on the metabolic characteristics of the tissue (see Chapter 3).

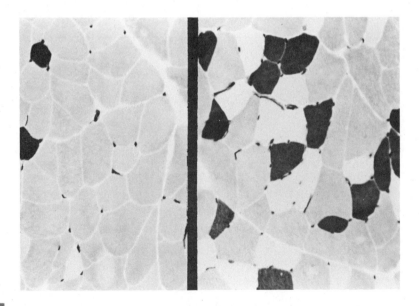

FIG. 1-8   Comparison of muscle fiber staining procedures in which different pH incubations are used. The left panel illustrates the results of an acid incubation (pH = 4.3). In this case, white fibers stain white and red fibers stain dark. The right panel illustrates an alkaline incubation (pH = 10.6). In the second case, white fibers (FG) stain dark and red fibers (SO) stain light. This panel also identifies intermediate (FOG) fibers, seen as the gray areas.

Perhaps the best way to demonstrate the functional differences of the fibers in the Peter and others[21] classification is to compare their various capacities. Figure 1-9 compares *SO, FOG,* and *FG fibers* with regard to speed of contraction, aerobic capacity (producing energy with oxygen), and anaerobic capacity (producing energy without oxygen). The metabolic significance of the various fiber types is discussed in Chapter 3. In that chapter fiber types are related to the biochemical pathways which produce energy for muscular contraction, aerobic and anaerobic. The important point is made that when we want to improve our capacity for using various fibers, we do so, at least partly, by improving the mechanisms which provide energy to those fibers.

Figure 1-10 shows a series of pictures that illustrate the muscle biopsy procedure used to collect samples for fiber identification. A local anesthetic is injected (panel A) into the area where a small incision will be made with a scalpel. The biopsy needle is inserted through the incision into the muscle (panel B). In this example, suction is being used to increase the size of the sample extracted. The end of the needle surrounds a small piece of tissue, which is cut and held within the needle. Next, the biopsy needle is withdrawn (panel C). Finally, the sample is removed from the needle, frozen in liquid nitrogen, and later analyzed (panel D).

	Speed of contraction	Aerobic capacity	Anaerobic capacity
Slow, oxidative (SO)	Slow	High	Low
Fast, oxidation glycolytic (FOG)	Fast	Medium	Medium
Fast, glycolytic (FG)	Fast	Low	High

FIG. 1-9   **Comparison of slow, oxidative (SO); fast, oxidative, glycolytic (FOG); and fast, glycolytic (FG) fiber types.**

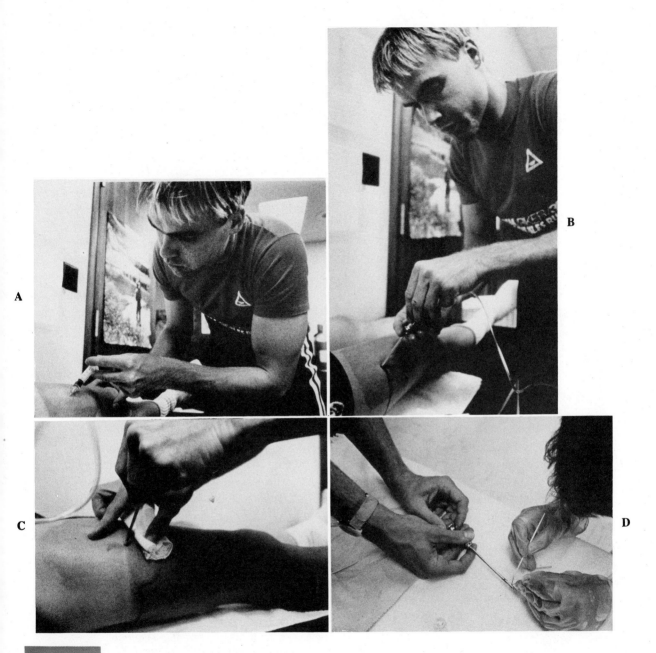

FIG. 1-10   The muscle biopsy procedure used to extract a sample of muscle tissue. Panel *A* shows a local anesthetic being injected into the area where a small incision will be made with a scalpel. The biopsy needle is inserted through the incision into the muscle (panel *B*). Suction is used to increase the size of the sample extracted. The biopsy needle is withdrawn with the muscle sample within (panel *C*). Finally, the muscle sample is removed from the needle, frozen in liquid nitrogen, and later analyzed (panel *D*).

Fiber type differences within and between individuals

It should be clear from the preceding discussion that muscles are mixed, that is, they contain examples of all types. We can take an example from biopsy data on the vastus lateralis (thigh) muscle. On the average both men and women show about 52% ST in this muscle. The variability is high, so that some athletes, like elite marathoners, may display ST percentages greater than 90%. Again, using the same muscle, men and women would show, on the average, 33% FOG and 14% FG. This means that if muscle is broadly classified into two categories, ST and FT, humans are on the average about 50-50. This is also seen in the gastrocnemius (calf), deltoid (shoulder), and biceps brachii (arm). The practical conclusion of these data is that humans, both men and women, tend to have mixed fiber characteristics in these muscles. However, wide variations are also noted, which might help explain why certain people excel in certain events.

Exceptions to the rule just stated would be noted for two other muscles. The soleus (calf) is 25% to 40% higher in ST characteristics than other leg muscles. Also, the triceps (arm) is 10% to 30% higher in FT characteristics than other arm muscles. It seems that the function of certain muscles is more specific, that is, a predominate type is present. Other muscles, noted above, are suited for both endurance and speed activities.

Fiber types and athletic performance

You would predict from the characteristics displayed in Figure 1-5 that endurance athletes, such as marathoners, would have a predominance of SO fibers in leg muscles. Also, you would most likely predict that sprinters would show an abundance of FG fibers. Such is indeed the case. Investigators at Ball State University found that elite distance runners had 79% ST in the vastus lateralis muscle, which was a significantly higher percentage than in untrained men (57.7%).[8] Sprinters have been shown to have a high percentage of FT fibers. Thus, it appears that elite endurance and sprint performers may be genetically advantaged by a predominance of slow- or fast-twitch fibers, respectively. It is generally agreed that the number of fibers is genetically determined. Currently, scientists are debating the possibility of altering fiber type through training. Growing evidence supports the hypothesis that characteristics can be changed, especially fast- to slow-twitch transitions.[22]

Figure 1-11 demonstrates the results of experiments conducted by Tesch, in which two groups with high (67%) and low (21%) percentages of fast-twitch fibers were compared on a muscular endurance task. Subjects were asked to exert force during 100 knee extensions at an angular velocity of 180 degrees per second. An *isokinetic* (constant speed) *strength* instrument was used to measure force (the Cybex II). The graph shows two distinctly different patterns of fatigue (or endurance), particularly after 25 contractions. Subjects with high fast-twitch percentages fatigued more rapidly, that is, they displayed less muscular endurance. In contrast, those with a lower fast-twitch percentage, and presumably a high slow-twitch percentage, showed less fatigability and more endurance. These data can easily be reproduced by comparing a sprinter and a marathoner on a similar test. The student should be reminded that the absolute strength (*not* expressed as a percentage of initial value) of these athletes would be quite different. The sprinter would undoubtedly be much stronger in the unfatigued state. The metabolic, or energy producing, implications of these findings are further discussed in Chapter 3.

Contrary to our intuitive predictions, however, throwers and high jumpers do not show a preponderance of FT fibers, that is, compared to sprinters. Saltin and others[25] suggest that one explanation for this may be that these sports require single efforts performed very quickly. The high degree of muscular coordination required may be better synchronized by ST fibers.

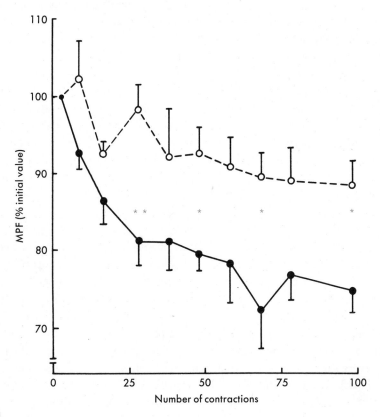

FIG. 1-11   Illustration of power production (mean power frequency, *MPF*) over 100 maximal knee extensions. The upper line *(open circles)* is the response of a group with low fast-twitch fiber area (21%), that is, high slow-twitch fiber percentage. The lower line *(closed circles)* represents the data from a group with high fast-twitch area (67%), that is, low slow-twitch fiber percentage. The response of the fast-twitch group illustrates higher fatigability. Differences between groups are denoted with * = p < .05 and ** = p < .01. (From Tesch, P.: Muscle fatigue in man with special reference to lactate accumulation during short term intense exercise, Acta Physiol. Scand. *480:*44, 1980.)

Hyperplasia

As mentioned earlier, the number of muscle fibers we have is genetically determined. However, it has been interesting to speculate about the growth of new fibers *(hyperplasia)* to explain performance changes observed in the highly trained athlete. This is especially true in certain athletic groups, such as weight lifters. Scientists have tried to provide objective evidence on this matter. Most researchers counted fibers before and after training, from cross-sectional samples of a muscle. Using this method, some have observed what they thought to be evidence of an increase in fibers. However, Gollnick and others,[13] using this method and a method by which single fibers were counted in the same tissue sample, found no evidence of hyperplasia. Since, contrary to popular opinion, a single fiber can exhibit branching, it is possible to make a cross-sectional cut of a fiber through both the main fiber trunk and its branch. This would make it appear as if two fibers existed, when in reality there was only one. Therefore, only single fiber counts should be used to study the hyperplasia question.

Hypertrophy

Although the number of muscle fibers we have appears to be genetically determined, we can increase the size of muscle fibers. Increasing the cross-sectional dimension of muscle fibers is called *hypertrophy*. Hypertrophy is stimulated by working the muscle fibers against an overload. Increasing the cross-sectional dimension of muscle fibers is closely related to their ability to exert force. This process is discussed in more detail in later chapters.

THE ROLE OF CONNECTIVE TISSUE

Connective tissue, mostly collagen, surrounds, intertwines, and forms a bony connection for muscle tissue. Two elastic connective tissue components are important to our understanding of muscle contraction and relaxation. One of these, the *parallel elastic component,* runs parallel with the muscle fibers. The other, the *series elastic component,* is located in the tendons at the end of the muscle fibers. These elastic fibers do not contract but can have a pronounced effect on the contractile process. It has been hypothesized that the parallel elastic component of muscle may act like a compressed spring which stores mechanical energy for subsequent contractions. For example, one can jump higher after placing the muscle under stretch. The series elastic component plays a role in the relaxation phase of muscle contraction. After actin and myosin separate with the removal of calcium, resting muscle length is restored with the aid of this component. For example, the series elastic component is stretched when muscle fibers contract. When the cross-bridges disconnect, this component brings the fibers back to resting length.

THE COACH AND THE TEACHER AS SPORTS SCIENTIST

Most of us who have been athletes, or who appreciate athletic activity, view sport and exercise on a wholistic level. We appreciate the beauty and power of the whole athletic act without giving much thought to the underlying subcellular mechanisms. To transfer this orientation to physiology requires an intense desire to discover ways, as a teacher, coach, or scientist, to improve performance. An understanding of the elastic properties of muscle, for example, may help lead to the discovery of improved jumping methods. Teaching and coaching are both an art and a science that demand, in one respect, the presentation of known material in innovative ways and, conversely, the solving of performance problems having no immediate textbook answer. Like the physician, the sports scientist must treat his ''patient'' by developing highly refined diagnostic and prescriptive skills. To develop these skills we must learn more about what lies beneath the skin and how it operates.

SUMMARY

Whole muscle is made up of bundles of fibers called fasciculi. Each fiber is surrounded by a membrane sheath, the sarcolemma, and consists of many myofibrils. The sarcoplasmic reticulum (SR) surrounds the myofibrils with both longitudinal and transverse tubules. Transverse (T) tubules provide a link between the cell membrane and the muscle cell. When a nervous stimulus is applied to a muscle fiber, the impulse travels through the T tubules, causing the SR to release calcium. Calcium release is the first step in the shortening of muscle known as contraction.

Muscle fibers have a striated appearance depending on the dispersion of two muscle proteins, actin and myosin. The basic descriptive unit of the striations is the sarcomere. The sarcomere runs between two anatomical lines called Z lines and consists of combinations of actin and myosin. Actin makes up thin filaments that extend from Z lines to form the I band. The A band is formed by the overlapping of the thin filaments with the thick filaments (myosin). The H zone is where only thick filaments are located. Cross-bridges protrude from the myosin filaments and connect at the appropriate time with the actin filaments, pulling them inward toward the center of the sarcomere. This movement, or shortening of the sarcomere, is the process called contraction.

To explain shortening, muscle physiologists have proposed a hypothesis known as the sliding filament hypothesis. This states that when at rest, myosin cross-bridges are inhibited from binding with actin because of a secondary muscle protein called troponin. However, when calcium is released from the SR, this inhibitory effect is eliminated. Thus, adenosine triphosphate located on the cross-bridge heads breaks down, with the aid of the enzyme myosin ATPase, which releases the energy necessary for the cross-bridges to pull the actin filaments inward.

Fibers can be classified according to their functional characteristics: their speed of contraction, aerobic capacity, and anaerobic capacity. One classification system designates three types: slow, oxidative (SO); fast, oxidative, glycolytic (FOG); and fast, glycolytic (FG). Endurance athletes are more likely to have primarily SO fibers, whereas sprint athletes are likely to have primarily FG fibers. During tests requiring repeated maximal contractions, athletes with higher SO percentages show far less fatigability than those with predominately FG fibers.

Connective tissue surrounding muscle fibers aids muscular contraction. The parallel elastic component, which runs parallel to muscle fibers, acts to store energy for subsequent contractions. Energy is stored in the form of mechanical energy, as in a compressed spring. The series elastic component aids in returning muscle fibers to their resting length after contraction.

KEY TERMS

fiber the cylindrical cell, ranging in length from 2 to 50 mm, which makes up skeletal muscle.

fiber type muscle fibers are characterized (typed) according to their contractile speed (fast or slow) or metabolic capacities (oxidative or glycolytic).

hyperplasia change in tissue cross section caused by growth of new fibers.

hypertrophy the increased cross-sectional dimension of the muscle fiber.

sarcomere the basic contractile unit in the muscle fiber.

sliding filament hypothesis the proposition that explains how protein filaments within the sarcomere move to cause muscle fiber contraction.

REVIEW QUESTIONS

1. Briefly explain the location and function of the following anatomical structures: mitochondria, sarcoplasmic reticulum, transverse tubules.

2. List the four contractile proteins and explain their spatial proximity.

3. What causes skeletal muscle to have a striated appearance?

4. Describe the changes in the various sarcomere components during muscle contraction.

5. Describe the process by which calcium releases the actin binding sites for coupling with myosin.

6. Explain the action of the cross-bridges and the movement of the contractile proteins during isometric and eccentric contraction.

7. Why are the characteristics of the FG fiber useful to the sprinter?

8. Why are the characteristics of the SO fiber useful to the long-distance runner?

9. Describe the variability within individuals in fiber type percentages.

10. Can fiber type be changed by training? Can the biochemical characteristics of fiber types be changed by training?

11. What is hyperplasia and can it be scientifically proven to exist?

REFERENCES

1. Becker, W.M.: Energy and the living cell: an introduction to bioenergetics, New York, 1977, J.B. Lippincott Co.

2. Bendall, J.R.: Muscles, molecules and movement: an essay in the contraction of muscles, New York, 1974, American Elsevier Publishing Co., Inc.

3. Buchthal, F., and Schmalbruch, H.: Contraction times and fibre types in intact human muscle, Acta Physiol. Scand. **79:**435, 1970.

4. Burke, R.E., and Edgerton, V.R.: Motor unit properties and selective involvement in movement. In Wilmore, J.H., and Keogh, J.F., editors: Exercise and sport science reviews, vol. 3, New York, 1975, Academic Press, Inc.

5. Carlson, B.M., and Faulkner, J.A.: The regeneration of skeletal muscle fibers following injury: a review, Med. Sci. Sports Exerc. **15:**187, 1983.

6. Cavagna, G.M.: Storage and utilization of elastic energy in skeletal muscle. In Hutton, R.S., editor: Exercise and sport sciences reviews, vol. 5, Santa Barbara, Calif., 1977, Journal Publishing Affiliates.

7. Clarkson, P.M., Johnson, J., Dextradeur, D., and others: The relationship among isokinetic endurance, initial strength level, and fiber type, Res. Q. Exerc. Sport **53:**15, 1982.

8. Costill, D.L., Fink, W.J., and Pollock, M.L.: Muscle fiber composition and enzyme activities of elite distance runners, Med. Sci. Sports Exerc. **8:**96, 1976.

9. Fournier, M., Ricci, J., Taylor, A.W., and others: Skeletal muscle adaptation in adolescent boys: sprint and endurance training and detraining, Med. Sci. Sports Exerc. **14:**453, 1982.

10. Gergely, J.: The mechanism of muscle contraction. In Sanadi, D.R., editor: Chemical mechanisms in bioenergetics, American Chemical Society Monograph No. 172, 1976.

11. Gollnick, P.D., Armstrong, R.B., Saubert, C.W., and others: Enzyme activity and fiber composition in skeletal muscle of untrained and trained men, J. Appl. Physiol. **33:**312, 1972.

12. Gollnick, P.D., Sjodin, B., Karlsson, J., and others: Human soleus muscle: a comparison of fiber composition and enzyme activities with other leg muscles, Pflugers Arch. **348:**247, 1974.

13. Gollnick, P.D., Timson, B.F., Moore, R.L., and others: Muscular enlargement and number of fibers in skeletal muscles of rats, J. Appl. Physiol. **50:**936, 1981.

14. Huxley, H.E.: The structural basis of muscular contraction, Proc. R. Soc. London, Ser. B **178:**131, 1971.

15. Huxley, H.E.: The double array of filaments in cross-striated muscle, J. Biophys. Biochem. Cytol. **3:**631, 1957.

16. Komi, P.V., and Karlsson, J.: Physical performance, skeletal muscle enzyme activities, and fiber types in monozygous and dizygous twins of both sexes, Acta Physiol. Scand. **105** Suppl. **462:** 1979.

17. Komi, P.V., and Tesch, P.: EMG frequency spectrum, muscle structure, and fatigue during dynamic contractions in man, Eur. J. Appl. Physiol. **42:**41, 1979.

18. Larsson, L.: Physical training effects on muscle morphology in sedentary males at different ages, Med. Sci. Sports Exerc. **14:**203, 1982.

19. Merton, P.A.: How we control the contraction of our muscles, Sci. Am. **226:**30, 1972.

20. Mommaerts, W.F.H.M.: Excitation and conduction. In Ross, G., editor: Essentials of human physiology, Chicago, 1978, Year Book Medical Publishers, Inc.

21. Peter, J.B., Barnard, R.J., Edgerton, V.R., and others: Metabolic profiles of three fiber types of skeletal muscle in guinea pigs and rabbits, Biochemistry **11:**2627, 1972.

22. Pette, D.: Activity-induced fast to slow transitions in mammalian muscle, Med. Sci. Sports Exerc. **16:**517, 1984.

23. Prince, F.P., Hikida, R.S., and Hagerman, F.C.: Human muscle fiber types in power lifters, distance runners, and untrained subjects, Pflugers Arch. **363:**19, 1976.

24. Salleo, A., Anastasi, G., LaSpada, G., and others: New muscle fiber production during compensatory hypertrophy, Med. Sci. Sports Exerc. **12:**268, 1980.

25. Saltin, B., Henriksson, J., Jansson, E., and others: Fiber types and metabolic potentials of skeletal muscles in sedentary man and endurance runners. In Milvy, P., editor: The marathon: physiological, medical, epidemiological and psychological studies, vol. 301, New York, 1977, The New York Academy of Sciences.

26. Smith, D.S.: Muscle, New York, 1972, Academic Press, Inc.

27. Tesch, P.: Muscle fatigue in man with special reference to lactate accumulation during short term intense exercise, Acta Physiol. Scand. **480:**44, 1980.

28. Thorstensson, A., and Karlsson, J.: Fatigability and fibre composition of human skeletal muscle, Acta Physiol. Scand. **98:**318, 1976.

SUGGESTED READINGS

Becker, W.M.: Energy and the living cell: an introduction to bioenergetics, Philadelphia, 1977, J.B. Lippincott Co.

Bendall, J.R.: Muscles, molecules and movement: an essay in the contraction of muscles, New York, 1974, American Elsevier Publishing Co., Inc.

Hoyle, G.: Muscles and their neural control, New York, 1983, John Wiley & Sons.

Huxley, H.E.: The structural basis of muscular contraction, Proc. R. Soc. **178:**131, 1971.

Merton, P.A.: How we control the contraction of our muscles, Sci. Am. **226:**30, 1972.

Saltin, B., Henricksson, J., Nygaard, E., and others: Fiber types and metabolic potentials of skeletal muscles in sedentary man and endurance runners. In Milvy, P., editor: The marathon: physiological, medical, epidemiological and psychological studies, vol. 301, New York, 1977, The New York Academy of Sciences.

CASE STUDY 1

STUDENT: I was thinking about the need of certain fiber type characteristics to excel at certain sports. What happens if I want to try out for the cross-country team and I only have 50% SO fibers? If I train hard can I get to 75%?

PROFESSOR: First, let me say that if you want to be a cross-country runner, do it. Don't worry about your fiber percentages. But, second, if you weren't born with a high percentage of SO fibers, don't be disappointed if you don't excel at long-distance running. In fact, be happy that you have a plausible explanation for your performance capacity. As time goes on, you may want to find an activity that better suits your capacity.

This is a common conversation between athletes and coaches, or students and teachers, when fiber type information becomes known. Komi and Karlsson[16] have studied monozygotic (identical) and dizygotic (fraternal) twins of both sexes. Their work confirmed that ST fiber distribution is definitely genetic. Also, they found that the variability in muscular power among individuals, as measured by a timed stair-running test, has a high genetic component. However, muscular strength, measured by maximal isometric knee extensions, was not related to inheritance. Therefore, athletes can improve their performance capabilities by increasing their strength, but those without a high percentage of ST fibers may be limited by their genetic makeup.

It does appear, however, that changes are possible within the FT classification. Studies by Prince and others[23] indicate that long-distance running can shift fibers from FG to FOG and weight training can cause the reverse, that is, shift from FOG to FG. It should be pointed out that the shift from FG to FOG fibers is not likely to produce an elite distance runner. New data indicate that high-intensity aerobic training alters the metabolic status of fibers. Therefore, conversion of the aerobic potential of muscle fibers may be possible.

Likewise, the biochemical characteristics of a specific muscle fiber can be changed by training, making it possible to perform more efficiently. For example, Fournier and others[9] found changes in certain muscle enzymes and noted that these changes were specific to the type of training (sprint or endurance) and to the type of fiber (fast or slow). Specifically, sprint training altered enzyme activity in fast fibers and endurance training produced enzyme changes in slow fibers.

It should also be mentioned that other factors, such as aerobic power and anaerobic threshold (discussed later), are related to running performance and may be partly independent of fiber type. Therefore, although fiber type is important to running capacity, it is not the only important factor.

CASE STUDY 2

STUDENT: Excuse me but I'm confused! I'm in your exercise physiology class but I don't know why. I want to be a basketball coach. Today you were talking about muscle fibers, sarcomeres, and sliding filaments. How will that ever help me win a basketball game? I don't care how muscles get the ball into the basket. I just care that they do.

Undergraduate students preparing to be teachers, and/or coaches, and studying exercise physiology often wonder about the relevance of learning about cellular muscle structure and function. To solve this problem for yourself you must examine your expectations. Many times we enter physical education intrigued by wholistic performance (playing a baseball game) and focused on the external manipulation of the student (teaching how to hit). Learning how the body works to cause successful movement is a new orientation. Students enter medicine interested in wholistic cures but with the understanding that the solution of medical problems requires a thorough understanding of bodily function and a need for skills to search out the most efficient solutions. Sport and exercise problems are not a matter of life and death, but they do often require more than a superficial functional understanding of the movement itself. Teachers and coaches need problem-solving skills that, like the physician's, are based on how the body works.

Students and athletes are deluged with media information about the effects of exercise and sport on their bodies. They ask very sophisticated questions and are not placated by nonscientific responses. It is common for students to inquire, for example, about what happens to cause muscles to grow during training, or for new coaches to be thrust into a sport in which they have little experience or about which little training information is available. One approach to solving such problems is through basic cellular understanding. You have one level of understanding if you know that hitting a baseball requires strength. You have another if you can provide a simple answer about improvement in the anaerobic capacity of FG fibers. Yet another level of understanding is required to design a training program that considers the energy pathways typically used in the sport. Knowledge provides independence.

chapter 2

ROLE OF THE NERVOUS SYSTEM IN MUSCULAR CONTRACTION

MAJOR LEARNING OBJECTIVE

Nervous control of muscle fiber contraction is a complex process. The nervous system may be the site of some fatigue.

■ Learning motor skills is a function of producing adaptation in the nervous system.

APPLICATIONS

Early learning behavior requires the learner to "think" of every movement before its execution. The skilled performer bypasses complex pathways to "visualize" the general pattern of the movement rather than the component parts.

■ Pedagogy should stress the facilitation of the transition from concentration on component parts to concentration on the general pattern of the movement.

THE purpose of this chapter is to explain how the nervous system delivers messages to skeletal muscles. The first chapter dealt with the contractile properties of skeletal muscle. Except for a reference to the role of nervous stimulation in releasing calcium from the SR, little was mentioned about the nervous system. It is important to bear in mind that sport and exercise require muscles to receive "instructions" to execute properly. The tennis serve, for example, is a voluntary act that demands precise and high-speed messages to muscles so that the racket can propel the ball into the service court. The fact that even the world's best tennis players cannot accomplish this task every time demonstrates the complexity of performance that is demanded of our athletes and their muscle function. However, accomplishing this task at all is evidence of the precision of neuromuscular coordination.

 ## ORGANIZATION OF THE NERVOUS SYSTEM

The first matter to be dealt with is a review of the organization of the nervous system. To fully understand nervous control we should remind ourselves about the *central nervous system* (brain and spinal cord), the *peripheral nervous system,* and the *autonomic nervous system*. In addition, we need to familiarize ourselves with the functional units that make up these systems: the neuron, neuromuscular junction, motor unit, and reflex arc. The brain serves as the control tower monitoring incoming and outgoing messages, and integrates information about the current status of the organism with information that has been previously stored. The spinal cord functions as a conduit through which ascending and descending cables pass and exit at appropriate levels. More about the central nervous system is discussed later in the chapter. The peripheral nervous system provides the connective link between the spinal cord and sites in the body's periphery (for example, the muscles). Although the autonomic nervous system does not directly influence muscle contraction, its effect on visceral function, such as the heart and blood vessels, indirectly supports the contractile process.

Peripheral nervous system

The peripheral nervous system is made up of 12 pairs of *cranial nerves* and 31 pairs of *spinal nerves*. Spinal nerves interact directly with skeletal muscles and provide the stimulus necessary for muscle contraction. Spinal nerves can be subdivided into four categories:
1. Somatic afferent—carry sensations from the periphery to the spinal cord. These sensations are both exteroceptive (pain, temperature, touch, and pressure) and proprioceptive (arising from muscles, tendons, and joint capsules).
2. Visceral afferent—carry sensations from mucous membranes, glands, and blood vessels.

3. Somatic efferent—communicate from the spinal cord to skeletal muscles.
4. Visceral efferent—communicate from the spinal cord to smooth muscle and glandular tissue.

Although it is helpful to think of this categorization, it would be incorrect to think that nerve fibers have specialized characteristics depending on function. In fact, each nerve is a collection of nerve fibers that conduct both *afferent* (sensory) and *efferent* (motor) *impulses*. Nerve fibers have the ability to conduct in both directions and from any stimulus (sensory or motor). They do exhibit specificity, however; they actually conduct in only one direction. Specificity arises from the fiber's termination. Fibers terminating in skeletal muscle are motor specific (they conduct toward the muscle only), whereas fibers arising from pain receptors in the skin and terminating in the spinal cord, for example, are sensory specific (impulse travels from receptor to cord). Another factor limiting the specificity of nervous fibers is that whereas nervous impulses can theoretically travel in both directions, in fact, nerve *synapses* (the connective links between nerve fibers) will allow conduction of impulses in only one direction. Thus, nerve fibers terminating in skeletal muscle serve a motor function only.

The neuron. The basic unit of the nervous system is the *neuron* (Figure 2-1). The neuron consists of the *cell body, dendrites,* and *axon*. Circuitry necessary to stimulate muscles in the foot may require several neurons connected by synapses. Conversely, a motor nerve leaving the spinal cord can terminate the muscle level without synapsing. The cell body of motor nerves is located in the ventral horn of the spinal cord, whereas sensory nerves terminate in the dorsal horn (Figure 2-2). The axon of the motor nerve continues unbranched until it nears its muscular destination, where it divides into a number of branches.

Axons can be covered by a fatty sheath known as the *myelin sheath* or can be unmyelinated. Myelinated axons have higher conduction velocities. Nodes called the *nodes of Ranvier* are located about every 0.5 mm along the sheath of myelinated fibers. Impulses are conducted from node to node, a process known as *saltatory conduction*. The very fast velocity of saltatory conduction results from an instantaneous passage of electrical current from one node to the next. A sheath, consisting of *Schwann cells*, surrounds the myelin sheath. Schwann cells are glial cells that insulate the axon and facilitate conduction velocity. The junction of two Schwann cells forms the nodes of Ranvier. Only axons that are encased in Schwann cells can regenerate following injury. Figure 2-3 describes the structure of an axon.

The neuromuscular junction. Axons terminate in muscle tissue in a structure known as a motor endplate or a neuromuscular junction (Figure 2-4). Axons travel within muscle, branch, and embed themselves within muscle fibers. The neuromuscular junction can be observed on slightly raised portions of the muscle. Within this raised portion is an invagination called a *synaptic cleft*. In FT fibers the cleft is identified by numerous folds in the sarcolemma. ST fibers do not exhibit as many, or as deep, synaptic clefts. Presum-

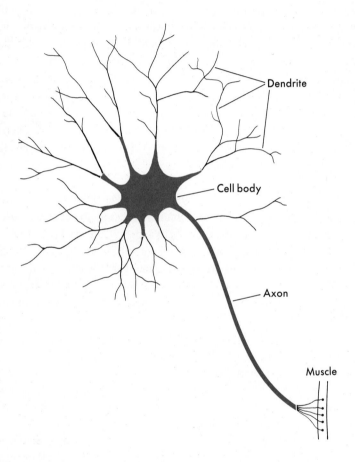

FIG. 2-1 The neuron. The neuron terminates in the muscle on one or more muscle fibers. It should be noted that there is only one nerve junction for each fiber.

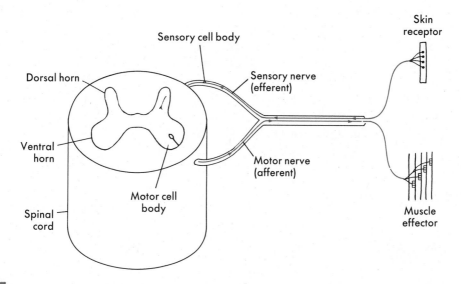

FIG. 2-2   **Location of sensory and motor nerve fibers in the spinal cord.**

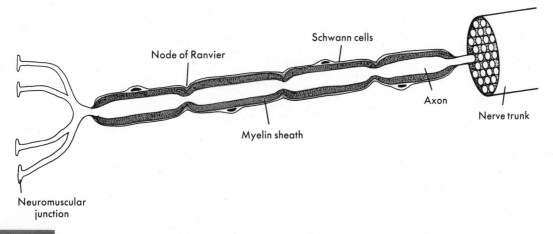

FIG. 2-3   **The structure of the axon.**

ably, this characteristic is related to muscle twitch velocity, that is, more synaptic clefts associated with greater velocity.

The motor unit. One motor nerve and all the muscle fibers that it innervates are referred to as a *motor unit*. Depending on the complexity of the function of a particular muscle, as few as 10 or as many as 2000 muscle fibers may be involved. As more intensity or tension is required to complete a task, such as continuing a task under fatiguing conditions or lifting heavier and heavier objects, additional motor units can be recruited to promote continuance. The relationship between the number of motor units recruited and force produced is hyperbolic, that is, greater force is produced as recruitment level increases. This relationship is illustrated as follows:

% Recruitment	% Maximum force
25	5
50	20
70	50
90	80
100	100

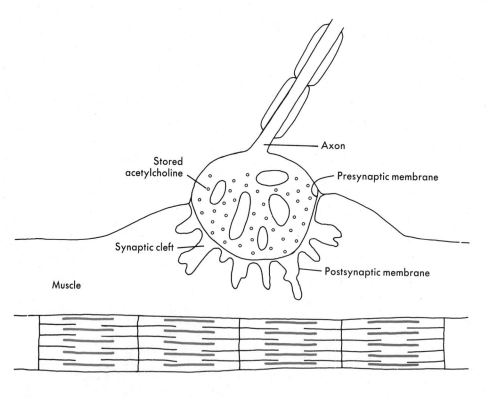

FIG. 2-4 The neuromuscular junction.

Even though whole muscle may be mixed relative to fiber type, one motor neuron always innervates fibers of the same type, that is, SO, FOG, or FG. For light tasks, in which few motor units are recruited, predominantly SO fibers are recruited. As the need for additional recruitment increases, FOG fibers are brought into action. With heavy demands FG fibers enter. Thus, fiber types are entered as a function of increased recruitment in the following way:

$$SO \rightarrow FOG \rightarrow FG$$

Axon diameters are smaller in slow motor units and, as would be expected, have slower conduction velocities.

The reflex arc. Sensory nerves that originate in the periphery, such as temperature receptors in the skin, terminate in the dorsal root of the spinal cord. Sensory nerves providing messages from their periphery and motor nerves capable of stimulating skeletal muscle activity provide the primary structures for what is known as the *reflex arc*. The classical reflex arc, seen in the *stretch reflex*, is monosynaptic, that is, a sensory nerve axon needs only one synapse with the cell body of a motor nerve (Figure 2-5). Other, more complex

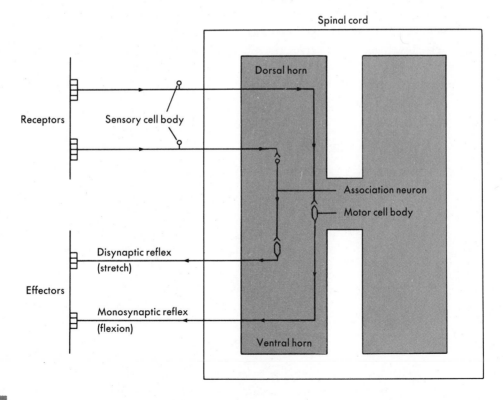

FIG. 2-5   **The reflex arc with examples of monosynaptic and disynaptic reflexes.**

reflexes require two or more synapses within the spinal cord. For example, a disynaptic reflex like the *flexion reflex* (your response to touching a hot stove) uses a small interconnecting neuron within the spinal cord called an *association neuron*.

■   ■   ■

Sport and exercise require voluntary movement. It is clear that higher brain centers transmit messages via descending tracts to the necessary levels of the spinal cord, where the message is transferred to the appropriate spinal nerve for delivery to muscle fibers. More information about brain anatomy and function appears later in this chapter.

Autonomic nervous system

One final description is necessary for a complete structural picture of the nervous system. The autonomic nervous system controls the function of the viscera. This is accomplished through the innervation of organs from the two branches: *parasympathetic* and *sympathetic* branches of the autonomic nervous system. Both of these branches are under the control of higher brain centers. The parasympathetic branch, also known as the craniosacral branch because of the positioning of its ganglia, is, in general, inhibitory. For example, this branch acts to slow the rate of the heart. However, in specific cases, as in digestion, this branch stimulates. *Acetylcholine* is the chemical transmitter at the nerve endings of the parasympathetic branch. The sympathetic branch, also known as the thoracolumbar branch, is, in general, facilitatory and releases *norepinephrine* at its nerve endings. Sympathetic nerves, for example, increase the rate of the heart. Sympathetic nerves can also be inhibitory. Since the continued functioning of skeletal muscle requires precise blood flow control, contractile phenomena are indirectly affected by autonomic function.

EXCITATION AND CONDUCTION IN MOTOR NERVE AND SKELETAL MUSCLE FIBERS

The sequence of events from the stimulation of a motor nerve to the development of muscle tension occurs as follows:

Motor nerve action potential → Propagation at neuromuscular junction →
Muscle action potential →
Excitation and cross-bridge coupling → Muscle tension development

This section deals with the development of action potentials in nerve and muscle (essentially the same mechanisms) and the propagation of the nervous impulse across the neuromuscular junction.

Nerve and muscle action potentials

When a nerve or muscle is stimulated above threshold (minimal stimulus for response), the passage of an impulse causes a change in electrical potential along the cell membrane. This change in potential is recorded as a spike and is called the *action potential.* The stimulus can be hormonal, thermal, mechanical, electromagnetic, or chemical. It should be remembered that both fibers comply with the *all or none law,* that is, they respond maximally or not at all. Another way of stating the all or none law is that the magnitude of the response is not dependent on the intensity of the stimulus but on local conditions. Figure 2-6 illustrates the basic elements of impulse propagation along the axolemma (sarcolemma in muscle). The action potential of a cell membrane is measured as a potential difference between two electrodes. The method of recording membrane action potentials is also shown in Figure 2-6. In a laboratory preparation, nerve tissue can be stimulated from an external source. A recording electrode is placed inside and another outside the nerve axolemma, so that changes in polarity can be observed.

During a state of rest (resting potential) the outside of the membrane is electrically positive compared to the inside. (Technically the inside is negative as compared to the outside which is neutral, that is, 0.) Likewise, sodium (Na^{++}) and chloride (Cl^-) ions predominate on the outside whereas potassium (K^+) ions predominate on the inside. When the membrane is adequately stimulated, the impulse is propagated by a progressive *depolarization* of the membrane, that is, the potential reverses, with the inside becoming electrically positive. This is caused by the influx of Na^{++} and Cl^- ions. As the impulse passes, the membrane returns to its resting polarized state (repolarization). Diffusion of K^+ ions to the outside of the membrane, carrying positive charges, creates repolarization.

Several additional terms are important to understand. A *subthreshold stimulus* is one that is too small to cause an action potential. Two or more subthreshold stimuli can combine to cause an action potential. This phenomenon is called *summation.* If two or more *suprathreshold* stimuli arrive at the muscle in rapid succession, the responses fuse to

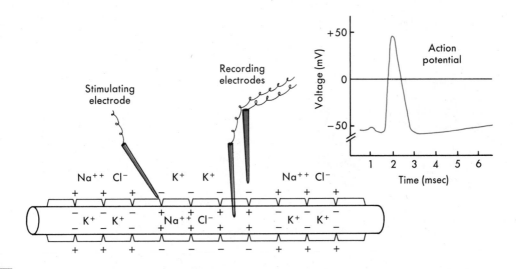

FIG. 2-6   **Electrical conduction of the nerve impulse. Resting action potential shown in the inset is −80 mV.**

create *tetanus*. The tetanic response is greater than that of a single stimulus alone (see Figure 2-7). After a membrane is stimulated there is the *refractory period,* during which the membrane cannot respond (absolute) or can only respond with a very intense stimulus (relative). *Facilitation* is a term used to explain the process of aiding the transmission of an action potential. *Inhibition* of the nervous stimulus can also occur, that is, an action potential can be prevented from continuing.

Neuromuscular transmission

Next, we address the question of the transmission of the impulse across the neuromuscular junction. For some time this transmission was explained by the so-called *electrical theory,* that is, simple electrical conduction across the synaptic gap. However, more recent evidence supports the *chemical theory*—that neuromuscular transmission is accomplished by the action of the chemical acetylcholine (ACh). ACh acts to both facilitate and inhibit an action potential. Knowledge of how ACh can, at one time, inhibit and, at another, facilitate is incomplete. Other neurotransmitter substances may be involved in inhibition. ACh is synthesized by motor nerves and is stored there. The nerve impulse causes the release of ACh from its storage sites. Following release, ACh diffuses across the synaptic cleft and reacts with receptive sites on the muscle fiber. This causes a change in the *endplate potential* (EPP). When the EPP reaches a critical level an action potential is initiated in the muscle fiber. The enzyme *acetylcholinesterase* is thought to remove ACh from the neuromuscular junction.

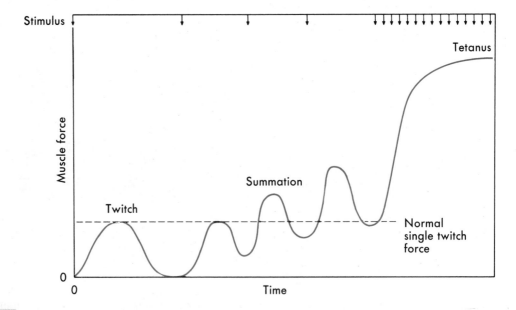

| **FIG. 2-7** | **Tension-time diagram illustrating a muscle twitch response, summation, and tetanus.** |

Fatigue, defined as the reduction or termination of muscular performance, can be caused by changes in the neuromuscular junction. For example, the junction can no longer transmit the impulse. This transmission failure is thought to be associated with a reduction in ACh. Many other hypotheses concerning the site of fatigue have been proposed. For instance, fatigue may rest within the muscle or within the motor neuron. Current views point to the muscle contraction mechanism as the site of fatigue during muscular exercise.

Practical summary. We return our attention to the tennis player with whom we began this chapter. The message to serve the ball proceeds down the spinal cord to the levels associated with appropriate movements over the whole body. On stimulation of the appropriate motor nerves with suprathreshold stimuli, impulses are propagated from the spinal cord into the somatic efferent system. Reaching the neuromuscular junction, the synapse is "jumped" and muscle fibers are stimulated. The stimulus is propagated down T tubules, thereby setting off the cross-bridge coupling mechanisms and causing increases in muscle tension. Considering the many muscles involved, all requiring slightly different tension productions and all precisely synchronized, it is truly amazing that the ball can be kept in the service court.

FACTORS RELATED TO MUSCLE CONTRACTION

Human movement involves the regulation of the length, force, and velocity of muscle fibers. Before we can discuss how control of movement takes place, it is helpful to illustrate the relationships between these factors. First, the force produced by a muscle is systematically related to its length (Figure 2-8). The greatest force is produced when the muscle is fixed at resting length. Increasing or decreasing length will lessen resulting force production. This is due to maximal actin-myosin overlap occurring at resting length. This means that maximal force production of the quadriceps should occur at full knee extension. However, in the intact human with muscles attached across joints, maximal functional force is achieved at an angle closer to 120 degrees than 180 degrees. Second, a muscle that is not supporting a load can contract most rapidly. As muscle velocity is reduced, force productivity can increase (Figure 2-9). For example, greatest force productivity is achieved with no velocity, that is, isometric contraction. Lastly, for any contraction, velocity is greatest when the initial muscle length is resting length.

As mentioned previously, muscle force is graded by additional recruitment of motor units. In addition, however, muscle force is affected by the signal intensity arriving from the nervous system. When the same number of muscle fibers are stimulated, greater force is produced when the rate of stimulation (pulses/second) is increased.

CONTROL OF MOVEMENT

Physical activity requires muscles to perform a diverse range of functions. For example, muscles must be able to perform the most precise and finely controlled tasks imaginable, but show equal capability to develop maximal tension in events requiring minimal control. What control mechanisms are required to allow such great diversity in muscular function?

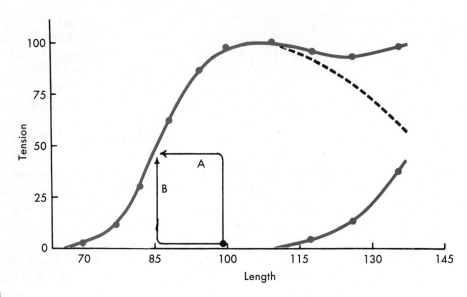

FIG. 2-8   Length-force diagram. (From Dowben, R.M.: Contractility, with special reference to skeletal muscle. In Mountcastle, V.B., editor: Medical physiology, ed. 14, St. Louis, 1980, The C.V. Mosby Co.)

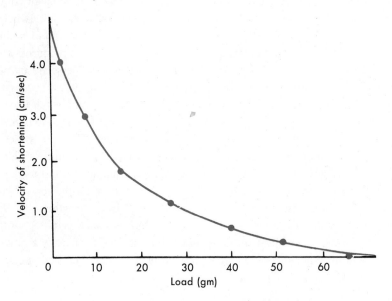

FIG. 2-9   Force-velocity diagram. (From Dowben, R.M.: Contractility, with special reference to skeletal muscle. In Mountcastle, V.B., editor: Medical physiology, ed. 14, St. Louis, 1980, The C.V. Mosby Co.)

Peripheral control

Control of muscular contraction in the periphery involves *proprioception.* That is, proprioceptive organs provide information about the state of muscles, tendons, and joints. Proprioception uses a system of feedback that helps to control contraction. There are two classes of proprioceptors. First, the joint receptors control position sense and, therefore, provide information to the conscious mind. Second, the muscle receptors control muscle sense, called *kinesthesis,* an unconscious process. Position sense should be further explained as knowledge of the dynamics of limb and whole body movement, for example, the angle of the knee as the foot strikes a soccer ball. Muscle sense, in contrast, refers to the ability of muscle to sense its own contractile properties, that is, length and tension. In doing so, muscle detects when more tension is required, and a stimulus is then sent to the spinal cord which, in turn, stimulates muscle to contract more intensely. Through the same mechanism, contraction can be inhibited when additional stretch might be damaging.

The structures that provide peripheral proprioceptive information are *muscle spindles, Golgi tendon organs, pacinian corpuscles,* and *Ruffini receptors.* The first two structures are related to muscle sense, whereas the latter two are related to position sense.

Muscle spindles are located in parallel with the extrafusal muscle fibers (skeletal muscle fibers) and, therefore, respond to movements made by these fibers. Two to 12 intrafusal fibers wrapped by a sheath constitute a muscle spindle. Intrafusal fibers are of two types, *nuclear bag fibers* and *nuclear chain fibers.* These fibers respond to the stretching of extrafusal fibers by sending messages to the spinal cord concerning the degree of stretch. As soon as the muscle shortens, spindles are automatically released from stretch and return to a resting state. Spindle response is made possible by the presence of two sensory nerve end organs within the spindle sheath. *Annulospiral* end organs wrap around both nuclear bag and nuclear chain fibers and respond primarily to static stretch. Muscle spindles are supplied by *gamma efferent* nerves that make up approximately one-third of the nerves entering muscle. (Two-thirds of the nerves are motor neurons, *alpha efferent,* that supply the extrafusal fibers.) When muscle is stretched by the application of a resistance (load), muscle spindles supply information about how much contraction will be necessary according to the resistance present. In other words, muscle spindles facilitate muscle contraction (Figure 2-10). Muscle spindles also work in a reflex manner. When the muscle is suddenly stretched, the impulse is carried to the spinal cord and is directed back to the muscle via a single synapse. The muscle contracts in response (Figure 2-5).

Golgi tendon organs are located in muscles at their junction with tendons. This location means that these organs are arranged in series with ten to twenty extrafusal fibers. They are stimulated by changes in tension produced by active stretching or muscle shortening. These changes in tension provide information about the strength of the contraction and, more importantly, about when the tension is too great. Golgi tendon organs act to inhibit contraction or protect muscles from injury.

Figure 2-11 illustrates the elements and interactions of the peripheral control system. In this system the *muscle* appears as the controller of movement and the *load* as the system controlled. The *tendon organs* and *spindles* act as transducers, that is, they monitor force, length, and velocity, respectively. The regulation of these factors provides feedback that modifies the efferent signal to muscle. "Instructions" arrive from the central nervous system in the form of alpha and gamma signals. Alpha signals are faster because they directly activate muscles. Conversely, gamma signals must activate spindles first. To provide coordinated control, the systems that monitor length, velocity, and force function simultaneously. Interneurons in the spinal cord modulate the force feedback response.

Fatigue of muscle offers an interesting example of how the peripheral control system works. As fatigue sets in, muscular force production is decreased. The alpha neurons,

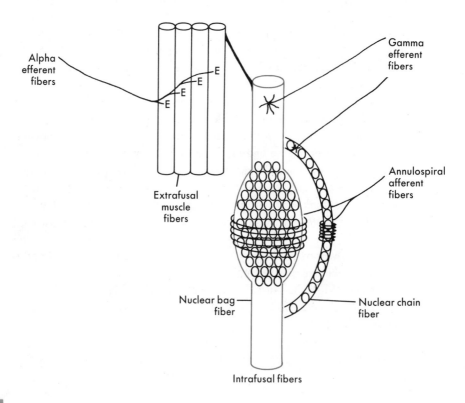

FIG. 2-10   The components of a muscle spindle.

which normally receive inhibitory signals from the tendon organs to conserve force production, now receive fewer inhibitory signals. Thus, more motor units can be recruited to increase force production.

As mentioned, pacinian corpuscles and Ruffini receptors are involved with providing information about body position. Both are found within joints and, in addition, pacinian corpuscles are found in the sheaths of tendons and muscles.

Central control

Complex human movement requires conscious control from higher brain centers. At present scientists have not been able to identify what might be called a "command center." We do know, however, a fair amount about how the "commands" are executed.[6] To begin to understand these mechanisms the student should be familiar with three systems: the *pyramidal system*, the *extrapyramidal system*, and the *proprioceptive-cerebellar system*. The major components of these systems appear in Figure 2-12.

The pyramidal system originates in the *motor cortex* of the brain. Its cell bodies synapse with motor neurons in the spinal cord and innervate those muscles involved in specific movements. The pyramidal pathway is a slow conducting system with about 1 million fibers at lengths up to 1 meter. The motor cortex is *not* oriented to specific

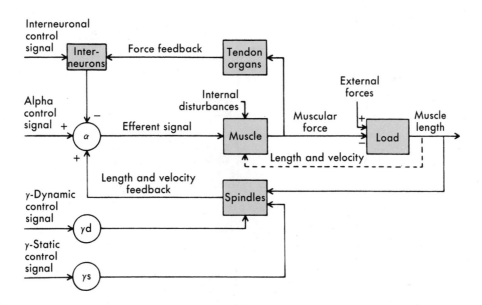

FIG. 2-11   The components and interactions of the peripheral control system. (From Houk, J.: Feedback control of muscle: a synthesis of the peripheral mechanisms. In Mountcastle, V.B., editor: Medical physiology, ed. 13, St. Louis, 1974, The C.V. Mosby Co.)

muscles but to movements. It is thought that early learning of motor skills trains this system.

General movement patterns and highly skilled movements are thought to originate in the extrapyramidal system. This system has its origins in the premotor cortex of the cerebral cortex. Instead of synapsing directly with motor neurons, this system goes through the *motor nuclei,* the *pons,* and the *cerebellum.* The skilled performer does not have to think of every movement before its execution but is aware of the general pattern. A quarterback, for example, does not have to think to cock the arm, transfer the weight to the back foot, extend the arm, etc. Instead, the whole pattern is completed without conscious awareness of the individual parts.

Kinesthetic information, concerning muscle sense, is received from the periphery and integrated with voluntary commands. Kinesthetic fibers end in the thalamus, cortex, and cerebellum.

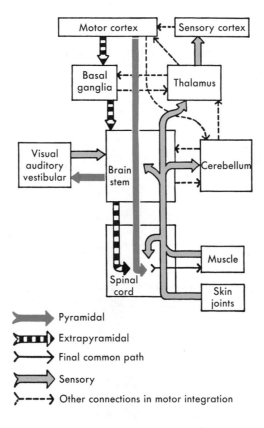

Central control of movement with special reference to the pyramidal and extrapyramidal systems. (From Zierler, K.L.: Mechanism of muscle contraction and its energetics. In Mountcastle, V.B., editor: Medical physiology, ed. 13, St. Louis, 1974, The C.V. Mosby Co.)

SUMMARY

This chapter has addressed the question of how the nervous system delivers messages to skeletal muscle. To answer this question, the structure and function of the nervous system were explained. Two predominate pathways, the pyramidal and extrapyramidal, carry messages from the brain to the spinal cord. These pathways carry impulses from the brain concerning specific movements and general movement patterns, respectively. The impulses descend the spinal cord and exit into the peripheral nervous system. Axons of motor neurons exit the spinal cord, may or may not synapse with other nerve fibers, and finally terminate in an effector organ, such as skeletal muscle. The impulse is propagated by means of saltatory conduction from one node of Ranvier to another along the nerve axon. On reaching the neuromuscular junction, the impulse causes the release of ACh, which enables continued transmission. If the impulse is suprathreshold, it will create an action potential in the muscle fiber. Action potentials are propagated as a result of the movement of sodium, chloride, and potassium ions in and out of the fiber, accompanied by a change in fiber polarity. A motor nerve axon may branch to many muscle fibers, and this is referred to as a motor unit. When increases in contractile intensity are required, more than one motor unit is called into action. Movement is controlled in the periphery by proprioceptors that feed back information about the position, length, and tension of muscles.

KEY TERMS

afferent refers to neurons that carry sensory impulses from the periphery to the spinal cord.

all-or-none law the law stating that when either a muscle or a nerve fiber is stimulated above threshold, it will respond maximally.

efferent refers to neurons that carry motor impulses from the spinal cord to an effector organ in the periphery, that is, skeletal muscle.

motor unit a single motor neuron (efferent) and all the muscle fibers that it innervates.

neuromuscular junction the anatomical site at which the neuron's axon terminates in muscle tissue. Also called the motor endplate.

neuron the basic anatomical unit of the nervous system. It consists of a cell body, dendrites, and an axon.

proprioception the peripheral control process by which feedback is provided concerning position, length, and tension in muscles, tendons, or joints.

reflex arc an anatomical unit that conducts impulses via an afferent neuron through the spinal cord and directly into an efferent neuron, producing an involuntary response in an effector organ.

synapse an anatomical unit that serves as the connective link between neurons.

REVIEW QUESTIONS

1. Diagram a reflex arc. Be sure to label all of the important anatomical components.

2. Describe the anatomy of the nodes of Ranvier. How do the nodes contribute to accelerated nerve conduction?

3. If a motor unit conforms to the all-or-none law, how is muscle contraction graded, that is, how can the muscle correctly respond to greater and greater external loads?

4. What fiber type is used for tasks requiring manual manipulation only?

5. What chemical transmitters are released at the nerve endings of the two branches of the autonomic nervous system? What effect does each have on heart rate?

6. Discuss the ionic interchange during membrane depolarization and repolarization.

7. What is the interrelationship of acetylcholine and acetylcholinesterase in the process of neuromuscular transmission?

8. To what do muscle spindles respond, and by what mechanism do they control muscle function?

9. To what do Golgi tendon organs respond, and by what mechanism do they control muscle function?

10. Give examples of the involvement of the pyramidal and extrapyramidal systems in early and advanced learning.

REFERENCES

1. Bendall, J.R.: Muscles, molecules and movement, New York, 1974, American Elsevier Publishing Co., Inc.

2. Burke, R.E., and Edgerton, V.R.: Motor unit properties and selective involvement in movement. In Wilmore, J., and Keogh, J., editors: Exercise and sport science reviews, New York, 1975, Academic Press, Inc.

3. Carlson, B.M., and Faulkner, J.A.: The regeneration of skeletal muscle fibers following injury: a review, Med. Sci. Sports Exerc. **15:**187, 1983.

4. Edgerton, V.R., Roy, R.R., Gregor, R.J., and others: Muscle fiber activation and recruitment. In Knuttgen, H.G., Poortman, J., and Vogel, J.A., editors: Biochemistry of exercise, Champaign, Ill., 1983, Human Kinetics Publishers, Inc.

5. Guyton, A.C.: Physiology of the human body, ed. 6, Philadelphia, 1984, Saunders College Publishing.

6. Hakkinen, K., and Komi, P.V.: Electromyographic changes during strength training and detraining, Med. Sci. Sports Exerc. **15:**455, 1983.

7. Henneman, E.: Spinal reflexes and the control of movement. In Mountcastle, V.B., editor: Medical physiology, St. Louis, 1979, The C.V. Mosby Co.

8. Henneman, E.: Peripheral mechanisms involved in the control of muscle. In Mountcastle, V.B., editor: Medical physiology, ed. 13, vol. 2, St. Louis, 1974, The C.V. Mosby Co.

9. Jacob, S.W., and Francone, C.A.: Structure and function in man, Philadelphia, 1965, W.B. Saunders Co.

10. Merton, P.A.: How we control the contraction of our muscles, Sci. Am. **226:**30, 1972.

11. Moritani, T., Nagata, A., and Muro, M.: Electromyographic manifestations of muscular fatigue, Med. Sci. Sports Exerc. **14:**198, 1982.

12. Nilsson, J., Tesch, P., and Thorstensson, A.: Fatigue and EMG of repeated fast voluntary contractions in man. Acta Physiol. Scand. **101:**194, 1977.

13. Sale, D.G., MacDougall, J.D., Upton, A.R.M., and others: Effect of strength training upon motoneuron excitability in man, Med. Sci. Sports Exerc. **15:**57, 1983.

14. Stephens, J.A., and Taylor, A.: Fatigue of maintained voluntary muscle contraction in man, J. Physiol. **220:**1, 1972.

15. Tribe, M.A., and Eraut, M.R.: Nerves and muscle, Cambridge, 1977, Cambridge University Press.

SUGGESTED READINGS

Merton, P.A.: How we control the contraction of our muscles, Sci. Am. **226:**30, 1972.

Tribe, M.A., and Eraut, M.R.: Nerves and muscle, Cambridge, 1977, Cambridge University Press.

CASE STUDY 1

I see from my window a young boy, probably 7 or 8 years old, repeatedly throwing a ball on the roof of his house and catching it as it rolls off. Contrary to his parents' view, who think he "never gets tired," he can experience fatigue like any adult. It would take him many throws before fatigue would set in, and most likely he would first become bored. Someday, though, when returning from a cross-country run or finishing a strenuous basketball practice, he will face the "demon" we know as fatigue.

Fatigue has indeed been somewhat of a "demon" for scientists. We know that something is taking place in people from their verbal accounts of fatigue, and we can even measure a decline in gross performance. It is another matter entirely, however, to provide a specific physiological explanation.

Our lack of answers does not stop athletes from asking "why." Perhaps no athlete has ever "fully" exerted himself during competition every time. If we knew more about what causes fatigue, we might be able to develop techniques for decreasing its effects. Of course, realistically we must remember that as soon as we help athletes get past one fatigue barrier, they will face a new, higher fatigue threshold. Fatigue and high-level performance are perhaps a permanent part of the human condition.

Continued.

Broadly stated, the sites of fatigue in the periphery of the body may have three origins, as listed here:

1. Motor neuron
2. Neuromuscular junction
3. Muscle fiber

Possible causes of fatigue in the muscle fiber might involve nutrition, circulation, electrolyte balance, muscle pH, etc. For example, muscle fibers may be depleted of fuel, deprived of adequate circulation, depleted of calcium, or high in lactic acid concentration, to cite just a few possible causes of fatigue. We leave a more detailed description of muscle fiber fatigue to future chapters. The nervous system may also be a possible site of fatigue.

Students can be both afraid and fascinated by fatigue. Even though it is temporary, the pain and discomfort of fatigue can be worrisome. What do you tell students who, by your urging, experience sensations duplicated only in the symptoms of serious disease?

Honestly we don't have all the answers. It appears, however, that the motor neuron is an unlikely site of fatigue. Nerve-muscle preparations demonstrate that the nerve is capable of a great deal of stimulation without fatigue.

The neuromuscular junction, on the other hand, may be the site of some fatigue. Stevens and Taylor[14] found that electromyographic (muscle) activity declined during sustained maximal isometric contractions. This decline was attributed to the decrease in nerve propagation across the neuromuscular junction. However, Nilsson, Tesch, and Thorstensson[12] showed that, during repeated maximal isokinetic contraction, declines in muscle strength (torque) were not accompanied by declines in the electromyograph (EMG). (The EMG records electrical activity of muscles through electrodes either placed on the surface or embedded within the muscle. As more motor units are added in a particular movement the electrical activity is proportionately elevated.) Such data locate the site of fatigue as more probably in the muscle fiber itself.

This apparent confusion is evidence for the complexity of the task, and the probability that there is more than one type of fatigue. We do know that both physiological and subjective fatigue decline with training; thus, we have a positive result to assure participants, as well as an understanding of the general location of our "blood, sweat, and tears."

P.S. The boy's ball got stuck on the roof and he disappeared into the house. Somebody is going to have to do something about roofs. They are often very difficult to play with.

CASE STUDY 2

Students concerned with the teaching and learning of motor skills often ask about the physiological basis of learning. The answer to this question, to the extent that we know it, lies within the nervous system. Exercise physiologists have not considered this topic to be within the boundaries of their subdiscipline. Instead, this has been a topic of study for those in motor learning, particularly those interested in motor control. However, the frequency of this question from students has demanded a response.

First, it is essential to know that learning, both cognitive and motor, is one of the most complex of human behaviors. The search for the physiological basis of learning is ongoing. Second, because of the problems encountered when studying the human nervous system, motor control scientists have turned to the animal model so that variables may be more easily controlled and understood. Thus, we have very little direct human data.

We can view learning as a physiological system that displays feedback characteristics. In a sense, this means that the human learns from itself, or that moving segments "feed back" information to modify the movement in progress. For example, kinesthetic sense helps the tennis player to adjust the serve in progress to adapt to small environmental or opponent changes.

Athletes have sometimes been described as being all "reflex." The "good hands" of the shortstop or the "quick reflexes" of the halfback are descriptions based on observed behavior that the layman attributes to simple reflex. These comments inaccurately simplify the mechanism underlying outstanding athletic performance. Fast athletic responses are not explained by peripheral stimulus—synapse in the spinal cord—or contractile response. Most likely, these responses originate in the brain, having been stimulated by appropriate visual, auditory, and/or tactile stimuli. Impulses travel through the extrapyramidal system to elicit these highly skilled movements. So quick and accurate are these movements that it would be easy to pass them off as "unthinking" spinal cord responses. Our current knowledge of the subject indicates otherwise, however.

Part of the beauty of watching a beginner improve motor skills involves his process of reducing movements to the most essential, what we sometimes call "making it look easy." The beginner executes many more movements than required. Early learning is a process that uses the pyramidal system. Each segment of the new movement must be visualized sequentially. It seems as if the beginner's "computer" is searching for the correct circuitry to select during each segment of the skill. The movement is put together piece by piece. As choices are made and reinforced by successful responses, there is no further necessity for computer search. The responses become "locked in," so that smooth, efficient movements result.

chapter 3

ROLE OF ENERGY METABOLISM IN MUSCULAR CONTRACTION

MAJOR LEARNING OBJECTIVE
One aerobic (oxygen) and two anaerobic
(ATP-PC and lactate) systems are involved in
providing energy for muscular contraction.

APPLICATIONS
Training for a sport should involve stressing the
correct metabolic pathway(s). Identify the
specific ''energetics'' of the sport (frequency,
duration, and intensity of specific movements),
determine whether the movements stress aerobic
and/or anaerobic pathways and design training
dimensions that stimulate the appropriate
pathway(s).

CHAPTERS 1 and 2 discussed the physical process by which muscle fibers contract and how contraction is linked to the nervous system. This chapter provides an understanding of how energy is produced within the body for muscular contraction.

The immediate source of energy for muscular contraction is *adenosine triphosphate* (ATP). Without it, energy would not be available for binding the thick with the thin filaments and for sliding the thin filaments to the center of the sarcomere. The process by which humans produce ATP is crucial to our understanding of how we move freely and efficiently during exercise and sports performance.

Superficially, energy metabolism may seem to be of only academic interest. Of what practical importance is an understanding of ATP production to a teacher or coach? The thesis of this chapter is that this material may be of the greatest practical value.

Understanding the interaction between the food we eat and the energy produced is the beginning of understanding the role of nutrition in exercise and sport. (Chapter 4 deals with this subject more specifically.) You will often find yourself in the role of nutritional counselor to athletes and interpreter of books and articles on the subject of sports nutrition. It is not your role to be a nutritionist, but a basic understanding will enable you to separate fact from myth.

Teachers and coaches in most public schools must develop their own training programs, sometimes with little personal experience with the sport in question. Training programs that develop performance fitness are largely a matter of improving the system that produces energy for that activity. For example, energy for cross-country skiing comes from a different system than that for swimming a 50 meters race. Knowledge of energy systems will provide the physiological principles that will aid in the development of training programs.

FOOD IS THE GENESIS

People in Western civilization tend to regard the intake of food in a rather passive manner. That is not to say that we treat it indifferently. The proliferation of the fast-food business pointedly emphasizes our consumptive tendencies. Our passivity is displayed by our general lack of understanding of what constitutes adequate nutrition and how nutrition regulates our bodily function.

Elite athletes, due to their competitive nature, constantly search for ways to gain a performance advantage. Smart athletes understand the relationship between the intake of nutrients and performance and eat accordingly. In most cases, however, faddism without functional benefits is more common than sound knowledge. The first step toward making smart decisions about nutrition is acquiring an understanding of how food "makes" energy for performance.

Carbohydrate, fat, and protein in our food are broken down through digestion to forms that can be used by muscle cells to synthesize ATP either *anaerobically* (without oxygen) or *aerobically* (with oxygen). Figure 3-1 illustrates this complex process in simple terms. The means by which carbohydrate, fat, and protein are prepared for use are dealt with later. First, we should start with the end of the process, cellular production of ATP.

CELLULAR PRODUCTION OF ATP

ATP liberates energy for muscular contraction when it splits to form *adenosine diphosphate* (ADP) and *inorganic phosphate* (P_i). To become viable again, another phosphate must be added to ADP (resynthesis of ATP). This P_i is provided by the breakdown of a substance *phosphocreatine* ($PC \rightarrow C + P_i$), which is available to a limited extent in muscle cells. Thus, we have the first of the two primary mechanisms by which ATP is synthesized anaerobically. (Again, no intake of oxygen is required.) The process of adding P_i to ADP is known as *phosphorylation*.

The next anaerobic mechanism involves the metabolic process known as *glycolysis*. Technically, this means that one molecule of glucose is broken down to pyruvic acid with a net production of two molecules of ATP. This occurs directly if glucose (or other monosaccharides such as fructose) is present within the cell, for example, if blood glucose has been delivered from the liver. A number of enzymes act as catalysts in the glycolytic pathway. Among these enzymes, several play important roles in the internal control of glycolysis. These are hexokinase, phosphofructokinase (PFK), pyruvate kinase, and lactate dehydrogenase. For example, PFK is a rate-limiting enzyme, that is, the rate of

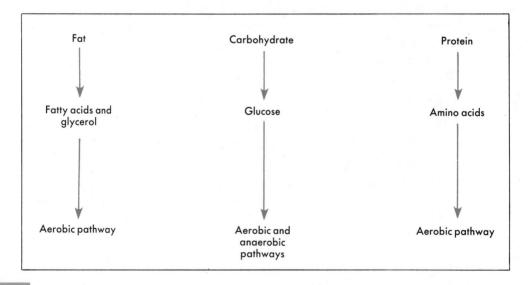

FIG. 3-1   Relationship of food consumed to metabolic pathways used for the production of energy.

glycolysis is dependent on PFK supply. Another means of obtaining glucose within the cell is by *glycogenolysis*. Glycogenolysis refers to the process of the breakdown of *glycogen,* the storage form of glucose, to glucose. If glucose and glycogen are not available, as in long-duration work or starvation, glycolysis is not possible. By implication, this also means that the production of ATP via the glycolytic pathway is not possible with fat and protein. One exception to this rule occurs when amino acids are degraded to glucose or glycogen in the liver by a process known as *gluconeogenesis*. Still, glucose is the substrate used to produce ATP anaerobically. Figure 3-2 illustrates the glycolytic pathway and its relationship with the aerobic pathway.

    Lactic acid and *alanine* are both end products of anaerobic metabolism and are dealt with later in detail. It is sufficient to say, at this point, that when anaerobic metabolism continues unabated, the production and use of lactic acid become out of balance and lactic acid enters the bloodstream in great quantities. This phenomenon has led many researchers to link this substance to the fatigue associated with short-duration, high-intensity exercise. *Pyruvic acid,* which is the final step of glycolysis, is also the first step in the

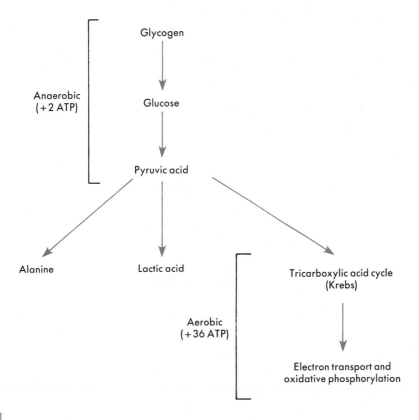

FIG. 3-2   Glycolysis and its relationship to the aerobic pathway.

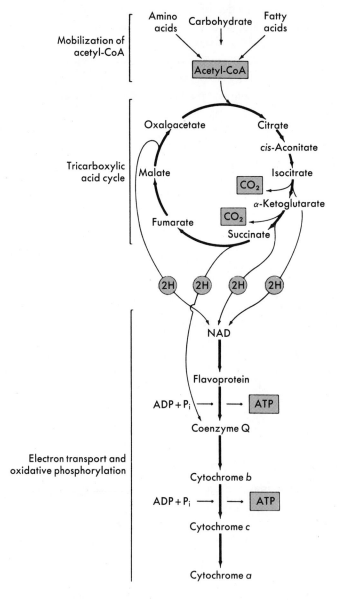

FIG. 3-3   Pathway of aerobic metabolism. (From Lehninger, A.L.: Short course in biochemistry, New York, 1973, Worth Publishers, Inc.)

aerobic metabolism of carbohydrate. Pyruvic acid is further broken down to *acetyl-CoA* and enters the *tricarboxylic acid (Krebs) cycle,* producing two ATP molecules, CO_2, H ions, (shown in Figure 3-3 as hydrogen atoms [2 H]), and electrons. (Fat and protein in the form of fatty acids and amino acids can also be degraded to acetyl-CoA to enter the tricarboxylic acid cycle.) As these electrons are chemically transported to oxygen to form water, ATP is phosphorylated with a net gain of 36 ATP molecules. Therefore, the entire aerobic process produces 38 ATP molecules (including the two produced during glycolysis). Figure 3-3 illustrates the pathway of aerobic metabolism. Another convenient way of depicting the aerobic breakdown of carbohydrate appears as follows:

$$C_6 H_{12} O_6 + 6 O_2 + 38 ADP + 38 P \rightarrow 6 CO_2 + 6 H_2O + 38 ATP$$

Therefore, the muscle cell has three alternative metabolic mechanisms to produce ATP:

Anaerobic

1. Resynthesis of ATP from the breakdown of PC.
2. Breakdown of glucose to form pyruvic acid and ultimately lactic acid.

Aerobic

3. Breakdown of acetyl-CoA from carbohydrate, fat, and protein to form CO_2 + H_2O + ATP.

SOURCES OF ENERGY
Carbohydrates

Depending on the chemical structure, ingested carbohydrate can be *monosaccharide, disaccharide,* or *polysaccharide*. However, only monosaccharides can be absorbed by the epithelial lining of the small intestine. This step is important in the digestion process because here the monosaccharide is converted to free glucose for entry into the bloodstream and transport to the liver and other organs. As an example, let us examine the carbohydrate content of a bowl of cereal with sugar, milk, and fruit. This combination contains all three carbohydrates. Cereal grains (starch) are polysaccharides, sugar (sucrose) and milk (lactose) are disaccharides, and the fruit (fructose) is an example of a monosaccharide. Therefore, the cereal, sugar, and milk must be converted to monosaccharides before they can enter the lining of the small intestine.

This conversion process is referred to as *hydrolysis*. Hydrolysis begins in the mouth with the secretion of an enzyme called *amylase* in the salivary fluid. Again, amylase contained in pancreatic juices continues the hydrolytic process in the small intestine.

Following the conversion of the monosaccharide to free glucose in the small intestine, the glucose enters the blood where most of it is transported to the liver. What happens in the liver? First, free glucose is converted to *glucose-6-phosphate*. (Glucose is catalyzed by the enzyme hexokinase to form glucose-6-phosphate [G-6-P]. G-6-P serves as a substrate for glycogen synthesis.) Next, one of the following alternatives occurs, depending on the need:

1. Reconversion of free glucose for transport in the blood to skeletal muscles and other organs.
2. Oxidation in the tricarboxylic acid cycle and electron transport system to form ATP for use in liver function.
3. Conversion to glycogen for liver storage.
4. Degradation to acetyl-CoA for conversion to fatty acids for transport through the blood to fat cells for storage.

Glucose transported to muscle cells can be immediately converted to G-6-P for use in glycolysis if energy is required, or to muscle glycogen if immediate use is not necessary. During exercise, when muscle cells require more energy, liver glycogen can be reconverted to blood glucose for transport to the tissues in need. Likewise, fatty acids formed from carbohydrate conversion in the liver can go directly to muscle cells in need. Similarly, fat can be converted to fatty acids for transport in the blood to muscle cells during exercise.

During exercise, blood glucose level rises or remains constant, depending on the intensity of the exercise, and it will not fall except in prolonged exercise such as marathon running. The supply of glucose during exercise is made possible principally by glycogenolysis in the liver but, in addition, by glucose stored in muscle (glycogen). In the case of very short-duration exercise, or in the early stages of any exercise, energy for muscular work can be supplied by anaerobic sources within muscle (ATP-PC). Exercise lasting more than 5 minutes, however, requires glucose and free fatty acid delivery to muscle cells from liver and fat tissue supplies. The course of blood glucose released from the small intestine is illustrated in Figure 3-4.

Fat (lipids)

Fat can be found in various forms in the body but all forms contain the basic lipid building blocks, fatty acids. *Phospholipids* serve as a primary structural component of cellular membranes and blood plasma. *Lipoproteins* serve as a transport mechanism to

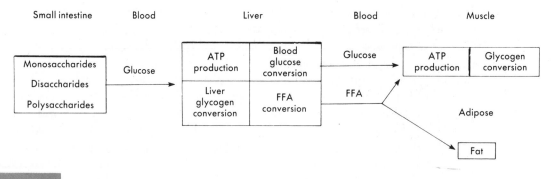

FIG. 3-4   Course of blood glucose released from the small intestine.

carry lipids from the small intestine to the liver and from the liver to fat cells. Two lipoproteins involved in this process, low-density lipoprotein (LDL) and very low-density lipoprotein (VLDL), are said to be high-risk factors for coronary heart disease. High-density lipoprotein (HDL) is thought to be involved in the breakdown of cholesterol, and current research relates high levels of this lipoprotein to protection from heart disease. *Triglycerides* serve as the storage form of lipids in fat cells. When hydrolyzed, triglycerides are converted to fatty acids that serve as fuel for energy production in muscle cells.

Consumed fat in the diet must be further digested in the small intestine so that lipid can be absorbed into the bloodstream. This is accomplished by the enzyme *lipase,* secreted by the pancreas, and by bile acids. Lipase hydrolyzes lipid-producing monoglycerides, glycerol, and fatty acids. These substances enter the epithelial lining of the small intestine and are reconstituted to form triglycerides. Triglycerides, along with cholesterol and glycerol, are then encased in particles called *chylomicrons* that are released into the lymphatic system. Thus, most lipid is released into the blood via the lymph.

When lipids reach the liver they are used in the following ways:

1. Synthesis of lipoproteins for transporting lipid for storage in fat cells.
2. Degradation to acetyl-CoA to produce ATP in the tricarboxylic acid cycle or for conversion to ketone bodies (produced from the breakdown of fats) that can be used as fuel for the tricarboxylic acid cycle in other tissues.
3. Degradation to fatty acids and bound to serum albumin to pass to peripheral tissues.

Most fuel storage in the human body is accomplished by fat storage. Of the fat stored, 98% is stored in adipose tissue and 2% in the muscle cells. (A smaller but critical amount of fuel is stored as glycogen in the liver and muscles.) Muscle cells can use lipid as a fuel by receiving either free fatty acids or ketone bodies from the liver, by receiving free fatty acids stored as fat, or by using fat stored in muscle tissue.

During rest, the major fuel for energy production is lipid. When short-duration, very intense exercise is engaged in, for example, a 100 meter dash, the only practical mechanism for energy production is anaerobic—from stored ATP and resynthesis by PC or lactate production through glycolysis. (Actually, a small percentage is most likely supplied aerobically.) Since glucose is the only fuel usable in the glycolytic process, lipid would not be employed. During light and moderate exercise that can be carried out over a long duration (up to approximately 50% $\dot{V}O_2$ max), the predominate fuel is lipid. In contrast, during heavy exercise, exceeding 90% $\dot{V}O_2$ max, the predominate fuel is glycogen. At work intensities around 50% to 60% $\dot{V}O_2$ max, lipid still remains the predominate fuel. Between 60% and 90% the contribution of glycogen grows. During very long-duration exercise, such as marathon running, the fuel is predominately carbohydrate until muscle and liver glycogen are depleted from the fibers in use. At this point, stored fat and protein are the only source of fuel in the fibers. It should be remembered that elite marathon runners compete at intensities greater than 80% $\dot{V}O_2$ max.

Protein

Protein intake serves as the source of *amino acids* for the maintenance of cellular structure and as fuel for energy production. Amino acids are the basic building blocks of protein. Until recently, protein was thought to contribute very little to exercise energy production. Now evidence indicates that as much as 10% of the exercise energy requirements may be provided by protein.

Protein hydrolysis begins in the stomach with the addition of the enzyme *pepsin*. Further breakdown to amino acids is accomplished in the small intestine by proteolytic enzymes found in pancreatic juices.

Entering the bloodstream from the small intestine as amino acids, protein is transported to the liver. Amino acids are processed in the liver in the following ways:

1. Pass directly through and enter the bloodstream again for transport throughout the body.
2. Are used for protein synthesis in liver structure.
3. Undergo gluconeogenesis, that is, are converted to pyruvate and then to glycogen.
4. Are degraded to acetyl-CoA, which can be converted to fatty acids or may enter the tricarboxylic acid cycle for production of energy for the liver.

Therefore, protein can be used as a source of energy for muscular work through gluconeogenesis or the conversion of amino acid to acetyl-CoA and free fatty acids. Likewise, a small amount of amino acids can be oxidized directly in the muscle.

Additional sources

Figure 3-5 illustrates what is known as the *Cori cycle*. Simply stated, this process converts lactic acid, produced in the muscle under anaerobic conditions, into liver glycogen that in turn can be converted to blood glucose for use by muscle cells as a fuel. Although this is a process that occurs during recovery from exercise to replenish food

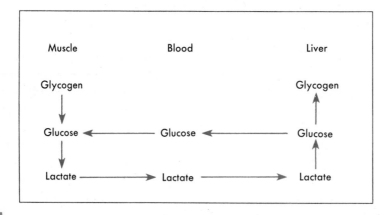

FIG. 3-5   Cori cycle.

stores, it is also possible to use this mechanism during exercise. Marathon runners who produce lactate in the early stages of a competitive race may use this lactate as a fuel later in the race. Presumably, the Cori cycle is used for this process. However, this mechanism may be limited by reduced liver blood flow during exercise. It should be stated that some tissues can oxidize lactate directly.

Another interesting possible source of energy results from the production of *alanine* (see Figure 3-2). Although the exact role of alanine in energy metabolism is uncertain, it is known to be an amino acid produced during glycolysis. Alanine plays an important role in protein synthesis but it is unlikely that this would be the purpose of alanine production during exercise. Alanine is stored in skeletal muscle and is probably released only during starvation or long-term exercise. In such a case, the alanine would be carried in the bloodstream to the liver, where it would be converted to glucose by gluconeogenesis and returned to the muscle cells.

HORMONAL REGULATION OF ENERGY METABOLISM

Certain aspects of energy metabolism that can be regulated internally (within the cell) do not require an outside influence. For example, the need for small increases in cellular energy production can be met by appropriate increases in cellular enzyme synthesis. The rate-limiting nature of the enzyme PFK (glycolysis), mentioned previously, is a case in point. However, there is also need for external control to ensure the integrity of the cell. Control requires the involvement of the autonomic nervous system and the endocrine system.

In times of emergency, during what is sometimes called the *flight-fright-fight syndrome,* there is need for a fast reacting body response. So fast, in fact, that this response is sometimes referred to as a "reflex." Actually, the autonomic nervous system, specifically the sympathetic branch, mediates this response. The sympathetic nervous system, under stress conditions, stimulates the adrenal medulla to secrete epinephrine and norepinephrine (catecholamines). Epinephrine acts to mobilize free fatty acids, glycogen, and glucose. Thus, energy is provided to appropriately respond to the stress. It might be mentioned here that the parasympathetic branch of the autonomic nervous system is responsible for resting functions.

Physiological regulation of metabolism might best be explained by a loose analogy with the purpose and mechanisms of the home thermostat. When the room temperature falls below a set point, the furnace is electronically signaled to turn on. As soon as the set temperature is reached, the furnace turns off. Regulation of energy metabolism requires a thermostat to detect need and to stimulate appropriate corrective actions.

This thermostatic function in the human takes place in the anterior pituitary, the master gland, whose secretions stimulate appropriate endocrine glands that, in turn, secrete hormones (see Figure 3-6). These hormones catalyze reactions in muscle and fat tissue that facilitate energy production. The two endocrine glands that are the most important to energy regulation are the *adrenal medulla* and the *pancreas*. The hormones secreted by these glands are epinephrine, and glucagen and insulin, respectively.

PURPOSE

Fat cells release FFA to muscle
tissue for ATP production

Cellular phosphorylase breaks
down glygogen for ATP production

Cellular phosphorylase breaks
down glygogen for ATP production

Insulin inhibits effects of
Epinephrine and Glucagon

Fat cells release FFA to muscle
tissue for ATP production

Insulin promotes blood glucose
and amino acid uptake and
synthesis of FFA from Aceytl CoA

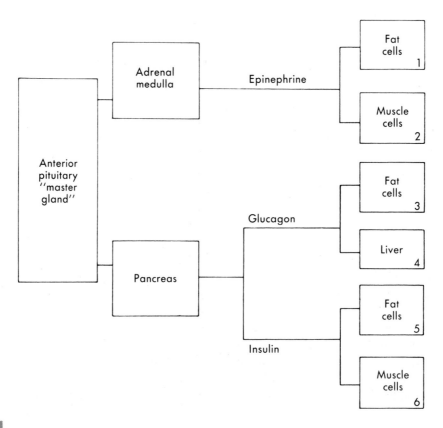

FIG. 3-6   Hormonal regulation of energy metabolism. Purpose: *1*, fat cells release FFA to muscle tissue for ATP production; *2*, cellular phosphorylase breaks down glycogen for ATP production; *3*, fat cells release FFA to muscle tissue for ATP production; *4*, cellular phosphorylase breaks down glycogen for ATP production; *5*, insulin inhibits effects of epinephrine and glucagon; *6*, insulin promotes blood glucose and amino acid uptake and synthesis of FFA from acetyl-CoA.

Phosphorylase is an enzyme that plays an important role in the breakdown of glycogen to glucose for use as a fuel for muscular exercise. During periods when sudden movement is required, the adrenal medulla is stimulated to release epinephrine. Epinephrine initiates a series of biochemical reactions that stimulate cellular phosphorylase.

Epinephrine serves an additional role as a chemical messenger to adipose tissue when energy is in demand. In this role, epinephrine initiates a series of reactions that ultimately result in the enzyme lipase catalyzing stored fat to form free fatty acids for use as a fuel for muscular exercise.

Glucagon is secreted by the pancreas when blood glucose levels fall below a certain threshold. The role of glucagon is to stimulate phosphorylase to break down liver glycogen to glucose. Thus, depleted blood glucose concentrations can be restored. Glucagon, like epinephrine, is a chemical messenger to fat cells. It also stimulates lipase to break down fat stores.

Insulin is another pancreatic hormone but, in contrast to glucagon, it is released when blood glucose levels are too high. Insulin travels to muscle tissue where it facilitates the uptake of glucose. Insufficient insulin release in the diabetic patient often necessitates the injection of insulin to control blood glucose levels. Insulin also serves to inhibit the effects of epinephrine and glucagon on fat cells; that is, fat cells under the influence of epinephrine and glucagon would normally release fatty acids for muscle ATP production. In this way, insulin further keeps blood glucose levels from rising too high by inhibiting fatty acid release, that is, glucose does not have to compete with fatty acids for tissue use.

During exercise, the pancreas generally decreases the production of insulin and increases that of glucagon. This has the effect of promoting the breakdown of glycogen and fat stores and preventing insulin from having an inhibiting effect on blood glucose levels.

Three other hormones, not shown in Figure 3-6, should be mentioned. *Growth hormone,* another anterior pituitary secretion, is released on command from the hypothalamus to stimulate protein synthesis and fat metabolism. The adrenal medulla secretes two *glucocorticoids,* cortisol and cortisone, and two *mineralocorticoids,* aldosterone and deoxycorticosterone. Aldosterone is discussed in detail in a subsequent chapter related to kidney function. Cortisol participates in metabolic control during exercise by stimulating the release of amino acids and mobilizing fat for energy metabolism. The *thyroid hormones,* thyroxine (T_4) and triiodothyronine (T_3), are secreted in response to the release from the pituitary of thyroid-stimulating hormone. These hormones also stimulate metabolism.

RELATIONSHIP OF SPORTS PERFORMANCE AND TRAINING TO METABOLIC PATHWAYS OF ENERGY PRODUCTION

In review, energy for muscular contraction is produced either aerobically or anaerobically. Anaerobic energy production can occur from two subsystems: ATP-PC and glycolysis. Aerobic energy is produced via the tricarboxylic acid cycle and the electron transport system. How do these systems relate to training for, and participation in, various sports?

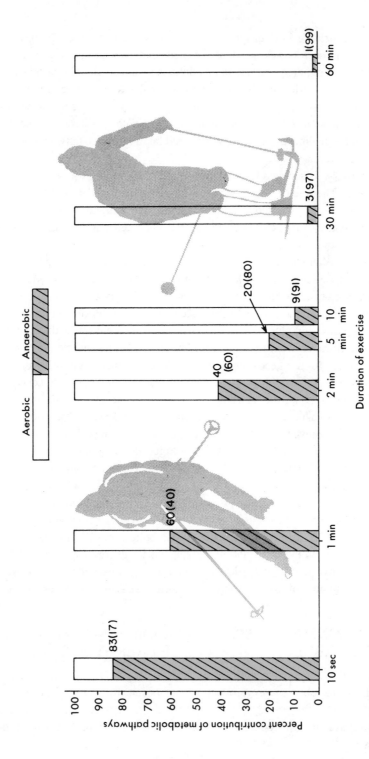

FIG. 3-7 Relationship of participation of metabolic pathways to duration of exercise.

Earlier in this chapter, differences in training were referred to between cross-country skiing and 50 meter swimming. Obviously, the medium is different and so is the motor skill. The reference to difference, however, was based on the energy systems used. The same contrast could be made between alpine skiing and cross-country skiing or between 50 meter swimming and 500 meter swimming. Alpine skiing requires maximal efforts over a very short period of time. Karlsson and others have observed very high lactic acid levels following alpine skiing competition. This would indicate that training for this sport should stress exercise that stimulates the glycolytic process. On the other hand, very little lactic acid is accumulated during cross-country skiing. Therefore, aerobic pathways should be trained in preparation for this event. So that the example is not overstated, it should be acknowledged that very few sports are purely anaerobic or aerobic. For example, hill climbing during cross-country skiing is quite anaerobic and must be considered when training this type of athlete. Figure 3-7 illustrates the relationship of participation by metabolic pathways to duration of exercise.

An analysis of the intensity, duration, and specific demands of a sport can lead to an understanding of the metabolic pathways that provide energy. In turn, this information can be used to establish appropriate training programs.

SUMMARY

Understanding energy metabolism provides a basis for helping athletes with their nutritional problems, as well as helping in the development of appropriate training programs. Carbohydrate, fat, and protein in our food are broken down through digestion to forms that can be used by muscle cells to synthesize ATP either anaerobically (without oxygen) or aerobically (with oxygen).

ATP for muscular contraction is made available by phosphorylation of ADP through the addition of an inorganic phosphate from the breakdown of PC to C + P_i; by glycolysis, which degrades glycogen to pyruvate and, in the absence of oxygen, to lactic acid; and aerobically by breaking down pyruvate to acetyl-CoA, which enters the tricarboxylic acid cycle and the electron transport system.

Carbohydrate in food takes the form of monosaccharides, disaccharides, and polysaccharides. Digestion breaks down ingested carbohydrate so that glucose can be released from the small intestine to the blood. Glucose travels to the liver where it can be stored as liver glycogen, used as energy for liver work, sent to muscle tissue and other organs, or degraded to free fatty acids. Carbohydrate is the only source of fuel for glycolysis and, combined with lipids, provides fuel for muscular contraction in a proportion depending on the duration and intensity of the exercise.

Digested lipids in the form of fatty acids enter the bloodstream from the small intestine and travel to the liver where they are used to synthesize lipoproteins, produce ATP in the tricarboxylic acid cycle, or form free fatty acids for delivery to peripheral tissues. Muscle cells can use lipid as a fuel by receiving either free fatty acids or ketone bodies from the liver, by receiving free fatty acids stored as fat, or by using fat stored in muscle tissue.

Although it is possible to use protein as a fuel for muscular contraction, its contribution is small compared to those of carbohydrate and fat. Alanine is a protein by-product of glycolysis stored in skeletal muscle and may be used in long-term exercise.

Lactic acid produced during anaerobic glycolysis is also a fuel for exercise metabolism. Lactate can be converted in the liver to blood glucose and returned to muscle as a fuel.

In addition to internal cellular mechanisms that regulate energy metabolism, hormones exert an influence over this process. For example, epinephrine, produced by the adrenal medulla, and glucagon and insulin, produced by the pancreas, strongly influence the production of ATP by their effect on fat cells, muscle cells, and the liver.

KEY TERMS

adenosine triphosphate (ATP) a high-energy phosphate bond that serves as the immediate source of energy for muscle contraction.

aerobic literally, "with oxygen"; refers to one of two metabolic systems that produce ATP for muscle contraction. The other system is anaerobic.

amino acids the basic chemical building blocks of protein in food.

anaerobic literally, "without oxygen"; refers to one of two metabolic systems that produce ATP for muscle contraction. The other system is aerobic.

epinephrine a hormone secreted by the adrenal medulla that stimulates ATP production by its action on fat and muscle cells.

fatty acids one of the basic chemical building blocks of fat in food. Fatty acids are used as a fuel for aerobic metabolism.

glucagon a hormone secreted by the pancreas that stimulates ATP production by its action on fat cells and the liver.

glucose a monosaccharide carbohydrate used as a fuel for aerobic and anaerobic metabolism.

glycogen the storage form of glucose.

glycolysis the anaerobic process by which glycogen is broken down to lactic acid to produce ATP for muscular contraction.

insulin a hormone secreted by the pancreas that promotes the uptake of blood glucose and amino acid by the cells. This hormone also inhibits the effects of epinephrine and glucagon.

Krebs cycle also known as the tricarboxylic acid cycle; describes the mechanism by which carbohydrate, fat, and protein are degraded to carbon dioxide, hydrogen ions, and electrons. The electrons are subsequently transported to oxygen, forming water and energy (ATP).

lactic acid an end product of anaerobic glycolysis.

percentage of maximal oxygen consumption (% $\dot{V}o_2$ max) a measurement unit used to express the intensity of physiological effort. For example, exercising at 50% $\dot{V}o_2$ max would demonstrate an exercise intensity one-half of one's maximal ability to consume oxygen.

phosphocreatine a substance found in limited quantities in muscle cells that when broken down anaerobically provides inorganic phosphate necessary to reconstitute ATP.

phosphorylation the process by which inorganic phosphate is provided so that adenosine triphosphate can be reconstituted from adenosine diphosphate.

REVIEW QUESTIONS

1. What are the two mechanisms by which energy is produced anaerobically? Explain the process of phosphorylation in each case.

2. Describe in detail the link between anaerobic glycolysis and the aerobic metabolic pathway.

3. Describe the electron transport system. What are the end products of the Krebs cycle and the electron transport system?

4. Describe the means by which carbohydrate can be stored in the liver and muscle cells for subsequent use during exercise.

5. What is the predominate fuel for producing energy during marathon running? What are the implications of this knowledge given the body's ability to store energy?

6. Describe the mechanism(s) by which lactic acid may be used as a fuel for muscular exercise.

7. What would be the adaptive advantage of stimulating the adrenal glands during a frightening experience?

8. What metabolic systems must be trained to improve sprint and endurance athletes? What elements of these systems do you hypothesize to be altered by physical training?

REFERENCES

1. Bergstrom, J., Hermansen, L., Hultman, E., and others: Diet, muscle glycogen and physical performance, Acta Physiol. Scand. **71**:140, 1967.

2. Costill, D.L., Sparks, K., Gregor, R., and others: Muscle glycogen utilization during exhaustive running, J. Appl. Physiol. **31**:353, 1971.

3. Deshaies, Y., and Allard, C.: Serum high-density lipoprotein cholesterol in male and female Olympic athletes, Med. Sci. Sports Exerc. **14**:207, 1982.

4. Essen, B.: Intramuscular substrate utilization during prolonged exercise. In Milvy, P., editor: The marathon: physiological, medical, epidemiological and psychological studies, vol. 301, New York, 1977, The New York Academy of Sciences.

5. Farrell, P.A., Wilmore, J.H., Coyle, E.F., and others: Plasma lactate accumulation and distance running performance, Med. Sci. Sports **11**:338, 1979.

6. Felig, P., and Wahren, J.: Amino acid metabolism in exercising man, J. Clin. Invest. **50**:2703, 1971.

7. Felig, P.: Amino acid metabolism in exercise. In Milvy, P., editor: The marathon: physiological, medical, epidemiological and psychological studies, vol. 301, New York, 1977, The New York Academy of Sciences.

8. Galbo, H., Richter, E.A., Hilsted, J., and others: Hormonal regulation during prolonged exercise. In Milvy, P., editor: The marathon: physiological, medical, epidemiological and psychological studies, vol. 301, New York, 1977, The New York Academy of Sciences.

9. Gollnick, P.D.: Biochemical adaptations to exercise: anaerobic metabolism. In Wilmore, J.H., editor: Exercise and sport sciences reviews, New York, 1973, Academic Press, Inc.

10. Gollnick, P.D.: Free fatty acid and turnover and the availability of substrates as a limiting factor in prolonged exercise. In Milvy, P., editor: The marathon: physiological, medical, epidemiological and psychological studies, vol. 301, New York, 1977, The New York Academy of Sciences.

11. Gollnick, P.D., and King, D.W.: Energy release in the muscle cell, Med. Sci. Sports **1**:23, 1969.

12. Hartley, L.H., Mason, J.W., Hogan, R.P., and others: Multiple hormonal responses to graded exercise in relation to physical training, J. Appl. Physiol. **33**:602, 1972.

13. Holloszy, J.O.: Biochemical adaptations to exercise: aerobic metabolism. In Wilmore, J.H., editor: Exercise and sport sciences reviews, New York, 1973, Academic Press, Inc.

14. Hultman, E., Bergstrom, J., and McLennan-Anderson, N.: Breakdown and resynthesis of phosphorylcreatine and adenosine triphosphate in connection with muscular work in man, Scand. J. Clin. Lab. Invest. **19**:56, 1967.

15. Karlsson, J., Nordesjo, L.O., Jorfeldt, L., and others: Muscle lactate, ATP, and CP levels during exercise after physical training in man, J. Appl. Physiol. **33**:199, 1972.

16. Lehninger, A.L.: Short course in biochemistry, New York, 1973, Worth Publishers, Inc.

17. Lemon, P.W.R., and Nagle, F.J.: Effects of exercise on protein and amino acid metabolism, Med. Sci. Sports Exerc. **13**:141, 1981.

18. Mackie, B.G., Dudley, G.A., Kaciuba-Uscilko, H., and others: Uptake of chylomicron triglycerides by contracting skeletal muscle in rats, J. Appl. Physiol. **49**:851, 1980.

19. Miller, J.M., Coyle, E.F., Sherman W.M., and others: Effect of glycerol feeding on endurance and metabolism during prolonged exercise in man, Med. Sci. Sports Exerc. **15**:237, 1983.

20. Paul, P., and Holmes, W.L.: Free fatty acid and glucose metabolism during increased energy expenditure and after training, Med. Sci. Sports **7**:176, 1975.

21. Tesch, P., Larsson, L., Eriksson, A., and others: Muscle glycogen depletion and lactate concentration during downhill skiing, Med. Sci. Sports **10**:85, 1978.

22. Tran, Z.V., Weltman, A., Glass, G.V., and others: The effects of exercise on blood lipids and lipoproteins: a meta-analysis of studies, Med. Sci. Sports Exerc. **15**:393, 1983.

23. Wahren, J.: Glucose turnover during exercise in man. In Milvy, P., editor: The marathon: physiological, medical, epidemiological and psychological studies, vol. 301, New York, 1977, The New York Academy of Sciences.

24. Winder, W.W.: Control of hepatic glucose production during exercise, Med. Sci. Sports Exerc. **17**:2, 1985.

SUGGESTED READINGS

Becker, W.M.: Energy and the living cell: an introduction to bioenergetics, Philadelphia, 1977, J.B. Lippincott Co.

Lehninger, A.L.: Bioenergetics: the molecular basis of biological energy transformations, ed. 2, New York, 1971, W.A. Benjamin, Inc.

Lehninger, A.L.: Short course in biochemistry, New York, 1973, Worth Publishers, Inc.

Sanadi, D.R., and Wohlrab, H.: Chemical reactions in oxidative phosphorylation. In Sanadi, D.R., editor: Chemical mechanisms in bioenergetics, ACS Monograph 172, Washington, D.C., 1976, American Chemical Society.

CASE STUDY 1

The following is typical of phone calls I have received from football coaches.

COACH: Hello! Professor? This is Coach Anderson. Randy Johnson, our starting tight end, is in your exercise physiology class. He's been telling the coaching staff that you don't think we should be eating steak as a pregame meal. We've been eating steak for years and our record shows it hasn't hurt us any.

PROFESSOR: It looks like we've had some miscommunication. Let's see if I can straighten things out. First, my teaching was not meant to disrupt or interfere in any way with your coaching. What I was trying to illustrate to the class was the relationship between the energy needs of various sports and how athletes eat to support those energy needs. Steak is a perfectly good food for replenishing calories lost in practice and for the protein needs of the body. However, using steak to supply the energy requirements for a football game is another matter. It is likely that only a small percentage of the energy used to perform in a football game comes from protein. Football uses primarily carbohydrate as a fuel for muscular work. With an adequate daily diet, which your players receive at the "training table," there is virtually no possibility that the carbohydrate the players have stored in their bodies will be depleted in a game.

COACH: Hold on! You mean to say that those pregame steaks had nothing to do with winning games?

PROFESSOR: I'm afraid that's the case. I'm not saying that the overall calories and nutrients in the total meal did not serve an important purpose. What I am saying is that the pregame steak is not supplying energy for work during the game.

COACH: O.K., let me get this straight. What you're saying is that just a normal balanced meal is most likely as good as any specialized meal.

PROFESSOR: That's right.

COACH: Well, I'll be. We've certainly poured a lot of money down the drain with pregame steaks over the years.

PROFESSOR: That may not be true. What I've told you is what the meal is not doing, not that the meal should necessarily be replaced.

COACH: I've got it! Thanks a lot. See you on Saturday.

This conversation illustrates a minor point perhaps, but it uncovers a major problem involving the many myths that exist in sport concerning the proper nutritional care of the athlete. Teachers and coaches can play a major role in reducing further misunderstanding by their knowledge of how energy is produced for performing muscular contraction.

CASE STUDY 2

A young teacher came by my office the other day. She had just been asked to coach a junior high school soccer team. She was excited about the prospect but at the same time slightly panicked.

TEACHER: The rules are clear to me and I think I can teach the basic skills I learned from the soccer coaching class, but I've never really played the game.

PROFESSOR: Are you worried about the strategy of the game?

TEACHER: No! No! I need to know how I get the players in shape. I know that's a big part of the game and all I ever trained for was the swimming team.

This problem, in various forms, is quite typical of the new teacher's experience. The solution to the problem requires some analysis of the game itself. What do the players do? What are the energy dynamics of the players?

At the risk of being too simplistic, let's try to describe the ''energetics'' of soccer players. First, they are generally moving at all times. Even when not directly involved with the ball they are walking or jogging. After receiving a pass, moving the ball up the field may not require great bursts of energy. Likewise, short passing does not require moves much more strenuous than running itself. However, several situations require fairly short maximal efforts, for instance, when a free ball is kicked into your area and it is necessary to gain control before the opponent. Tackling an opponent is also a high-energy task. A goal kick is an example of a very short but very intense movement.

Obviously, the coach will have to conduct a much more thorough analysis. For our purposes we have identified enough of the energy dynamics to illustrate the point.

From your understanding of the material in this chapter you should be able to help this teacher. Is soccer an aerobic or anaerobic sport? The correct answer is *both*. The continuous movement makes soccer generally aerobic. The fairly short but highly intense running, of perhaps 1 minute at most, involves anaerobic activity, producing lactic acid. The very short and very intense movements, such as in kicking, are also anaerobic, but of the ATP-PC type.

Therefore, it would be reasonable for a coach to estimate the proportion of the time spent in performing aerobic and anaerobic movements and use that as a guide for designing a training program to get the team in shape. Certainly the movements should be as specific as possible. A combination of very short sprints, up to 10 seconds (ATP-PC); longer sprints, up to 440 and 880 meters (lactic acid); and long, slow, distance running, up to several miles (aerobic), would be appropriate.

This analysis does not provide an exact daily or specific practice session program but it does offer a few guidelines for developing the program. A summary of these guidelines is as follows:

1. Analyze the ''energetics'' of the sport.
2. Determine the metabolic nature of the movements (aerobic and/or anaerobic).
3. Design training durations and intensities that will stimulate the correct metabolic pathways.

chapter 4

INTERACTION OF DIETARY INTAKE AND MUSCLE FUNCTION

MAJOR LEARNING OBJECTIVE
The predominant fuel for light to moderate exercise (<50% of maximum) is fat and for moderate to heavy exercise (>50% of maximum) is carbohydrate. The food we eat and store as glycogen, fatty acids, and protein is related to performance in, and recovery from, certain physical activities.

APPLICATIONS
Long-duration sports may be limited by the body's capacity to store glycogen. Short-duration sports use carbohydrate preferentially with little chance of depletion.

AMONG its several functions, the food we eat is metabolized to form ATP for muscular contraction. Muscle work results in the production of heat. Thus, measurement of heat production is a reflection of food metabolized to form energy. Heat is measured in calories. Both the food we eat and the exercise we perform can be evaluated in caloric terms. Therefore, both energy intake and energy expenditure can be studied with the same unit. The teacher and coach need to understand the interaction of energy intake and energy expenditure in order to make nutritional recommendations to athletes. In other words, they need to know how much the athlete expends in order to suggest an adequate caloric intake. This chapter will not address the issue of which foods we eat. The goal is not meal planning for athletes, but rather helping the student understand the concept of calories, how they are measured, and how many are required for various activities.

This chapter also discusses the effect of diet on muscle function. The fuel we use during exercise and how we might improve exercise capacity and recovery from exercise by choosing correct nutrients are discussed.

ENERGY INTAKE AND EXPENDITURE

The average person is not usually concerned with energy utilization at the tissue level. On the other hand, the concept of energy, especially as measured by the caloric value of food, has become almost a fetish for the weight-conscious public. ATP is largely an unknown term but "light" and "low cal" have become common terminology in Western culture. Energy expenditure is also a common concern, and physical educators are often asked how many calories will be expended by this or that activity. Energy intake and expenditure are at the forefront of public consciousness, and teachers and coaches should be completely familiar with their interrelatedness.

The calorie

The term "calorie" used by lay people is incorrect because a "calorie" is really a *large calorie,* 1,000 times larger than a *kilocalorie* (kcal). A kilocalorie is what people are actually referring to when they use the term "calorie," and it is the term used most often in nutritional literature. The kilocalorie is the amount of heat required to raise the temperature of 1 kilogram of water 1° C, from 14.5° C to 15.5° C.

It is important to recognize the caloric equivalences of different forms of energy. For example, the chemical energy of food can be shown to be equivalent to the mechanical energy of physical exercise as well as to stored chemical energy, such as body fat. So we can speak of the calorie value of the food we eat, the exercise we perform, and the fat we store. A pound of stored fat contains approximately 3,500 kilocalories. The accepted international unit for expressing energy is the kilojoule (kJ). One kilojoule equals 0.239 kilocalories. Therefore, 3500 kilocalories is equal to 14,644 kilojoules.

Measurement of caloric energy

Calorimetry is the measurement of heat production. If we want to determine the energy produced from the combustion of food, we measure the calories used or the heat produced. When heat is measured directly, the technique is called *direct calorimetry*. An example is the use of the *bomb calorimeter* to determine the caloric value of food samples. Food is placed in a chamber and combusted, and the resulting heat production is measured. Human calorimeters are also used for measuring heat production. As the person sits or exercises within a chamber, sensitive thermocouples (measurement device) record the change in temperature brought about by the metabolism of food or by the exercise being performed.

It is difficult to measure energy production and utilization directly at the cellular level. However, calorimetry gives us a gross record of energy use. Perhaps the most practical method of measuring heat exchange in humans is by *indirect calorimetry*. The principle here is that we can calculate the amount of heat produced if we know how much oxygen is used in breaking down carbohydrate, fat, and protein to form ATP. Listed here are the kilocalories produced when 1 liter of oxygen is used by persons eating certain diets:

5.047 kcal—Carbohydrate diet

4.863 kcal—Mixed diet

4.686 kcal—Fat diet

4.600 kcal—Protein diet

Less oxygen is used in the production of a unit of ATP than is used in fat and protein metabolism. Measurement of oxygen consumption, because of its practicality, is a widely used method of examining energy utilization in humans. Examples of both direct and indirect calorimetry are shown in Figure 4-1.

It is often useful to broadly discriminate between the nutrients being used during exercise. The *respiratory exchange ratio* (R) is used for this purpose. R is the ratio of carbon dioxide produced to oxygen consumed. When pure carbohydrate is being used for energy we see an R value of 1.0. This value compares to 0.7 for fat and 0.8 for protein. Since R values can be increased by increasing carbon dioxide production during lactate buffering, they should be interpreted carefully.

How to determine caloric requirements

Life itself implies the use of energy. Even lying or sitting quietly involves work by body tissues and requires energy. When we perform muscular work to move ourselves from place to place or to play in strenuous games, energy requirements increase drastically.

The chemical changes in the body that maintain life are referred to as *metabolism*. Metabolism is measured in calories used per unit of body size or weight during a specific amount of time. *Basal metabolic rate* (BMR) refers to the minimum amount of energy expenditure needed to maintain life. Measurements are recorded after an overnight 12-hour fast while the person is lying at rest. BMR measurement involves recording calories used during a specific amount of time. Since larger persons have a higher BMR, values are expressed in terms of either square meters of body surface or kilograms of body weight per day. The BMR is approximately 50% of the daily energy expenditure and is 10% lower in females. It also decreases with age. This shift with age is thought to be because of the greater percentage of body composition taken up by fat with increasing years. The BMR for healthy adults averages 1600 to 1800 kilocalories in males and 1200 to 1450 kilocalories in females. This difference is accounted for by differences in body composition between the sexes.

Most human activity occurs above the basal level and is about 10% higher than the BMR. *Resting metabolic rate* (RMR), where the subject is at rest but clearly not in a basal state, is expressed in kilocalories per hour per kilogram of body weight and averages between 0.8 and 1.4.[8] Values for women are 10% to 20% lower. RMR is recorded during a resting state but not under strict basal conditions (lying at rest after a specified amount of sleep and following a fast). The following are average daily RMR values for men and women:

	Kilocalories		Hours		Body weight (kg)		Daily resting metabolism (kcal)
Men	1.0	×	24	×	70 (154 lb)	=	1680
Women	0.9	×	24	×	58 (128 lb)	=	1253

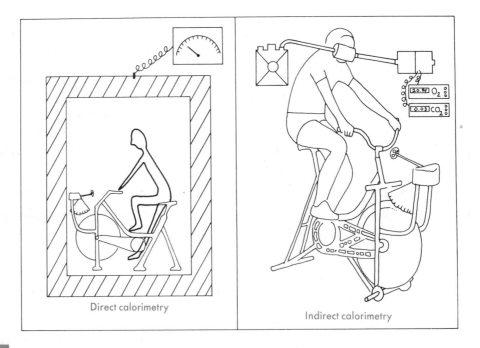

Direct calorimetry

Indirect calorimetry

FIG. 4-1   **Measurement of human energy production by direct (heat production) and indirect (oxygen consumption) calorimetry.**

The RMR values (kcal/h/kg) vary with body weight and also with fat percentage. Table 4-1 contains the values that are used to make such adjustments.

Several techniques are available for estimating the caloric cost of daily muscular work. One way is to keep a daily log of physical activity and match the activity with average caloric values. Table 4-2 contains examples of average caloric values for several sports. For example, jogging three 10-minute miles has a caloric cost of approximately 318 kilocalories (10.6 kcal × 30 min).

It is time consuming and expensive to measure oxygen consumption over an entire day of activity. Another less exact procedure involves adding to the resting metabolism a percentage increase based on the intensity of the activity performed.[8] For example, a woman engaging in moderate activity has an estimated daily energy requirement of 1320 kilocalories, plus an additional requirement of 990 kilocalories (75% of 1320), for a total requirement of 2310 kcal/day.

Work classification	Work description	Additive factor
Very light	Sitting most of the day, studying, talking, about 2 hours of standing	Add 30%
Light	Typing, teaching, shop work, laboratory work, some walking	Add 50%
Moderate	Walking, housework, gardening, carpentry, light industry, little sitting	Add 75%
Strenuous	Unskilled labor, forestry work, skating, outdoor games, dancing, little sitting	Add 100%

TABLE 4-1 ‖‖‖ RESTING ENERGY METABOLISM (KCAL/H/KG) FACTORS FOR ADULTS ACCORDING TO BODY WEIGHT AND COMPOSITION*

Men	Women	% Fat	Weight in kilograms								
			50	55	60	65	70	75	80	85	90
Thin		5	0.99	1.06	1.12	1.19	1.26	1.32	1.39	1.46	1.53
Average		10	0.94	1.01	1.08	1.14	1.21	1.28	1.34	1.41	1.48
Plump	Thin	15	0.89	0.96	1.03	1.09	1.16	1.23	1.30	1.36	1.43
Fat	Average	20	0.84	0.91	0.98	1.05	1.11	1.18	1.25	1.31	1.38
	Plump	25	0.80	0.86	0.93	1.00	1.07	1.13	1.20	1.26	1.33
	Fat	30	—	0.81	0.88	0.95	1.02	1.08	1.15	1.21	1.28

Adapted from Bogert, L.J., Briggs, G.M., and Calloway, D.H.: Nutrition and physical fitness, ed. 2, Philadelphia, 1984, W.B. Saunders Co.

*To use this table, the factor listed in the table must be multiplied times 24 (hr/day) and again times the body weight (kg) to determine a daily RMR. For example, a thin woman (15% fat) weighing 55 kg would have a RMR/day of 1267 kcal (.96 × 24 × 55).

Digesting food requires energy. This factor alone causes an increase in the metabolic rate following a meal. This increase is referred to as *specific dynamic action* (SDA). For a balanced meal, including protein, fat, and carbohydrate, the SDA amounts to about 10% of the BMR. The SDA has to be taken into consideration when calculating caloric expenditure. It is estimated that if your energy needs are 2,400 kcal/day, you need to take in at least 2,640 kcal/day (an extra 10%) to account for the SDA.

Residual energy expenditure following exercise is difficult to determine and is often

TABLE 4-2 ‖‖‖ CALORIC COSTS OF VARIOUS SPORTS

Sport	Caloric cost (kcal/min)
Climbing	10.7-13.2
Cycling	
5.5 mph	4.5
9.4 mph	7.0
13.1 mph	11.1
Dancing	3.3-7.7
Football	8.9
Golf	5.0
Gymnastics	
Balancing	2.5
Abdominal exercises	3.0
Trunk bending	3.5
Arm swinging and hopping	6.5
Rowing	
51 strokes/min	4.1
87 strokes/min	7.0
97 strokes/min	11.2
Running	
Short distance	13.3-16.6
Cross-country	10.6
Tennis	7.1
Skating (fast)	11.5
Skiing	
Moderate speed	10.8-15.9
Uphill, maximum speed	18.6
Squash	10.2
Swimming	
Breaststroke	11.0
Backstroke	11.5
Crawl (55 yard/min)	14.0
Wrestling	14.2

Reprinted by permission of the American Alliance of Health, Physical Education, Recreation, and Dance, 1900 Association Dr., Reston, Va., 1980, The Alliance.

neglected when determining caloric requirements. We usually think of providing energy for exercise but forget that energy must be produced for the recovery process as well. The metabolic rate can be well above the resting level for many minutes and even hours following exercise. This is important to remember when using exercise as a weight control technique or when planning caloric replacement for athletes undergoing heavy training. It is common, for example, for a football player in training to consume 5,000 kcal/day. If we assume the player's normal intake is 3,000 kcal/day, we have an additional 2,000 kcal/day expended because of football practice. Dividing 2,000 by 3 hours (time spent in football practice) results in a caloric utilization of 666 kcal/hour or 11.1 kcal/min. This caloric expenditure may be a normal variant of the average (8.9 kcal/min) presented in Table 4-2, but it might also be accounted for by the added energy expenditure of recovery from hard training. Of course the intensity of play greatly affects residual energy expenditure. For example, the beginner who does not expend as much energy at play will also expend far less residual energy than the experienced player performing under intense competitive conditions.

Growing children require more calories than would be estimated by their physical activity. The following data from a study of a group of moderately active children illustrate this point.[1] It can be seen that caloric expenditure rises during the growth period and falls as growth slows down.

	Age (yr)	Weight (kg-lb)	Height (cm-in)	(kcal)	Calories (kcal · kg⁻¹)
Boys	10-12	35-77	140-55	2500	71.4
	12-14	43-95	150-59	2700	62.8
	14-18	59-130	170-67	3000	50.8
	18-22	67-147	175-69	2800	41.8
Girls	10-12	35-77	142-56	2250	64.3
	12-14	44-97	155-61	2300	52.3
	14-16	52-114	157-62	2400	46.2
	16-18	54-119	160-63	2300	42.6
	18-22	58-128	163-64	2000	34.5

This chart is a general guide and applies only to moderately active children. Children participating in athletics would require additional calories.

Mechanical work efficiency

Mechanical work efficiency is the ratio of mechanical work performed divided by total energy expended, minus resting energy expenditure.

$$\text{Net efficiency} = \frac{\text{Work performed}}{\text{Total energy expended} - \text{Resting energy expenditure}}$$

Human work efficiency is not greater than 25%. For example, if a certain amount of walking requires 250 kilocalories of mechanical work, but 1,000 kilocalories of energy are expended, the efficiency of that work is 25%. The remaining 75% of the energy is released as heat. Thus, for performing work, at least four times more fuel must be supplied than is required for the work itself. If we were 100% efficient, no excess heat would be produced, and we would need to eat only enough to perform the work.

Work efficiency is influenced by endurance and fatigue, as well as several other factors. Improved exercise biomechanics requiring less physical work should improve efficiency. Another important factor influencing work efficiency is heat production and removal. Cooling the body requires energy. The great amount of heat produced by the body during exercise requires an effective thermoregulatory system. Mechanisms by which heat dissipates from the body are discussed in Chapter 10.

Energy value of food

As mentioned previously, caloric values for various foods can be determined by calorimetry. Results of such analyses are available in most nutrition texts. It is also possible to calculate the caloric content of a food if you know the weight and caloric value of each constituent. The calculation for milk is presented here:

$$4.9 \text{ g carbohydrate}/100 \text{ g milk} \times 4 \text{ kcal/g} = 19.6 \text{ kcal}$$
$$4.7 \text{ g fat}/100 \text{ g milk} \times 9 \text{ kcal/g} = 33.3 \text{ kcal}$$
$$3.5 \text{ g protein}/100 \text{ g milk} \times \underline{4 \text{ kcal/g} = 14.0 \text{ kcal}}$$
$$66.9 \text{ kcal}$$

Thus, 100 grams of milk contains 66.9 kilocalories. An 8-ounce glass of milk weighs 224 grams, and therefore it contains 163 kilocalories (66.9×2.44).

EFFECT OF DIET ON MUSCLE FUNCTION

The six most important nutrients for the body are carbohydrate, fat, protein, water, vitamins, and electrolytes. The latter three nutrients are dealt with in other chapters. Our concentration here will be on the role of carbohydrate, fat, and protein in the production of energy for muscle function.

Fuel use during exercise

Perhaps the earliest study dealing with fuel for exercise was the study published in 1920 by Krogh and Lindhard.[30] They used R to examine the contribution of carbohydrate and fat to energy yield in exercise. Their work suggested that the proportion of carbohydrate and fat used in exercise may be a matter of substrate supply. The studies of Christensen and Hansen,[9-13] performed using the same technique followed, and over the years these have served as the basis for our understanding of carbohydrate and fat utilization during prolonged, exhaustive exercise, that is, high-intensity aerobic exercise. To summarize their results:

1. The higher the work load the greater the proportion of energy that comes from carbohydrate.
2. Those consuming diets high in carbohydrate used a higher proportion of carbohydrates for energy during exercise than did those consuming high-fat diets.

3. Endurance increased in those consuming high-carbohydrate diets and decreased in those consuming high-fat diets.
4. When subjects on either high-fat or high-carbohydrate diets became fatigued, a high proportion of energy had been coming from fat.

Later study confirmed this work. Subjects were asked to exercise at 25%, 50%, and 80% of their maximum oxygen consumption ($\dot{V}O_2$ max).[20] ($\dot{V}O_2$ max is a measure of working capacity. Percentages of this measure are often used to compare exercise intensities when subjects have differing capacities.) R was 0.87, 0.90, and 0.93, respectively (see Figure 4-2). Again, this study indicates that as exercise intensity increases and R rises toward 1.0 a greater proportion of the energy comes from carbohydrate. Likewise, another investigation found a relatively low R when subjects rode a bicycle ergometer at a low submaximal load (300 kilogram-meter/min) for 30 minutes.[24] These data support fat as the most important substrate for low-level, submaximal exercise. (The R value is also used as an

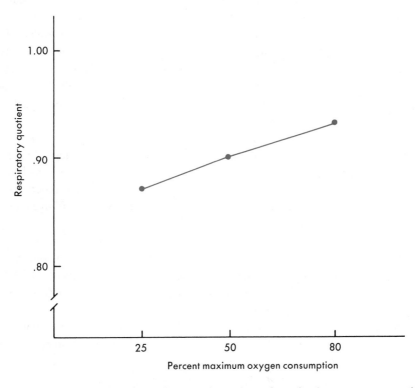

FIG. 4-2   The relationship between the increase in percent of maximal oxygen consumption (intensity of exercise) and the respiratory exchange ratio (R). An increase in R illustrates an increased reliance on carbohydrate metabolism. (From Hermansen, L., Hultman, E., and Saltin, B.: Muscle glycogen during prolonged severe exercise, Acta Physiol. Scand. *71:*129, 1967.)

estimate for the onset of blood lactate accumulation, since the R rises with increased carbon dioxide production. During intense exercise, increased carbon dioxide production reflects the need to buffer lactic acid and is not necessarily related to the food being burned.) Low-level exercise may be the exercise of choice when weight loss is the primary objective.

Over the last 20 years examination of the contributions of various fuels by muscle biopsy has become possible.[2] Small samples of muscle tissue can be excised so that local metabolism can be followed. A great deal of attention has been given to the storage, depletion, and repletion of carbohydrate in muscle (glycogen) with this technique. We know, for example, that muscle glycogen content varies between muscles (9.98 g/100 g of muscle in the deltoid muscle compared to 1.40 g/100 g of muscle in the quadriceps) and that little variation occurs over a day when subjects eat and work as usual.[23]

A study of both trained and untrained subjects who rode a bicycle ergometer to exhaustion, with several 20-minute bouts at 77% $\dot{V}_{O_2}$ max (aerobic), showed a close relationship between muscle glycogen used and R.[20] In another study the vastus lateralis muscle was biopsied as subjects pedalled a bicycle ergometer six 1-minute sprints, at 150% $\dot{V}_{O_2}$ max (anaerobic). (Here 150% refers to a calculation of an equivalent of oxygen consumption, not oxygen consumption per se.[20]) Results showed that not only was glycogen depleted in this anaerobic exercise, but fast-twitch (FT) fibers were depleted first. This contrasts with prolonged aerobic exercise where slow-twitch (ST) fibers are depleted first. *Glycogen depletion* following marathon running has been found to be highest in ST fibers (70%) compared to a 20% depletion in FT fibers.[29]

It is important to note that although fat stores in adipose tissues are, for all practical purposes, unlimited, carbohydrate reserves need to be protected because of their relative low quantity. The maximum quantity of glycogen stored in the liver and muscle is probably no higher than 800 g.[31] Since the highest rate of glycogen use reported to date is 4 g/100 g of muscle,[4] it can be readily seen that prolonged exercise of large muscles can consume stored glycogen quickly.

It is clear that at low exercise intensities energy for muscle contraction is derived mostly from fat. As exercise intensity increases, so does the contribution of carbohydrate to the energy needs of muscle. Carbohydrate becomes the predominant fuel at exercise intensities between 50% and 70% $\dot{V}_{O_2}$ max. At approximately 85% to 90% $\dot{V}_{O_2}$ max most energy is derived from carbohydrate.

Recent evidence has confirmed that as much as 10% of exercise metabolism is supported by protein. Heretofore, the contribution of protein was thought to be more limited. Research is being conducted that should shed more light on the interrelation of carbohydrate, fat, and protein contributions to exercise metabolism.

Muscle glycogen and exercise capacity

When we consider the importance of a substrate, carbohydrate, for example, we think not only of its contribution to energy requirements but also of whether its depletion is a limiting factor for exercise capacity. It has been noted that since muscle glycogen is so completely depleted when subjects exercise to exhaustion at 75% to 80% $\dot{V}_{O_2}$ max that muscle glycogen must be a limiting factor to exercise capacity.[22] In addition, high correlations have been reported between total work time in exhaustive aerobic tasks and the amount of stored muscle glycogen before exercise.[23] Reduction of glycogen is dependent on the intensity rate at which one is working.[22]

The relationship of glycogen depletion and exercise time is depicted in Figure 4-3.[4] Both trained and untrained subjects rode a bicycle ergometer intermittently to exhaustion at 76% and 79% $\dot{V}_{O_2}$ max, respectively. Biopsies for determination of muscle glycogen were taken every 20 minutes. Both groups depleted glycogen stores significantly over time, with a tendency for more to be depleted in untrained than in trained subjects.

It has been noted that even though glycogen is depleted quickly at high work loads, R decreases very little.[22] This indicates that carbohydrate is still being supplied but from sources other than muscle glycogen. Liver glycogen is a potent source of carbohydrate, so it is likely that liver glycogen is converted to glucose, which travels to the tissues in the blood to be used for muscle metabolism. This suggests that muscle glycogen may not be

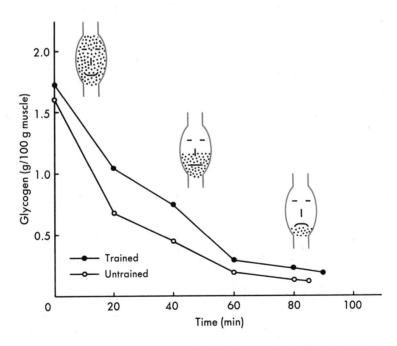

FIG. 4-3   The depletion of glycogen stores in trained and untrained subjects during long-duration exercise. (Adapted from Bergstrom, J., Hermansen, L., Hultman, E., and others: Diet, muscle glycogen and physical performance, Acta Physiol. Scand. *71:*140, 1967.)

the only factor limiting exercise capacity but that some other factor, such as blood glucose level, is also involved.

Depletion of muscle glycogen is definitely an important factor in continuance of prolonged exercise. However, the extent to which other factors are critical and how they interact with muscle glycogen depletion has not been fully elucidated.

Diet and aerobic performance

Since the importance of muscle and liver glycogen stores to prolonged exercise has been established, we must ask whether it is possible to manipulate these stores through diet. Can we increase the body's storage capacity for carbohydrate and thereby increase endurance performance?

It has been shown that muscle glycogen storage can be increased by depleting the stores through exhaustive exercise and then providing a carbohydrate-rich diet.[5] Such depletion is localized in the exercised muscles and does not occur in unused muscles. Glycogen resynthesis is not accomplished when a fat and protein diet follows exercise and when the carbohydrate diet is not preceded by hard exercise. Also, it has been observed that a carbohydrate-free diet preceding the carbohydrate-rich diet further enhances glycogen storage. After a carbohydrate diet, glycogen storage has been found to be 3.70 g/100 g of muscle compared with the normal range of 0.95 to 2.0 g/100 g of muscle.[4]

How does increased glycogen storage affect performance? Investigators had subjects pedal to exhaustion on a bicycle ergometer at 75% $\dot{V}O_2$ max under three dietary conditions: mixed diet, high-fat and protein diet, and high-carbohydrate diet.[4] The following is a summary of their findings. "Before" and "After" refer to before and after exercise. Muscle biopsies were performed to determine muscle glycogen amounts.

Mixed diet			Fat and protein diet			Carbohydrate diet		
Before	After	Exercise	Before	After	Exercise	Before	After	Exercise
(g/100 g muscle)		time (min)	(g/100 g muscle)		time (min)	(g/100 g muscle)		time (min)
1.93	0.20	125.8	0.69	0.19	58.8	3.70	0.45	189.3

It is easy to see the strong relationship between initial glycogen storage and exercise time. This and other studies have led to the popular use by endurance athletes of what has become known as *carbohydrate loading*. Following exhaustive exercise to deplete muscle glycogen the athlete follows a regimen of 3 days on a carbohydrate-poor diet (high fat and protein) and then 3 days on a carbohydrate-rich diet immediately preceding competition. Recent evidence indicates that equal success can be achieved with the exhaustive exercise and the carbohydrate-rich diet phase only.

In a similar study, the effects of a mixed diet were compared with both high-fat and high-carbohydrate diets during exhaustive exercise at both 50% and 70% $\dot{V}O_2$ max.[40] Results appear as follows:

	50% $\dot{V}O_2$ max Percent contribution from carbohydrate			70% $\dot{V}O_2$ max Percent contribution from carbohydrate		
	Beginning	End	Average	Beginning	End	Average
Mixed diet	47	37	40	64	47	53
High-fat	44	23	35	54	30	48
High-carbohydrate	61	44	50	68	51	60

The contribution of carbohydrate to energy yield increases with the intensity of exercise. Carbohydrate metabolism does not predominate in those on any of the diets until exercise intensities reach or exceed 50% $\dot{V}O_2$ max. The greatest carbohydrate yield occurs with the high-carbohydrate diet and the lowest with the high-fat diet. As exercise proceeds to exhaustion (beginning vs. end) fat metabolism again predominates. At 70% $\dot{V}O_2$ max the high-carbohydrate diet resulted in the longest performance times. Most marathon performances are run at or slightly above this level (at about 85% $\dot{V}O_2$ max). These data indicate that performance time may be better at the 50% level with the high-fat diet. This may have implications for ultramarathoners, who reduce exercise intensity to sustain the longer performances of 50 and 100 mile runs. Caution should be used regarding recommendation of carbohydrate overloading procedures. Medical evidence suggests that kidney function may be compromised by repeated overloading.

In summary, it has been shown that diet and exercise, when properly manipulated, do enhance glycogen storage in muscle. In addition, this enhancement improves performance time, especially at or above 70% $\dot{V}O_2$ max. Recent evidence indicates that equal benefits can be achieved without the carbohydrate-free portion of the "loading" procedure. It should be noted that persons participating in events that last less than 45 to 60 minutes probably will not benefit from loading, since little muscle glycogen depletion occurs during short periods of exercise. For example, a 10 kilometer runner would probably benefit more from a mixed diet.

Diet and anaerobic performance

Studies investigating short-term, highly intense exercise have shown that ATP and PC stores in muscle are the primary energy sources.[28,29] During the execution of maximal isometric contraction (a good example of short-term maximal anaerobic exercise) ATP is 20% depleted and PC is about 80% depleted. Only a small portion of muscle glycogen is used, and lactate production is high.[6] Neither ATP nor glycogen appears to be a limiting factor; but lack of phosphate and failure of continued glycolysis because of the accumulation of lactate do seem to interfere with performance.

When exercise is anaerobic, such as sprinting, performed at 150% $\dot{V}O_2$ max, glycogen is depleted from muscle fibers. But the glycogen is selectively depleted, first from those most recruited during anaerobic exercise, the FT fibers.[20] Very little glycogen is depleted from ST fibers during anaerobic exercise.

Researchers have examined responses to short-term maximal exercise after diet, after prolonged exercise, and after combined aerobic and anaerobic exercise.[27-29] In all cases an isokinetic apparatus (Cybex II) was used to measure muscle torque. The short-term exercise consisted of continuous maximal contractions at $180°/sec^{-1}$ for 1 minute. The highest torque produced, peak torque, is a measure of strength, whereas the difference between peak torque and torque produced at the end of the minute is a measure of muscle fatigue. In the diet experiments, subjects were fed either carbohydrate-free or carbohydrate-rich diets. Muscle glycogen, as expected, was significantly depleted by the former

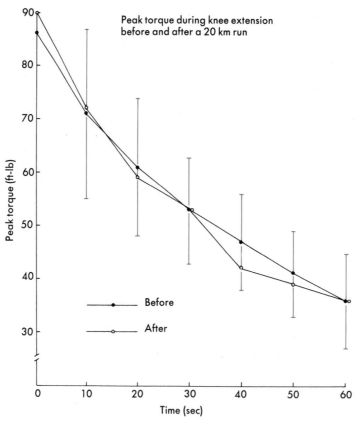

FIG. 4-4 Peak torque (strength) during a 1-minute maximal isokinetic contraction task before and after a 20 km (12 mile) run. There was no significant difference between trials. (From Noble, B.J., Kraemer, W.J., and Fleck, S.J.: Muscle strength and endurance following long distance running. [In press.])

and increased by the latter. Neither diet significantly affected peak torque or fatigue.

Following a marathon run, which depletes primarily ST fibers of muscle glycogen, peak torque was not affected, but the muscle was found to be significantly more fatigued.[29] Figures 4-4 and 4-5 show the results of a similar study with similar findings.[38] Long-distance runners ran 20 kilometers (12 miles) at race pace on a treadmill. Before and after the run, subjects performed a 60-second endurance test of repeated maximal extensions and flexions. Peak torque was not affected by the run, but total work (area under the extension/flexion force curve) was significantly reduced. Results were attributed to a

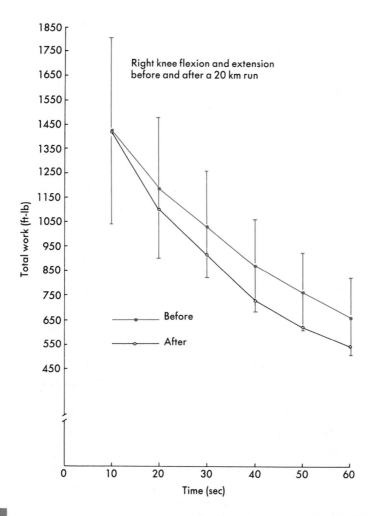

FIG. 4-5   **Total work (muscular endurance) during a 1-minute maximal isokinetic contraction task before and after a 20 km (12 mile) run. Endurance significantly decreased following the prolonged work. (From Noble, B.J., Kraemer, W.J., and Fleck, S.J.: Muscle strength and endurance following distance running. [In press.])**

decreased capacity to hold tension and a greater reliance on FT fibers because of glycogen depletion in ST fibers.

In this third set of experiments subjects ran at maximum pace for 75 minutes, cycled for 30 minutes at 70% $\dot{V}_{O_2}$ max, performed three bouts of maximal isokinetic contractions, and cycled five repeated maximum bouts of 1 minute each. This regimen was designed to deplete both ST and FT fibers of muscle glycogen. In fact, following this exercise ST fibers were 80% depleted and FT were 78% depleted. Both peak torque and torque decline were significantly reduced with this exercise.

Dietary intervention alone does not seem to be sufficient to affect anaerobic performance of the type used in the experiments just discussed. When ST fibers alone are depleted in marathon running, strength is not affected, since expression of strength is primarily a FT fiber activity; however, in the 1-minute task, where more FT fibers are depleted, muscle shows both a decline in strength and an increase in fatigue during a short-term anaerobic task.

These studies represent only a beginning to our understanding of anaerobic exercise, but they do illustrate some important points. It appears that a rested anaerobic athlete cannot be helped by the manipulation of muscle glycogen with either high- or low-carbohydrate diets. A normal mixed diet is sufficient. Athletes should not precede muscular endurance tasks with exhausting aerobic exercise. A weight lifting regimen, for example, may not be compatible with prior exhaustive running. Athletes who perform both maximal contractions and longer term endurance activities, such as soccer players, probably deplete both fiber types during the course of play. Preliminary studies of soccer players have shown this to be true.[28] Therefore, coaches should train to increase both capacities, aerobic and anaerobic. Further studies are needed to examine the effect of diet following exhaustive anaerobic exercise.

Feeding before and during exercise

A pregame meal should not be confused with total athletic nutrition.[43] Too often coaches place emphasis on the period 12 to 24 hours before competition but neglect overall nutrition. With young athletes training daily at higher and higher energy levels, not only during the season but in the off-season as well, it is imperative that nutrition be attended to long before the pregame meal. It may be that the athlete is so badly depleted of necessary nutrients that the best of meals could not help at that time. Even though pregame meals have been shown to be ineffective in improving performance (excluding carbohydrate loading), many nutritional myths still exist. For a thorough review of all aspects of athletic nutrition the student is referred to the excellent book by Williams.[43] For the most part, pregame meals are thought to have little effect on athletic performance when the athlete has been consuming a normal diet.

Since we know that carbohydrate plays an important role in aerobic exercise above 50% $\dot{V}_{O_2}$ max and that glycogen stores are limited, it seems plausible that providing glucose just before or during aerobic exercise may be beneficial. Investigators had subjects run or cycle for 30 minutes at 60% to 72% $\dot{V}_{O_2}$ max before and after ingestion of glucose (31.8 g in 300 ml of water).[14] They concluded that "the relatively minor role of oral glucose in carbohydrate oxidation indicates that glucose feedings during prolonged exercise are of limited importance for muscle metabolism." However, they suggest that glucose feedings may prevent depletion of liver glycogen by increasing blood glucose levels. Other researchers have examined the effects of glucose ingestion at higher exercise intensities (80% and 100% $\dot{V}O_2$ max).[16] Performance time at 80% $\dot{V}O_2$ max was decreased by 19% (from 53.2 to 43.2 minutes) with glucose ingestion compared with exercise when water only was allowed. No differences were observed at 100% $\dot{V}O_2$ max. This experiment indicates that the glucose supplement at 80% $\dot{V}O_2$ max increased the rate of carbohydrate oxidation and impeded the mobilization of free fatty acids.

Several commercial glucose solutions are commonly used during endurance activities. One study compared Gatorade, Breaktime, Body Punch, and water to determine how quickly each cleared the stomach after ingestion.[15] If a substance does not clear the stomach, it cannot provide metabolic support. Subjects ingested 400 milliliters of each solution and 15 minutes later stomach contents were aspirated. Although there was no significant differences between three of the preparations, Gatorade was found to be significantly less effective in stomach clearance (35% to 40% remained). This result was attributed to the higher concentration of glucose (4.5 g%) in Gatorade. Glucose concentration in supplemental drinks should not exceed 2.5 g% to empty the stomach effectively. Furthermore, endurance athletes should attend to their water replacement needs first. If glucose levels are critical, as in marathon running, the glucose concentrations of fluid supplements must be kept low. It should also be noted that glucose supplementation 30 minutes before performance may increase insulin levels, which could result in hypoglycemia during exercise.

Repletion of muscle glycogen

We know that hard exercise can deplete muscle fibers of glycogen stores. How quickly and by what means can these stores be repleted *(glycogen repletion)?* This question is especially relevant to the coach planning hard practices and developing nutritional strategies for athletes participating in tournaments or following schedules that allow little time between events.

To give us some perspective on this problem it is valuable to examine the response of animals to exhaustive exercise.[42] Rats swam to exhaustion, and muscle and liver glycogen were measured before exercise and periodically for 48 hours after exercise. A significant reduction in glycogen was observed in FT and ST fibers, as well as in the liver immediately after exercise. Glucose solution was added by stomach tube immediately after exercise and again after 1 hour. Animals also ate regular food as desired during the entire postexercise experimental period. Glycogen was restored to the liver before it was restored in muscle tissue. Within muscle tissue, FT fibers were replenished more quickly than were ST fibers. These data provide a pattern of glycogen resynthesis when adequate replacement is available and consumed.

Repletion of glycogen in human muscle tissue was studied after 2 hours of hard work.[39] So that both fiber types would be depleted, during the first hour subjects engaged in endurance exercise, and during the second hour they performed repeated maximum bouts on a bicycle ergometer. Two hours after exercise subjects began consuming a carbohydrate-rich diet. Glycogen levels dropped from 125 mmol $\cdot$ kg^{-1} before exercise to 22 mmol $\cdot$ kg^{-1} immediately after exercise. They were not fully repleted until 46 hours after exercise. The increase occurred in both fibers but, as with the rat tissue, FT fibers were replenished faster. Resynthesis appears to begin almost immediately; however, other authors observed no significant increase until 60 minutes after exercise.[33] Since resynthesis appears to occur before feeding, it can be hypothesized that the increase is explained either by endogenous carbohydrate or by gluconeogenesis from protein or lactate.

Further investigation was conducted using laboratory animals to study glycogen repletion from endogenous stores after depletion by exhaustive continuous and intermittent exercise.[18] Following exercise skeletal muscle and liver were 94% and 97% depleted, respectively. There was no significant difference in glycogen depletion between continuous and intermittent work. Food intake was restricted for 4 hours after exercise to examine whether endogenous stores could explain immediate repletion. Endogenous substances were not able to restore glycogen in muscle and liver. After the 4-hour fast the animals were fed and by 24 hours after exercise a glycogen supercompensation was observed. It appears that food intake is necessary for repletion.

Other investigators examined repletion of glycogen in human muscle following anaerobic work. Six subjects rode a bicycle ergometer at 140% $\dot{V}O_2$ max at 1-minute intervals to exhaustion. Two hours after exercise three subjects consumed a mixed diet and three consumed a mixed diet plus additional carbohydrate. No significant differences were found between groups. Biopsies taken 0, 2, 5, 12, and 24 hours after exercise revealed that repletion was 28%, 39%, 53%, 67%, and 102%, respectively of preexercise amounts (see Figure 4-6). It was concluded that complete recovery can be accomplished in 24 hours and that the rate of resynthesis cannot be accelerated by a high-carbohydrate diet.

Of what benefit is this research to the teacher and coach? The following are a few practical implications of these investigations:

1. FT fibers are repleted first; therefore those activities that utilize these fibers primarily can be repeated sooner after depletion than ST fiber activities, that is, sprinting can be repeated before endurance work.

2. There seems to be no difference in depletion whether the exhaustive exercise is continuous or intermittent. Thus, whether athletes are trained with one method or with the other, coaches must attend to repletion.

3. Although resynthesis of carbohydrate begins immediately, before refeeding, complete repletion cannot occur without feeding. Again, the coach should begin a feeding regimen as soon as eating can be easily tolerated, for example, 2 hours after exercise.

4. Repletion of carbohydrate cannot be accelerated above that supplied by a mixed diet. Depleted athletes should be encouraged to begin eating a mixed diet as soon as possible. A high fat and protein diet is contraindicated. Repletion may not be complete for up to 1 week.

5. With a correct diet, repletion may occur as early as 12 or as late as 46 hours. However, most evidence indicates that at least 24 hours is necessary to replenish muscle fibers and liver with carbohydrates.

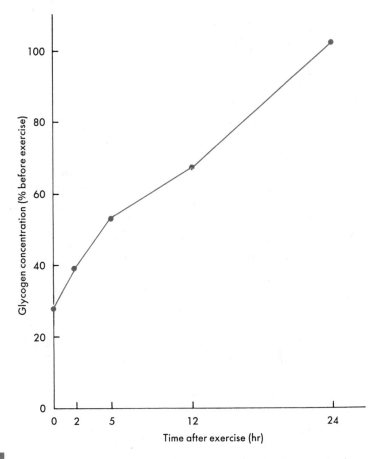

FIG. 4-6   Glycogen resynthesis following exhaustive exercise at 140% $\dot{V}_{O_2}$ max. (Adapted from MacDougall, J.D., Ward, G.R., Sale, D.G., and others: Muscle glycogen repletion after high intensity intermittent exercise, J. Appl. Physiol. *42:*129, 1977.)

The effect of training on fuel utilization

If it is possible to spare glycogen stores during prolonged exercise by using fat instead, performance may be improved. Several studies have examined this question by studying trained and untrained muscle. For example, trained and untrained subjects were compared while riding to exhaustion on a bicycle ergometer after several 20-minute bouts at 77% $\dot{V}_{O_2}$ max.[22] The untrained group had lower muscle glycogen levels at the end of each 20-minute bout. It is suggested that trained subjects can rely on fat metabolism for a longer period of time, thus sparing the glycogen stores. Similar results were observed in a study of seven physically fit and eight less fit subjects. Each rode for 4 hours at 30% $\dot{V}_{O_2}$ max. Results revealed that 14% of the fuel utilization came from carbohydrate in the fit group, compared with 25% carbohydrate utilization by the less fit group. This result, obtained at low, submaximal exercise, supports the previous observation that subjects who are more fit utilize more fat.[41]

Additional support for glycogen "sparing" is indicated by a high correlation (-0.79) between the rate of release of free fatty acids and increases in lactic acid.[25] Fat metabolism seems to be inhibited by lactic acid. Since untrained subjects produce more lactic acid at lower, submaximal levels, they are more dependent on glycogen stores. Further investigation[37] has shown that the skeletal muscle of trained human subjects has a greater capacity to release free fatty acids from adipose tissue.[25]

SUMMARY

The calorie, or kilocalorie as it is more correctly known, is the unit of measurement for both the energy we gain from the food we eat and for the expenditure of energy for maintenance of body processes. Since it is important to monitor the type of nutrient that is used in energy production, and it is not always convenient to biopsy muscle tissue, the respiratory exchange ratio (R) is often measured as an estimate of energy substrate. An R of 1.0 reflects combustion of pure carbohydrate, and an R of 0.7 reflects combustion of pure fat.

Daily energy requirements can be calculated by determining the basal metabolic rate (BMR); estimating daily activity level; correcting calculations to account for the effects of specific dynamic action (SDA) of food; and considering the residual energy requirements for recovery from hard physical training. Additional calories must be included during growth to account for this process.

It is apparent that the human body is not 100% efficient. We must eat more food than is required to account for the actual physical work being accomplished. In fact, maximum mechanical efficiency of the body is only 25%. The remaining 75% of the energy consumed is released as heat.

Early studies examined fuel utilization during exercise by measuring R. At rest and during light exercise up to 50% $\dot{V}_{O_2}$ max, the predominant fuel is fat. After 50% $\dot{V}_{O_2}$ max carbohydrate is the predominant fuel. At exercise intensities of 85% to 90% $\dot{V}_{O_2}$ max, nearly all energy used is derived from carbohydrate.

When diet is manipulated by "carbohydrate loading" and exhaustive exercise is performed to deplete muscle glycogen, a supercompensation of muscle glycogen storage occurs. This supercompensation results in a significant increase in aerobic exercise time (at or above 70% $\dot{V}O_2$ max).

Similar dietary intervention does not seem to enhance performance in short-term anaerobic tasks, even though muscle glycogen is significantly increased on a carbohydrate-rich diet. Muscle strength is not affected by prolonged endurance running in which ST fibers are depleted of muscle glycogen, but the rate of fatigue, in a 1-minute test of continuous maximal contractions in which FT fibers are predominantly used, is significantly increased. When both ST and FT fibers are depleted through exercise, both strength and fatigue are affected.

Glucose is an important precursor of energy production, and the depletion of blood glucose and other carbohydrate stores may be critical for prolonged aerobic performance. Glucose supplementation has been studied and increased blood glucose concentrations have been shown to affect performance time adversely. Additionally, commercial glucose solutions with high concentrations of glucose do not clear the stomach easily, and thus do not provide immediate metabolic support.

Replenishment of glycogen to depleted muscle fibers requires dietary intervention. Both mixed and carbohydrate-rich diets will accomplish repletion in 24 hours.

Trained aerobic athletes appear to have the ability to ''spare'' carbohydrate. These athletes rely more on fat metabolism during exercise than do untrained persons, which may improve performance in which muscle glycogen depletion is critical.

KEY TERMS

basal metabolic rate the minimal energy expenditure necessary to maintain life.

calorimetry a means of determining caloric values by measurement of heat produced, either through direct combustion of food samples or through measurement of changes in temperature brought about by the metabolism of food.

glycogen depletion the removal of carbohydrates from storage in muscle tissue or liver resulting from long-duration, high-intensity exercise.

glycogen repletion the process of restoring carbohydrates in muscle tissue or liver following long-duration, high-intensity exercise.

kilocalorie (kcal) the unit of measure used to describe both energy intake and energy expenditure.

metabolism the chemical changes within the body that provide energy and maintain life.

respiratory exchange ratio (R) the ratio of carbon dioxide produced and oxygen consumed used as a measure of nutrient use.

specific dynamic action an increase in metabolic rate associated with the digestion of food.

REVIEW QUESTIONS

1. Compare the terms direct and indirect calorimetry. Discuss the interrelationship between heat production, oxygen consumption, and the respiratory exchange ratio.

2. Why is basal metabolic rate lower in females, and why does it decline with age?

3. Why is residual energy expenditure important when calculating caloric intake requirements of athletes in training?

4. Diagram the contributions of fat and carbohydrate to exercise metabolism as they vary according to exercise intensity. In other words, plot the percentage of contribution (0% to 100%) of each fuel on the vertical axis, using a dotted line to represent fat contribution and a solid line to represent carbohydrate contribution, and the percentage of maximal oxygen consumption ($\dot{V}o_2$ max) (0% to 100%) on the horizontal axis. Where do the two lines (fat and carbohydrate) cross?

5. Discuss the effects of mixed, fat and protein, and carbohydrate diets on endurance time, that is, on aerobic performance.

6. Discuss specifically how glycogen is depleted from muscle fibers in both aerobic and anaerobic exercise.

7. Discuss the possible adverse effects of glucose supplementation during endurance performance.

8. Can glycogen depletion be replenished from endogenous stores? Approximately how long does it take to replenish glycogen and what conditions are necessary for this repletion?

9. What is meant by the term *glycogen sparing?*

REFERENCES

1. American Alliance of Health, Physical Education, Recreation, and Dance: Nutrition for athletes, Reston, Va., 1980, The Alliance.

2. Bergstrom, J.: Muscle electrolytes in man, determined by neutron activation analysis on needle biopsy specimens: a study on normal subjects, kidney patients and patients with chronic diarrhea, Scand. J. Clin. Lab. Invest. **14:**1, 1962.

3. Bergstrom, J.: Local changes of ATP and phosphorylcreatine in human muscle tissue in connection with exercise, Circ. Res. **20**(Suppl. 1):91, 1967.

4. Bergstrom, J., Hermansen, L., Hultman, E., and others: Diet, muscle glycogen and physical performance, Acta Physiol. Scand. **71:**140, 1967.

5. Bergstrom, J., and Hultman, E.: Muscle glycogen synthesis after exercise: an enhancing factor localized to the muscle cells in man, Nature **210:**309, 1966.

6. Bergstrom, J., and Hultman, E.: Nutrition for maximal sports performance, JAMA **221:**999, 1972.

7. Blair, S.N., Ellsworth, N.M., Haskell, W.L., and others: Comparison of nutrient intake in middle-aged men and women runners and controls, Med. Sci. Sports Exerc. **13:**310, 1981.

8. Bogert, L.J., Briggs, G.M., and Calloway, D.H.: Nutrition and physical fitness, ed. 11, Philadelphia, 1984, W.B. Saunders Co.

9. Christensen, E.H., and Hansen, O.: Zur methodik der respiratorischen Quotient-Bestimmungen in Ruhe und bei Arbeit, Skandinav. Arch. Physiol. **81:**137, 1939.

10. Christensen, E.H., and Hansen, O.: Untersuchungen Über die Verbrennungsvorgange bei langdaurender, schwerer Muskelarbeit, Skandinav. Arch. Physiol. **81**:153, 1939.

11. Christensen, E.H., and Hansen, O.: Arbeitsfahigkeit und Ernahrung, Skandinav. Arch. Physiol. **81**:160, 1939.

12. Christensen, E.H., and Hansen, O.: Hypolgykamie, arbeitsfahigkeit und ermudung, Scandinv. Arch. Physiol. **81**:172, 1939.

13. Christensen, E.H., and Hansen, O.: Respiratorischer Quotient und O_2-Aufnahme, Skandinav. Arch. Physiol. **81**:180, 1939.

14. Costill, D.L., Bennett, A., Branam, G., and others: Glucose ingestion at rest and during prolonged exercise, J. Appl. Physiol. **34**:764, 1973.

15. Coyle, E.F., Costill, D.L., Fink, W.J., and others: Gastric emptying rates for selected athletic drinks, Res. Q. **49**:119, 1978.

16. Foster, C., Costill, D.L., and Fink, W.J.: Effect of pre-exercise feedings on endurance performance, Med. Sci. Sports, **11**:1, 1979.

17. Foster, C., Costill, D.L., and Fink, W.J.: Gastric emptying characteristics of glucose and glucose polymer solutions, Res. Q. Exerc. Sports **51**:299, 1980.

18. Gaesser, G.A., and Brooks, G.A.: Glycogen repletion following continuous and intermittent exercise to exhaustion, J. Appl. Physiol. **49**:722, 1980.

19. Galbo, H., Holst, J.J., and Christensen, N.J.: The effect of different diets and of insulin on the hormonal response to prolonged exercise, Acta Physiol. Scand. **107**:19, 1979.

20. Gollnick, P.D., Armstrong, R.B., Sembrowich, W.L., and others: Glycogen depletion pattern in human skeletal muscle fibers after heavy exercise, J. Appl. Physiol. **34**:615, 1973.

21. Hargreaves, M., Costill, D.L., Coggan, A., and others: Effect of carbohydrate feedings on muscle glycogen utilization and exercise performance, Med. Sci. Sports Exerc. **16**:219, 1984.

22. Hermansen, L., Hultman, E., and Saltin, B.: Muscle glycogen during prolonged severe exercise, Acta Physiol. Scand. **71**:129, 1967.

23. Hultman, E.: Physiological role of muscle glycogen in man, with special reference to exercise, Circ. Res. **20**(Suppl. 1):99, 1967.

24. Issekutz, B., Birkhead, N., and Rodahl, K.: Effect of diet on work metabolism, J. Nutr. **79**:109, 1963.

25. Issekutz, B., Miller, H., Paul, P., and others: Aerobic work capacity and plasma FFA turnover, J. Appl. Physiol. **20**:293, 1965.

26. Ivy, J.L., Miller, W., Dover, V., and others: Endurance improved by ingestion of a glucose polymer supplement, Med. Sci. Sports Exerc. **15**:466, 1983.

27. Jacobs, I.: Lactate concentrations after short, maximal exercise at various glycogen levels, Acta Physiol. Scand. **111**:465, 1981.

28. Jacobs, I., Kaiser, P., and Tesch, P.: The effects of glycogen exhaustion on maximal, short time performance. Proceedings of the International Symposium on Sports Biology, Vierumaki, Finland, 1979, Human Kinetics Publishers, Champaign, Ill., 1982.

29. Jacobs, I., Kaiser, P., and Tesch, P.: Muscle strength and fatigue after selective glycogen depletion in human skeletal muscle fibers, Eur. J. Applied Physiol. **46**:47, 1981.

30. Krogh, A., and Lindhard, J.: Relative value of fat and carbohydrate as sources of muscular energy: with appendices on the correlation between standard metabolism and the respiratory quotient during rest and work, Biochem. J. **14**:290, 1920.

31. Karlsson, J., and Saltin, B.: Lactate, ATP and CP in working muscles during exhaustive exercise in man, J. Appl. Physiol. **29:**598, 1970.

32. Karlsson, J., Diamant, B., and Saltin, B.: Muscle metabolites during submaximal and maximal exercise in man, Scand. J. Clin. Lab. Invest. **26:**385, 1971.

33. Karlsson, J., and Saltin, B.: Oxygen deficit and muscle metabolites in intermittent exercise, Acta Physiol. Scand. **82:**115, 1971.

34. Lemon, P.W.R., and Nagle, F.J.: Effects of exercise on protein and amino acid metabolism, Med. Sci. Sports Exerc. **13:**141, 1981.

35. MacDougall, J.D., Ward, G.R., Sale, D.G., and others: Muscle glycogen repletion after high intensity intermittent exercise, J. Appl. Physiol. **42:**129, 1977.

36. McMurray, R.G., Wilson, J.R., and Kitchell, B.S.: The effects of fructose and glucose on high intensity endurance performance, Res. Q. Exerc. Sports **54:**156, 1983.

37. Mole, P., and Holloszy, J.: Exercise-induced increase in the capacity of skeletal muscle to oxidize palmitate, Proc. Soc. Exp. Biol. Med. **134:**798, 1970.

38. Noble, B.J., Kraemer, W.J., and Fleck, S.J.: Muscle strength and endurance following long distance running, presented at the Pan American Congress of Sports Medicine and Exercise, Miami, 1981.

39. Piehl, K.: Time course for refilling glycogen stores in human muscle fibers following exercise-induced glycogen depletion, Acta Physiol. Scand. **90:**297, 1974.

40. Pruett, E.D.R.: Fat and carbohydrate metabolism in exercise and recovery and its dependence upon workload severity, Oslo, Norway, 1971, Institute of Work Physiology.

41. Rahkila, P., Soimajarvi, J., Karvinen, E., and others: Lipid metabolism during exercise: respiratory exchange ratio and muscle glycogen content during 4 h bicycle ergometry in two groups of healthy men, II, Eur. J. Applied Physiol. **44:**245, 1980.

42. Terjung, R.L., Baldwin, K.M., Winder, W.W., and others: Glycogen repletion in different types of muscle and in liver after exhausting exercise, Am. J. Physiol. **226:**1387, 1974.

43. Williams, M.H.: Nutritional aspects of human physical and athletic performance, Springfield, Ill., 1976, Charles C Thomas, Publisher.

SUGGESTED READINGS

1. Bogert, L.J., Briggs, G.M., and Calloway, D.H.: Nutrition and physical fitness, ed. 11, Philadelphia, 1984, W.B. Saunders Co.

2. Bergstrom, J., and Hultman, E.: Nutrition for maximal sports performance, JAMA **221:**999, 1972.

3. Colsolazio, C.F., Johnson, R.E., and Pecora, L.J.: Physiological measurements of metabolic functions in man, New York, 1963, McGraw-Hill Book Co., Inc.

4. Kleiber, M.: The fire of life: an introduction to animal energetics, New York, 1961, John Wiley & Sons, Inc.

5. Lewis, S., and Gutin, B.: Nutrition and endurance, Am. J. Clin. Nutr. **26:**1011, 1973.

6. Mayer, J.: Human nutrition: its physiological, medical and social aspects, Springfield, Ill., 1979, Charles C Thomas, Publisher.

7. Williams, M.H.: Nutritional aspects of human physical and athletic performance, Springfield, Ill., 1976, Charles C Thomas, Publisher.

LABORATORY APPLICATION: DETERMINING DAILY CALORIE INTAKE

Many coaches are interested in determining the energy required for various sports so that they can make daily caloric intake recommendations to athletes. How can this be accomplished?

First, the student should be cautioned that we are talking about total calories only and not the nutritional content of those calories. Proper quantities of all necessary nutrients should be included in the athlete's diet. Also, the estimations provided here should not be viewed as error free. By necessity, some of the factors are averages and will not apply to every single athlete. The coach must monitor the body compositions of athletes (fat content as well as body weight) to evaluate the adequacy of the estimations. The values here will enable you to determine total daily energy expenditure for individual athletes.

1. Knowing the athlete's sex, body weight (in kilograms), and approximate fat percentage, calculate daily resting metabolic rate using Table 4-1.
2. Multiple the daily resting metabolic rate by 10% to calculate the SDA.
3. Estimate the energy cost of the sport by multiplying the kilocalories expended per minute (Table 4-2) by the number of minutes of practice. (Since residual energy expenditure is difficult to estimate, the best the coach can do is to monitor body weight for large fluctuations and make adjustments accordingly.)
4. Estimate total daily energy expenditure by adding the values from 1, 2, and 3 above.

Taking some hypothetical athletes we can now estimate their caloric needs.

Type of athlete: football player
Sex: male
Body weight: 90 kilograms (198 lb.)
Body fat: 10%*
Age: 17 years (average daily caloric requirement for age 17 is 3000 kilocalories)
Practice time: 2 hours per day
1. Daily resting metabolic rate
   1.48 kcal/hr/kg × 90 kg × 24 hr = 3197 kcal
2. SDA
   3197 kcal × 0.10 = 320 kcal
3. Energy cost of the sport
   8.9 kcal/min × 120 min = 1068 kcal
4. Total daily energy expenditure
   3197 + 320 + 1068 = 4585 kcal/day

---

*A simple method of calculating body fat can be found in Chapter 21.

Type of athlete: tennis player
Sex: female
Body weight: 50 kilograms (110 lb.)
Body fat: 15%
Age: 18 years (average daily caloric requirement for age 18 is 2000 kilocalories)
Practice time: 2 hours per day

1. Daily resting metabolic rate
   0.89 kcal/hr/kg $\times$ 50 kg $\times$ 24 hr = 1068 kcal
2. SDA
   1068 kcal $\times$ 0.10 = 107 kcal
3. Energy cost of the sport
   7.1 kcal/min $\times$ 120 min = 852 kcal
4. Total daily energy expenditure
   1068 + 107 + 852 = 2027 kcal/day

Type of athlete: cross-country runner
Sex: male
Body weight: 65 kilograms (143 lb)
Body fat: 10%
Age: 14 years (average daily caloric requirements for age 14 is 2700 kilocalories)
Practice time: 2 hours per day

1. Daily resting metabolic rate
   1.14 kcal/hr/kg $\times$ 65 kg $\times$ 24 hr = 1778 kcal
2. SDA
   1778 kcal $\times$ 0.10 = 178 kcal
3. Energy cost of the sport
   10.6 kcal/min $\times$ 120 min = 1272 kcal
4. Total daily energy expenditure
   1778 + 178 + 1272 = 3228 kcal/day

As mentioned previously, these values are not error free, but they can serve as a starting point for the coach as he or she guides the athlete to an energy intake that matches expenditure.

CASE STUDY

The following is a conversation between a professor of physiology and a high school volleyball coach attending a summer school course in exercise physiology.

COACH: I've read that diet can be an effective method of improving performance in prolonged exercise. Can "carbohydrate loading" be helpful to volleyball players under certain circumstances?

PROFESSOR: First, we have to know what metabolic pathway is used in volleyball. Is volleyball an aerobic or an anaerobic sport?

COACH: Well, it's probably both. I would say that 70% to 80% is anaerobic, that is, it uses both ATP-PC and lactate, and the rest is aerobic.

PROFESSOR: Do you think that muscle glycogen plays a major role in energy production?

COACH: I'm not sure, but glycolysis undoubtedly plays some role in energy metabolism, both in the production of lactic acid and as a substrate for Krebs cycle activity.

PROFESSOR: I agree. Muscle glycogen is utilized, but how much the muscle fibers are depleted is another question. Remember the study by Jacobs that found a carbohydrate-rich diet had no effect on maximal isokinetic strength or endurance curves.

COACH: But that was with no prior exercise. When Jacobs studied exercise that depleted both fast-twitch and slow-twitch fibers, both strength and endurance were affected.

PROFESSOR: What needs to be done is a study of the effects of a high-carbohydrate diet after fast-twitch fibers have been depleted by strenuous anaerobic exercise. However, such an experiment may not be practical for volleyball, since fast-twitch fibers may not be depleted either by practice or by competition, and you usually have plenty of time to replete glycogen stores.

COACH: Our practices are getting more intense all the time, and we don't think much about tapering before games. Could the accumulation of many hard practices, inadequate diet, and the close proximity between practice and games affect performance? Also, in tournaments we can play up to nine games if we make the finals.

PROFESSOR: Your point is well taken. What you suggest is probable, but we need to substantiate it with experimental data. You may want to try some field research on your own.

PART TWO

CARDIORESPIRATORY FUNCTION

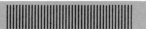

chapter 5

MAXIMAL AEROBIC AND ANAEROBIC POWER

MAJOR LEARNING OBJECTIVE

Aerobic capacity is measured by determining maximal oxygen consumption ($\dot{V}_{O_2}$ max). Success in long-duration (aerobic) sports is associated with a high $\dot{V}_{O_2}$ max, which has a high genetic component.

■ Anaerobic capacity is a function of the ability of the ATP-PC and lactate systems to produce energy. Short-duration, high-intensity sport athletes have high anaerobic capacities. This capacity has a high genetic component.

APPLICATIONS

Evaluation of aerobic and anaerobic capacities can help the coach or clinician and help the athletes select sports that conform to their individual capacities.

■ Simple arm and leg ergometer tests can be used in a field setting to predict these capacities.

THE second section of this book focuses on cardiorespiratory function. Simply stated, this section describes the process by which environmental air is taken into the lungs, exchanged with the blood and body tissues, and returned to the lungs for removal. Aerobic metabolism requires the intake of oxygen, transport in the blood, and uptake by the cells. Understanding of this process requires knowledge of pulmonary function, gas transport in the blood, and the role of the heart as a blood pump.

The question of human capacity for production of energy is of both practical and theoretical importance. This section addresses this question by examining the capacity of both aerobic and anaerobic systems.

When humans push themselves to the limits of available capacity, body systems are disrupted, that is, homeostasis is disturbed. This section also discusses the role of the kidney in homeostatic maintenance during exercise and sport.

In previous chapters, aerobic and anaerobic metabolism have been cited extensively. For the most part, these references have been limited to properties of muscle tissue regarding the production of energy. For example, slow-twitch fibers have been referred to as primarily aerobic fibers. These fibers are rich in mitochondria and oxidative enzymes that promote ATP production by the Krebs cycle and electron transport system. On the other hand, fast-twitch fibers have been referred to as primarily anaerobic fibers, that is, the capacity of these fibers to produce ATP by glycolysis is great.

What is the capacity of the aerobic and anaerobic processes to produce energy for exercise? This chapter examines this capacity in relation to the oxygen transport system.

AEROBIC POWER

The ability of humans to perform work or exercise is best examined by determining capacity. Just as you cannot adequately describe a glass without measuring its holding capacity, you cannot thoroughly describe human function without describing its capacity to perform work or exercise. What is the exercise aerobic capacity of humans? As soon as a term like capacity is introduced, questions are raised as to its quantification. Can capacity really be measured? The answer is probably not. We can estimate capacity but not measure it as such. Therefore, our terminology should reflect what we can actually measure. The term *power of the aerobic,* or *anaerobic, system* is more accurate and actually reflects what is measured, that is, the rate of aerobic or anaerobic energy use.

First, we need to define the term. *Aerobic power* is the maximal amount of oxygen that can be consumed per minute during maximal exercise. In exercise physiology literature, several terms are used synonymously with aerobic power. One, maximal oxygen consumption, refers directly to the variable measured. For ease of description, this term is abbreviated $\dot{V}O_2$ max. Another term, *aerobic capacity,* as previously mentioned, is nebulous and unquantifiable. Aerobic power is perhaps the more precise term because it most accurately expresses the terms of its calculation. That is, $\dot{V}O_2$ max is expressed in volume (liters) per unit of time (minute). Technically, this is an expression of power. When $\dot{V}O_2$ is expressed as $L \cdot min^{-1}$, the purpose of the expression is to describe the absolute power of the cardiorespiratory system. Often it is advantageous to speak of $\dot{V}O_2$ max relative to the amount of tissue that must be supplied. In this case the most common unit is ml/kg of body weight $\cdot min^{-1}$. This unit is best suited for making comparisons between athletic groups or between athletes and nonathletes or trained and untrained people. Still another unit of expression describes oxygen consumption relative to lean body mass (LBM) or the fat-free weight that is served. Because fat is not served by the oxygen transport system, it is often appropriate to make direct comparisons between active tissue served.

Early studies

Modern scientific documentation of aerobic power can be traced back to the early 1900s. In 1923, Hill and Lupton[28] showed that maximal oxygen consumption was variable among individuals. The following year Hill and others[26] reported that maximal oxygen consumption was important to prolonged exercise, that is, those who have higher $\dot{V}O_2$ max values perform better in endurance activities. Herbst[22] studied the response of oxygen consumption to increasing speed and found that oxygen consumption reached a point where additional increases in speed could no longer elicit an increase in oxygen consumption. This finding led to the establishment of the criterion for the measurement of aerobic power, that is, a maximal plateau value that cannot be increased with further work.

Measurement of aerobic power

During World War II, extensive scientific attention was given to the study of the "important components of physical performance."[67] It was clear that tests developed to that point had been biased by motivational and physical skill factors. Attempts to solve the measurement problem led to the development of testing procedures that, in various forms, are still used today.[67] Following is a summary of the results of these classical studies:
1. Using a constant treadmill speed (7 mph) and increasing work load by increasing treadmill grade (2.5% per stage) is more satisfactory than the reverse.
2. Oxygen consumption should be measured during the final minute (1:45 to 2:45) of a 3-minute stage, since a steady state has been reached in that time. (NOTE: Oxygen consumption does not increase to the need immediately but requires a period of time to reach equilibrium.)
3. The increase in oxygen consumption associated with any increase in a grade of 2.5% is $300 \text{ ml} \cdot min^{-1}$. $\dot{V}O_2$ max is attained when an increase in grade results in an increase in oxygen consumption no greater than $150 \text{ ml} \cdot min^{-1}$.
4. All persons (males) can easily run at 7 mph.
5. A light meal (750 kcal) does not have an adverse effect on $\dot{V}O_2$ max.
6. High room temperature can significantly reduce $\dot{V}O_2$ max measurements.
7. The entire procedure has a test-retest reliability of 0.95.

TABLE 5-1 ‖‖‖ BRUCE TREADMILL GRADED EXERCISE TEST PROTOCOL*

Stage	Duration (min)	Speed (mph)	Grade (%)	MET	$\dot{V}O_2$ (ml/kg · min^{-1})
I	3	1.7	10	4.0	14.0
II	3	2.5	12	6.6	23.1
III	3	3.4	14	10.0	35.0
IV	3	4.2	16	14.2	49.7
V	3	5.0	18	16.1	56.4

From Bruce, R.A., and McDonough, J.R.: Stress testing in screening for cardiovascular disease, Bull. N.Y. Acad. Med. **45:**1288, 1969.
*Since 1 MET is equal to 3.5 ml/kg · min^{-1}, the $\dot{V}O_2$ for any stage can be estimated by multiplying 3.5 times MET.

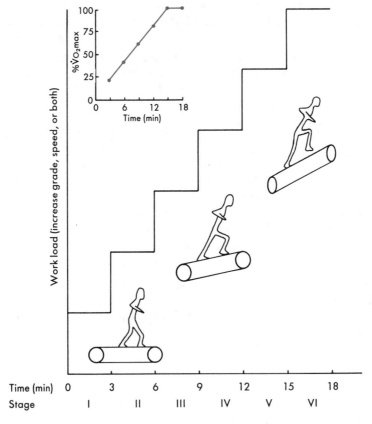

FIG. 5-1   Common treadmill graded exercise test protocols. The inset shows the rise in $\dot{V}O_2$ with time in a graded protocol.

Various laboratories have made adaptations to this procedure depending on the available equipment, group tested, and experimental purpose. Figure 5-1 illustrates the common characteristics of most treadmill test protocols, that is, the tests are graded with each stage lasting about 3 minutes.

A common procedure for studying aerobic power of both normal and patient populations is the Bruce protocol[8] (see Table 5-1). This protocol begins at a relatively light load (5 *MET,* which means 5 times the resting metabolic rate) and increases the work load every 3 minutes by increasing both the speed and the grade. Modifications have recently been made in this protocol for use with various patient populations.

The technical aspects of the measurement of oxygen consumption are not necessary for our present discussion; however, it may be helpful for the student to be able to have a mental picture of the process. Figure 5-2 illustrates a typical apparatus for measuring oxygen consumption. Basically, the following pieces of equipment are necessary:

1. Flowmeter to record the volume of air inspired (or expired) by the subject. (Since air volume is affected by both temperature and pressure, both air temperature and barometric pressure must be recorded simultaneously with the air volume so that necessary corrections can be made.)
2. Respiratory valve to direct air from the flowmeter (or room) to the subject with each inspiration and out to an air trap during exhalation.
3. Air trap or other device that will hold expired air long enough for it to be sampled and analyzed.
4. Oxygen and carbon dioxide analyzers to measure the percentage of the expired gases.

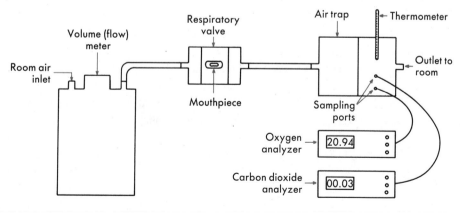

FIG. 5-2   **Typical open system apparatus for measuring oxygen consumption.**

Oxygen consumption can then be calculated for any collection period by using the following equation:

$$\dot{V}_{O_2} \text{ (L} \cdot \text{min)} = \frac{\text{Volume of gas (L} \cdot \text{min)}}{100} \times \text{true } O_2$$

True O_2 is the number of milliliters of oxygen consumed for every 100 milliliters of air inspired (or expired). Since the amount of air inspired equals that expired only when the ratio of CO_2 production/O_2 consumption is equal to 1.0, the direct reading of oxygen percentage cannot be used. Thus, true O_2 corrects the oxygen concentration for differences in volume between the inspired and expired sides. True O_2 is calculated as follows:

$$\text{True } O_2 = \% \, N_2 \text{ (inspired)} \times 0.265 - \% \, O_2 \text{ (expired)}$$

Simply stated, to measure oxygen consumption you must record the volume of air inspired (or expired) and the percentages of O_2 and CO_2 in that air.

Another format for discussing the calculations of oxygen consumption is presented as follows:

$$\dot{V}_{O_2} = \dot{V}_{O_2} \text{ inspired} - \dot{V}_{O_2} \text{ expired}$$

$$\dot{V}_{O_2} \text{ inspired} = \text{Ventilation}_{\text{inspired}} \times 0.2093$$

$$\dot{V}_{O_2} \text{ expired} = \text{Ventilation}_{\text{expired}} \times O_2 \text{ expired}$$

Carbon dioxide is measured because a 1:1 ratio exists between oxygen consumption and carbon dioxide production only at a respiratory exchange ratio of 1.0.

Specificity of measurement

Over the years, exercise physiologists have used several testing modes for determining aerobic power. The most common have been the step test, bicycle ergometer, and treadmill. There has always been discussion among researchers concerning the comparability of values obtained in different laboratories when different testing instruments have been used. The following material examines some of the various tests and methods that have been used prevalently.

Twelve subjects were tested on a treadmill and again on a step test.[35] $\dot{V}_{O_2}$ values were 48.3 and 48.0 ml/kg $\cdot$ min^{-1}, respectively. The small difference in $\dot{V}_{O_2}$ values and the high correlation between the tests (0.95) indicates that either method could be used effectively. The practicality of the step test may be outweighed by the lack of flexibility in changing work load.

In another instance, treadmill and bicycle tests were compared in separate experiments, with bicycle $\dot{V}_{O_2}$ values found to be lower than treadmill $\dot{V}_{O_2}$ values (9.9%, 12.4%, and 5.0%).[5,36,48] Results on the bicycle test are affected by a lower muscle mass involvement, a bias toward heavier subjects, and perhaps an advantage to those with stronger legs. However, when maximal leg force and various leg composition factors were taken into consideration, these variables could not fully account for the differences between treadmill and bicycle tests.[36]

In another case, muscle mass involvement was tested by comparing a treadmill test with two bicycle tests, one seated and the other standing.[38] The standing test, which involves additional muscle mass (vs seated), elicited $\dot{V}O_2$ max values significantly higher than the seated test, but still significantly lower than the treadmill values, which presumably involve even more muscle mass. If the goal was to achieve the highest values possible in a normal group of subjects, the treadmill would be the instrument of choice.

Interest in measuring the aerobic power of rowers has stimulated the development of rowing ergometers. One such ergometer was compared to a bicycle ergometer.[15] Although $\dot{V}O_2$ max was higher on the rowing apparatus, the difference was not significant.

Swimming tests for $\dot{V}O_2$ max have also been developed. Some investigators[5] found tethered swimming test results to be 14% lower in $\dot{V}O_2$ max than those from the treadmill; however, others[42] tested highly trained college swimmers and found no difference. The specificity of the test may be of greater importance to the highly trained athlete. To examine this hypothesis, swimmers were tested on the treadmill and also on a tethered swimming test, before and after a swimming training program.[41] A significant increase was noted following training in the swimming test and no difference observed in the treadmill test. It appears that the specific power of the sport is best analyzed by selecting tests that engage the specifically trained muscle fibers.

Another study examined the $\dot{V}O_2$ max testing-specificity hypothesis.[66] Skiers, rowers, and cyclists were tested on the treadmill (uphill) and in tests that were specifically related to their sports. All three groups showed slightly higher values in tests that most nearly duplicated their sport specialization. Again, if the aerobic power of a highly trained athlete is in question, a test that is specifically related to the sport is preferable. With untrained subjects, of all the testing instruments available, the treadmill is probably the test of choice.

Aerobic power of athletes

If aerobic power is, in fact, a significant component in endurance performance, it seems plausible that values would be higher in aerobically trained athletes. Figure 5-3 shows the differences observed among various male athletic groups.* (Aerobic/anaerobic sport refers to the fact that neither energy system is clearly dominant.) It can be readily seen that aerobic athletes have the highest aerobic powers. Even recreational runners show powers greater than most combined aerobic/anaerobic sport athletes. The data in the middle group in Figure 5-3 should be interpreted in only the broadest sense. Sample groups will vary from one study to another, making the ranking of sports relative to aerobic power debatable. The point is that athletic groups, broadly considered, can be categorized according to the average aerobic power values that characterize the participants.

A comprehensive analysis has been made of world-class distance runners.[57] Distance runners were subdivided into middle-long distance runners (3 to 6 milers) and marathon

*References 4, 9, 12, 21, 30, 45, 46, 60, 72.

runners, and each was compared to an untrained group. The average training mileage for the two running groups was 45.4 and 100.7 miles per week, respectively. Table 5-2 compares these groups in $\dot{V}O_2$ max, % ST fibers, LDH (a glycolytic enzyme), SDH (an oxidative enzyme), and % fat. No difference in $\dot{V}O_2$ max was found between the running groups. Even though aerobic power is a predictor of athletic success within the total population, within an elite group of runners, all of whom were higher than 70 ml/kg · min⁻¹, prediction of success from aerobic power alone is not possible. For more accurate predictions, muscle tissue characteristics must be evaluated. For example, the middle-long distance runners had a significantly lower percentage of ST fibers and SDH, an oxidative enzyme involved in the Krebs cycle. As expected, no differences were observed between groups in LDH. An interesting individual difference was observed in Don Kardong, who finished fourth in the 1976 Olympic marathon. His ST fiber percentage was only 50%. However, on further analysis it was determined that he had a high percentage of FOG fibers that resulted in a total aerobic potential of 75%.

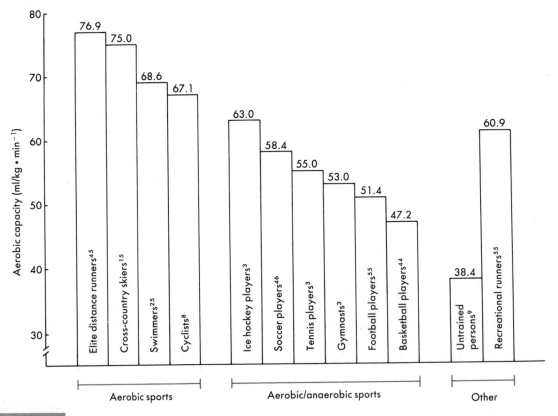

FIG. 5-3   **Aerobic power of various athletic groups.**

Aerobic power is higher in aerobic athletes than in other athletic groups and untrained persons. However, within a group of elite aerobic athletes, aerobic power is not predictive of success.

Aerobic power and genetic influence

In 1929, Holzinger[31] developed a technique to determine the heritability of biological traits by studying twins. The technique has been used by investigators to analyze the genetic contribution to aerobic power. For example, it has been estimated that 93% of aerobic power is under genetic influence, and that although aerobic power is trainable, there is a genetic ceiling on improvement.[39] Recently, findings of a series of studies that compared monozygous (identical) and dizygous (fraternal) twins were reported.[33] One study revealed no significant genetic contribution to either aerobic power or oxidative enzymes. However, ST fiber percentage had a high genetic influence, 99.6% for males and 92.2% for females. The discrepancy in the aerobic power results reported in these studies may be due to the fact that the latter study[40] failed to control socioeconomic, health, and physical activity factors between groups. Because of the discrepancy in aerobic power findings, it is not possible to be certain, but because of the ST fiber results, it is likely that successful performance in aerobic sports is largely a matter of inheritance.

Aerobic power in relation to sex

$\dot{V}_{O_2}$ max does not differ between boys and girls before puberty. However, after puberty, females exhibit values (L $\cdot$ min^{-1}) that are 25% to 30% below those of males.[1] Figure 5-4 broadly illustrates the distributions for males and females (average age = 21.1 and 19.6) entering the American military service.[71] It can be seen that the two distributions (ml/kg $\cdot$ min^{-1}) overlap, so that some females approach the average for males, and some males are below the average for females. The mean difference is 25%. When aerobic power is expressed in L $\cdot$ min^{-1}, not taking into account body weight differences, the difference is even greater (39%). However, correcting values for lean body mass, that is, for active tissue, the aerobic power differences are half those expressed in ml/kg $\cdot$

TABLE 5-2 |||||| COMPARISON OF MIDDLE-LONG DISTANCE RUNNERS, MARATHON RUNNERS, AND AN UNTRAINED LEAN GROUP ON $\dot{V}_{O_2}$ MAX, % ST FIBERS, LDH ACTIVITY, SDH ACTIVITY, AND % FAT

	$\dot{V}_{O_2}$ max	% ST	LDH	SDH	% Fat
Middle-long distance	78.8	61.8*	78.8	17.7*	5.0
Marathon runners	74.1	79.0	74.1	21.6	4.3
Untrained	54.2*	57.7*	54.2*	6.4*	8.2

*Significantly different from marathon runners (p < .05)

min^{-1}. It seems obvious that the body composition differences between the sexes account for some of the sex difference in $\dot{V}O_2$ max. In addition, heart size and red blood cell concentration are likely contributing factors.

Prediction of aerobic capacity

In 1954, Astrand and Ryhming[3] published a report that included a nomogram for predicting $\dot{V}O_2$ max from one submaximal exercise heart rate (HR). The prediction was based on the assumed linearity between the increase in $\dot{V}O_2$ and HR. Other researchers followed with similar prediction techniques.[42,43] Such techniques were attractive for several reasons, particularly their practicality in a field setting. Studies that compared actually measured $\dot{V}O_2$ max with predicted $\dot{V}O_2$ max showed that the predictions, in fact, underpredicted by 15% to 20%. Underpredictions were caused by the lack of linearity between $\dot{V}O_2$ and HR at near-maximal exercise loads (see Figure 5-5). Prediction techniques assumed that the researcher could simply extrapolate a submaximal $\dot{V}O_2$/HR line out to the maximal HR, and $\dot{V}O_2$ max could be directly predicted. Since $\dot{V}O_2$ continues to rise after HR reaches a maximum, an underprediction occurs.

In an attempt to achieve even greater simplicity, a group of researchers developed equations for predicting $\dot{V}O_2$ max from submaximal ratings of perceived exertion (RPE).[54] (See Chapter 10 for a further explanation of this variable.) The equation for females is $\dot{V}O_2$ max (L · min^{-1}) = $-0.902 + 0.163$ (RPE). Using perceived exertion (RPE = 19), the error between actual and predicted $\dot{V}O_2$ max values was only +2%, 2.146 vs 2.195 (see Figure 5-6). HR (190) was used as a predictor for comparative purposes with a resulting error of -14%, 2.146 vs 1.839. Perhaps the reason that the RPE prediction works so well in predicting a fairly complex phenomenon like $\dot{V}O_2$ max is that this variable represents a "gestalt" of many sensations caused by many underlying physiological processes. The

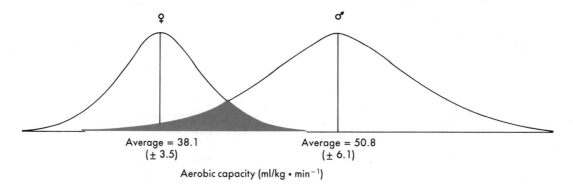

Average = 38.1   Average = 50.8
(± 3.5)   (± 6.1)

Aerobic capacity (ml/kg · min^{-1})

FIG. 5-4   **Frequency distributions of aerobic power for men and women entering the American military service. (Developed from Vogel, J.A., Ramos, M.U., and Patton, J.F.: Comparisons of aerobic power and muscle strength between men and women entering the U.S. Army, Med. Sci. Sports 9:58, 1977.)**

simplicity of recording RPE in field settings makes it an attractive possibility for prediction purposes. Although additional investigations are required, presumably a single, steady state, submaximal load on a bicycle would suffice to achieve an RPE rating necessary to make the prediction.

Perhaps the 12-minute (1.5 mile) run test has the highest field validity of any measure of $\dot{V}O_2$ max. Results of this test, easily attained, are highly related to laboratory results in a large segment of the population, healthy children through adults.

Aerobic power is a complex phenomenon. Attempts to predict it from submaximal HR tests have not proved to be accurate. Multiple regression studies, using several predictor

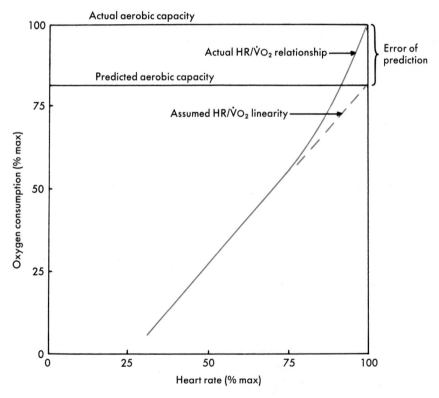

FIG. 5-5   The relationship of oxygen consumption and heart rate with specific reference to the prediction of $\dot{V}O_2$ max. To predict $\dot{V}O_2$ max from submaximal heart rate the assumption is made that the HR/$\dot{V}O_2$ relationship remains linear to maximal levels. However, since the HR/$\dot{V}O_2$ relationship is no longer linear at near-maximal heart rates, an error in prediction is made.

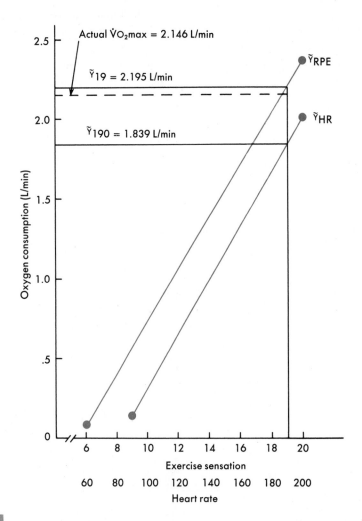

FIG. 5-6   Prediction of $\dot{V}O_2$ max from perceived exertion *(RPE)* and heart rate *(HR)* in a group of females. (From Noble, B.J., Maresh, C.M., and Ritchey, M.: Comparison of exercise sensations between females and males, Med. Sci. Sports *14:*175, 1981.)

variables, have proven accurate but, in general, laboratory equipment is required. The search for a simple but accurate field test of aerobic capacity continues. However, if broad classification is desired, existing methods do allow fairly accurate ranking ($\pm 10\%$).

Limiting factors

What limits the body's ability to consume oxygen? In other words, what accounts for the increase in $\dot{V}O_2$ max that occurs from aerobic training? The following equation indicates both the factors involved and their interrelationship:

$$\begin{array}{cccc} O_2 \text{ Consumption} = & \text{HR} & \times \text{ Stroke volume} \times \text{ Arteriovenous oxygen difference} \\ (\text{ml} \cdot \text{min}^{-1}) & (\text{beats} \cdot \text{min}) & (\text{ml} \cdot \text{beat}) & (\text{mg} \cdot 100 \text{ ml blood}) \end{array}$$

The first two factors, *heart rate* and heart *stroke volume,* when multiplied together, equal *cardiac output* (ml of blood/min). Thus, the equation can also be stated: Cardiac output $\times$ Arteriovenous oxygen difference. The latter term is also referred to as *oxygen extraction* to indicate the amount of oxygen that has been extracted from the arterial blood as it passes by the muscle cells. We can add the word *maximal* to all the terms of the equation to help us understand what limits aerobic power. Research indicates that changes in maximal cardiac output account for approximately 50% of the changes observed in $\dot{V}O_2$ max following training. The other 50% is associated with increases in oxygen extraction by the muscle cells.[29] This view has been challenged, suggesting that $\dot{V}O_2$ max is limited by the metabolic capacity of the muscle tissue, that is, O_2 is available so the source of the maximal plateau of oxygen consumption lies in the muscle itself.[32] If this argument were true, $\dot{V}O_2$ max could be raised by increasing either muscle mass involvement during the maximal test or the O_2 concentration available to muscle. Yet another author states that "available evidence argues strongly against this concept."[62] Although explanation of the physiological phenomena that account for the cardiovascular changes responsible for $\dot{V}O_2$ max remains incomplete, it seems clear that O_2 extraction increases in muscle, that is, 80% to 85% of available O_2 is extracted from the blood at $\dot{V}O_2$ max; and blood flow to nonexercising tissue decreases, thus increasing perfusion of active muscle. That is, there is a redistribution of cardiac output. The predominant view of exercise scientists is that cardiac output and oxygen extraction are the ultimate limiting factors for change in $\dot{V}O_2$ max. In other words, most think both central (cardiac) and peripheral (extraction) factors are responsible for changes in $\dot{V}O_2$ max.

Dynamics of oxygen consumption during exercise

Aerobic exercise is by necessity submaximal. When we think of performing aerobically, we think of prolonged exercise. It is not possible to maintain a performance, such as a marathon run, at $\dot{V}O_2$ max. This is due to the interaction of the aerobic and anaerobic pathways at the high levels of exercise necessary to elicit $\dot{V}O_2$ max. In other words, the pace that will stimulate a runner to exhibit maximal aerobic power will have a large anaerobic component as well. To sustain marathon performances, it is necessary to decrease pace to a level that stimulates a lower level of $\dot{V}O_2$. One group of scientists cite

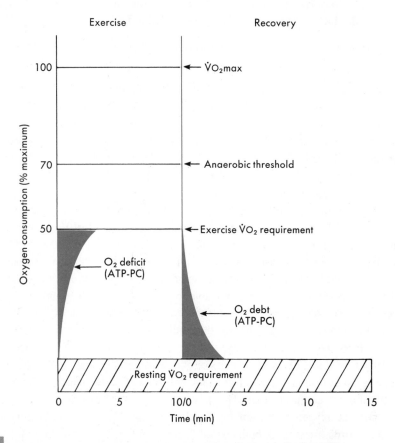

FIG. 5-7 Oxygen consumption during exercise (50% $\dot{V}_{O_2}$ max) and recovery with special reference to oxygen deficit and oxygen debt. This figure illustrates the classical interpretation of oxygen debt developed by A.V. Hill. OBLA refers to onset of blood lactate accumulation.

"fractional utilization" of oxygen consumption and suggest that good runners have the ability to perform at higher fractions (percentages) of $\dot{V}_{O_2}$ max.[13] Usually marathoners race at 85% of $\dot{V}_{O_2}$ max or below, depending on the individual. Obviously, with two runners with the same $\dot{V}_{O_2}$ max, the one able to run at a higher fraction of aerobic power would be the better runner. Oxygen requirements during prolonged exercise depend on the interaction of exercise duration and intensity. For example, the work intensity (% $\dot{V}_{O_2}$ max) that can be sustained over an entire workday is no higher than 50% $\dot{V}_{O_2}$ max. As the work load demand increases, so does the oxygen consumption, but the work load must be manipulated up and down depending on exercise duration so that exercise can be sustained.

Figure 5-7 illustrates a number of points concerning oxygen consumption dynamics during exercise. First, it should be remembered that the baseline for exercise oxygen consumption is the resting oxygen requirement, not zero. Second, oxygen consumption does not rise immediately to meet the exercise requirement. This transition requires 2 to 3 minutes. During this period, the exercise $\dot{V}_{O_2}$ requirement is not accounted for by the oxygen consumption. The difference between these two values is referred to as the *oxygen deficit*. During this period, additional energy is produced anaerobically by the ATP-PC system. Third, when oxygen consumption finally equals the exercise requirement, a *steady state* is said to exist, that is, supply and demand are equal. Fourth, in this example, submaximal exercise is being performed because the $\dot{V}_{O_2}$ requirement is below $\dot{V}_{O_2}$ max. In fact, the $\dot{V}_{O_2}$ requirement is only 50% of $\dot{V}_{O_2}$ max; therefore the exercise can be classified as predominately aerobic.

As mentioned in Chapter 3, an end product of glycolysis is lactic acid. Lactic acid begins to accumulate in the blood when production exceeds use in the cells. The point at which lactic acid begins to rise in the blood has been referred to as the *anaerobic threshold*. A preferable term is *onset of blood lactate accumulation* (OBLA), since lactate production probably does not exhibit a threshold as such. Fractional utilization, mentioned earlier, is related to the OBLA. The factor that determines the percentage of $\dot{V}_{O_2}$ max at which one can perform for long durations is the accumulation of lactic acid. It should be remembered that even though lactic acid begins to accumulate in the blood, it does not become problematic until the body's buffering system cannot any longer counteract the accumulation. (Buffering refers to the blood bicarbonate system that lessens the effect of lactic acid.) Therefore, OBLA as such is not critical, but the critical point is when accumulation exceeds buffering capacity.

To complete the picture, Figure 5-8 illustrates an anaerobic exercise in which the energy requirement is well above that which can be supplied totally by the aerobic pathway. Therefore, energy must be gained from anaerobic sources to meet the need. Since anaerobic sources are limited, it is difficult to continue such an exercise for very long. In this example, not only are ATP-PC stores used (transitional O_2 deficit), but also energy is produced from glycolysis, resulting in lactate accumulation. The replenishment of ATP-PC stores and the removal of lactate during the recovery period is considered in the next section. It should be pointed out, however, that Figure 5-8 represents the classical

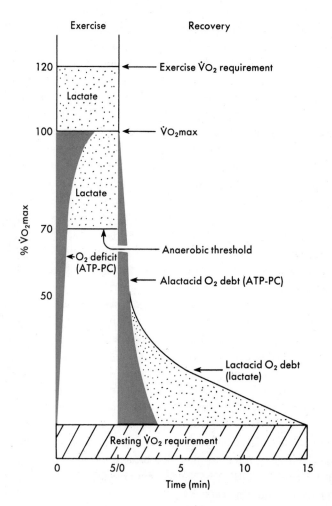

FIG. 5-8   Oxygen consumption during exercise (greater than $\dot{V}_{O_2}$ max) and recovery with special reference to oxygen deficit and oxygen debt (alactacid and lactacid).

view of *oxygen debt* and is not supported by current evidence, that is, the contribution of lactate to the *excess postexercise oxygen consumption* (EPOC).

Aerobic power summary

The first section of this chapter has been concerned with aerobic power. Aerobic power is defined as the maximal amount of oxygen that can be consumed per minute during maximal exercise. For comparative purposes, it is best to express aerobic power by taking body composition into consideration, that is, milliliters per kilogram of body weight per minute. Since aerobic power is related to the amount of muscle mass used, testing instruments that call on small quantities of muscle mass can result in a misleading value. It is best to test athletes on instruments that stimulate muscle fibers which have been trained. Athletes who are involved in prolonged physical activity display the highest aerobic powers, but it is not possible to predict success from aerobic power among elite aerobic athletes. Evidence is conflicting at this time, but it is likely that a considerable portion of aerobic power is inherited. Females have lesser aerobic powers than males due to a smaller body size, heart stroke volume, hemoglobin concentration, and mitochondrial density. Attempts to accurately predict aerobic power from submaximal heart rate have not been successful. Some evidence exists that perception of exertion may be a useful and practical predictor. Aerobic power appears to be limited by cardiac output and the ability of muscle tissue to extract oxygen from the blood. Oxygen consumption rises with the intensity of exercise. The ability to sustain oxygen consumption over time depends on the interaction of the exercise duration and intensity, that is, high intensity levels can only be sustained for a short period of time. Since oxygen consumption does not rise to meet the energy requirement immediately, anaerobic energy sources must be used even in light submaximal exercise (oxygen deficit). The added need is met by stored ATP-PC. When the exercise requirement is higher than the anaerobic threshold, additional energy is provided by glycolysis, resulting in the accumulation of lactic acid.

ANAEROBIC POWER

It is difficult to speak of aerobic and anaerobic pathways as completely independent within sports, as such. They are independent as physiological systems, but highly interrelated within the activity context. For most types of sports we speak of the two systems acting in concert, with one predominating. Even at the extremes of endurance and sprint activities, it is inaccurate to speak of a single energy pathway in use. With that knowledge in mind, we look at the anaerobic pathway more closely.

What is *anaerobic power?* Anaerobic power is the maximal ability of the anaerobic systems (ATP-PC + lactic acid) to produce energy. Unlike aerobic power, which can be measured in a rather straightforward manner, anaerobic power requires the measurement of two systems.

Even after the most strenuous exercise, ATP stores are depleted to only 40% of resting levels. However, after the same exercise PC is nearly depleted. Therefore, apparently, the availability of PC limits short-term heavy exercise.[19] Exclusive use of the ATP-PC system probably is possible only in high-intensity activities that last less than 6 seconds.[7]

An exercise that requires maximal use of the lactic acid system can last no longer than 40 to 60 seconds.[45] As mentioned earlier lactate does not begin to accumulate in the blood, that is, reach OBLA, until exercise intensity reaches about 50% $\dot{V}_{O_2}$ max, when it increases exponentially (see Figure 5-9). The OBLA point seems to be higher for aerobically trained athletes. Only during very heavy exercise does the lactic acid system predominate (>85% $\dot{V}_{O_2}$ max), and the duration of this exercise is very limited.

Figure 5-10 illustrates the rise of lactic acid levels in the muscle and blood with increasing work loads.[53] Both levels rise exponentially with very little lactate increase at low loads and greater increases at high loads. There has been speculation whether a relationship exists between lactate concentrations in the muscle, where it is created, and its accumulation in the blood, where it is usually measured. Investigators have

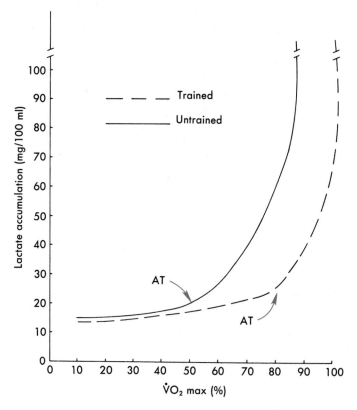

FIG. 5-9 The relationship of lactic acid accumulation and % $\dot{V}_{O_2}$ max with special reference to the onset of blood lactate accumulation (OBLA) and the difference between trained and untrained groups.

found significant and relatively high correlations (0.74) between muscle and blood lactate levels.[34,53] Still, this correlation indicates that approximately 45% of the variability in muscle lactate level is not accounted for by measured changes in blood lactate level.

Measurement of anaerobic power

The ATP-PC system requires invasive techniques (biopsy) for direct measurement. Therefore, the potential of this system is usually estimated indirectly by measuring *peak anaerobic power output* and is expressed as a rate per unit of time. Margaria and others[44] have developed a test that measures peak anaerobic power output (kg-m $\cdot$ sec^{-1}). Subjects run 6 meters from the bottom of a stairway, ascending one step at a time. Time is recorded between the third and ninth steps. If we know the vertical distance climbed between the

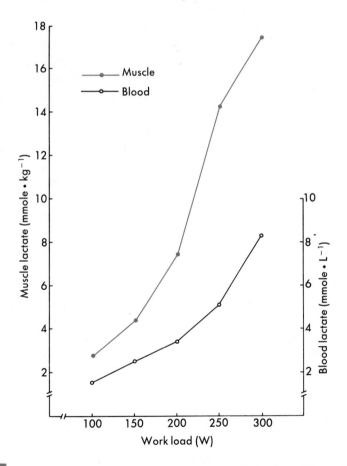

FIG. 5-10　The relationship of muscle and blood lactate accumulation and work load. (From Noble B.J., Borg, G., Jacobs, I., and others: A category-ratio perceived exertion scale: relationship to blood and muscle lactates and heart rate, Med. Sci. Sports Exerc. *15:*523, 1983.)

third and ninth steps (D), the weight of the subject (W), and elapsed time (t), we can compute power (P).

$$P \text{ (kg-m} \cdot \text{sec}^{-1}) = \frac{W \text{ (kg)} \times D \text{ (m)}}{t \text{ (sec)}}$$

The lactate system can be measured invasively by taking a blood sample and measuring its lactate concentration. To determine the capacity for lactate accumulation, it must be measured at its maximal rate. This requires an exercise intensity that exceeds $\dot{V}O_2$ max levels and is sustained for as long as possible.

Isokinetic equipment (Cybex) is also used for an indirect measure of anaerobic power.[69] The test usually involves having the subject perform maximal contractions at a designated angular velocity (for example, $180° \cdot \text{sec}^{-1}$) over a set period of time (1 minute), or for a set number of contractions (50). *Torque* is measured with each contraction. Since torque declines over time, or number of contractions, the amount of decline is a measure of the fatigability of muscle, also called *anaerobic decay*. High absolute torque and rapid decline are characteristic of a high FT fiber muscle and high fatigability. In contrast, lower absolute torque and a less rapid decline are characteristic of a high ST fiber muscle and low fatigability. Since the twitch characteristics of muscle also identify the predominate energy pathway, we can broadly determine anaerobic power with such a test. Investigators have found that in exercise of the type just described, lactate concentrations were lowest in muscles richest in ST fibers, and highest in muscles richest in FT fibers.[68] Also, FT fibers were characterized by a high concentration of LDH. The characteristics of predominately FT fiber muscles make them particularly adaptable to anaerobic activity. Thus, their faster fatigue pattern with repeated contractions is predictable (see Figure 1-6, Chapter 1), that is, the greater the decline, the greater is the anaerobic power. Conversely, a smaller decline is associated with higher aerobic power.

Peak anaerobic power output of athletes

Peak anaerobic power output (ATP-PC) has been studied in several groups of athletes on the national teams of India.[70] Figure 5-11 shows the results observed in several of the groups (bicycle ergometer). Those with the ability to make quick, explosive movements in basketball and soccer had the highest power outputs. The lower power output value for the women field hockey players was probably because of body size differences. As expected, sprinters' power outputs were significantly higher than long-distance runners'.

Oxygen debt

Oxygen debt is a hypothesis developed by A.V. Hill and others[26] to explain EPOC,[17] which was defined earlier. This hypothesis was later adapted to account for the different rates of oxygen consumption during the postexercise recovery period.[46] Two new terms were created, *alactacid* and *lactacid oxygen debt* (see Figure 5-8). The alactacid debt refers to the early, fast phase when oxygen consumption rapidly declines immediately after exercise. Lactacid debt is associated with the so-called slow phase when oxygen consumption gradually declines toward preexercise values. The most controversial aspect of these designations is the explicit causal relationship assumed between EPOC and lactate conversion.[17] Presumably, the slow phase is involved with ATP-PC reconstitution (alactacid), and the fast phase accounts for lactate conversion (lactacid). Little evidence supports this.[17] However, oxygen consumption is increased above resting values after exercise. Why this increase, and how is it related to lactate? The EPOC in Figure 5-8 declines, but the relationship to lactate production and postexercise conversion is in question.

Lactate-tracer studies indicate that lactate is primarily oxidized to carbon dioxide and water during the postexercise period.[17] This finding is contrary to the prediction of the classical "O_2 debt" hypothesis, which states that most lactate formed during exercise is converted to glycogen. Why, then, is oxygen consumption increased after exercise? Gaesser and Brooks[17] have proposed several possibilities:

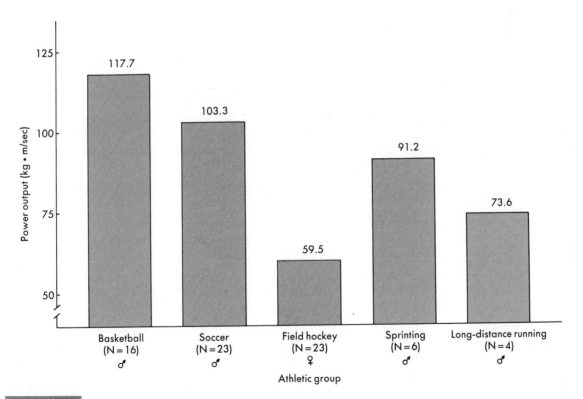

FIG. 5-11 Anaerobic power output in various athletic groups. (Developed from the data of Verma, S.K., Mohindroo, S.R., and Kansal, D.K.: The maximal anaerobic power of different categories of players, J. Sports Med. *19:*55, 1979.)

1. The dynamics of PC resynthesis, during *both* slow and fast phases of oxygen consumption, correspond closely to postexercise oxygen consumption.
2. EPOC may be related to the increase in catecholamines (epinephrine and norepinephrine), thyroxine, and glycocorticoids (cortisol and cortisone), which are known to increase metabolism.
3. Calcium may be related to EPOC due to its stimulating effect on mitochondrial respiration.
4. Perhaps the most important possibility is the known effect of increased body temperature on oxygen consumption.

Although we know that lactate levels and oxygen consumption are elevated immediately following exercise and decline in a known relationship, their interrelationship is *not* causal. The challenge to scientists is to understand this interrelationship through research.

Anaerobic exercise and fatigue

Continuous maximal contractions lead to rapid fatigue. Fatigue is defined as the inability to continue to exercise at the same intensity, or the decline of force production of muscle. Investigators have observed a decrease in the electromyogram (EMG) during maximal isometric contractions of the first dorsal interosseous muscle of the hand.[65] It was stated that these data pointed to the neuromuscular junction as the site of fatigue. However, other researchers, using repeated maximal isokinetic contractions of the vastus lateralis muscle, observed only minor EMG changes when the muscle was fatigued.[52] These data suggest some local factor in muscle as the site of fatigue. Moreover, the location of this fatigue was primarily in FT fibers. The apparent conflict between these investigations may be due to the differences in type of contraction (isometric or isokinetic), size of the involved muscles (small or large), and the number of involved motor units (few or many). What factors within muscle might account for fatigue?

As mentioned previously, at complete exhaustion, PC stores are approximately at zero, whereas ATP is still at 60% to 70% of resting values. It appears that the limited supply of PC is the limiting factor for continued contraction in short-term exercise.[19]

The following steps reduce skeletal muscle performance during maximal exercise:[23]

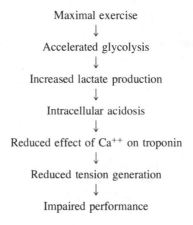

Maximal exercise
↓
Accelerated glycolysis
↓
Increased lactate production
↓
Intracellular acidosis
↓
Reduced effect of Ca^{++} on troponin
↓
Reduced tension generation
↓
Impaired performance

We know that the production of ATP by glycolysis results in the production of lactic acid. Very high levels of lactate within muscle following maximal exercise have been reported.[34] These cause a rapid decline in both muscle pH and blood pH.[19] Phosphofructokinase (PFK) is the rate-limiting enzyme in the glycolytic pathway and is known to be inhibited by low pH.[23] Low pH may also inhibit further production of ATP anaerobically, thus causing muscle fatigue. It has been suggested that increased H ion concentration caused by high lactate production may decrease the effect of Ca^{++} on troponin, thus reducing tension generation.[23] Although it is tempting to accept this very plausible explanation, the problem of muscle fatigue is not completely solved. Considerably more experimental evidence is required to provide indisputable validation.

Peak anaerobic power output and genetic influence

Muscular strength and power have been included in genetic studies of monozygous and dizygous twins.[40] Muscular strength, measured as maximal isometric knee extension, did not show a significant between-twin variation between the two twin types. Therefore, there is no high heritability estimate for this variable. Power was estimated by the Margaria stair-running test[44] and recorded in kg-meters/sec. Here, significant variability between the twins was observed between male twin groups. The heritability estimate was 97.8, indicating a very high genetic component. It appears that whereas muscular strength is highly susceptible to training, muscular power (ATP-PC) is less susceptible because of the genetic influence.

Anaerobic power summary

Anaerobic power can be defined as the maximal ability of the anaerobic systems (ATP-PC + lactic acid) to produce energy. The ATP-PC system can be measured directly, but it requires invasive techniques (muscle biopsy). Indirectly, this system can be estimated by recording peak power output (kg-meters $\cdot$ sec^{-1}) over a short period of time, less than 10 seconds. The ability of the lactate system can be indirectly estimated by pedaling at a maximal rate for 30 seconds on a bicycle ergometer (Wingate test) or by performing continuous maximal contractions for 60 seconds on an isokinetic device. Such a test characterizes what can be called anaerobic decay or the decline of peak power output over time. EPOC, previously explained by the *oxygen debt* hypothesis developed by A.V. Hill and later modified, has been found to be inadequate. EPOC is not related to lactate conversion as predicted by the hypothesis. It has been suggested that fatigue during anaerobic exercise may be related to the accumulation of lactic acid, which decreases pH, in turn inhibiting glycolysis and decreasing the effect of Ca^{++} on troponin, which reduces tension generation. Peak anaerobic power output (ATP-PC) has been found to have a very high genetic component (97.8).

KEY TERMS

aerobic power the maximal amount of oxygen that can be consumed per minute during maximal exercise.

anaerobic decay the decline of peak anaerobic power output with repeated maximal contractions over time (usually <60 seconds). This measurement is said to indirectly estimate the capacity of the lactic acid system.

anaerobic power the maximal ability of the anaerobic systems (ATP-PC and lactic acid) to produce energy.

excess postexercise oxygen consumption (EPOC) oxygen consumption greater than resting values recorded during the recovery period following exercise.

isokinetic exercise exercise in which the angular velocity of muscle contraction is held constant.

onset of blood lactate accumulation (OBLA) the point at which lactic acid concentration begins to increase in the blood.

oxygen debt a term that has been used to explain the excess postexercise oxygen consumption.

peak anaerobic power output an indirect measurement of the ATP-PC system in which the highest production of power (kg-m $\cdot$ sec^{-1}) is recorded during maximal exercise over a short period of time (<10 seconds).

total anaerobic power output synonymous with anaerobic power output, reflecting the actions of both the ATP-PC and the lactic acid systems, specifically associated with the total production of power over a 30-second period (Wingate test).

torque production of angular force, for example, in an isokinetic test.

REVIEW QUESTIONS

1. What criterion should be met to ensure a reliable determination of aerobic power? How might untrained and trained subjects differ in their fulfillment of this criterion?

2. What testing mode would be appropriate for the determination of aerobic power if you wanted to compare runners, cyclists, and swimmers? Why?

3. Describe the characteristics of soccer that demonstrate the need for participants to display both aerobic and anaerobic power.

4. If aerobic power is primarily determined genetically, what is the role of training for endurance athletes?

5. Discuss those factors that limit the expression of aerobic power. How can we account for changes in aerobic power with training?

6. During the initial stage of aerobic exercise, before reaching steady state, we contract an oxygen deficit. Where do we gain the energy needed to sustain exercise during this period?

7. What do we think happens to OBLA with appropriate training? From what you know about aerobic and anaerobic systems, how can you account for this change?

8. Describe the difference between peak anaerobic power output and anaerobic decay.

9. What is the current thinking concerning the explanation of excess postexercise oxygen consumption?

10. How is lactic acid accumulation related to muscle fatigue?

REFERENCES

1. Alexander, J.F., Liang, M.T., Stull, G.A., and others: A comparison of the Bruce and Liang equations for predicting $\dot{V}o_2$ max in young male adults, Res. Q. Exerc. Sports **55**:383, 1984.

2. Astrand, I., and Astrand, P.: Aerobic work performance: a review. In Astrand, I., and Astrand, P., editors: Environmental stress, New York, 1978, Academic Press, Inc.

3. Astrand, P., and Rhyming, I.: A nomogram for calculation of aerobic capacity (physical fitness) from pulse rate during submaximal work, J. Appl. Physiol. **7**:218, 1954.

4. Astrand, P., and Rodahl, K.: Textbook of work physiology, ed. 2, New York, 1977, McGraw-Hill, Inc.

5. Astrand, P., and Saltin, B.: Maximal oxygen uptake and heart rate in various types of muscular activity, J. Appl. Physiol. **16**:977, 1961.

6. Bar-Or, O.: A new anaerobic capacity test: characteristics and applications, Brasilia, 1978, Twenty-first World Congress in Sports Medicine.

7. Bergstrom, J., Harris, R.C., Hultman, E., and others: Energy-rich phosphagens in dynamic and static work. In Pernow, B., and Saltin, B., editors: Muscle metabolism during exercise, New York, 1971, Plenum Press.

8. Bruce, R.A., and McDonough, J.R.: Stress testing in screening for cardiovascular disease, Bull. N.Y. Acad. Med. **45**:1288, 1969.

9. Burke, E.R., Cerny, F., Costill, D., and others: Characteristics of skeletal muscle in competitive cyclists, Med. Sci. Sports **9**:109, 1977.

10. Cade, R., Conte, M., Zauner, C., and others: Effects of phosphate loading on 2,3-diphosphoglycerate and maximal oxygen uptake, Med. Sci. Sports Exerc. **16**:263, 1984.

11. Clarkson, P.M., Kroll, W., and McBride, T.C.: Plantar flexion fatigue and muscle fiber type in power and endurance athletes, Med. Sci. Sports Exerc. **12**:262, 1980.

12. Costill, D.L., Fink, W.J., and Pollock, M.L.: Muscle fiber composition and enzyme activities of elite distance runners, Med. Sci. Sports **8**:96, 1976.

13. Costill, D.L., Thomason, H., and Roberts, E.: Fractional utilization of the aerobic capacity during distance running, Med. Sci. Sports **5**:248, 1973.

14. Costill, D.L., and Winrow, E.: Maximum oxygen intake among marathon runners, Arch. Phys. Med. Rehabil. **51**:317, 1970.

15. Cunningham, D.A., Goode, P.B., and Critz, J.B.: Cardiorespiratory response to exercise on a rowing and bicycle ergometer, Med. Sci Sports **7**:37, 1975.

16. Dolgener, F.A.: Prediction of maximal aerobic power in untrained females, R.Q. **49**:20, 1978.

16a. Fox, E.L., and Mathews, D.K.: The physiological basis of physical education and athletics, ed. 3, Philadelphia, 1981, Saunders College Publishing.

17. Gaesser, G.A., and Brooks, G.A.: Metabolic bases of excess post-exercise oxygen consumption: a review, Med. Sci. Sports Exerc. **16**:29, 1984.

18. Gergley, T.J., McArdle, W.D., DeJesus, P., and others: Specificity of arm training on aerobic power during swimming and running, Med. Sci. Sports Exerc. **16**:349, 1984.

19. Gollnick, P.D., and Hermansen, L.: Biochemical adaptations to exercise: anaerobic metabolism. In Wilmore, J.H., editor: Exercise and sport sciences reviews, New York, 1973, Academic Press, Inc.

20. Hagan, R.D., Smith, M.G., and Gettman, L.R.: Marathon performance in relation to maximal aerobic power and training indices, Med. Sci. Sports Exerc. **13**:185, 1981.

21. Hanson, J.S.: Maximal exercise performance in members of the U.S. Nordic ski team, J. Appl. Physiol. **35:**592, 1973.

22. Herbst, R.: Der Gasstoffwechsel als mass der koperlichen Leistungsfahigkeit. I. Mitteilung: Die Bestimmung des Sauerstoffaufnamevermogens beim Gesunden, Deut. Arch. Klin. Med. **162:**33, 1928.

23. Hermansen, L.: Effect of acidosis on skeletal muscle performance during maximal exercise in man, Bull. Eur. Physiopathol. Respir., **15:**229, 1979.

24. Hermiston, R.T., and Faulkner, J.A.: Prediction of maximal oxygen uptake by a stepwise regression technique, J. Appl. Physiol. **30:**833, 1971.

25. Hickson, R.C., Rosenkoetter, M.A., and Brown, M.M.: Strength training effects on aerobic power and short-term endurance, Med. Sci. Sports Exerc. **12:**336, 1980.

26. Hill, A.V., Long, C.N.H., and Lupton, H.: Muscular exercise, lactic acid, and the supply and utilization of oxygen, I-III. Proc. R. Soc. Lond. **96:**438, 1924.

27. Hill, A.V., and Lupton, H.: The oxygen consumption during running, J. Physiol. **56:**32, 1922.

28. Hill, A.V., and Lupton, H.: Muscular exercise, lactic acid, and the supply and utilization of oxygen, Q. J. Med. **16:**135, 1923.

29. Holloszy, J.O.: Adaptation of skeletal muscle to endurance exercise, Med. Sci. Sports **7:**155, 1975.

30. Holmer, I., Lundin, A., and Eriksson, B.O.: Maximum oxygen uptake during swimming and running by elite swimmers, J. Appl. Physiol. **36:**711, 1974.

31. Holzinger, K.J.: The relative effect of nature and nurture influences on twin differences, J. Ed. Psychol. **54:**231, 1929.

32. Kaijser, L.: Limiting factors for aerobic muscle performance, Acta Physiol. Scand. Suppl. **346:**1, 1970.

33. Kanstrup, I-L., and Ekblolm, B.: Blood volume and hemoglobin concentration as determinants of maximal aerobic power, Med. Sci. Sports Exerc. **16:**256, 1984.

34. Karlsson, J.: Lactate and phosphagen concentrations in working muscle of man, Acta Physiol. Scand. Suppl. **358:**1, 1971.

35. Kasch, F.W., Phillips, W.H., Ross, W.D., and others: A comparison of maximal oxygen uptake by treadmill and step test procedures, J. Appl. Physiol. **31:**1387, 1966.

36. Katch, F.I., McArdle, W.D., and Pechar, G.S.: Relationship of maximal leg force and leg composition to treadmill and bicycle ergometer maximum oxygen uptake, Med. Sci. Sports **6:**38, 1974.

37. Katch, V.L., and Weltman, A.: Interrelationship between anaerobic power output, anaerobic capacity, and aerobic power, Ergonomics **22:**325, 1979.

38. Kelly, J.M., Serfass, R.C., and Stull, G.A.: Elicitation of maximal oxygen uptake from standing bicycle ergometry, Res. Q. Exerc. Sport **51:**315, 1980.

39. Klissouras, V.: Heritability of adaptive variation, J. Appl. Physiol. **31:**338, 1971.

40. Komi, P.V., and Karlsson, J.: Physical performance, skeletal muscle enzyme activities, and fiber types in monozygous and dizygous twins of both sexes, Acta Physiol. Scand. Suppl. **462:**1, 1979.

41. Magel, J.R., Foglia, G.F., McArdle, W.D., and others: Specificity of swim training on maximum oxygen uptake, J. Appl. Physiol. **38:**151, 1975.

42. Magel, J.R., and Faulkner, J.A.: Maximum oxygen uptakes of college swimmers, J. Appl. Physiol. **22:**929, 1967.

43. Margaria, R., Aghemo, P., and Rovelli, E.: Indirect determination of maximal O_2 consumption in man, J. Appl. Physiol. **20:**1070, 1965.

44. Margaria, R., Ahgemo, P., and Rovelli, E.: Measurement of muscular power (anaerobic) in man, J. Appl. Physiol. **21:**1662, 1966.

45. Margaria, R., Cerretelli, R.P., and Mangili, F.: Balance and kinetics of anaerobic energy release during strenuous exercise in man, J. Appl. Physiol. **19:**623, 1964.

46. Margaria, R., Edwards, H.T., and Dill, D.B.: The possible mechanism of contracting and paying the oxygen debt and the role of lactic acid in muscular contraction, Am. J. Physiol. **106:**687, 1933.

47. Reference deleted in proofs.

48. McArdle, W.D., and Magel, J.R.: Physical work capacity and maximum oxygen uptake in treadmill and bicycle exercise, Med. Sci. Sports **2:**118, 1970.

49. Miles, D.S., Critz, J.B., and Knowlton, R.G.: Cardiovascular, metabolic, and ventilatory responses of women to equivalent cycle ergometer and treadmill exercise, Med. Sci. Sports Exerc. **12:**14, 1980.

50. Murase, Y., Kobayashi, K., Kamei, S., and others: Longitudinal study of aerobic power in superior junior athletes, Med. Sci. Sports Exerc. **13:**180, 1981.

51. Nagle, F.J., Richie, J.P., and Giese, M.D.: $\dot{V}o_2$ max responses in separate and combined arm and leg air-braked ergometer exercise, Med. Sci. Sports Exerc. **16:**563, 1984.

52. Nilsson, J., Tesch, P., and Thorstensson, A.: Fatigue and EMG of repeated fast voluntary contractions in man, Acta Physiol. Scand. **101:**194, 1977.

53. Noble, B.J., Borg, G., Jacobs, I., and others: A category-ratio perceived exertion scale: relationship to blood and muscle lactates and heart rate, Med. Sci. Sports Exerc. **15:**523, 1983.

54. Noble, B.J., Maresh, C.M., and Ritchey, M.: Comparison of exercise sensations between females and males, Med. Sport **14:**175, 1981.

55. Parkhouse, W.S., and McKenzie, D.C.: Possible contribution of skeletal muscle buffers to enhanced anaerobic performance: a brief review, Med. Sci. Sports Exerc. **16:**328, 1984.

56. Parr, R.B., Wilmore, J.H., Hoover, R., and others: Professional basketball players: athletic profiles, Phys. Sports Med. **6:**77, 1978.

57. Pollock, M.L.: Submaximal and maximal working capacity of elite distance runners. I. Cardiovascular aspects, Ann. N.Y. Acad. Sci. **301:**310, 1977.

58. Prud'homme, D., Bouchard, C., LeBlanc, C., and others: Sensitivity of maximal aerobic power to training is genotype-dependent, Med. Sci. Sports Exerc. **16:**489, 1984.

59. Quirk, J.E., and Sinning, W.E.: Anaerobic and aerobic responses of males and females to rope skipping, Med. Sci. Sports Exerc. **14:**26, 1982.

60. Raven, P.B., Gettman, L.R., Pollock, M.L., and others: A physiological evaluation of professional soccer players, Br. J. Sports Med. **10:**209, 1976.

61. Ready, A.E., and Quinney, H.A.: Alterations in anaerobic threshold as the result of endurance training and detraining, Med. Sci. Sports Exerc. **14:**292, 1982.

62. Rowell, L.B.: Human cardiovascular adjustments to exercise and thermal stress, Physiol. Rev. **54:**75, 1974.

63. Seals, D.R., and Mullin, J.P.: $\dot{V}O_2$ max in variable type exercise among well-trained upper body athletes, Res. Q. Exerc. Sport **53**:58, 1982.

64. Siconolfi, S.F., Cullinane, E.M., Carleton, R.A., and others: Assessing $\dot{V}O_2$ max in epidemiological studies: modification of the Astrand-Rhyming test, Med. Sci. Sports Exerc. **14**:335, 1982.

65. Stephens, J.A., and Taylor, A.: Fatigue of maintained voluntary muscle contraction in man, J. Physiol. (Lond.) **220**:1, 1972.

66. Stromme, S.B., Ingjer, F., and Meen, H.D.: Assessment of maximal aerobic power in specifically trained athletes, J. Appl. Physiol. **42**:833, 1977.

67. Taylor, H.L., Buskirk, E., and Henschel, A.: Maximal oxygen intake as an objective measure of cardio-respiratory performance, J. Appl. Physiol. **8**:73, 1955.

68. Tesch, P., Sjodin, B., Thorstensson, A., and others: Muscle fatigue and its relation to lactate accumulation and LDH activity in man, Acta Physiol. Scand. **103**:413, 1978.

69. Thorstensson, A., Grimby, G., and Karlsson, J.: Force velocity relations and fiber composition in human knee extensor muscles, J. Appl. Physiol. **40**:12, 1976.

70. Verma, S.K., Mohindroo, S.R., and Kansal, D.K.: The maximal anaerobic power of different categories of players, J. Sports Med. **19**:55, 1979.

71. Vogel, J.A., Ramos, M.U., and Patton, J.F.: Comparisons of aerobic power and muscle strength between men and women entering the U.S. Army, Med. Sci. Sports **9**:58, 1977.

72. Wilmore, J.H., Parr, R.B., Haskell, W.L., and others: Football pros' strength—and CV weaknesses—charted, Phys. Sports Med. **4**:44, 1976.

73. Wyndham, C.H.: Submaximal tests for estimating maximum oxygen intake, Can. Med. Assoc. J. **96**:736, 1967.

SUGGESTED READINGS

Gollnick, P.D., and Hermansen, L.: Biochemical adaptations to exercise: anaerobic metabolism. In Wilmore, J.H., editor: Exercise and sports sciences reviews. New York, 1973, Academic Press, Inc.

Hermansen, L.: Effects of acidosis on skeletal muscle performance during maximal exercise in man, Bull. Eur. Physiopath. Resp. **15**:229, 1979.

Holloszy, J.O.: Adaptation of skeletal muscle to endurance exercise, Med. Sci. Sports **7**:155, 1975.

Rowell, L.B.: Human cardiovascular adjustments to exercise and thermal stress, Physiol. Rev. **54**:75, 1974.

Saltin, B.: Aerobic work capacity and circulation at exercise in man: with special reference to the effect of prolonged exercise and/or heat exposure, Acta Physiol. Scand. **62**(suppl. 230):1, 1964.

LABORATORY APPLICATION: PREDICTION OF $\dot{V}O_2$ MAX

A simple prediction of $\dot{V}O_2$ max that does not require an exhaustive effort by subjects is an ongoing goal for scientists. However, as with many other complex processes, it is difficult to achieve accurate prediction with a single variable. Several studies have developed equations that predict $\dot{V}O_2$ max from multiple variables (multiple regression studies). Two such equations have been derived for active and inactive males[24]:

Active

$$\dot{V}_{O_2} \text{ max (L} \cdot \text{min}^{-1}) = -2.966 - 0.031 \text{ (age)} + 0.026 \text{ (FFW)} - $$
$$0.013 \text{ (HR)} + 25.4 \text{ (F}_{ECO_2}) + 0.330 \text{ (V}_{T_2}) - 8.77 \text{ (}\Delta R)$$

FFW—Fat free weight.

HR—Heart rate recorded during 8% stage of a progressive treadmill test (4.2 mph).

F_{ECO_2}—Fraction of expired carbon dioxide between minutes 8 and 9 of the treadmill test.

V_{T_2}—Pulmonary tidal volume at 0% grade on the treadmill test.

R—Rate of change of the respiratory exchange ratio between 1 and 2 minutes and between 8 and 9 minutes.

Inactive

$$\dot{V}_{O_2} \text{ max (L} \cdot \text{min}^{-1}) = 3.619 - 0.022 \text{ (age)} - 0.033 \text{ (FFW)} - 2.587 \text{ (R)} + 0.253 \text{ (V}_{T_9})$$

R—Respiratory exchange ratio between minutes 8 and 9 of the treadmill test.

V_{T_9}—Tidal volume during 8% stage of the treadmill test.

The correlations between the observed and predicted $\dot{V}_{O_2}$ max in the study that developed these equations was 0.90. This means that $\dot{V}_{O_2}$ max can be reasonably predicted from the submaximal treadmill test. The test protocol consists of the following: continuous walking beginning at 0% grade and a speed of 4.2 mph; after 2 minutes the treadmill is raised to 2% for 2 minutes; then the grade is increased 1%/min to a maximum of 20%. Thus, a predictive test would not have to exceed the 8% stage. Assuming that equipment is available, such a test would prove useful in groups for which a maximal test might prove too expensive. Of course, any prediction must be viewed as an approximation rather than an exact estimate. Such predictions can be used to broadly classify individuals regarding physical fitness but would not be suitable for characterizing elite athletes.

Another equation has been developed for college age women that requires a treadmill but no sophisticated measurement equipment.[16] The experimental test used 3-minute stages at a constant speed of 150 m/min (approximately 5.6 mph) with the grade increasing by 2.5% per stage beginning at 0%. However, the prediction equation for the first 3-minute stage was equal to ($\pm 1\%$) the 15-minute time point (stage 5). Therefore, stage 1 is all that is necessary for predictive purposes.

$$\dot{V}_{O_2} \text{ max (L} \cdot \text{min}^{-1}) = -0.005 \text{ (HR)} + 0.0546 \text{ (BW)} - 0.0654 \text{ (\% fat)} + 0.7394$$

HR—Heart rate recorded during the third minute of the first stage.

BW—Body weight in kilograms.

LABORATORY APPLICATION: ESTIMATION OF ANAEROBIC POWER OUTPUT

An anaerobic test (Wingate test) has been developed that proposes to estimate the potential of both the ATP-PC and the lactate systems. The test, which can be used for either arms or legs only, uses maximal exercise for 30 seconds on the bicycle ergometer.

Revolutions are monitored every 5 seconds during the test. The peak output (revolutions/5 seconds), which usually occurs in the first two 5-second periods, reflects the peak power and is referred to as *peak anaerobic power output*. The following table indicates the suggested resistance (in kilipond [kp]) settings to be used on a Monark bicycle ergometer for various body weights:

Body weight (kg)	Arm setting (kp)	Leg setting (kp)
20—24.9	1.25	1.75
25—29.9	1.5	2.0
30—34.9	1.75	2.5
35—39.9	2.0	3.0
40—44.9	2.25	3.25
45—49.9	2.5	3.5
50—54.9	2.75	4.0
55—59.9	3.0	4.25
60—64.9	3.25	4.75
65—69.9	3.5	5.0
70—74.9	3.95	5.5
75—79.9	4.0	5.75
80—84.9	4.25	6.25
>85	4.5	6.5

Peak anaerobic power output is computed by multiplying the kp setting times the peak number of revolutions (per 5-second interval) times 6 meters. For example, a 70 kg subject who produced a maximum of 10 revolutions during one 5-second period would have a power output of 330 kg-m/5 sec (5.5 kp $\times$ 10 $\times$ 6).

The overall output over 30 seconds is said to be an index that reflects the rate of glycolysis and is called *total anaerobic power output*. In other words, the total test is a measure of both the ATP-PC and the lactate systems. If the same subject generated 50 revolutions in 30 seconds, the anaerobic capacity would be 1650 kp-m/30 sec (5.5 $\times$ 50 $\times$ 6).

CASE STUDY 1

From the information provided in this chapter you should have formed in your mind physiological profiles of typical aerobic and anaerobic athletes. There is no *typical* athlete, since many individual differences can be displayed even within the same athletic group. But, for the sake of argument, let's see if we can identify the characteristics of a hypothetical aerobic athlete. Let's assume that a highly trained runner comes to our laboratory and wants to know ''what makes him tick.'' What would we find?

First, we should include tests that evaluate both aerobic and anaerobic energy pathways. Here is a sequence of tests and test variables that should meet our objectives:

1. Due to sport specificity, the aerobic test should be conducted on a treadmill and should involve running rather than walking. The test should be divided into stages, with each succeeding stage representing a higher work load. The variables to be tested would be as follows:

    a. $\dot{V}O_2$ taken at each stage until exhaustion.

    b. Lactic acid level from a blood sample taken at each stage until exhaustion.

    c. Lactic acid level from a blood sample taken following the exercise to detect maximal accumulation.

2. To determine *peak anaerobic power output* and *anaerobic decay* we will administer a 1-minute isokinetic test in which maximal knee extensions are continuously repeated at $180° \cdot sec^{-1}$. The following variables will be measured from this test:

    a. Peak anaerobic power output recorded during the first two 5-second periods of the test (greatest number of repetitions in 5 seconds).

    b. Anaerobic decay measured by the decline in the muscle torque response from the beginning to the end of the 1-minute test. In other words, this test measures the decline of anaerobic power output over 1 minute.

3. A muscle biopsy of the vastus lateralis muscle will be taken before and after the aerobic capacity test to determine the following:

    a. Fiber type distribution.

    b. Muscle pH.

    c. Oxidative enzyme use.

Here is a table of the results:

Variable	Quantitative response	Qualitative response
Aerobic power (ml/kg $\cdot$ min^{-1})	71.3	High
OBLA (% $\dot{V}O_2$ max)	85.0	Very high
Maximal lactate concentration (mg/100 ml)	95.0	Moderately high
Peak anaerobic power output (kg-m/5 sec)	150.0	Low
Anaerobic decay (% of initial value)	90.0	Low
ST fibers (%)	80.0	High
Muscle pH	6.8	Moderately low
Succinate dehydrogenase (SDH)	21.6	High

Continued.

Compared to some elite American marathon runners, the aerobic capacity of our hypothetical runner is not extremely high, but compared to the normal population, a value of 71.3 must be considered significant. The point at which this runner began to accumulate lactate (anaerobic threshold) was 85% of $\dot{V}O_2$ max, which is very high. Such a value is comparable to that of Frank Shorter (elite American marathoner) who has an exceptional ability to run at a high percentage of aerobic capacity without accumulating lactate. A maximal lactate of 95 mg/100 ml is respectable, but does not indicate a great ability to tolerate lactic acid. As long as this runner stays below the anaerobic threshold, no problems are encountered, but above this level a low tolerance for anaerobic work is exhibited.

This conclusion is also confirmed by the rather low absolute value for power output and the power decay over 1 minute. This latter measure, which declined to only 90% of the initial value, is a typical response of an athlete with a high percentage of ST fibers. This response demonstrates low fatigability and low anaerobic capacity. The 80% ST fiber composition further confirms this profile. Some anaerobic athletes are known to be able to drive blood pH, and presumably muscle pH as well, to levels around 6.5. This athlete's pH of 6.8 again indicates the lack of ability to withstand a highly acidic internal environment. The final variable, SDH, completes the picture of a highly trained aerobic athlete with a high level of this oxidative enzyme.

These data should help you, and the runner, to understand "what makes him tick" but I want to caution you against developing firm stereotype profiles of certain athletic types. This always results in confusion when you observe an athlete with a high performance capacity who does not conform to preconceived values. But please use this case study as a guide to understanding physiological characteristics of aerobic athletes.

CASE STUDY 2

   How can anaerobic power testing be used in the selection and training of anaerobic athletes? It should be obvious that anaerobic power is a specific and independent measure. Therefore, unless anaerobic athletes have a significant aerobic component in their sport, performance cannot be predicted or evaluated by aerobic capacity. Sports such as volleyball, gymnastics, soccer, basketball, sprinting, and baseball require an anaerobic test for selection of athletes and evaluation of training changes. When faced with a selection or evaluation problem, the first task for the coach is to determine which of the two anaerobic

Continued.

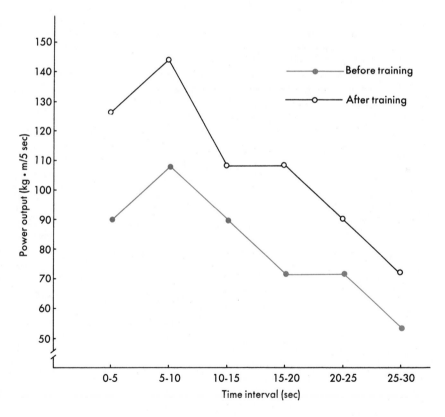

FIG. 5-12   Estimation of anaerobic capacity (Wingate test) of a gymnast before and after specific anaerobic training.

components or both are involved in the sport. The following list will provide a speculative guide[46]:

Sport	Percent anaerobic involvement	
	ATP-PC	Lactic acid
Volleyball	90	10
Gymnastics	90	10
Soccer (forwards)	80	20
Basketball	85	15
Sprinting (100 m)	98	2
Baseball	80	20

Let's take a gymnast as an example. Gymnastics has a very high ATP-PC component (90%). It is an interesting sport in that it can be anaerobic for both arms (bars, side horse) and for the arms and legs (vaulting, free exercise). Probably the problem of selection in gymnastics is esoteric in that many children start this sport at an early age, when capacity is not a primary issue, and by the time they reach a high school program, past performance is the main selection criterion. However, the coach may want to confirm the potential of an athlete or use testing as a means of finding a solution to a performance problem. For example, the coach may have been working hard with an athlete without noticeable results. Anaerobic testing may be an appropriate approach in this case. Continuing this line of thought, we can use as an example a side horse specialist. Since this activity involves the arms exclusively, in terms of weight bearing, and lasts no longer than about 30 seconds, the Wingate test for arms would be appropriate. If the athlete's body weight is 55 kg (121 lb), the arm setting on the ergometer would be 3.0 kp. Figure 5-12 illustrates the response of this athlete (power output in kp-m/5 sec) to this 30-second test. The curve with the closed circles shows the response to the initial test. Peak power output is 108 kp-m/5 sec with total power output (30 seconds) equal to 486 kp-m/30 sec. At this time we have no norms for total power output so the best we can do is to compare performance within the same individual between time periods. Care should be taken to ensure that practice is given on the apparatus so that learning does not bias the measurement. The open circle curve in Figure 5-12 shows a follow-up test after a period of anaerobic training. It can be seen that both peak power output and total power output have improved 25% in each case. This may result from specific training on the side horse or a combination of specific and nonspecific but related training, like hand walking or weight training. Presumably, as anaerobic power increases, so will the ability to sustain the weight-bearing component of the side horse. Therefore, testing of anaerobic power can be a valuable tool for the coach.

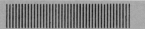 **chapter 6**

PULMONARY FUNCTION

MAJOR LEARNING OBJECTIVE

Minute ventilation increases with exercise intensity and after the initial transient period is primarily controlled by carbon dioxide production. Above the onset of blood lactate accumulation (OBLA), that is, with exercise intensities greater than 50% $\dot{V}_{O_2}$ max, minute ventilation increases out of proportion to the need for oxygen intake.

APPLICATIONS

Talking during exercise above the anaerobic threshold (OBLA) is virtually impossible. Breathlessness during the early seconds of exercise is related to the transient lag before the steady state.

■ A "talk test" is a valuable tool to keep exercise intensity below the anaerobic threshold. Beginning exercisers often quit early because they equate this breathlessness with inability to adapt.

LAVOISIER[49] was the first scientist to recognize the relationship between respiratory exchange and metabolism. He quantitatively measured both oxygen consumption and carbon dioxide production and cited their connection to the internal combustion of food. Oxygen and carbon dioxide transport within the body can be subdivided into three parts for the purpose of description: exchange of respiratory gases between the environment and the lung (pulmonary function); gas exchange and transport in the blood; and use and production of respiratory gases in the cell. The last function has been fundamentally described in previous chapters. Gas transport in the blood is the subject of the next chapter. This chapter is concerned with pulmonary function.

How does oxygen enter into the body so that ultimately it can be used in aerobic metabolism? Also, how do we relieve ourselves of the carbon dioxide produced in the body both as an end product of aerobic metabolism and as the result of the buffering of lactic acid?

TABLE 6-1 |||||| COMMONLY USED PULMONARY FUNCTION TERMS, SYMBOLS, AND ABBREVIATIONS

Gas		Blood	
V	gas volume	Q	volume of blood
$\dot{V}$	gas volume/unit time	$\dot{Q}$	volume of blood/unit time
P	gas pressure	a	arterial blood
F	fractional concentration (percentage) of a gas	v	venous blood
f	respiratory frequency (breaths/unit time)	c	capillary blood
D	diffusing capacity		
R	respiratory exchange ratio ($\dot{V}_{CO_2}/\dot{V}_{O_2}$)		
V_E	ventilatory equivalent ($O_2 = \dot{V}_E/\dot{V}_{O_2}$)		
STPD	Standard temperature pressure dry ($0°$ C, 760 mm Hg, dry)		
BTPS	Body temperature pressure saturated (with water vapor)		
I	inspired gas		
E	expired gas		
A	alveolar gas		
T	tidal gas		
D	dead space gas		
B	barometric		

To understand pulmonary function literature and follow the material presented in this chapter, we must become acquainted with the terminology of the pulmonary physiologist. Table 6-1 introduces some of the common symbols and abbreviations used in pulmonary physiology.

FUNCTIONAL ANATOMY, RESPIRATORY MECHANICS, AND LUNG VOLUMES

Ventilation of the lung is brought about by the chest cage acting as a pump. The inspiratory and expiratory muscles attached to the chest cage cause it to change volume, and the lungs passively follow. This process can be initiated unconsciously, as during rest, or changed by will, as in voluntary hyperventilation. The purpose of this section is to describe the anatomical structures responsible for the ventilation of the lung. Through its pulmonary function, the body is attempting to accomplish the following[87]:

1. Alternately create supraatmospheric and subatmospheric pressures in the lung. Therefore, a pressure difference is established with the atmosphere, causing air to enter and leave the lungs.
2. Mix inhaled air with the air already in the lung. This will increase the alveolar O_2 tension (P_{AO_2}) and decrease the alveolar CO_2 tension (P_{ACO_2}).
3. Exchange oxygen and carbon dioxide with the blood.

Functional anatomy

The pulmonary system can be broadly divided into two units: *conducting airways* and *gas exchange regions*. Conducting airways include the mouth and/or nose, pharynx, larynx, trachea, and the first 16 branches of the bronchial tubes. No gas exchange takes place in the conducting airways, and they are characterized by the presence of cartilaginous support and smooth muscle. The functional unit of the lung is the respiratory bronchiole, with the *alveoli* arising from it. This unit represents the seventeenth through the twenty-fourth branches of the bronchi and is responsible for exchanging air with the blood.[93] Figure 6-1 illustrates the anatomical units of the gas exchange region. The blood and air are separated at the alveolar membrane by the endothelium of the pulmonary capillary and by the thin epithelium of the alveolar walls (1 micrometer). The pulmonary system contains about 140 ml of blood in about 1000 miles of capillaries.[73] The total alveolar surface area is 70 m², representing some 300 million alveoli.[90] During a state of rest the blood transit time through the lung is about 0.75 second, and during exercise about 0.34 second.[73]

Respiratory mechanics

During *inspiration,* respiratory muscles cause an enlargement of the chest cavity. The diaphragm and the external intercostal muscles are the major muscles of inspiration. The phrenic nerve innervates the diaphragm, causing it to contract (descend). At the same time, the external intercostal muscles, innervated by thoracic motor nerves, raise the rib cage upward and outward.[93] By increasing the size of the lung, the pressure in the alveoli decreases to −3 mm Hg with respect to the atmosphere. This negative pressure pulls atmospheric air down the conducting airways into the alveoli. As air enters the lung, pressure rises until alveolar pressure equals atmospheric pressure ($\Delta = 0$ mm Hg), at which time inspiration stops.[38] During exercise, as the demand for ventilation increases, the role of the external intercostal muscles increases. In addition, at high rates of ventilation, the scalenes, sternocleidomastoids, and trapezius act as accessory muscles to the external respiration process.

During *expiration* of low ventilatory volumes, the process is reversed due to the passive recoil of the chest cavity. The decrease in lung size increases alveolar pressure to +3 mm Hg, which aids the flow of air back into the atmosphere. Expiration stops when alveolar pressure equals atmospheric pressure ($\Delta = $ mm Hg).[38] Abdominal muscles and internal intercostal muscles aid the expiratory process during forced expiration.

The rib cage is lined with a membrane called the *parietal pleura*. Similarly, the lungs

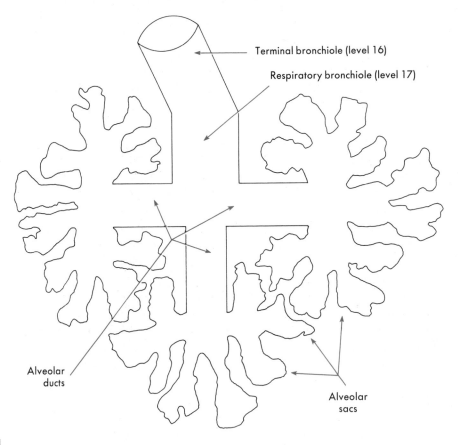

Terminal bronchiole (level 16)

Respiratory bronchiole (level 17)

Alveolar ducts

Alveolar sacs

FIG. 6-1   Anatomical units of the gas exchange region of the lungs: respiratory bronchiole, alveolar ducts, and alveolar sacs.

are lined with a membrane called the *visceral pleura*. The space between these two membranes is called the *intrapleural space*, which has a pressure referred to as the *intrapleural pressure*. This pressure remains below both the atmospheric pressure and the alveolar pressure. The pressure differential remains constant at −5 mm Hg, but the absolute pressure values rise with expiration and fall with inspiration. Lungs exhibit a collapsing tendency that provides the stimulus for the negative intrapleural pressure. Because the rib cage offers resistance to the continued recoil, the lungs do not completely collapse at expiration.[38] The relationship between alveolar and intrapleural pressures is illustrated in Figure 6-2.

It is interesting to note that failure to exhale while surfacing during scuba diving can result in the rupture of the alveoli (pneumothorax). The alveoli rupture into the pleura with collapse of the lung. The negative pressure created in the intrapleural space, with respect to the alveoli, will then cause the alveolar air to rush into the space.

Lung volumes

Air entering the lungs can be thought of as a column extending from the mouth and nose down to the alveoli. It should be obvious that only the air reaching the alveoli can be exchanged and that not all of the air inhaled reaches the alveoli. The space in the conducting airways where air is not exchanged is referred to as *anatomical dead space*. Therefore, alveolar volume (V_A) is equal to tidal volume (V_T), the amount taken from the atmosphere on inspiration, minus dead space volume (V_D).[48]

$$V_A = V_T - V_D$$

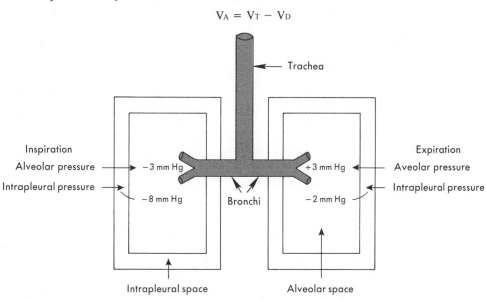

FIG. 6-2   **The relationship among atmospheric, alveolar (intrapulmonary), and intrapleural pressures. Positive and negative numbers refer to pressure differences from atmospheric pressure, that is, 0 mm Hg means that the pressure equals atmospheric pressure.**

Since V_T averages about 500 ml at rest, and average anatomical dead space is 150 ml, the alveolar volume for a single breath is about 350 ml. (A rule of thumb for predicting anatomical dead space is that $V_D = 2.22$ ml · kg^{-1} body weight.[68]) The anatomical dead space can double during exercise due to dilation of the airways.

Figure 6-3 shows average lung volumes and their relationship to one another. For example, *total lung capacity* (5.97 L) is the sum of *residual volume* (1.19 L) and *vital capacity* (4.78 L).[42] Residual volume is the air that remains in the lungs after a maximal expiration. This volume is critical, since it shows that not all pulmonary air is exchanged with the atmosphere, even after a maximal expiration. Vital capacity is the volume of air expired with a maximal forced expiration following a maximal inspiration. *Tidal volume* is the amount of air inspired or expired with each breath. It is approximately 12% of the vital capacity at rest and can be as high as 50% of the vital capacity during heavy exercise.[47] After a normal tidal excursion during quiet breathing, it is possible to inspire and expire still more air. Therefore, some capacity for inspiration and expiration is held in reserve. These volumes are called the *inspiratory reserve volume* and the *expiratory reserve volume*. Note that the sum of tidal volume, inspiratory reserve volume, and

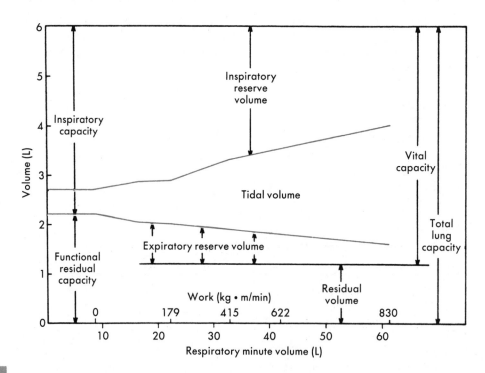

FIG. 6-3   Average lung volumes and their relationship to one another. (From Lambertson, C.J.: The lung: physical aspects of respiration. In Mountcastle, V.B., editor: Medical physiology, ed. 14, vol. 2, St. Louis, 1979, The C.V. Mosby Co.)

expiratory reserve volume is equal to vital capacity.[17,42] As exercise intensity increases, tidal volume increases to meet the body's needs and, in turn, the reserve volumes decrease.

The total air exchanged with the atmosphere per minute is referred to as *minute ventilation*. This value varies from about 6.0 L at rest to 150 to 170 L during heavy exercise.[72] Minute ventilation can be described as follows:

$$\dot{V}_E \ (L \cdot min^{-1}) = V_T \times f$$

With a breathing frequency of 12 breaths/min and a tidal volume of 500 ml, the minute ventilation would be 6.0 L. This value does not include a correction for dead space, so it should be remembered that minute ventilation is not equal to alveolar ventilation.

PHYSIOLOGY OF THE LUNG

Alveolar gas composition

From the standpoint of gas exchange with the blood, the alveolar air is the most important. With each breath, fresh atmospheric air must be mixed with the air that remains in the lungs, so that the concentration of oxygen is sufficient to load the blood. As inspiration begins, the first gas to reach the alveoli will be dead space gas remaining from expiration, thus alveolar CO_2 tension will increase and alveolar O_2 tension will decrease initially. Following this initial transient phase, as fresh air ventilates the alveoli, the reverse response occurs (decreased P_{ACO_2} and increased P_{AO_2}). During expiration, alveolar air shows an increase in alveolar CO_2 tension and a decrease in alveolar O_2 tension, due to continued metabolic carbon dioxide production and oxygen consumption. Initially, expired air measured at the mouth will be more like atmospheric air than alveolar air, since dead space air is exchanged first.

Gas percentages, partial pressures, and pressure gradients

The concentration of atmospheric gases is 20.94% for oxygen, 0.03% for carbon dioxide, 79.03% for nitrogen, and insignificant quantities of other gases. The ability of a gas to move across the body's membranes (diffusion) depends on favorable gradients for movement, because gas moves from higher to lower concentrations. Gradients (concentration differences) are measured in terms of partial pressure differences. *Dalton's law of partial pressures* states that the pressure exerted by a mixture of gases is equal to the sum of the individual (that is, partial) pressures exerted by each gas.[93] Therefore:

$$P_B = P_{O_2} + P_{CO_2} + P_{N_2}$$

The partial pressure of a dry gas is equal to the fractional concentration (F) of the gas multiplied by the total barometric pressure. For example, at sea level:

$$P_{O_2} = \frac{20.94\%}{100} \times 760 \text{ mm Hg} = 159 \text{ mm Hg}$$

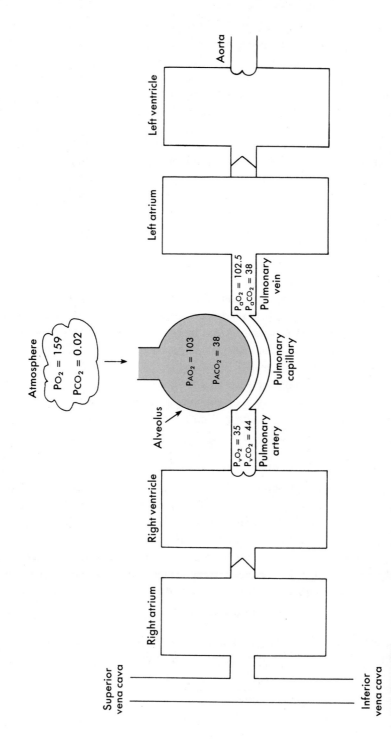

Partial pressures (mm Hg) of oxygen and carbon dioxide in the atmosphere, alveoli, and blood before (pulmonary artery) and after (pulmonary vein) passage through the pulmonary capillaries. (Data from Pace, W.R.: Pulmonary physiology in clinical practice, Philadelphia, 1970, F.A. Davis Co.)

FIG. 6-4

The sum of the partial pressures of the atmospheric pressures of atmospheric air can be expressed as follows:

$$760 \text{ mm Hg} = 159 \text{ mm Hg } (P_{O_2}) + 0.2 \text{ mm Hg } (P_{CO_2}) + 601 \text{ mm Hg } (P_{N_2})$$

It should also be remembered that atmospheric air can be saturated with water, and water exerts a pressure (P_{H_2O}). The effect of water vapor tension on respiratory gas volumes is discussed in a subsequent section (Measurement of pulmonary function).

Since atmospheric air mixes with air under metabolic influence, gas concentrations and, therefore, partial pressures change at the alveolar level. Figure 6-4 illustrates this point and presents the partial pressures for oxygen and carbon dioxide that exist between the alveoli and the pulmonary capillaries. It can be seen that a favorable gradient exists for the transfer of oxygen (P_{AO_2} = 103 mm Hg vs P_{VO_2} = 35 mm Hg) into the blood and carbon dioxide (P_{ACO_2} = 38 mm Hg vs P_{VCO_2} = 44 mm Hg) into the lung.[66] Also, note the equilibrium between alveolar gas pressures and those in arterial (pulmonary vein) blood, which is a sign of adequate ventilation and exchange.

Pulmonary diffusion

For the most efficient diffusion to take place across the alveolar-capillary membrane, it is not only necessary to have adequate alveolar ventilation, but also the pulmonary capillaries must be perfused with blood. In other words, there must be an adequate *ventilation/perfusion ratio*. If, for example, the alveoli are not adequately ventilated, hypoxia can occur, that is, decreased arterial O_2 tension. If pulmonary blood flow is not sufficient, hypercapnea can occur, that is, increased arterial CO_2 tension. However, even in normal individuals, the ventilation/perfusion ratio is only 0.85 at rest.[48] This occurs because some blood travels through the unventilated portions of the lung.[10] When any portion of the lung receives circulation but is not ventilated, or vice versa, this area is referred to as *physiological dead space*.

Assuming a normal ventilation/perfusion ratio exists, adequate membrane permeability is required for gases to diffuse. In certain disease states, such as pulmonary edema, in which fluid collects in the intermembrane space, diffusion is much more difficult and, if the edema is not treated, the disease can be life threatening.

Diffusing capacity of the lung is defined as the total amount of gas passing between the pulmonary air and the capillary blood per minute.[48] Diffusion is dependent on three factors. First is the diffusion constant of the gas. For example, carbon dioxide diffuses more slowly than oxygen in the gas phase, but carbon dioxide is more soluble in water (24 times). Therefore, oxygen diffuses more readily in the lung and carbon dioxide combines more readily in plasma, that is, carbon dioxide crosses the capillary-alveolar membrane more readily. The second factor to be considered is the diffusion surface area. The greater the surface area, the greater is the diffusion. The third factor is the rate of gas transfer. The greater the pressure gradient, the faster is the diffusion.[93]

It should be remembered that diffusion involves more than spanning the alveolar-capillary membrane. Oxygen, for example, must travel through the blood plasma, enter the wall of the erythrocyte, and pass though the intracellular fluid to combine with hemoglobin. This process is discussed in Chapter 7.

Diffusion capacity for oxygen can be calculated by the following formula[48]:

$$D_{O_2} = \frac{\text{Total } O_2 \text{ uptake (ml } \cdot \text{ min}^{-1})}{\text{Mean } P_{AO_2} - \text{Mean } P_{CO_2}}$$

Table 6-2 shows that diffusion capacity increases with increasing exercise levels up to moderate exercise.[82] During exercise, alveolar ventilation increases out of proportion to blood flow in the pulmonary capillary. However, even during maximal exercise, diffusion capacity is not a limiting factor but blood flow (cardiac function) limits further exercise.[48] That is, the ability of the body to exchange gas between the lung and blood is functioning efficiently at the time when exercise is terminated due to fatigue.

Measurement of pulmonary function

The measurement of gas volumes is governed by what are known as the *gas laws*. Two of the more important gas laws are[93]:

Boyle's law—at constant temperature, the volume of a gas is inversely related to its pressure.

Charles' law—at constant pressure, the volume of a gas is directly proportional to its absolute temperature.

It is also important to remember that a gas saturated with water vapor, such as expired air, takes up more volume than if it were dry. Therefore, to compare gas volumes measured under various conditions, they must be corrected to standard conditions. Expired ventilation volumes are usually reported as *body temperature pressure saturated* (BTPS)[48]:

$$\text{Observed volume (L } \cdot \text{ min}^{-1}) \times \frac{273^\circ \text{ (Kelvin) } - 37^\circ \text{ C (body temperature)}}{273 - T \text{ (gas temperature)}}$$

$$\times \frac{760 \text{ mm Hg (sea level } P_B) - WVT \text{ (water vapor tension at observed temperature)}}{760 - 47 \text{ (WVT at } 37^\circ \text{ C)}}$$

This correction standardizes ventilation to a condition of normal body temperature (37° C); sea level pressure (760 mm Hg); and being fully saturated with water vapor. Gas volumes need to be corrected so that values from different laboratories or values recorded under different environmental conditions can be compared. Carbon dioxide production and oxygen consumption are expressed as *standard temperature pressure dry* (STPD).[18]

$$\text{Observed volume (L } \cdot \text{ min}^{-1}) \times \frac{\text{Barometric pressure } - WVT}{760} \times \frac{273}{273 + \text{Ambient temperature}}$$

For example:

$$50.0 \times \frac{760 - 22.4 \text{ (at } 24^\circ \text{ C)}}{760} \times \frac{273}{273 + 24}$$

$$50.0 \times \quad 0.971 \quad \times \quad 0.919$$

$$\underline{44.6} \text{ L } \cdot \text{ min}^{-1} \text{ (}\dot{V}_E \text{ STPD)}$$

TABLE 6-2 |||||| THE RELATIONSHIP BETWEEN DIFFUSION CAPACITY
(ml · min^{-1}/mm Hg) AND EXERCISE LEVEL ($\dot{V}o_2$ ml · min^{-1}), AND
OXYGEN TENSION (mm Hg)*

Exercise level ($\dot{V}o_2$ ml/min)	Oxygen tension (mm Hg) Pulmonary capillary	Alveoli	Diffusion capacity (ml · min^{-1}/mm Hg)
861	35.5	50.0	57
1,298	35.0	54.0	69
1,820	35.0	55.0	91

*From Turino, G.M., Bergofsky, E.H., Goldring, R.M., and others: Effect of exercise on pulmonary diffusing capacity, J. Appl. Physiol. **18**:447, 1963.

In addition to the pulmonary volumes mentioned previously, two other volumes measured by spirometric methods are especially important in detecting *chronic obstructive pulmonary disease* (COPD). COPD includes diseases such as bronchitis and emphysema, which are marked by obstruction of expiratory flow. To evaluate these diseases it is common to measure *maximal breathing capacity* (MBC) and *forced expiratory volume* (FEV). To evaluate these:

MBC—The subject breathes maximally into a collecting chamber for 12 seconds and the total volume is recorded, multiplied by five, and reported in liters per minute, BTPS.[66] The normal value for MBC is between 125 and 170 L · min^{-1}.[18]

FEV—After inspiring maximally, the subject expires maximally into a spirometer and a percentage of total vital capacity expired over a specified period of time is reported, usually 1 second (FEV$_{1.0}$). The normal value for FEV$_{1.0}$ is 83%.[18]

Oxygen cost of breathing

The respiratory system, like any other system, uses oxygen to perform work. The cost depends on the *compliance* of the lungs and chest wall, their distensibility, and *conductance*, the flow of air through the conducting airways. In COPD patients, altered lung compliance and conductance can greatly increase the oxygen cost of breathing. During heavy exercise in normal individuals, the cost of contracting the respiratory muscles may be as high as 10% of the oxygen consumption.[78] For example, with an oxygen consumption of 5000 ml · min^{-1}, the oxygen cost of breathing could be 500 ml · min^{-1}. Otis and others[65] estimate the cost of breathing in normal individuals at rest to be 0.5 to 1.0 ml of oxygen per liter of pulmonary ventilation.

VENTILATORY RESPONSE TO EXERCISE

During exercise, pulmonary ventilation must meet the metabolic requirements. If ventilation is inadequate (hypoventilation), there will be a buildup of carbon dioxide, which can lead to an increase in arterial CO_2 tension (respiratory acidosis). Conversely, if ventilation exceeds metabolic requirements (hyperventilation), arterial CO_2 tension will decrease (respiratory alkalosis). Both situations impair cell function.[85] That is, under conditions of acidosis and alkalosis, the subject can only continue exercise for a limited period of time.

Steady state exercise response

Below the OBLA, pulmonary ventilation rises to a steady state. The dynamics of this rise have been the subject of scientific inquiry since Geppert and Zuntz (1888)[34] attempted to explain the rapid increase in ventilation with the onset of exercise. Several authors have described the characteristics of the ventilatory rise to the steady state.[72,85,91] Phase I is a rapid rise associated with the start of exercise, phase II is a slower rise, and steady state ventilation is referred to as phase III. During exercise below OBLA, both tidal volume and frequency increase, although tidal volume increases more. After phase I, the steady state is reached within approximately 3 minutes. Above OBLA, phase II will last longer, and, in fact, in some instances no steady state may be reached.[85] Longer phase II and failure to achieve steady state are both related to a large production of carbon dioxide. The phases are illustrated in Figure 6-5.[85]

Graded exercise response

Let us examine the dynamics of ventilation during a test such as the Bruce test (see Chapter 5), which incrementally increases exercise intensity until exhaustion. From pre-

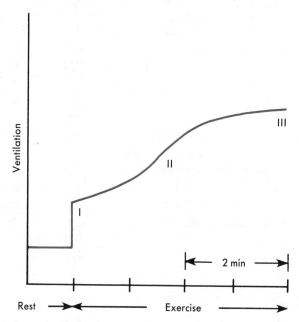

FIG. 6-5   The rise of pulmonary ventilation during steady state exercise. Phase I is the rapid rise associated with the start of exercise. Phase II is the slower rise, and steady state ventilation is called phase III. (Reprinted from Wasserman, K.: Breathing during exercise, N. Engl. J. Med. *298:*780, 1978.)

vious discussion, we know that $\dot{V}_{O_2}$ rises linearly with exercise intensity. What response can we expect from $\dot{V}_{CO_2}$ under similar circumstances?

We know from Chapter 4 that the contribution of carbohydrate to energy production increases with increasing exercise intensity. This results in an increase in respiratory quotient, that is, $\dot{V}_{CO_2}$ meets or exceeds $\dot{V}_{O_2}$, bringing the ratio to 1.0 or above. (When we discuss the exchange of respiratory gases, the respiratory quotient is called the *respiratory exchange ratio* and is designated R). Thus, the ratio increases with more and more carbon

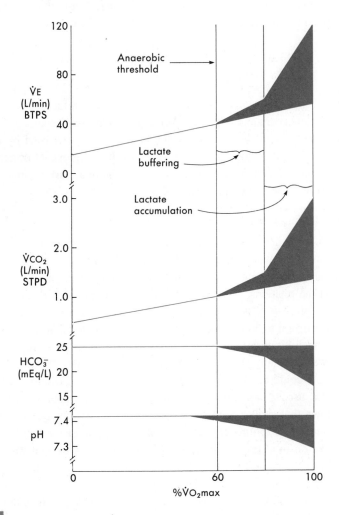

FIG. 6-6   The response of pulmonary ventilation ($\dot{V}_E$), carbon dioxide production ($\dot{V}_{CO_2}$), bicarbonate (HCO_3^-), and blood acidity (pH) above and below the anaerobic threshold during graded exercise (various percentages of $\dot{V}_{O_2}$ max). (Reprinted, by permission of the New England Journal of Medicine [*298*:780, 1978].)

dioxide produced relative to oxygen consumed. You would expect that $\dot{V}CO_2$ and $\dot{V}O_2$ would not be linearly related at higher exercise intensities. That is, indeed, the case. The loss of linearity occurs at the OBLA. It is interesting to note that pulmonary ventilation ($\dot{V}E$) responds similarly to $\dot{V}CO_2$, that is, $\dot{V}E$ no longer rises linearly with $\dot{V}O_2$ after the OBLA. These relationships are illustrated in Figure 6-6.[85] It should be noted that the increase in R is not causally related to carbohydrate use. The increased carbon dioxide production results from the accumulation of lactate acid and its buffering.

Immediately after the OBLA, the accumulation of lactic acid is buffered by the bicarbonate (HCO_3^-) system. That is, since the increase in H^+ ion concentration is buffered, there is only an insignificant decline in pH. The bicarbonate system response is shown as follows:

$$H^+ + HCO_3^- \rightarrow H_2O + CO_2$$

However, excess carbon dioxide is produced in the buffering process. During this period of lactate buffering, $\dot{V}E$ and $\dot{V}CO_2$ increase at the same rate because of the body's need to relieve itself of the additional carbon dioxide. Further increases in exercise intensity result in the significant accumulation of lactic acid, which cannot be compensated by bicarbonate. Therefore, a metabolic acidosis is created as shown by a significant decrease in pH. At the same time, bicarbonate declines as does Pa_{CO_2}. The relationships among $\dot{V}E$, $\dot{V}CO_2$, HCO_3^-, and pH are also shown in Figure 6-5.

Prediction of OBLA from pulmonary ventilation

Because the OBLA (sometimes inappropriately referred to as the anaerobic threshold) may be an important measure of performance capacity, especially in the endurance athlete, scientists have taken an interest in its prediction by noninvasive procedures. The prediction is based on the relationship between pulmonary ventilation ($\dot{V}E$) and oxygen consumption ($\dot{V}O_2$), which is no longer linear at higher exercise intensities. Supposedly, the $\dot{V}E$ rises out of proportion to $\dot{V}O_2$ at the point of lactate accumulation. Detection of what was called the anaerobic threshold (AT), which we will refer to as OBLA, from pulmonary measures was originally presented by Wasserman and McIlroy[86] in 1964. They proposed that the OBLA could be predicted by the point at which an increase in R was observed. Their method used a breath-by-breath analysis system to monitor changes in R.[87] Later, it was shown that similar results could be found by less complicated procedures.[21] It was discovered that abrupt changes in $\dot{V}E$ and $\dot{V}CO_2$ provided a valid indirect method of detecting the onset of lactic acid accumulation. In other words, it was stated that lactic acid begins to accumulate at the point that $\dot{V}E$ and $\dot{V}CO_2$ are no longer linear with $\dot{V}O_2$.

The attractiveness of noninvasively detecting OBLA from changes in pulmonary ventilation ($\dot{V}E$) has been matched by a concern for its reliability. Although mean group data usually provide a definitive breakpoint in the linearity of $\dot{V}E$ and $\dot{V}O_2$, such breakpoints are often difficult to identify with individuals. For example, in one study of 10 subjects, only 6 "demonstrated easily, defined breakpoints."[80] Test-retest reliabilities of only 0.72 to 0.77[21] have been reported. When evaluating pulmonary ventilation as a function of time during the graded exercise test, the estimation can vary from 15 to 30 seconds. Intrasubject and interinvestigator discrepancies make the use of pulmonary ventilation as a predictor of OBLA questionable.

In addition, many investigators argue that lactic acid response does not exhibit a threshold. My own research supports the theory that lactic acid increases in a continuous hyperbolic fashion from rest. The rate of production is very low at low exercise intensities and high at high exercise intensities. For those who do accept a definite inflection point, for example, at 4 mmol of lactic acid, the term *OBLA* may be a better choice. This term does not necessitate a point of contention as to whether the muscle is functioning anaerobically before the inflection point. Other researchers, in an attempt to accommodate the scientific debate, prefer a term like *ventilatory threshold* or *inflection point*. The debate, although waning, will most likely continue for a few years. It is important for the student to remember three points:

1. There may be a lactic acid inflection point, or OBLA.
2. There is a ventilatory inflection point.
3. Although these two points sometimes coincide, there is no reason to think that this phenomenon is always causal.

PULMONARY FUNCTION IN ATHLETES

The question is often asked whether trained athletes are distinguishable from untrained persons in pulmonary or respiratory response to exercise. We learned in the last chapter that $\dot{V}O_2$ max, for example, is limited by cardiac output and oxygen extraction at the tissue level. It would not seem, then, that it would be advantageous to increase pulmonary function.

Whether or not improved pulmonary function provides a clear advantage, endurance athletes have been shown to have greater forced vital capacity (FVC) and total lung capacity (TLC) than untrained persons (see Figure 6-7).[69] It stands to reason that the training of respiratory muscles would offer a positive advantage to the expression of certain pulmonary volumes.

A study compared the breathing efficiency of endurance athletes and nonathletes.[56] Subjects exercised on the treadmill at 33% $\dot{V}O_2$ max. The endurance athletes had significantly lower values for ventilatory equivalent for oxygen ($\dot{V}E/\dot{V}O_2$), carbon dioxide ($\dot{V}E/\dot{V}CO_2$), and alveolar CO_2 tension than the nonathletes (see Figure 6-8). These results indicate that the trained athletes were more efficient, that is, they required less ventilation for each liter of oxygen consumed or carbon dioxide produced. Endurance athletes appear to have a relative insensitivity to the factors that stimulate increased breathing during exercise.

Pulmonary diffusing capacity (D) has been studied in young, competitive swimmers (age 10 to 16 years[84]) and was found to be significantly related to age, height, weight, and body surface area, indicating that as these athletes grew, their ability to diffuse respiratory gases improved. These researchers also found that the best prediction of D was physical working capacity (kg-m · kg body weight) at a heart rate of 170 (PWC_{170}). This finding supports earlier work that found a correlation of 0.92 between D and PWC_{170}.[41]

In summary, endurance-trained athletes show greater forced vital capacity and total lung capacity than untrained persons. Endurance athletes also show an improved breathing efficiency at low submaximal exercise compared to nonathletes. Pulmonary diffusing capacity increases with age, body size, and training and can be predicted from PWC_{170}.

REGULATION OF EXERCISE VENTILATION (HYPERPNEA)

What is *regulation?* The simplest analogy is the feedback model of the thermostat. A set point is determined, above and below which the temperature requires control. When temperature is below the set point, this information is sensed and the furnace is given the instruction to produce heat. When the temperature reaches or exceeds the set point, the furnace is again instructed to turn off.

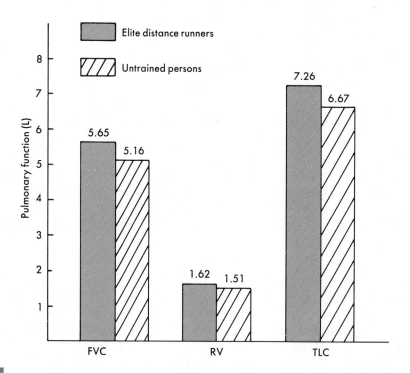

FIG. 6-7 Differences in forced vital capacity (FVC), residual volume, and total lung capacity (TLC) between elite distance runners and untrained persons. (Data from Raven, P.B.: Pulmonary function of elite distance runners. In Milvy, P., editor: The marathon: physiological, medical, epidemiological and psychological studies, *301*, New York, 1977, N.Y. Acad. Sci.)

During rest, pulmonary ventilation exhibits inherent rhythmicity. Clusters of neurons, located in the medulla of the brain stem, are loosely referred to as the *respiratory center* (in fact, there is more than one center). During inspiration, the inspiratory neurons fire, stimulating the phrenic and intercostal nerves. During expiration, the expiratory neurons inhibit the inspiratory neurons from firing.[93] For pulmonary ventilation to be under control, it must exactly match metabolic need. That is, as metabolic needs vary, the respiratory center (thermostat) needs to be informed so that it can turn pulmonary ventilation on and off.

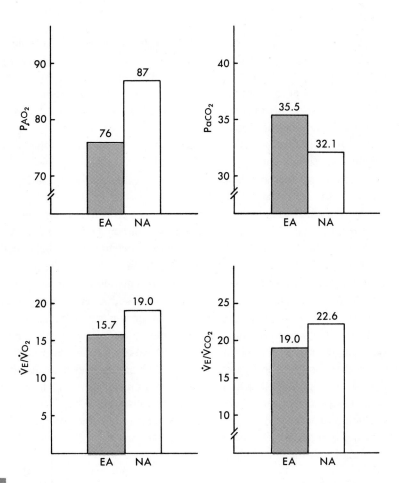

FIG. 6-8   Differences in ventilatory equivalent for oxygen ($\dot{V}_E/\dot{V}_{O_2}$), carbon dioxide ($\dot{V}_E/\dot{V}_{CO_2}$), alveolar partial pressure of oxygen (P_{AO_2}), and arterial partial pressure of carbon dioxide (P_{aCO_2}) between endurance athletes (EA) and nonathletes (NA). Both groups exercised at 33% $\dot{V}_{O_2}$ max. (Data from Martin, B.J., Sparks, K.E., Zwillich, C.W., and others: Low exercise ventilation in endurance athletes, Med. Sci. Sports *11:*181, 1979.)

Respiratory control is a much more complicated process during exercise than during rest. The exact mechanism of control of exercise hyperpnea is not completely understood. This section briefly reviews the voluminous work done that has attempted to address the question of how respiratory regulation functions during exercise.

When exercise hyperpnea is under control, we see a relative constancy in arterial CO_2 tension (Pa_{CO_2}), arterial O_2 tension (Pa_{O_2}), and arterial H^+ ion concentration. Below the OBLA, these variables remain controlled. We saw earlier that pulmonary ventilation ($\dot{V}_E$) rises proportionally with $\dot{V}_{CO_2}$, but this relationship is not causative. What does stimulate ventilatory control?

Control below the OBLA

Two hypotheses have been proposed (see Figure 6-9), the first of which is the *neurogenic hypothesis,* which states that during muscle contraction, a message to increase ventilation is sent directly, via the nervous system, to the brain stem. It is thought that the rapid response of phase I at the beginning of exercise could not be accounted for by a blood-borne stimulus. It seems that the primary stimulus is neurogenic, with carbon dioxide flow back to the lungs as secondary.[43,44]

Second, the *humoral hypothesis* has also been proposed, which states that as muscle metabolism increases, certain chemicals initially carried in the venous blood eventually reach reflex receptor sites that stimulate ventilation. During phases II and III, carbon dioxide returned to the lungs can account for the increased ventilation and control of arterial blood but the exact cause is uncertain. In one experiment, skeletal muscle was maintained in a resting state while increasing amounts of carbon dioxide were delivered to the lungs.[97] The resulting isocapnic hyperpnea lends credence to the humoral hypothesis. The humoral hypothesis is also referred to as the *CO_2 flow theory.*[89] This hypothesis claims that the neurogenic hypothesis is not the only explanation for the fast response in phase I. It is proposed that an increase in cardiac output and a decrease in ventilation/perfusion ratio would lead to an increase in arterial CO_2 tension and hydrogen ions, which could then stimulate a rapidly responding chemoreceptor to increase ventilation. Since the carotid bodies (chemoreceptor located in carotid arteries) are too far downstream to act fast enough, another site needs to be identified. No such site has yet been identified.

Both hypotheses support the skeletal muscle as the source of the ventilatory stimulus, but argue for an independent means of transmission. Dempsey and others[24] state that "despite the conflicting data and many unknowns still remaining, the 'primary' drive to breathe emanating from a changing tissue metabolic rate resides in either the 'CO_2 flow' or neurogenic schools of thought or their combination."

Control above the OBLA

Above the OBLA is the additional problem of decreasing arterial pH. Since the buffering of lactic acid with HCO_3^- results in increased carbon dioxide production, it is necessary for pulmonary ventilation to increase beyond the metabolic need so that arterial

CO_2 tension ($Paco_2$) is controlled. Such control is observed until a point halfway between the OBLA and $\dot{V}O_2$ max, that is, $Paco_2$ is reduced in proportion to the reduction of HCO_3^-, which maintains a normal pH.[92] Above that level, respiratory compensation is not possible. Control of ventilation above the OBLA is linked to the carotid bodies, which are sensitive to changes in gas tension. Patients have been studied who had their carotid bodies removed to treat their asthma.[88] During strenuous exercise, which produced metabolic acidosis, ventilation failed to increase to provide compensation. Therefore, the carotid bodies have been identified as acting in concert with other factors to control exercise hyperpnea.

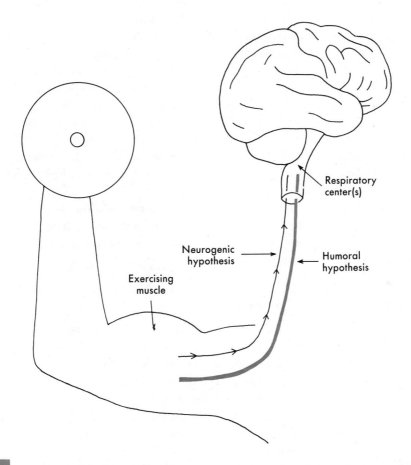

FIG. 6-9 Illustration of the two primary hypotheses to explain exercise hyperpnea below the "anaerobic threshold" (OBLA). Both hypotheses support exercising muscle as the source of the ventilatory stimulus. The neurogenic hypothesis argues that the stimulus is transmitted to the respiratory center(s) in the brain stem via the nervous system. The humoral hypothesis proposes that the stimulus is transmitted through the blood.

GENETIC INFLUENCE ON PULMONARY VENTILATION

In 1948, Monge[62] stated that ''athleticism must be the norm for the survival of man in the high altitudes.'' This statement was made because of observed similarities between athletes and high-altitude natives in hypoxic ventilatory drive. Specifically, both groups have a greatly reduced need to breathe under low partial pressure conditions, for example, altitude. Thus, investigators have been interested in whether this response in athletes is genetic or produced by physical training.

Thirteen endurance athletes at the University of Colorado were studied to determine whether Monge's suggestion was correct.[13] All athletes and a comparison group of nonathletes were studied under hypoxic and hypercapnic conditions at rest, and under hypoxic conditions during exercise. Hypoxic and hypercapnic drives in athletes at rest were 35% and 47% lower than nonathletes. However, no differences were found during exercise. In a later study, athletes and nonathletes were compared at equal relative work loads (33% and 66% $\dot{V}O_2$ max).[57] Investigators found that athletes have a lower rate of exercise pulmonary ventilation ($\dot{V}E$) per unit of metabolic rate. Parents and siblings of elite distance runners were tested, and these sedentary relatives also had a low ventilatory response to hypoxia.[77] In addition, resting ventilatory response to hypercapnia was studied in trained swimmers and their families.[75] A decreased hypercapnic response was found in both groups. These studies strongly support a genetic influence. Apparently, genetic influences can be modified by severe environmental stress, such as high altitude exposure.[72]

An unresolved question involves determining what advantage a low exercise $\dot{V}E$ might provide for endurance athletes. Some authors suggest that low exercise $\dot{V}E$ may be advantageous due to the lower work of breathing in athletes or to the correlation between $\dot{V}E$ and the perception of effort during exercise.[56]

PULMONARY DISEASE
Chronic obstructive pulmonary disease

There are two pathologic conditions usually associated with the term chronic obstructive pulmonary disease (COPD): *chronic bronchitis* and *emphysema*. In the United States, COPD ranks sixth among those diseases that limit physical activity.[83]

The basic symptom of chronic bronchitis is a chronic cough caused by the increase in secretion of sputum. As the disease advances, there is a decrease in vital capacity,[16] inequality in the ventilatory/perfusion ratio,[33] an increase in arterial CO_2 tension,[7] and a decrease in arterial O_2 tension.[32] In emphysema, destruction of elastic tissue results in narrower airways, which increase airflow resistance.[17]

With respect to testing these patients, the treadmill is recommended because the subject's ventilatory response is less than with the bicycle ergometer at equivalent $\dot{V}O_2$ levels. Several authors[27,71] have identified two distinct responses among COPD patients: those of ''fighters'' and ''nonfighters.'' The fighters increase exercise ventilation so that arterial CO_2 tension can be maintained and the nonfighters do not. Because dyspnea is so great in all COPD patients, exercise testing is usually limited by symptoms rather than physiological limitations.

Exercise programs can be beneficial for COPD patients. With training, symptoms are lessened[1] and improved tolerance to submaximal exercise occurs.[59] This effect can be explained by improved physical fitness, which results in reduced physiological strain after training. Unless these patients remain physically active, they begin a spiraling decline marked by dyspnea, inactivity, and further dyspnea.

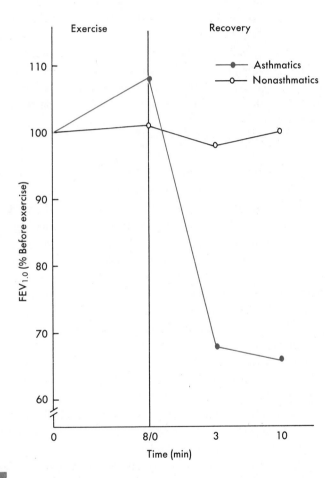

FIG. 6-10 Exercise-induced changes in $FEV_{1.0}$ following 8 minutes of exercise in asthmatics and nonasthmatics. (Data from Morton, A.R., Fitch, K.D., and Hahn, A.G.: Physical activity and the asthmatic, Phys. Sports Med. *9:*51, 1981.)

Asthma

Another devastating pulmonary disease, affecting almost 8 million Americans, is *asthma*. This disease affects 2.1 million children under the age of 17.[3] Since exercise can induce asthmatic symptoms in almost every asthmatic, it is important for the teacher and coach to recognize its symptoms and to understand possible remedial approaches.

Asthma attacks are marked by what is known as bronchospasm. That is, the bronchi become constricted by a combination of factors: the contraction of smooth muscle surrounding the bronchi; the swelling of bronchial tissue; and the collection of mucus along the walls of the bronchi. The exact causative mechanism is not known, but the onset of symptoms is related to certain irritants such as tobacco smoke, animal dander, and cold air. Exercise-induced asthma (EIA) has been proposed to be due to several causes, but the most widely accepted hypothesis involves the cooling of the airways.[22] The cooling is said to cause the release of bronchoconstrictive mediators.

Figure 6-10 illustrates EIA in asthmatics following 8 minutes of exercise. Five to 10 minutes after exercise, $FEV_{1.0}$ drops to 65% to 70% of preexercise values, indicating increased airway obstruction.[63] The EIA is usually spontaneously relieved within 15 to 60 minutes. Several effective bronchodilator drugs are now available that can both reduce and prevent bronchospasm.

SUMMARY

The pulmonary system can be broadly divided into two units: conducting airways and gas exchange regions. Gas exchange takes place only in the most distal structures, that is, respiratory bronchioles, alveolar ducts, and alveolar sacs. The total alveolar surface area is 70 m^2, representing some 300 million alveoli. The diaphragm and external intercostal muscles are the major muscles of inspiration. As the chest expands, the pressure in the lungs drops, drawing in atmospheric air. During heavy exercise, accessory muscles aid inspiration. Expiration is largely a passive recoil of the lungs that ends when alveolar pressure equals atmospheric pressure. Intrapleural pressure remains below alveolar and atmospheric pressure because of the tendency of the lungs to collapse. Collapse is not possible because of equal and opposite resistance offered by the rib cage.

The space in the conducting airways where air is not exchanged is referred to as anatomical dead space. Since this air cannot be exchanged, it must be subtracted from tidal volume, the amount taken from the atmosphere, to compute alveolar ventilation. Total lung capacity is the sum of the residual volume, the amount of air remaining in the lungs following expiration, and the vital capacity, maximal expiration following maximal inspiration. The total air exchanged with the atmosphere per minute is referred to as minute ventilation. Minute ventilation varies from about 6.0 L at rest to about 150 to 170 L during heavy exercise. Minute ventilation is equal to tidal volume (V_T) times breathing frequency (f).

Diffusion of respiratory gases between alveoli and capillary blood depends on pressure gradients. Gradients are measured in terms of partial pressure differences. For example, the partial pressure of oxygen in the alveoli is about 103 mm Hg, compared to pulmonary capillary pressure of 35 mm Hg. This differential ensures movement of oxygen into the blood. Even during maximal exercise, diffusion capacity of the lung is not a limiting factor, but cardiac function limits further exercise. Expired ventilation is reported by standardizing the measures to body temperature (37° C), sea level barometric pressure (760 mm Hg), and saturated or body temperature pressure saturated volumes (BTPS). Carbon dioxide production and oxygen consumption are expressed as standard temperature pressure dry (STPD). The oxygen cost of breathing ranges from 0.5 to 1.0 ml of oxygen per liter of pulmonary ventilation.

Carbon dioxide production and pulmonary ventilation increase linearly with oxygen consumption until the onset of blood lactate accumulation (OBLA). After the OBLA, carbon dioxide is produced out of proportion to oxygen consumption, and $\dot{V}_{CO_2}$ and $\dot{V}_E$ are no longer in a linear relationship with oxygen consumption. Following the OBLA, excess carbon dioxide is produced because lactic acid accumulation is buffered by bicarbonate, releasing carbon dioxide of nonmetabolic origin. Below the OBLA, pulmonary ventilation rises to a steady state in three phases. Phase I is a rapid rise associated with the start of exercise. Phase II is the slower rise to phase III, which is called steady state ventilation.

Despite considerable scientific interest in what has been called the anaerobic threshold and its prediction from pulmonary ventilation, its reliability has been recently questioned. Endurance athletes have been shown to have a greater forced vital capacity and total lung capacity compared to untrained persons. Also, endurance athletes have been found to breathe less under hypoxic and hypercapnic conditions at rest and at equal relative work loads during exercise, compared to nonathletes. Studies have linked this response with a genetic influence rather than one acquired through training.

Two main hypotheses have been proposed to explain ventilatory control during exercise below the OBLA. The first is the neurogenic hypothesis, which has been prompted by the very rapid response of ventilation at the beginning of exercise. Therefore, because a humoral response would be too slow, it is hypothesized that stretched muscles directly stimulate the respiratory center in the brain stem through the nervous system. The second hypothesis is the humoral hypothesis. During phases II and III, carbon dioxide returned to the lungs is said to account for the increased ventilation and the control of carbon dioxide, oxygen, and pH in the arterial blood. Both hypotheses suggest that skeletal muscle is the source of the ventilatory stimulus but argue for an independent means of transmission. Much more research is needed to fully understand the regulation of pulmonary ventilation during exercise.

Above the OBLA, decreasing arterial pH must be controlled. In fact, pH is controlled until a point about halfway between OBLA and $\dot{V}_{O_2}$ max. Carotid bodies have been linked to this control mechanism.

KEY TERMS

dyspnea difficult or labored breathing.
hypercapnia excess carbon dioxide content in the blood.
hyperoxia excess oxygen content.

hyperpnea increase in depth and rate of breathing as with exercise.

hyperventilation increased air in the lungs above normal. Can lead to respiratory alkalosis due to washing out of carbon dioxide from the blood.

hypocapnia low carbon dioxide content in the blood.

hypoventilation decreased air in the lungs below normal. Can lead to respiratory acidosis due to retention of carbon dioxide in the blood.

hypoxia low oxygen content.

isocapnia normal carbon dioxide content.

normoxia normal oxygen content

REVIEW QUESTIONS

1. Describe the respiratory mechanics responsible for resting inspiration and expiration.

2. Explain the difference between minute ventilation and alveolar ventilation.

3. Is diffusing capacity a limiting factor during maximal exercise? Explain.

4. Explain the difficulty in achieving a steady state pulmonary ventilation above the OBLA relative to the bicarbonate buffering system.

5. What is responsible for the identification of a ventilatory inflection point?

6. Briefly describe the control of exercise hyperpnea above and below the OBLA.

7. What are the symptoms of chronic bronchitis and emphysema and how might they be alleviated through physical training?

8. How can a physical educator aid an asthmatic patient to adapt to an exercise program and the probable occurrence of bronchospasm?

REFERENCES

1. Alpert, J.S., Bass, H., Szues, M.M., and others: Effects of physical training on hemodynamics and pulmonary function at rest and during exercise in patients with chronic obstructive pulmonary disease, Chest **66:**647, 1974.

2. American Academy of Pediatrics: The asthmatic child and his participation in sports and physical education, Pediatrics **45:**150, 1970.

3. American Lung Association: How to control asthma, Superstuff Self-help Program, New York, 1981, The American Lung Association.

4. American Lung Association: What every physical educator should know about asthma, New York, 1979, The American Lung Association.

5. Anderson, S.D.: Drugs affecting the respiratory system with particular reference to asthma, Med. Sci. Sports Exerc. **13:**259, 1981.

6. Asmussen, E.: Exercise and the regulation of ventilation, Circ. Res. **20**(suppl.):1132, 1967.

7. Astin, T.W.: The relationship between arterial blood oxygen saturation, carbon dioxide tension, and pH and airway resistance during 30% oxygen breathing in patients with chronic bronchitis with airway obstruction, Am. Rev. Respir. Dis. **102:**382, 1970.

8. Bender, P.R., and Martin, B.J.: Maximal ventilation after exhausing exercise, Med. Sci. Sports Exerc. **17:**164, 1985.

9. Bernard, T.E., Kamon, E., and Franklin, B.A.: Estimation of oxygen consumption from pulmonary ventilation during exercise, Hum. Factors **21**:417, 1979.

10. Bouhuys, A.: The physiology of breathing, New York, 1977, Grune and Stratton, Inc.

11. Brooks, G.A.: Response to Davis' manuscript, Med. Sci. Sports Exerc. **17**:19, 1985.

12. Brooks, G.A.: Anaerobic threshold: a review of the concept and directions for future research, Med. Sci. Sports Exerc. **17**:22, 1985.

13. Bryne-Quinn, E., Weil, J.V., Sodal, I.E., and others: Ventilatory control in the athlete, J. Appl. Physiol. **30**:91, 1971.

14. Buono, M.J., Constable, S.H., Morton, A.R., and others: The effect of an acute bout of exercise on selected pulmonary function measurements, Med. Sci. Sports Exerc. **13**:290, 1981.

15. Buono, M.J., and Roby, F.B.: Acid-base metabolic and ventilatory responses to repeated bouts of exercise, J. Appl. Physiol.: Respir. Environ. Exerc. Physiol. **53**:436, 1982.

16. Carilli, A.D., Denson, L.J., Rock, F., and others: The flow-volume loop in normal subjects and in diffuse lung disease, Chest **66**:472, 1974.

17. Comroe, J.H., and others: The lung, ed. 2, Chicago, 1962, Year Book Medical Publishers, Inc.

18. Consolazio, C.F., Johnson, R.E., and Pecora, L.J.: Physiological measurements of metabolic functions in man, New York, 1963, McGraw-Hill Book Co.

19. Davis, J.A.: Anaerobic threshold: review of the concept and directions for future research, Med. Sci. Sports Exerc. **17**:6, 1985.

20. Davis, J.A.: Response to Brooks' manuscript, Med. Sci. Sports Exerc. **17**:32, 1985.

21. Davis, J.A., Vodak, P., Wilmore, J.H., and others: Anaerobic threshold and maximal aerobic power for three modes of exercise, J. Appl. Physiol. **41**:544, 1976.

22. Deal, E.C., McFadden, E.R., Ingram, R.H., and others: Role of respiratory heat exchange in production of exercise-induced asthma, J. Appl. Physiol. **46**:467, 1979.

23. Dejours, P.: Control of respiration in muscular exercise. Handbook of physiology, section 3, Respiration **1**:1146, 1964.

24. Dempsey, J.A., Vidruk, E.H., and Mastenbrook, S.M.: Pulmonary control systems in exercise, Fed. Proc. **39**:1498, 1980.

25. Farrell, P.A., Maron, M.B., Hamilton, L.H., and others: Time course of lung volume changes during prolonged treadmill exercise, Med. Sci. Sports Exerc. **15**:319, 1983.

26. Favier, R., Desplanches, D., Frutoso, J., and others: Ventilatory and circulatory transients during exercise: new arguments for a neurohumoral theory, J. Appl. Physiol.: Respir. Environ. Exerc. Physiol. **54**:647, 1983.

27. Filley, G.F., Beckwith, H.J., Reeves, J.T., and others: Chronic obstructive bronchopulmonary disease. II. Oxygen transport in two clinical types, Am. J. Med. **44**:26, 1968.

28. Fitch, K.D., and Morton, A.R.: Specificity of exercise in exercise-induced asthma, Br. Med. J. **4**:577, 1971.

29. Fletcher, C.M., Jones, N.L., Burrows, B., and others: American emphysema and British bronchitis. A standardized comparative study, Am. Rev. Respir. Dis. **90**:1, 1964.

30. Folinsbee, L.J., Wallace, E.S., Bedi, J.F., and others: Exercise respiratory pattern in elite cyclists and sedentary subjects, Med. Sci. Sports Exerc. **15**:503, 1983.

31. Ford, A.B., and Hellerstein, H.K.: Estimation of energy expenditure from pulmonary ventilation, J. Appl. Physiol. **14**:891, 1959.

32. Gabriel, S.K.: Respiratory and circulatory investigations in obstructive and restrictive lung disease, Acta Med. Scand. **546:**1, 1972.

33. Gaxiano, D., Seaton, A., and Ogilvie, C.: Regional lung function in patients with obstructive lung diseases, Brit. Med. J. **5705:**330, 1970.

34. Geppert, J., and Zuntz, N.: Ueber die Regulation der Atmung, Arch. Ges. Physiol. **42:**189, 1888.

35. Godfrey, S.: Clinical variables of exercise-induced bronchospasm. In Dempsey, J.A., and Reed, C.E., editors: Muscular exercise and the lung, Madison, 1977, University of Wisconsin Press.

36. Graham, T.E., Wilson, B.A., Sample, M., and others: The effects of hypercapnia on the metabolic response to steady-state exercise, Med. Sci. Sports Exerc. **14:**286, 1982.

37. Green, J.F., and Sheldon, M.I.: Ventilatory changes associated with changes in pulmonary blood flow in dogs, J. Appl. Physiol.: Respir. Environ. Exerc. Physiol. **54:**997, 1983.

38. Guyton, A.C.: Physiology of the human body, Philadelphia, ed. 6, 1984, Saunders College Publishing.

39. Haber, P.S., Colebatch, H.J.H., Ng, C.K.Y., and others: Alveolar size as a determinant of pulmonary distensibility in mammalian lungs, J. Appl. Physiol.: Respir. Environ. Exerc. Physiol. **54:**837, 1983.

40. Jones, N.L.: Dyspnea in exercise, Med. Sci. Sports Exerc. **16:**14, 1984.

41. Holmgren, A.F., and Astrand, P.O.: DL and dimensions and functional capacities of the O_2 transport system in humans, J. Appl. Physiol. **21:**1463, 1966.

42. Kaltreider, N.L., Fray, W.W., and Philips, E.W.: Effect of age on total pulmonary capacity and its subdivisions, Am. Rev. Tuberc. **37:**662, 1938.

43. Kao, F.F., Michel, C.C., Mei, S.S., and others: Somatic afferent influence on respiration. Ann. N.Y. Acad. Sci. **109:**696, 1963.

44. Kao, F.F., Schlig, B., and Brooks, C.M.: Regulation of respiration during induced muscular work in decerebrate dogs, J. Appl. Physiol. **7:**379, 1955.

45. Katch, F.I., Freedom, P.S., and Jones, C.A.: Evaluation of acute cardiorespiratory responses to hydraulic resistance exercise, Med. Sci. Sports Exerc. **17:**168, 1985.

46. Kay, C., and Shephard, R.J.: On muscle strength and the threshold of anaerobic work, Int. Z. Angew. Physiol. **27:**311, 1969.

47. Lambertsen, C.J.: Physical and mechanical aspects of respiration. In Mountcastle, V.B., editor: Medical physiology, vol. 2, St. Louis, 1974, The C.V. Mosby Co.

48. Lambertsen, C.J.: The atmosphere and gas exchanges with the lungs and blood. In Mountcastle, V.B., editor: Medical physiology, vol. 2, St. Louis, 1974, The C.V. Mosby Co.

49. Lavoisier, A.L.: Experiences sur la respiration des animaux et sur les changements qui arrivent a l'air en passant par leurs poumons, Mem. de l'Acad. des Sci. **174:**185, 1777.

50. Levine, S.: Ventilatory response to muscular exercise. In Davies, D.G., and Barnes, C.D., editors: Regulation of ventilation and gas exchange, New York, 1978, Academic Press, Inc.

51. Lewis, B.M.: Measurement of arterial blood gases at the transition from exercise to rest, J. Appl. Physiol.: Respir. Environ. Exerc. Physiol. **54:**1340, 1983.

52. Londeree, B.R.: Anaerobic threshold training. In Burke, E.J., editor: Toward an understanding of human performance, Ithaca, 1977, Mouvement Publications.

53. Mahler, D.A., Moritz, E.D., and Loke, J.: Exercise performance in marathon runners with airway obstruction, Med. Sci. Sports Exerc. **13**:284, 1981.

54. Martin, B.J., Chen, H.-I., and Kolka, M.A.: Anaerobic metabolism of the respiratory muscles during exercise, Med. Sci. Sports Exerc. **16**:82, 1984.

55. Martin, B.J., and Sager, J.M.: Ventilatory endurance in athletes and non-athletes, Med. Sci. Sports Exerc. **13**:21, 1981.

56. Martin, B.J., Sparks, K.E., Zwillich, C.W., and others: Low exercise ventilation in endurance athletes, Med. Sci. Sports **11**:181, 1979.

57. Martin, B.J., Weil, J.V., Sparks, K.E., and others: Exercise ventilation correlates positively with ventilatory chemoresponsiveness, J. Appl. Physiol.: Respir. Environ. Exerc. Physiol. **45**:557, 1978.

58. Mead, J., and Loring, S.H.: Analysis of volume displacement and length changes of the diaphragm during breathing, J. Appl. Physiol.: Respir. Environ. Exerc. Physiol. **53**:750, 1982.

59. Mertens, D.J., Shephard, R.J., and Kavanagh, T.: Long-term exercise therapy for chronic obstructive lung disease, Respiration **35**:96, 1978.

60. Mickelson, T.C., and Hagerman, F.C.: Anaerobic threshold measurements of elite oarsmen, Med. Sci. Sports Exerc. **14**:440, 1982.

61. Milic-Emili, G., Petit, J.M., and Deroanne, R.: Mechanical work of breathing during exercise in trained and untrained subjects, J. Appl. Physiol. **17**:43, 1962.

62. Monge, M.C.: Acclimatization in the Andes, Baltimore, 1948, Johns Hopkins University Press.

63. Morton, A.R., Fitch, K.D., and Hahn, A.G.: Physical activity and the asthmatic, Phys. Sports Med. **9**:51, 1981.

64. Myhre, K., and Andersen, K.L.: Respiratory responses to static muscular work, Respir. Physiol. **12**:77, 1971.

65. Otis, A.B., Fenn, W.O., and Rahn, H.: The mechanics of breathing in man, J. Appl. Physiol. **2**:592, 1950.

66. Pace, W.R.: Pulmonary physiology in clinical practice, Philadelphia, 1970, F.A. Davis Co.

67. Powers, S.K., Dodd, S., Deason, R., and others: Ventilatory threshold, running economy and distance running performance of trained athletes, Res. Q. Exerc. Sport **54**:179, 1983.

68. Radford, E.: Ventilation standards for use in artificial respiration, J. Appl. Physiol. **7**:451, 1955.

69. Raven, P.B.: Pulmonary function of elite distance runners. In Milvy, P., editor: The marathon: physiological, medical, epidemiological and psychological studies, vol. 301, New York, 1977, The New York Academy of Sciences.

70. Ready, A.E., and Quinney, H.A.: Alterations in anaerobic threshold as the result of endurance training and detraining, Med. Sci. Sports Exerc. **14**:292, 1982.

71. Robin, E.D., and O'Neill, R.P.: The fighter versus the non-fighter. Control of ventilation in chronic obstructive pulmonary disease, AMA Arch. Environ. Health **7**:125, 1963.

72. Rotkis, K.C.: The other pink puffers or ventilation during exercise, Az. Med. **36**:184, 1979.

73. Roughton, F.J.W.: The average time spent by the blood in the human lung capillary and its relation to the rates of CO_2 uptake and elimination in man, Am. J. Physiol. **143**:621, 1945.

74. Rusko, H., Rahkila, P., and Karvinen, E.: Anaerobic threshold, skeletal muscle enzymes and fiber composition in young female cross-country skiers, Acta Physiol. Scand. **108**:263, 1980.

75. Saunders, N.A., Leeder, S.R., and Rebuck, A.S.: Ventilatory responses to carbon dioxide in young athletes: a family study, Am. Rev. Respir. Dis. **113:**497, 1976.

76. Scharf, S.M., Bark, H., Heimer, D., and others: "Second wind" during inspiratory loading, Med. Sci. Sports Exerc. **16:**87, 1984.

77. Scoggin, C.H., Doekel, R.D., Kryger, M.H., and others: Familial aspects of decreased hypoxic drive in endurance athletes, J. Appl. Physiol.: Respir. Environ. Exerc. Physiol. **44:**464, 1978.

78. Shephard, R.J.: The oxygen cost of breathing during vigorous exercise, Q. J. Exp. Physiol. **51:**336, 1966.

79. Sly, R.M., Harper, R.T., and Rosselot, I.: The effect of physical conditioning upon asthmatic children, Ann. Allergy **30:**86, 1972.

80. Stamford, B.A., Weltman, A., and Fulco, C.: Anaerobic threshold and cardiovascular responses during one- versus two-legged cycling, R.Q. **49:**351, 1978.

81. Tanaka, K., Matsuura, Y., Matsuzaka, A., and others: A longitudinal assessment of anaerobic threshold and distance-running performance, Med. Sci. Sports Exerc. **16:**278, 1984.

82. Turino, G.M., Bergofsky, E.H., Goldring, R.M., and others: Effect of exercise on pulmonary diffusing capacity, J. Appl. Physiol. **18:**447, 1963.

83. United States Department of Health, Education and Welfare: Monthly vital statistics report. Annual summary for the U.S. (births, deaths, marriages and divorces), Washington, D.C., 1967, U.S. Government Printing office.

84. Vaccaro, P., Zauner, C.W., and Updyke, W.F.: Resting and exercise respiratory function in well trained child swimmers, J. Sports Med. **17:**297, 1977.

85. Wasserman, K.: Breathing during exercise, N. Engl. J. Med. **298:**780, 1978.

86. Wasserman, K., and McIlroy, M.B.: Detecting the threshold of anaerobic metabolism in cardiac patients during exercise, Am. J. Cardiol. **14:**844, 1964.

87. Wasserman, K., Whipp, B.J., Koyal, S.N., and others: Anaerobic threshold and respiratory gas exchange during exercise, J. Appl. Physiol. **35:**236, 1973.

88. Wasserman, K., Whipp, B.J., Casaburi, R., and others: CO_2 flow to the lungs and ventilatory control. In Dempsey, J.A., and Reed, C.E., editors: Muscular exercise and the lung, Madison, 1977, University of Wisconsin Press.

89. Wasserman, K., Whipp, B.J., and Castagna, J.: Cardiodynamic hyperpnea: hyperpnea secondary to cardiac output increase, J. Appl. Physiol. **36:**457, 1974.

90. Weibel, E.R.: Morphometry of the human lung, Berlin, 1963, Springer-Verlag.

91. Whipp, B.J.: The hyperpnea of dynamic muscular exercise. In Hutton, R.S., editor: Exercise and sport sciences reviews, vol. 5, Santa Barbara, 1978, Journal Publishing Affiliates.

92. Whipp, B.J.: Tenets of the exercise hyperpnea and their degree of corroboration, Chest **73:**274, 1978.

93. Whipp, B.J.: The respiratory system. In Ross, G., editor: Essentials of human physiology, Chicago, 1978, Year Book Medical Publishers, Inc.

94. Wiley, R.L., and Lind, A.R.: Respiratory responses to sustained static muscular contractions in humans, Clin. Sci. **40:**221, 1971.

95. Williams, C.G., Wyndham, C.H., Kok, R., and others: Effect of training on maximum oxygen intake and on anaerobic metabolism in man, Int. Z. Angew. Physiol. **24:**18, 1967.

96. Wilmore, J.H., Vodak, P.A., Parr, R.B., and others: Further simplification of a method for determination of residual lung volume, Med. Sci. Sports Exerc. **12:**216, 1980.

97. Yamamoto, W.S., and Edwards, M.: Homeostasis of CO_2 during intravenous infusion of CO_2, J. Appl. Physiol. **15:**807, 1960.

SUGGESTED READINGS

Asmussen, E.: Exercise and the regulation of ventilation, Circ. Res. **20**(suppl.):1132, 1967.

Bouhuys, A.: The physiology of breathing, New York, 1977, Grune and Stratton, Inc.

Dempsey, J.A., and Reed, C.E.: Muscular exercise and the lung, Madison, 1977, University of Wisconsin Press.

Dempsey, J.A., Vidruk, E.H., and Mastenbrook, S.M.: Pulmonary control systems in exercise, Fed. Proc. **39:**1498, 1980.

Krogh, A.: The respiratory exchange of animals and man, New York, 1916, Longmans, Green and Co.

Levine, S.: Ventilatory response to muscular exercise. In Davies, D.G., and Barnes, C.D., editors: Regulation of ventilation and gas exchange, New York, 1978, Academic Press, Inc.

Wasserman, K.: Breathing during exercise, N. Engl. J. Med. **298:**780, 1978.

Whipp, B.J.: The hyperpnea of dynamic muscular exercise. In Hutton, R.S., editor: Exercise and sport sciences reviews, vol. 5, Santa Barbara, 1978, Journal Publishing Affiliates.

Whipp, B.J.: The respiratory system. In Ross, G., editor: Essentials of human physiology, Chicago, 1978, Year Book Medical Publishers, Inc.

CASE STUDY 1

During the 1984 Los Angeles Olympic Games, despite predictions to the contrary, there were no apparent smog-related injuries or performance decrements. Of course, for those events not requiring large pulmonary ventilations, for example, most submaximal events, symptoms associated with smog exposure are masked. In other words, small changes in pulmonary ventilation that may be functionally significant may not be perceived by the athlete or markedly alter performance. The overriding reason for the lack of difficulty in L.A., however, was probably the generally positive weather conditions over the Olympic competition period. (An Olympic record was set for both the women's [first ever] and men's marathon [2 hours, 9 minutes] events.) In addition to the weather, it should be mentioned that many Los Angeleans took advantage of this time of hectic activity to leave the city. The lack of significant traffic and resulting reductions in automobile emissions greatly improved the usually smog-ridden environment.

What are the significant contaminants in polluted air and how might they have affected physiological function? Polluted air contains oxidants including ozone (O_3), nitrogen dioxide (NO_2), and sulfur dioxide (SO_2). These oxidants are created when automobile emissions and industrial pollutants interact with environmental air. Generally, these pollutants create bronchoconstriction, similar to that observed in COPD patients. In fact, chronic exposure to a polluted environment is known to be related to the onset of emphysema. Bronchoconstriction, as described in this chapter, interferes with pulmonary gas exchange (oxygen and carbon dioxide) by increasing air resistance. Ozone, a major constituent of the pollution in our cities' overly "automobilized" environments, is known to increase respiration and decrease tidal volume with acute exposure. Carbon monoxide that competes, with success, with oxygen for sites on the hemoglobin molecule can seriously interfere with cardiopulmonary function. Cardiac patients must be very careful to remain indoors when oxidants are at a high level in the environment. Athletes might be advised to do the same.

As I ride my nonpolluting horse through the Wyoming/Colorado mountains and marvel at the clean Rocky Mountain air, I know that the air pollution problem is not going to go away easily. Los Angeles is not the only city with air pollution problems. Other competitions will be held in cities where the problem is not only speculated about but becomes a reality. Much more research is needed to discover the effects of short- and long-term exercise exposure to polluted environments. Even more, we need more internal combustion of food and fewer internal combustion engines.

CASE STUDY 2

The probability is quite high that a physical education teacher or athletic coach will have an asthmatic child in class or on a team. Of course, the effectiveness of bronchodilator medications, such as theophylline, cromolyn sodium, and the beta-2 agonists, makes it possible for most asthmatics to play strenuously and to compete without apparent symptoms. In some cases, you may not even know that one of your best athletes is asthmatic. The medications just listed are all legal for sanctioned sports competition, so there is no worry of disqualification. Obviously, it should be the obligation of the asthmatic child or the parents to inform you of the condition and how it is being controlled.

Constriction of the bronchi, referred to as bronchospasm or bronchoconstriction, marks the asthmatic attack. The constriction makes expiration difficult and often causes a wheezing sound. When symptoms are brought on by exercise, the condition is called exercise-induced asthma (EIA).

The following warning signals might alert you that a student in your class may be having problems[3]:

1. Anxious or scared look
2. Unusual paleness or sweating
3. Flared nostrils when the child tries to inhale
4. Pursed lips while breathing
5. Fast breathing
6. Vomiting
7. Hunched-over body posture; the child can't stand or sit straight and can't relax
8. Coughing when the child has no cold
9. Frequent clearing of the throat
10. Irregular breathing
11. Wheezing, however light
12. Noisy, difficult breathing

Even with the possibility of EIA, the American Academy of Pediatrics[2] recommends that the child with asthma should be advised to take part in school and recreational sports programs. The American Lung Association[4] advises physical educators to help the asthmatic child to learn to "listen to the body" so that exercise can be appropriately regulated. The child should ask three "checkpoint" questions:

1. Am I breathing too fast?
2. Is my heart beating too fast?
3. Am I wheezing?

Continued.

An asthmatic who has had good medical care and advice will recognize symptoms and know the proper self-care steps to control his condition. However, it is advisable for the teacher or coach to know how to help the asthmatic child if needed. Three steps should be taken when the child is wheezing moderately and has not reached a stage where only emergency medication will reverse the symptoms[4]:

1. During a bronchospasm, the muscles of the shoulders, abdomen, neck, chest, and upper back also become tense. This added tension further intensifies the episode. Therefore, it is necessary for the child to *relax*. Either a sitting or supine position should be taken, with arms hanging loosely or lying along the sides. The child should keep his eyes closed and breathe normally. Progressive relaxation techniques should be employed, starting with the lower body and working up to the scalp by alternately tensing and relaxing muscles to ensure relaxation.

2. During a bronchospasm, trapped air remains in the lungs. This should be removed. *Diaphragmatic breathing* will help to alleviate this situation. It is best to lie on the back with hands placed on the abdomen so that the child can feel his hands rise and fall with proper contraction of the diaphragm.

3. During a bronchospasm, *drinking warm liquids* (water, soup, or tea) helps to relax the muscles in the respiratory airways and helps to dislodge collected mucus.

When the symptoms disappear, the child should return to regular activities immediately.

What activities would you recommend as an exercise program for asthmatics? Gradual warm-up may prevent the development of EIA.[35] Morton and others[63] found that interval running (10 or 20 seconds coupled with 30 or 60 seconds of rest) was less asthmogenic than continuous running. Swimming is less asthmogenic than either running or cycling.[28] Increased aerobic fitness increases the exercise level at which asthmatic symptoms occur.[79]

In summary, exercise for the asthmatic is definitely *not* contraindicated. Asthmatic children, with proper self-care and body listening techniques, can prevent the onset of symptoms or control symptoms before they become severe. If necessary, bronchodilator medications are available to prevent and bring bronchospasm under control.

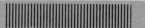 **chapter 7**

GAS
TRANSPORT

MAJOR LEARNING OBJECTIVE
The blood is almost fully saturated with oxygen at all levels of physical activity, from rest through maximal exercise. However, iron deficiency, high altitude, and hyperventilation can alter the dynamics of gas transport.

APPLICATIONS
Iron deficiency can hamper the oxygen-binding characteristics of hemoglobin. Increasing altitude lowers the partial pressure of oxygen (P_{O_2}), which makes hemoglobin binding problematic. Hyperventilation "blows off" carbon dioxide, making breath-holding easier.
■ Iron deficiency, especially in menstruating women, should be monitored closely. At low and moderate altitudes decreasing P_{O_2} is compensated for by increased minute ventilation. Prerace hyperventilation can increase the time before breathing becomes necessary during exercise.

AFTER the alveoli have been ventilated and gases have diffused across the alveolar-capillary membrane, the blood transports respiratory gases. Oxygen is loaded in the blood, transported, and unloaded at the tissues. Conversely, carbon dioxide is loaded at the tissues, transported, and unloaded at the pulmonary capillary. We can say that oxygen and carbon dioxide become *associated* with blood for the purpose of transport. On the other hand, oxygen and carbon dioxide become *dissociated* from blood when they reach their respective destinations. Thus, association of oxygen and dissociation of carbon dioxide occur at the pulmonary "station"; the reverse occurs at the tissue "station." This chapter deals with the role of blood in the processes of association and dissociation. Figure 7-1 illustrates the interaction of the pulmonary system, the cardiovascular system, and the tissues in gas transport.

OXYGEN TRANSPORT

Oxygen association

Oxygen becomes associated with blood for transportation to tissues by one of two processes. Oxygen can be (1) physically dissolved in the blood plasma or (2) bound with hemoglobin (Hb) in the red blood cell (RBC).

Gases dissolve in fluids according to *Henry's law,* which states that "the quantity of a gas that can dissolve in a fluid is equal to the product of the gas partial pressure and the solubility coefficient (a)."[16]

$$P_{O_2} \cdot a$$

The solubility coefficient for oxygen is 0.023 (ml $O_2 \cdot$ ml^{-1}) of blood per unit of atmospheric pressure. Therefore, at sea level:

$$0.023 \div 760 = 0.00003 \text{ ml } O_2 \cdot \text{ml}^{-1} \text{ blood mm Hg}$$

Since blood variables are usually expressed per 100 milliliters of blood, the quantity of oxygen that dissolves in arterial blood (with P_{O_2} at 100 mm Hg) is 0.3 ml $O_2 \cdot$ 100 ml^{-1} blood $(0.00003 \times 100 \times 100)$.[16]

Only a small percentage of the oxygen carried in blood travels dissolved in plasma. This is because, as just shown, the capacity for dissolving oxygen in blood is small. To illustrate this point, we can use an elite athlete as an example. A male endurance runner with extremely high aerobic power may be able to consume 6.0 L $O_2 \cdot$ min^{-1} at maximum. An equally high cardiac output ($\dot{Q}$) would be 30 L $\cdot$ min^{-1}. With a capacity for dissolving oxygen of 0.3 ml $\cdot$ 100 ml, this hypothetical athlete would need a cardiac output capacity of 2,000 L $\cdot$ min^{-1} to sustain a $\dot{V}_{O_2}$ max of 6.0 L $\cdot$ min^{-1}, that is, $\dfrac{6.0}{0.3} \times$ 100. It is obvious that another process is required to carry oxygen within the capacity of the heart to pump blood.

The most important process is the association of oxygen with hemoglobin to form *oxyhemoglobin,* as shown here:

$$O_2 + Hb \rightarrow HbO_2$$

This binding occurs rapidly, having a half-life of 0.1 seconds or less.[12] The process depends almost entirely on a favorable pressure gradient. If capillary P_{O_2} is less than that of alveolar P_{O_2}, the blood will load oxygen. Binding potential also varies with blood temperature, hydrogen ion (H^+) concentration, and carbon dioxide tension (P_{CO_2}). These factors will be discussed later in this chapter.

One molecule of hemoglobin contains four heme groups, each containing one molecule of iron. Since one molecule of iron can combine with one molecule of oxygen, one molecule of hemoglobin can combine with four molecules of oxygen. The *oxygen capacity of hemoglobin* can be computed by multiplying the grams of hemoglobin (per 100 ml of blood) by the amount of oxygen that can combine with 1 gram of hemoglobin (1.34

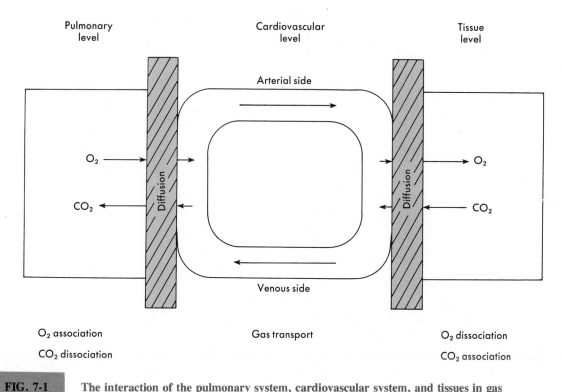

Pulmonary level	Cardiovascular level	Tissue level

Arterial side

$O_2 \longrightarrow$ Diffusion O_2

$CO_2 \longleftarrow$ Diffusion CO_2

Venous side

| O_2 association | Gas transport | O_2 dissociation |
| CO_2 dissociation | | CO_2 association |

FIG. 7-1   **The interaction of the pulmonary system, cardiovascular system, and tissues in gas transport.**

ml). An average value for hemoglobin is 15 g · 100 ml^{-1} blood (14 grams for females and 16 grams for males). Therefore:

$$15 \text{ g} \cdot 100 \text{ ml} \times 1.34 \text{ ml O}_2 = 20.1 \text{ ml O}_2 \cdot 100 \text{ ml}^{-1} \text{ blood}$$

With such a capacity, it would be possible for the hypothetical athlete mentioned earlier to manage O$_2$ consumption completely with hemoglobin binding, that is:

$$201 \text{ ml O}_2 \cdot \text{L blood} \times 30 \text{ L} \cdot \text{min } \dot{Q} = 6,030 \text{ ml O}_2 \cdot \text{min}^{-1}$$

Even with sufficient atmospheric oxygen, adequate pulmonary ventilation, and optimal diffusing capacity, hemoglobin does not become 100% saturated with oxygen. The proportion of hemoglobin bound with oxygen is called *percent saturation* (% So$_2$). For example, if oxygen is 19.5 ml · 100 ml in arterial blood returning from the lungs (about average for a person at rest), the percent saturation is:

$$\% \text{ So}_2 = \frac{\text{Hb O}_2}{\text{O}_2 \text{ capacity}} = \frac{19.5 \text{ ml} \cdot 100 \text{ ml}^{-1}}{15 \text{ g} \times 1.34} = \frac{19.5}{20.1} = 0.97$$

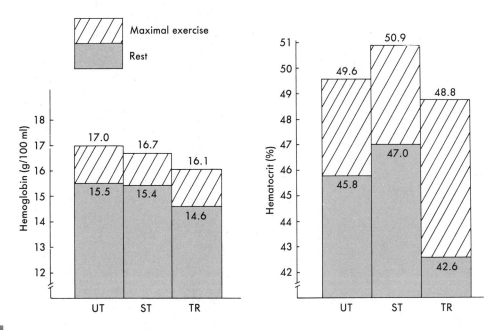

FIG. 7-2 **Hemoglobin and hematocrit values at rest and during the last minute of maximal exercise in untrained, semi-trained, and trained subjects. (Developed from the data of Braumann, K.M., Boning, D., and Trost, F.: Oxygen dissociation curves in trained and untrained subjects, Eur. J. Appl. Physiol. *42:*51, 1979.)**

Therefore, the So_2 of hemoglobin in arterialized blood in humans at rest is 97%. The practice of blood doping (reinfusion of red blood cells extracted earlier) for long-distance competition is an attempt to increase the So_2 of hemoglobin (see Chapter 19).

Oxygen association during exercise

The amount of hemoglobin and the hematocrit (Hct) (the percentage of the total blood volume occupied by red blood cells) are critical factors in O_2 association. Indeed, they are of paramount importance. Therefore, scientists have been concerned with how O_2 association in red blood cells might be compromised. Hemoglobin and hematocrit levels in the blood of subjects when at rest and during the last minute of maximal exercise were studied in three groups.[1] The results of this study are presented in Figure 7-2. Both hemoglobin and hematocrit levels increase with maximum exercise, largely because of hemoconcentration, that is, because of the shift of blood plasma volume. During exercise blood plasma shifts to the tissues, where it is needed to maintain water balance. A significant difference was noted between groups in both resting hemoglobin and hematocrit levels,

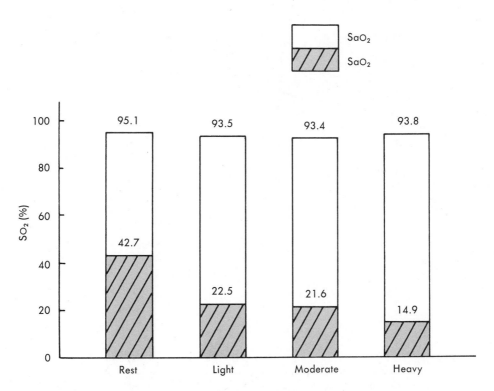

FIG. 7-3 Percent saturation of oxygen (So_2) in arterial and mixed venous blood at rest and during light, moderate, and heavy exercise. (Developed from the data of Thomson, J.M., Dempsey, J.A., Chosy, L.W., and others: Oxygen transport and oxyhemoglobin dissociation during prolonged muscular work, J. Appl. Physiol. *37:658*, 1974.)

with lower values appearing in the trained (TR) group. Although lower hematocrit levels mimic anemia, they are, in fact, caused by the greater amount of blood plasma, not by a reduction in red blood cells. This "athletic anemia" does not affect maximum aerobic power until hemoglobin drops to values of less than 12 g · 100 ml^{-1}.[3] Iron deficiency, a possible cause of low hemoglobin levels in athletes, is a growing concern of coaches, particularly those who coach women. If hemoglobin levels are compromised, functional capacity may be compromised.

Still another important factor in exercise performance is % So_2 of hemoglobin. Figure 7-3 illustrates the data of an investigation of % So_2 in persons at rest and during light, moderate, and heavy exercise.[14] Arterial saturation remained relatively constant between rest and heavy exercise (at greater than 90% $\dot{V}o_2$ max). The O_2 carrying capacity of blood rose slightly because of hemoconcentration during exercise. Despite declining O_2 concentration in mixed venous blood because of the increased metabolic requirements of tissues during exercise, arterial So_2 remained constant. This response indicates that blood So_2 is not a factor limiting maximum aerobic power.

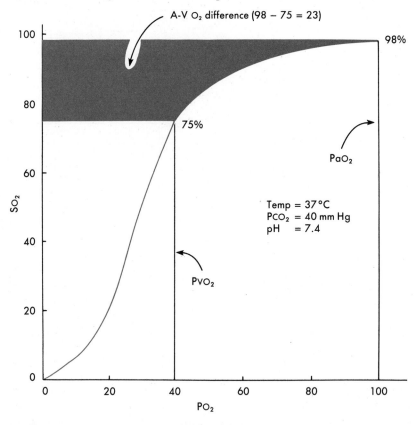

FIG. 7-4   **The oxyhemoglobin dissociation curve, that is, the relationship between percent saturation of oxygen (% So_2) and partial pressure of oxygen (Po_2).**

Oxygen dissociation

The equation $O_2 + Hb \rightarrow HbO_2$ is reversible. That is, $HbO_2 \rightarrow O_2 + Hb$. Oxygen dissociates from hemoglobin according to the metabolic requirements of tissues. As metabolism in the cell increases and cellular P_{O_2} is reduced, the process of dissociation is facilitated. Figure 7-4 depicts the *oxyhemoglobin dissociation curve*. This curve shows the relationship between the blood P_{O_2} and the hemoglobin S_{O_2}. Although this relationship can be altered by temperature, P_{CO_2}, and hydrogen ion (H^+) concentration (pH), the curve is depicted under standard conditions (temperature, 37° C; P_{CO_2}, 40 mm Hg; and pH, 7.4). In the arterial system, after oxygenation in the lungs, blood is approximately 98% saturated with oxygen and maintains a partial pressure of 100 mm Hg. When arterial blood reaches tissues and the pressure gradient between blood and tissues is high (100 to 40 mm Hg), oxygen dissociates quickly, leaving the O_2 saturation of mixed venous blood at approximately 75% during rest. (NOTE: Because the metabolic rates of various tissues differ, the percent saturation of venous blood coming from those tissues varies also. For ease of description, mixed venous blood values are usually reported.) The difference between arterial and mixed venous O_2 saturation is referred to as *A-V oxygen difference*. For example, when arterial blood is 98% saturated with O_2 and mixed venous blood is 75% saturated, the A-V oxygen difference is 23% (98% − 75% = 23%). Thus, 19.6 vol % of arterial O_2 − 15 vol % of venous O_2 = 4.6 ml $O_2 \cdot$ 100 ml^{-1} blood. What A-V O_2 difference indicates is the amount of oxygen extracted from blood by tissues. O_2 extraction increases markedly during heavy exercise. This increase is critical to aerobic metabolic capacity.

To understand the oxyhemoglobin dissociation curve completely, we should keep the concept of association in mind. (The curve, in fact, deals with association as well as dissociation.) If P_{O_2} is altered for any reason (for example, by altitude or pulmonary disease), arterial blood may be less saturated than normal. However, S_{O_2} declines slowly with decreasing P_{O_2}, and one has to go to very high altitudes, for example, before hypoxic effects are noticed. At P_{O_2} below approximately 60 mm Hg, the curve drops precipitously. Therefore, when P_{O_2} drops to low values, as it does in the blood of persons at high altitudes, oxygen dissociates from hemoglobin rapidly. In this situation, where functional capacity might otherwise be compromised, quick release of oxygen to tissues compensates for the drop in P_{O_2}. (A complete discussion of the effects of altitude appears in Chapter 12.)

Regardless of the atmospheric pressure, the top (flat) portion of the dissociation curve indicates loading of oxygen on hemoglobin molecules. The steep portion of the curve, at P_{O_2} levels associated with body tissues, indicates unloading of oxygen from hemoglobin.

Factors affecting oxygen dissociation during exercise

In addition to pressure gradient increases, three other factors influence O_2 dissociation during exercise. Blood temperature changes, concentrations of 2,3-diphosphoglycerate, and the Bohr effect also affect O_2 dissociation.

As blood temperature increases, the dissociation curve shifts to the right. This means that hemoglobin decreases its affinity for oxygen so that oxygen is released at a higher P_{O_2}. This response is favorable for the athlete because it facilitates release of oxygen to the tissues during exercise. It has been noted that although the oxyhemoglobin dissociation curve shifts to the right during exercise, it maintains the same slope.[9] This shift is often assessed by the measurement of P_{50}, the partial pressure at which the hemoglobin is 50% saturated with oxygen. Significant increases in P_{50} have been reported during maximal exercise[1,7] (see Figure 7-5). This means that the same % S_{O_2} is achieved at a higher P_{O_2}, that is, dissociation is facilitated. However, during intermittent exercise[13] and prolonged, submaximal exercise,[4,14] no significant changes were noted.

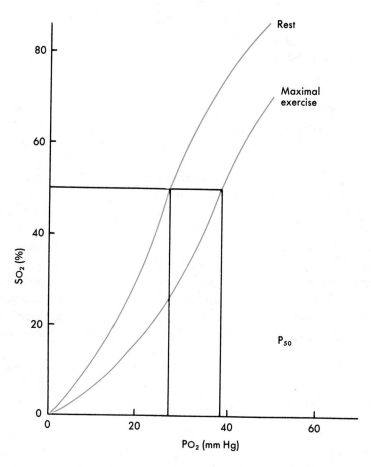

FIG. 7-5   Illustration of the right shift in the oxyhemoglobin dissociation curve during maximal exercise. A measure of shift is called P_{50} which refers to the partial pressure at which the hemoglobin is 50% saturated with oxygen.

The second factor that influences O_2 dissociation during exercise is *2,3-diphosphoglycerate* (2,3-DPG), an end product of metabolism in the red blood cell. Other phosphates, for example, ATP, are found in the red blood cell but their concentrations are relatively small. Increased concentrations of 2,3-DPG are thought to decrease binding affinity of hemoglobin for oxygen, (shown by the rightward shift of the dissociation curve). Significant increases in 2,3-DPG concentrations have been noted after maximal exercise,[1,7] with low P_{O_2}, with anemia, and with low cardiac output. During intermittent exercise[13] and submaximal exercise[14] no significant changes in 2,3-DPG were observed in untrained subjects. Small but significant changes in P_{50} and 2,3-DPG have been observed during endurance exercise in highly trained middle distance runners.[15] It appears that increases in 2,3-DPG are accompanied by increases in P_{50}, and that very intense exercise is usually required to produce 2,3-DPG changes.

A third factor that causes a shift to the right of the oxyhemoglobin dissociation curve is the *Bohr effect*. The Bohr effect results from increases in P_{CO_2} or decreases in pH that occur with certain types of exercise, that is, those activities in which it is common to exceed OBLA, such as in sprinting. As with the other factors mentioned earlier, the Bohr effect aids in the unloading of oxygen at the tissue level.

CARBON DIOXIDE TRANSPORT

Carbon dioxide association

Carbon dioxide associates with blood at the tissue level so that it can be transported to the lungs for exchange with the atmosphere. Several processes are involved in carbon dioxide transport. A general description of these processes is given in Figure 7-6.

About 10% of carbon dioxide leaving tissues reacts with and is carried in blood plasma. An insignificant amount (less than 1%) combines with plasma proteins to form *carbamino compounds*. As with oxygen, carbon dioxide (5% or half of that carried in the plasma) *physically dissolves* in the plasma, according to Henry's law. In mixed venous blood (P_{VCO_2} = 46 mm Hg), 1.38 mM of carbon dioxide is dissolved per liter of blood (solubility coefficient = 0.03 mM/L · mm Hg^{-1}).[16] The remaining carbon dioxide in plasma (5%) combines with water to form carbonic acid (H_2CO_3), which readily dissociates to bicarbonate and hydrogen ions (HCO_3^- and H^+). The carbon dioxide is carried mainly in the form of bicarbonate ions. A negligible amount (0.001%) is carried as carbonic acid. The hydrogen ions are buffered by plasma proteins as follows:

$$H_2O + CO_2 \rightarrow H_2CO_3 \rightarrow HCO_3^{-1} + H^+$$

The remaining 90% of the carbon dioxide leaving the tissues undergoes reactions within red blood cells. Some dissolves in cellular water (5%). About 21% of carbon dioxide molecules combine with the protein (globin) portion of the hemoglobin molecule to form carbamino compounds. This reaction produces oxygen, which can be returned to tissues for cell metabolism. Most carbon dioxide (63%) combines with water to form carbonic acid, which, as in plasma, dissociates to bicarbonate and hydrogen ions. The hydrogen ions are buffered by the hemoglobin.

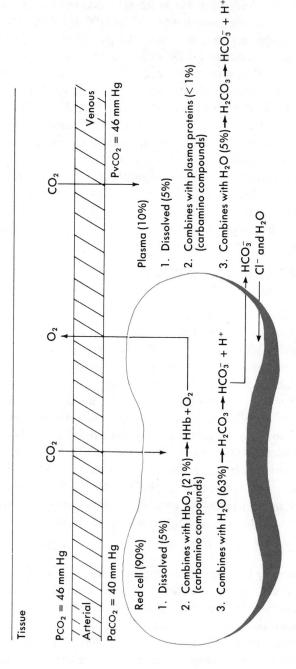

FIG. 7-6   **General description of the processes by which CO₂ produced in the tissues associates with blood passing through tissue capillaries.**

Bicarbonate ions account for a greater proportion of carbon dioxide association in red blood cells than in plasma because of the presence in red blood cells of the enzyme *carbonic anhydrase* (CA). Carbonic anhydrase serves as a catalyst in converting carbon dioxide and water into carbonic acid. Little carbonic anhydrase is present in plasma; thus, the reaction there proceeds very slowly. Blood spends approximately 1 second in the capillaries.[11] With carbonic anhydrase present in red blood cells this is adequate time for carbon dioxide association to occur. Without carbonic anhydrase in red blood cells, the process of loading carbon dioxide could take as long as 200 seconds.[11]

Although most carbon dioxide leaving tissues initially reacts with red blood cells, it is actually carried in the plasma. This is because as soon as bicarbonate ions are formed in red blood cells, they diffuse into the plasma. So, together with the bicarbonate ions formed in plasma, 90% of carbon dioxide is carried in plasma in the form of bicarbonate ions.[16] Diffusion of bicarbonate ions from red blood cells, if not for *chloride shift,* could cause an electrical imbalance. To prevent such an imbalance, chloride (Cl^-) diffuses into red blood cells to offset bicarbonate ion outflow. Water also moves into red blood cells to maintain osmotic equilibrium.

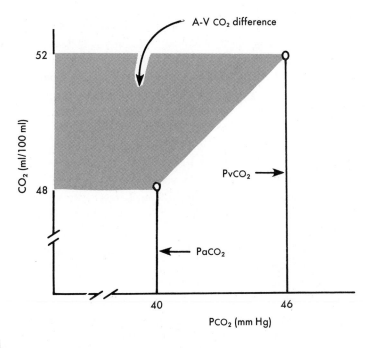

FIG. 7-7   The CO_2 dissociation curve.

Carbon dioxide dissociation

On reaching the lungs, carbon dioxide needs to dissociate from the blood, that is, returning from transport form (HCO_3^-) to gaseous form. The reaction that forms bicarbonate ions from carbon dioxide is a reversible reaction, enabling the release of carbon dioxide.

$$CO_2 + H_2O \rightleftarrows H_2CO_3 \rightleftarrows HCO_3^- + H^+$$

The relationship between carbon dioxide content of the blood and P_{CO_2} is linear throughout the physiological range[16] (see Figure 7-7). This means that carbon dioxide dissociates from the blood in direct proportion to P_{CO_2}.

SUMMARY

Oxygen and carbon dioxide associate with blood for the purpose of transport. Association occurs at the lungs for oxygen and at tissue sites for carbon dioxide. Conversely, oxygen and carbon dioxide dissociate from blood when they reach their destinations, at the tissues for oxygen and the lungs for carbon dioxide. Oxygen associates with blood by physically dissolving in plasma and combining with the iron portions of hemoglobin molecules in red blood cells. The oxygen-carrying capacity of blood can be computed by multiplying the grams of hemoglobin (per 100 ml blood) by the amount of oxygen that can combine with 1 gram of hemoglobin (1.34 ml). Thus, 15 g $\cdot$ 100 ml^{-1} $\times$ 1.34 = 20.1 ml O_2 $\cdot$ 100 ml^{-1} blood. The extent to which hemoglobin reaches its capacity for binding with oxygen is referred to as percent saturation (% S_{O_2}).

Both hemoglobin concentration and hematocrit (the percentage of total blood volume occupied by red blood cells) increase with maximal exercise. The increase is the result of hemoconcentration, that is, the shift of fluid from blood plasma to tissues. An iron-deficient diet can cause a reduction in performance capacity but hemoglobin has to drop to levels of less than 12 g $\cdot$ 100 ml^{-1} of blood for this to happen. Percent saturation of arterial blood is not altered between rest and heavy exercise, but saturation of venous blood declines as a result of increased extraction of oxygen by tissues.

Oxygen dissociates from hemoglobin in relation to changes in partial pressure of oxygen (P_{O_2}). In arterial blood, with P_{O_2} at 100 mm Hg, hemoglobin is approximately 98% saturated with oxygen. In venous blood, with P_{O_2} at 40 mm Hg, hemoglobin is approximately 75% saturated with oxygen. This difference in saturation levels is referred to as the A-V O_2 difference. The A-V O_2 difference varies with the metabolic requirements of tissues. The relationship between % S_{O_2} and P_{O_2}, as represented by the oxy-hemoglobin dissociation curve, is curvilinear. That is, at high P_{O_2} values, blood is slow to give up its oxygen, and the reverse is true at low P_{O_2} values. The dissociation curve shifts to the right with maximal exercise. This shift, which facilitates oxygen unloading, is caused by increases in blood temperature and by increased levels of 2,3-diphosphoglycerate (2,3-DPG), an end product of red blood cell metabolism. The Bohr effect (increased P_{CO_2} and decreased blood pH) also causes a shift of the curve to the right.

Three processes are involved in the association of carbon dioxide with blood, both in plasma and in red blood cells. In plasma, 5% of the total carbon dioxide transported is dissolved. Another 5% combines with water to form carbonic acid, which dissociates to bicarbonate (HCO_3^-) and hydrogen (H^+) ions, and less than 1% combines with plasma proteins to form carbamino compounds. In red blood cells, 5% of the carbon dioxide is dissolved, 21% combines with the protein portion of hemoglobin to form carbamino compounds, and 63% combines with water to form bicarbonate ions. After bicarbonate ions are formed in red blood cells they diffuse into and are transported by plasma. Carbon dioxide is converted to bicarbonate ions more rapidly in red blood cells than in plasma because of the presence in red blood cells of the enzyme carbonic anhydrase.

KEY TERMS

anemia a condition marked by a below normal red blood cell concentration.

association the act of combining.

A-V oxygen difference the difference in oxygen saturation between arterial and venous blood.

Bohr effect the shift of the oxyhemoglobin dissociation curve to the right as a function of increased Pco_2 and lower pH.

dissociation the act of separating.

hematocrit the percentage of red blood cells in blood.

hemoglobin complex iron-protein molecule important in the transport of oxygen and carbon dioxide in blood.

oxyhemoglobin chemical combination of oxygen with hemoglobin.

REVIEW QUESTIONS

1. Why is it necessary to transport oxygen in blood by a mechanism other than in solution in plasma?

2. Explain percent saturation of oxygen.

3. Describe "athletic anemia." What causes this condition?

4. Describe the relationship between % So_2 and Po_2 as it is represented on the oxyhemoglobin dissociation curve.

5. What three factors affect oxygen dissociation during exercise? How?

6. Describe the chloride shift during carbon dioxide dissociation.

REFERENCES

1. Braumann, K.M., Boning, D., and Trost, F.: Oxygen dissociation curves in trained and untrained subjects, Eur. J. Applied Physiol. **42**:51, 1979.

2. Cade, R., Conte, M., Zauner, C., and others: Effect of phosphate loading on 2,3-diphosphoglycerate and maximal oxygen uptake, Med. Sci. Sports Exerc. **16**:263, 1984.

3. Davies, C.T.M., Chukweumeka, A.C., and van Haaren, J.P.: Iron-deficiency anaemia: its effect on maximum aerobic power and response to exercise in African males aged 17-40 years, Clin. Sci. **44**:555, 1973.

4. Dempsey, J.A., Thomson, J.M., Forester, H.V., and others: HbO_2 dissociation in man during prolonged work in chronic hypoxia, J. Applied Physiol. **38**:1022, 1975.

5. Ehn, L., Carlmark, B., and Hoglund, S.: Iron status in athletes involved in intense physical activity, Med. Sci. Sports Exerc. **12**:61, 1980.

6. Frederickson, L.A., Puhl, J.L., and Runyan, W.S.: Effects of training on indices of iron status of young female cross-country runners, Med. Sci. Sports Exerc. **15**:271, 1983.

7. Klein, J.P., Forster, H.V., Stewart, R.D., and others: Hemoglobin affinity for oxygen during short-term exhaustive exercise, J. Appl. Physiol. **48**:236, 1980.

8. Lambertsen, C.J.: Transport of oxygen and carbon dioxide by the blood. In Mountcastle, V.B., editor: Medical physiology, ed. 14, vol. 2, St. Louis, 1980, The C.V. Mosby Co.

9. Miyamura, M., and Honda, Y.: CO_2 dissociation curves of oxygenated whole blood obtained at rest and in exercise, Eur. J. Applied Physiol. **39**:37, 1978.

10. Novosadova, J.: The changes in hematocrit, hemoglobin, plasma volume and proteins during and after different types of exercise, Eur. J. Applied Physiol. **36**:223, 1977.

11. Roughton, F.J.W.: The average time spent by the blood in the human lung capillary and its relation to the rates of CO_2 uptake and elimination in man, Am. J. Physiol. **143**:621, 1945.

12. Roughton, F.J.W., and Forster, R.E.: Relative importance of diffusion and chemical reaction rates in determining rate of exchange of gases in the human lung, with special reference to true diffusing capacity of pulmonary membrane and volume of blood in the lung capillaries, J. Appl. Physiol. **11**:290, 1957.

13. Shappell, S.D., Murray, J.A., Bellingham, A.J., and others: Adaptation to exercise: role of hemoglobin affinity for oxygen and 2,3-diphosphoglycerate, J. Appl. Physiol. **30**:827, 1971.

14. Thomson, J.M., Dempsey, J.A., Chosy, L.W., and others: Oxygen transport and oxyhemoglobin dissociation during prolonged muscular work, J. Appl. Physiol. **37**:658, 1974.

15. Taunton, J.E., Taunton, C.A., and Banister, E.W.: Alterations in 2,3-DPG and P_{50} with maximal and submaximal exercise, Med. Sci. Sports **6**:238, 1974.

16. Whipp, B.J.: The respiratory system. In Ross, G., editor: Essentials of human physiology, Chicago, 1978, Year Book Medical Publishers, Inc.

SUGGESTED READINGS

Lambertsen, C.J.: Transport of oxygen and carbon dioxide by the blood. In Mountcastle, V.B., editor: Medical physiology, ed. 13, vol. 2, St. Louis, 1974, The C.V. Mosby Co.

Whipp, B.J.: The respiratory system. In Ross, G., editor: Essentials of human physiology, Chicago, 1978, Year Book Medical Publishers, Inc.

CASE STUDY 1

A track athlete from UCLA joined us one summer in Laramie, Wyoming (altitude 7,200 feet) to work and run at the higher altitude. This young woman noticed that her long-distance runs were slower in Laramie than in coastal (sea level) Los Angeles. However, except for minor tiredness during the first few days, which could have been attributable to travel and time change, there were no symptoms related to the increase in altitude. Adaptation occurred quickly and for the most part was not noticed.

In a subsequent summer this same athlete joined us on Pike's Peak (altitude 14,100 feet) for a research project we were conducting on the effects of high altitude on exercise performance. She flew from Los Angeles to Denver, and drove immediately to Colorado Springs and up to the summit of Pike's Peak. Within a few hours she was completely incapacitated with symptoms of mountain sickness: nausea, dizziness, anorexia, and headache. The symptoms were not life threatening, but they were very uncomfortable. Within 2 to 3 days symptoms were reduced, and they had subsided completely in a week.

How is it that a person who travels from sea level to an elevation of 7,200 feet with no apparent symptoms develops acute mountain sickness with ascent to 14,100 feet? This problem, along with performance implications with altitude sojourns, will be addressed in detail in Chapter 12. It is sufficient to say, at this point, that definitive explanations for the causes of mountain sickness do not appear to be forthcoming. However, a simplistic explanation relating to the oxyhemoglobin dissociation curve can be given. Below are some descriptive characteristics of the three locations involved in this case.

	Elevation (feet)	P_B (mm Hg)	Atmospheric P_{O_2} (mm Hg)	S_{O_2} (%)
Los Angeles	0	760	159	95
Laramie	7,200	580	121	93
Pike's Peak	14,100	420	88	82

Elevation, barometric pressure, and atmospheric P_{O_2} in the atmosphere change in linear fashion; that is, as elevation increases the barometric pressure and atmospheric P_{O_2} go down proportionately. However, between Los Angeles and Laramie the arterial S_{O_2} declined only 2%, but increasing the elevation a comparable amount again (the ascent to Pike's Peak) brings an additional reduction of 11%. This 13% drop in S_{O_2} between Los Angeles and Pike's Peak places P_{O_2} on the steep portion of the oxyhemoglobin dissociation curve. The % S_{O_2} for Laramie, however, is represented on the upper part of the curve, showing that relatively large reductions in partial pressure result in only small reductions in % S_{O_2} at the lower altitude.

Although we can see that the partial pressure change precipitates the altitude symptomatology, we still know relatively little about the underlying physiological mechanisms. Possible explanations are suggested in Chapter 12.

Swimmers often hyperventilate before events. Universally, they will correctly tell you that they perform this maneuver to increase their breath-holding ability early in the race. In contrast, they tend to be universally incorrect in their explanation of the physiological cause of this ability. A typical answer is, "It increases my oxygen."

We know that arterial blood is almost completely saturated with oxygen, even with normal breathing. Thus, it is unlikely that voluntary hyperpnea (hyperventilation) raises arterial oxygen concentration appreciably. On the other hand, hyperventilation does increase the rate of alveolar carbon dioxide exchange with the atmosphere. This decreases alveolar carbon dioxide tension, increasing the gradient between the alveoli and the pulmonary capillary. Therefore, diffusion of carbon dioxide from blood increases. Because most carbon dioxide is carried as bicarbonate ions, carbon dioxide diffusion results in a decrease in both these and the hydrogen ions that formed when the bicarbonate ions were formed. Decreasing bicarbonate and hydrogen ions increases blood pH. This response creates *respiratory alkalosis*. Continuous, rapid hyperventilation increases the excitability of both the peripheral and the central nervous systems. This causes a tingling sensation in the extremities, and the lack of carbon dioxide as a stimulant for breathing can cause dizziness. After voluntary hyperventilation stops, the rate and depth of respiration are depressed until arterial carbon dioxide tension is brought back into equilibrium. During this period the stimulus for breathing is depressed. Thus, many swimmers can swim a lap without taking a breath.

The other side of the coin is hypoventilation (underbreathing). As you might expect, with this condition alveolar carbon dioxide tension rises. Because of the decreased pressure gradient arterial carbon dioxide tension rises also. This results in the increase of bicarbonate and hydrogen ions and the decrease of blood pH. This response is termed *respiratory acidosis*. Symptoms of this condition are increased rate and depth of respiration.

chapter 8

KIDNEY FUNCTION AND ACID-BASE BALANCE

MAJOR LEARNING OBJECTIVE

The kidneys play an impotant role in physiological homeostasis. For example, the kidneys are involved in maintaining body fluid balance. Increases in urine protein are found with increasing exercise intensity. This condition has been called ''athletic pseudonephritis.'' Blood has also been found in the urine of athletes, unrelated to trauma.

APPLICATIONS

Frequent ingestion of water before and during long-distance activities is suggested for maintenance of fluid balance. Race directors should provide fluids periodically over long-distance race courses.

"**L**A fixite du milieu interieur est la condition de la vie libre." This statement by Claude Bernard, nineteenth century physiologist, which established the concept of homeostasis in modern biology, also serves as an appropriate departure for a discussion of the kidneys. Indeed, the kidneys are responsible for maintaining internal equilibrium of the body fluids. Substances useful to bodily function need to be retained. Substances produced in excess or those that disturb homeostasis need to be eliminated. The function of the kidney is analogous to that of the offensive lineman in football. It "clears the way" so that the other organs can perform effectively. This chapter focuses on kidney function,

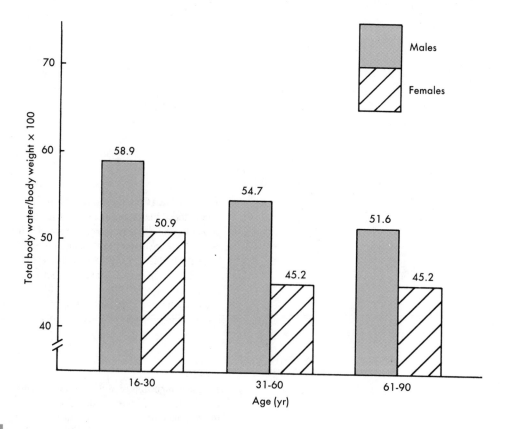

FIG. 8-1   Total body water, expressed as a percentage of body weight, with special reference to age and sex differences. (Data from Randall, H.T.: Fluid, electrolyte, and acid-base balance, Surg. Clin. North Am. *56:*1019, 1976.)

particularly in regard to kidney response to exercise. Special emphasis is also given to acid-base balance, in which the kidneys play an important role.

BODY FLUIDS AND THEIR CONSTITUENTS

Fluids in the body are contained in two primary fluid compartments.[31] The fluids of the *intracellular compartment* account for 30% to 40% of total body weight.[31] The fluids of the *extracellular compartment* account for about 20% of total body weight. The extracellular compartment comprises three subunits that contain (1) the fluids of the interstitial spaces, (2) the plasma, and (3) special fluids such as cerebrospinal and intraocular fluids. Figure 8-1 shows total body water, expressed as a percentage of total body weight, with special reference to age and sex differences. Differences are also related to body fat amounts. For example, females maintain a larger percentage of body weight as fat, which contains less water than muscle. The average male (70 kilograms body weight) has 42 liters of body water. Distribution of body water throughout the various fluid compartments is shown in Figure 8-2. Two thirds of body water is intracellular.

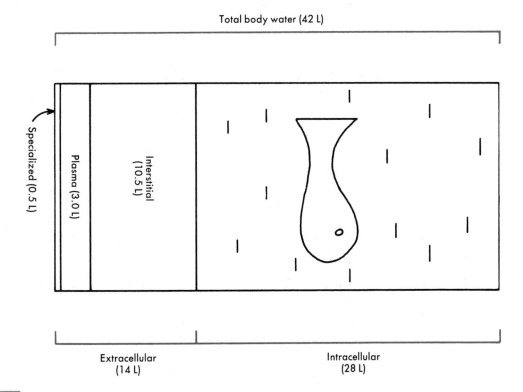

FIG. 8-2   Body water compartments and their volumes in the average male (70 kg body weight).

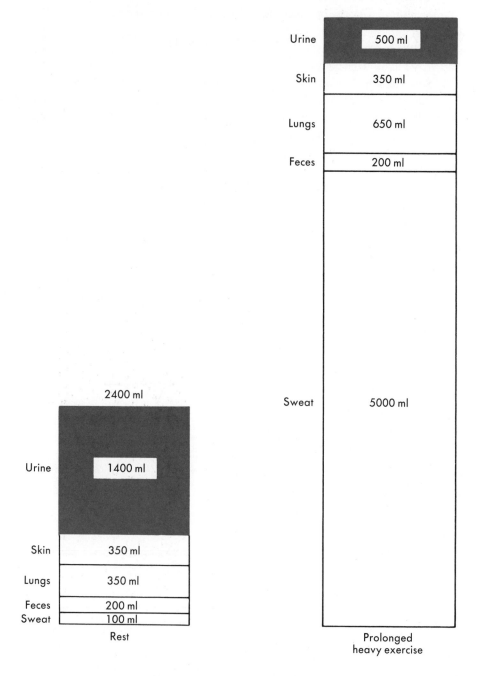

Urine	500 ml
Skin	350 ml
Lungs	650 ml
Feces	200 ml
Sweat	5000 ml

2400 ml

Urine	1400 ml
Skin	350 ml
Lungs	350 ml
Feces	200 ml
Sweat	100 ml

Rest

Prolonged
heavy exercise

FIG. 8-3   **Daily water loss at rest and during prolonged, heavy exercise. (Data from Guyton, A.C.: Textbook of medical physiology, ed. 6, Philadelphia, 1981, W.B. Saunders Co.)**

The electrical equilibrium of cells depends on a predominance of potassium (K^+) within cells and a predominance of sodium (Na^+) and chloride (Cl^-) in interstitial fluid. Both intracellular and interstitial fluid volumes depend on the *osmolality* of the fluids, that is, the number of particles contained in the solution. Osmolality is measured as the number of milliosmoles per kilogram of water in the solution. The average osmolality of body fluids is 285 mOsm $\cdot$ kg^{-1} water.[13] When osmolality of body fluids exceeds this amount, the normal kidney excretes high-osmolality urine, and when body fluid osmolality is lower than this amount, the kidney excretes low-osmolality urine.

To maintain water balance, the intake of water must equal output. We are reliant on our thirst mechanism for controlling intake. At rest, some water is lost from the body by evaporation from the skin and lungs (insensible water loss), by sweating, and in the feces. Most of the water lost is excreted by the kidneys. During prolonged heavy exercise, however, most water is lost through sweating[15] (see Figure 8-3).

FUNCTIONAL ANATOMY

Although the human body has two kidneys, they function as one and can be considered as such (Figure 8-4). Each kidney weighs about 150 grams. Kidney blood supply

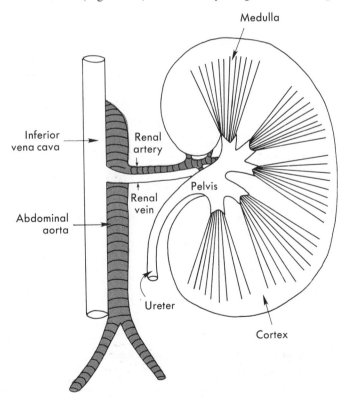

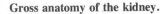 **FIG. 8-4**   **Gross anatomy of the kidney.**

arrives through the renal artery via the abdominal aorta. The basic anatomical unit of the kidney is the *nephron,* of which there are 1,200,000. No new nephrons develop after birth.[13] A nephron can be anatomically separated into the *glomerulus* (Figure 8-5) and the *tubular system* (Figure 8-6). The *glomerulus* is a tuft of capillaries separated by the *afferent arteriole* and the *efferent arteriole.* Between 20% and 25% (1,200 ml) of the cardiac output enters the kidneys per minute. Because the *glomerular membrane* has many pores, it is approximately 100 times more permeable than skeletal muscle.[27] The membrane is highly permeable to water and most particles (solutes), except protein, that body water carries. Water and solutes filter into *Bowman's capsule* and enter the tubular system. As shown in Figure 8-6, the tubular system consists of the *proximal tubules,* the *loop of Henle,* the *distal tubule,* and the *collecting tubule.* Emanating from the efferent arteriole is the *peritubular capillary,* which runs parallel to the tubular system. As the filtered fluid passes through the tubules, most of the water and some solutes are refiltered into the peritubular capillaries and transported out of the kidney via the venous system. The water and solutes that are not refiltered become urine travelling into the *kidney pelvis* and

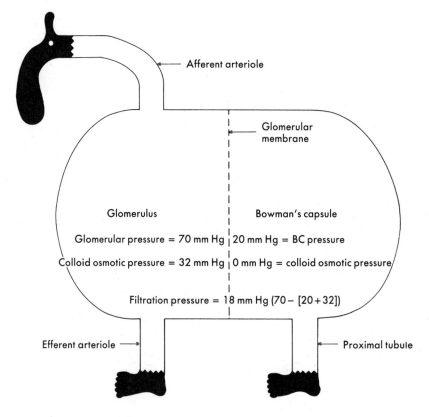

FIG. 8-5   **The glomerulus with special reference to the pressure gradient (filtration pressure) across the glomerular membrane.**

through the *ureter* to the *urinary bladder*. Retention and elimination of water and solutes depend on the body's needs. For example, virtually all of the glucose filtered by the kidney is reabsorbed and recirculated. On the other hand, creatinine, a by-product of protein metabolism that is not usable by the body, is completely excreted.

KIDNEY FUNCTION

Glomerulus

Blood enters the glomerulus through the afferent arteriole at the rate of about 1,200 ml · min⁻¹. In normal men, approximately 125 ml · min⁻¹ (180 L · day⁻¹) is filtered through the glomerular membrane. This value is about 10% less in women.[13] *Renal blood flow* (RBF) is a direct function of changes in arterial pressure and an inverse function of resistance in the afferent and efferent arterioles.[13] In other words, if arterial pressure increases, renal blood flow increases, and if arterial resistance increases, renal blood flow decreases.

The *glomerular filtration rate* (GFR) is directly proportional to filtration pressure. Filtration pressure is affected by glomerular capillary pressure, Bowman's capsule pressure, and colloid osmotic pressure (COP).[31] Filtration pressure is illustrated in Figure 8-5. Since colloid osmotic pressure is determined primarily by plasma proteins, and very few

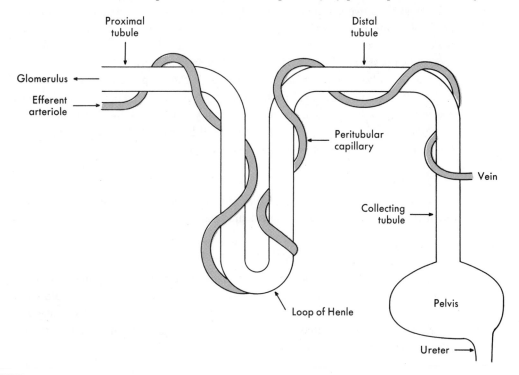

FIG. 8-6   The tubular system.

protein molecules can pass through the glomerular membrane, colloid osmotic pressure is essentially 0 in Bowman's capsule. However, the filtration pressure (18 mm Hg) and the porosity of the glomerular membrane allow water and dissolved plasma constituents to enter Bowman's capsule freely. If for some reason the afferent arteriole is constricted, there is a decrease in glomerular pressure, which reduces filtration pressure and, in turn, the amount of filtrate.

Tubular system

Of the 180 liters of filtrate entering the tubular system each day, a little over a liter is excreted as urine. Urine output varies directly with renal blood flow. For example, during exercise urine output decreases. This decrease is probably a result of the decrease in renal blood flow caused by sympathetic nerve stimulation, which constricts afferent arterioles, thus decreasing glomerular pressure.

Reabsorption occurs selectively throughout the tubular system. Glucose, protein, and amino acids are refiltered in the proximal tubules. *Electrolytes,* such as sodium, potassium, and chloride, are reabsorbed in all but the collecting tubules. Extracellular osmolality is controlled by production of urine with higher solute concentrations when electrolytes are in excess, and vice versa when electrolyte levels are low. Electrolytes must be reabsorbed by *active transport,* that is, through diffusion into peritubular capillaries by means of chemical "carrier" substances at the expense of energy. With the disappearance of electrolytes from tubular fluid, a large concentration gradient develops, causing water to be drawn passively into the peritubular capillaries as well.

In a 1923 classic experiment, Marshall and Vickers[26] proved that the tubules of the kidney also contain secretory mechanisms. The normal secretions of the tubules are creatinine, potassium, and hydrogen ions. These substances move out of the tubular epithelium into the tubules. This movement will be examined in subsequent sections in discussions of regulation of potassium and hydrogen ions.

Kidney function measurements

A test of kidney function is the measurement of *plasma clearance,* that is, the extent to which the kidney excretes unwanted substances.

$$\text{Plasma clearance} = \frac{\text{Amount of substance in urine (mg} \cdot \text{min}^{-1})}{\text{Amount of substance in plasma (mg} \cdot \text{ml}^{-1} \text{ plasma})}$$

Since glomerular filtration rate in humans cannot be measured directly with micropuncture techniques, indirect measurements must be made. A typical estimate measures *inulin clearance.* Inulin, a starch, is a diagnostic aid used specifically in testing glomerular filtration. Inulin is filtered by the glomerulus but is not reabsorbed, that is, the amount found in the urine is the amount filtered by the glomerulus.

$$\text{GFR} = \frac{\text{Amount of inulin in urine} \cdot \text{min}^{-1}}{\text{Concentration of inulin in plasma}}$$

Renal blood flow can be estimated by measuring the clearance of *p-aminohippurate* (PAH) after it has been injected intravenously. PAH is almost completely excreted by the kidney so that venous amounts approach 0.

The concentration of urine is often measured as specific gravity. Normal urine specific gravity is 1.010. Specific gravity for concentrated urine is approximately 1.035 and for dilute urine is about 1.001.

Regulation of electrolytes

Figure 8-7 illustrates the various theories suggested for explaining sodium regulation. When the concentration of sodium increases in extracellular fluid, the renal tubules decrease reabsorption of sodium so that its concentration increases in the urine. When the extracellular concentration is too low the opposite occurs. In the latter case, *aldosterone*,

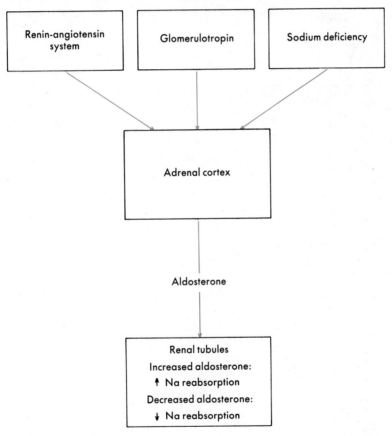

FIG. 8-7 The role of aldosterone in the regulation of sodium reabsorption: alternative theories. (Drawn from material in Guyton, A.C.: Physiology of the human body, ed. 6, Philadelphia, 1984, Saunders College.)

secreted by the adrenal cortex, acts on the renal tubules to cause increased reabsorption. Three theories have been offered to explain this *adrenal cortical response.*[16] One suggests that a sodium deficiency can act directly on the adrenal cortex. A second theory suggests that a sodium deficiency can cause midbrain structures to release *glomerulotropin* into the bloodstream, which stimulates the adrenal cortex to secrete aldosterone. A third theory purports that the *renin-angiotensin system* is involved. Sodium deficiency, according to this theory, causes the release of renin within the kidney. Renin leads to the formation of

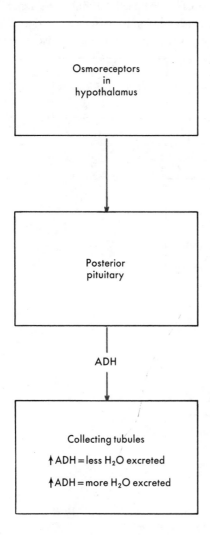

FIG. 8-8   **Control of ADH release from the posterior pituitary.**

angiotensin I and angiotensin II, which travel in the bloodstream to the adrenal cortex.

Regulation of potassium is secondary to regulation of sodium. When aldosterone increases reabsorption of sodium, it simultaneously decreases potassium reabsorption. It has also been found that potassium has a direct effect on the adrenal cortex.

Chloride (Cl^-) and bicarbonate ion regulation (HCO_3^-) are also secondary to sodium regulation. When sodium (Na^+) is refiltered, it leaves an electronegativity within the tubule. Therefore, for each sodium ion reabsorbed either a chloride ion or a bicarbonate ion is also refiltered. Which ion follows depends on the acid-base balance of the extracellular fluid. If the extracellular fluid is acidic, more HCO_3^- is reabsorbed.

Regulation of water balance

Water balance in the body is related to the kidneys' ability to concentrate urine. For instance, when the fluid compartments are filled with excess water, the kidneys produce dilute urine. When water is lacking, the kidneys produce highly concentrated urine. The permeability of the pores in the collecting tubule can be altered by the release of *antidiuretic hormone* (ADH). With water loss, the osmolality of body fluids increases. This increase is detected by osmoreceptors located in the hypothalamus (supraoptic and paraventricular nuclei), which, in turn, stimulate the posterior pituitary to release antidiuretic hormone (see Figure 8-8). Antidiuretic hormone causes the pores of the collecting tubule to become extremely permeable to water; thus, water is reabsorbed by the kidney, resulting in the excretion of concentrated urine. However, the *filtrate* that comes from the distal tubules is normally dilute because body water is normally plentiful. When there is an excess of body water, antidiuretic hormone release is inhibited. Thus, the permeability of the collecting tubules is reduced markedly, and urine remains dilute as it goes to the bladder.

KIDNEY RESPONSE TO EXERCISE

Exercise represents an interesting variant from the normal stress faced by the kidney. The body requires greater cardiac output during exercise to meet the energy requirements of working tissues. The kidney does not require a great blood flow, since it is not a major organ of exercise responses. But changes that take place in the body during prolonged exercise, like water and electrolyte losses, dictate a more than passive role for the kidney.

Renal blood flow and glomerular filtration rate

Renal blood flow has been studied mainly by measurement of PAH clearance. In short-term exercise renal blood flow decreases as exercise intensity increases[14] (see Figure 8-9). When heart rate is used as a measure of exercise intensity a negative correlation (−0.89) has been observed between the percentage decrease in renal blood flow during exercise and exercise heart rate. For example, at a heart rate of 150 the renal blood flow decreased to 62% of what it was at rest. This finding was confirmed during prolonged submaximal (45 minutes) and maximal exercise.[8] During 12-minute stints at 47%, 77%, and 100% of $\dot{V}O_2$ max, renal blood flow decreased by 32%, 54%, and 72%, respectively. When exercise time at 47% of maximum was extended to 90 minutes, no further decrease in renal blood flow (32%) was observed. It is clear that blood flow to the kidney is reduced during exercise. A decrease from 1,200 ml $\cdot$ min^{-1} at rest to 250 ml $\cdot$ min^{-1} during maximum exercise has been reported.[3] This decrease seems to be the result of constriction of both afferent and efferent arterioles.[33]

Practical summary. The research just presented shows that as exercise intensity increases, blood flow to the kidney decreases. Blood volume is shunted to other areas of the body more critical to exercise maintenance.

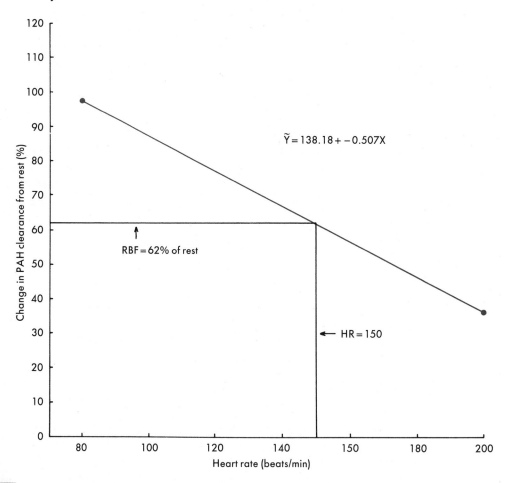

$$\tilde{Y} = 138.18 + -0.507X$$

RBF = 62% of rest

← HR = 150

Change in PAH clearance from rest (%)

Heart rate (beats/min)

FIG. 8-9   The relationship of change in renal blood flow (estimated from PAH clearance) and exercise heart rate. At an *HR* of 150 the renal blood flow is reduced to 62% of rest. (Regression line computed from data of Grimby, G.: Renal clearances during prolonged supine exercise at different loads, J. Appl. Physiol. *20:*1294, 1965.)

Although glomerular filtration also decreases with exercise, the decrease is less marked than that of renal blood flow. Glomerular filtration rate is fairly stable until heart rate reaches 150, at which point there is a greater, more significant decrease. A decrease of 30% has been reported with moderate and heavy exercise.[29] Since the decline of the glomerular filtration rate is less than the decline in renal blood flow, filtration must be protected because of the increase in filtration fraction. The increase in filtration fraction is probably caused by the balance in constriction between the afferent and efferent arterioles.[6] A larger decrease in glomerular filtration rate has been observed in dehydrated subjects.[32] Since most kidney experiments are conducted using hyperhydrated subjects, glomerular filtration rate studies may not be accurate.

Practical summary. The research just presented shows that filtering by the kidney is reduced during exercise. However, major reductions do not occur until moderate to heavy exercise intensities are reached, and even during heavy exercise the kidney continues to filter.

Urine flow

Urine flow decreases during and after exercise, but the rate is not predictable. This, again, may be caused by variable water loads of subjects in these experiments. A correlation of 0.78 between decreased exercise urine flow and decreased glomerular filtration rate has been reported.[6] Since glomerular filtration rate decreases significantly only during moderate or heavy exercise, one would not expect urine flow to decrease until then. One study, in fact, reported no antidiuretic effect until subjects were engaged in heavy exercise.[20] Only small amounts of water were given to subjects in this experiment to avoid hyperhydration, since hyperhydration stimulates antidiuresis.

Practical summary. Participants in endurance events who heed recommendations about water intake during prolonged exercise will probably experience the need to urinate during events. However, athletes participating in high-intensity, short-duration events will most likely not feel the need to urinate during exercise.

Electrolytes

Fourteen males were studied during 45-minute periods of submaximal bicycle ergometer exercise (supine).[7] Urinary sodium excretion decreased significantly during exercise. This decrease was about 50% of resting levels. Another similar investigation also noted a decrease in urinary sodium.[14] The decrease is thought to be associated with an increase in tubular reabsorption, which may be secondary to changes in the hormone aldosterone.[7] Sodium, chloride, and water excretion were found to be depressed 24 to 48 hours following 60 minutes of exercise at about 60% $\dot{V}O_2$ max.[10] This response was thought to be only partly related to aldosterone, since aldosterone levels returned to normal within 6 to 12 hours.

Changes in potassium excretion are apparently not consistent with changes in excretion of other electrolytes during exercise. No change in potassium excretion was reported with 45 minutes of submaximal supine exercise.[7] However, with heavy exercise, potassium excretion is known to increase. This inconsistency may be related to renal blood flow, that is, renal blood flow must decrease below a critical level.[6]

Practical summary. These studies indicate that athletes who sweat heavily during long periods of exercise need to be concerned with loss of electrolytes, especially sodium.

Urinary protein

Urinary protein increases following exercise have been reported for more than 100 years.[24] After discovering protein and other formed elements in the urine of a high percentage of football players, it was suggested that the response was similar to acute glomerular nephritis (acute inflammation of the glomerulae, marked by increased excretion of protein, cells, and other substances).[12] The condition was named, because of its

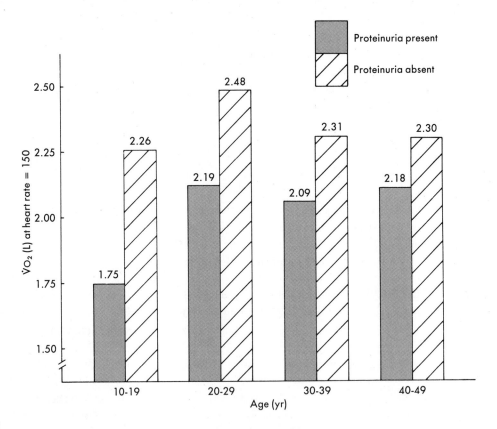

FIG. 8-10 $\dot{V}O_2$ at HR 150 in those who do and do not exhibit proteinuria in various age groups. (Data from Perlman, L.V., Cunningham, D., Montoye, H., and others: Exercise proteinuria, Med. Sci. Sports 2:20, 1970.)

transience, *athletic pseudonephritis*. To determine whether this condition is traumatic in origin, five groups, representing both contact and noncontact sport athletes, were studied.[1] The percentage of those showing urinary albumin (protein) varied between 70% and 100%. Track, a noncontact sport, showed the highest percentage, indicating that the response is unrelated to trauma. The condition normalizes 1 hour after short, heavy exercise and 10 hours after endurance work, specifically an 85 kilometer ski race.[9]

In another study the presence of urinary protein was measured before and after a maximal treadmill run in 499 males. Oxygen consumption at a heart rate of 150 ($\dot{V}O_2$ − 150) was found to be related to the occurrence of *proteinuria*. Subjects in all age groups showed proteinuria when exercising at 150% $\dot{V}O_2$ max (Figure 8-10). It has been found that proteinuria increases with exercise intensity,[20] and also that exercise proteinuria can be reduced with training.[5]

Increased glomerular membrane permeability and decreased tubular reabsorption were thought to be related to exercise proteinuria.[28] Investigators could find no evidence of change in tubular reabsorption but agreed that glomerular permeability for relatively large molecules (protein) is increased.[9] Because of significant correlations between protein excretion and glomerular filtration rate and between blood pH and decreased glomerular filtration rate, others propose that proteinuria is related to increased permeability of the glomerular membrane induced by increased blood acidity.[18]

Practical summary. Exercise proteinuria is not thought to be dangerous to the athlete, and the condition should not affect a player's eligibility to participate in a sport.

Urinary sediments

Urinary sediments consist of red blood cells, white blood cells, epithelial cells, crystals, and casts. Few sedimentary elements are found in normal urine. Figure 8-11 illustrates a study in which amounts of erythrocytes, leukocytes, and epithelial cells in urine were measured before and after a progressive bicycle ergometer test.[29] Increases were noted in all three cell types following exercise. Similar results have been reported following walking and jogging on treadmills.[21]

Several researchers have reported hyaline casts in urine after strenuous exercise.[1,17,21] Hyaline casts consist primarily of urinary glycoprotein (uromucoid), which originates in the kidney cortex.[29] As with proteinuria, kidney trauma has been suggested as a cause of hyaline casts, but no differences were found between amounts found in contact and noncontact sport athletes.[1] Renal biopsies performed on two patients showed abnormal urine following a strenuous bout of squat jumps.[17] Casts and tubular abnormalities were similar to but distinguishable from symptoms of acute glomerular nephritis.

Practical summary. The causes of postexercise urinary sedimentation are not completely understood, but the condition is not, in and of itself, thought to contraindicate activity participation.

Control of water balance during exercise

To achieve water balance during exercise, sodium and water excretion must be under precise control. Extracellular fluid volume is regulated by the excretion of sodium and water. When the osmolality of extracellular fluid decreases because of a loss of water, the change is detected by hypothalamic osmoreceptors, which, in turn, stimulate secretion of antidiuretic hormone. Aldosterone also regulates water balance by causing sodium reab-

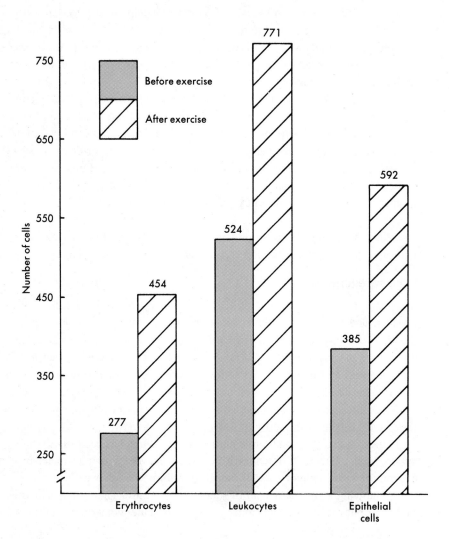

FIG. 8-11   Urinary sediments (erythrocytes, leukocytes, and epithelial cells) before and after progressive bicycle ergometer exercise. (Data from Poortmans, J.R.: Exercise and renal function. In Hutton, R.S., editor: Exercise and sports sciences reviews, vol. 5, Santa Barbara, 1977, Journal Publishing Affiliates.)

sorption, which causes water to be drawn passively into the capillaries. Thus, how aldosterone is controlled during exercise is an important concern of those involved in endurance sports and sports in which water loss is excessive, for instance, football players playing in hot climates.

Research shows that the renin-angiotensin system plays an important role in the control of aldosterone during exercise.[23,25] Renin activity was studied in six subjects each working at 40%, 70%, and 100% $\dot{V}O_2$ max on the bicycle ergometer.[23] Norepinephrine and epinephrine *(catecholamines)* levels were also measured. Figure 8-12 shows that both renin and norepinephrine were significantly increased with exercise at 70% and 100% $\dot{V}O_2$ max, but not at 40%. Epinephrine levels were not significantly changed at any exercise level. Because of the parallel response of renin and norepinephrine, a sympathetic catecholamine, the researchers suggested that renin activity may be related to sympathetic nervous system activity. The direct relationship between renin activity and exercise intensity has been confirmed.[25] It is believed that during exercise the sympathetic nervous system stimulates the kidney to produce renin and angiotensin II. Renin constricts the afferent arterioles to reduce renal blood flow, and angiotensin II stimulates the adrenal cortex to release antidiuretic hormone.[6,29]

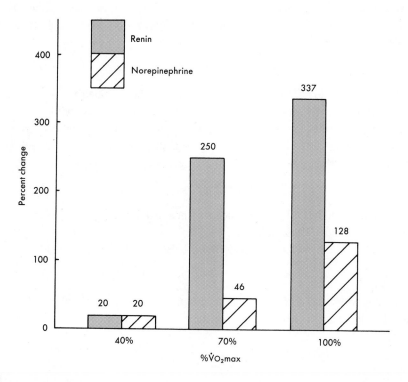

FIG. 8-12 Percent change in renin and norepinephrine at various exercise intensities. (Data from Kotchen, T.A., Hartley, L.H., Rice, T.W., and others: Renin, norepinephrine, and epinephrine responses to graded exercise, J. Appl. Physiol. *31:*178, 1971.)

Practical summary. Although the exact mechanisms by which the kidney controls water balance are not completely understood, the research shows that the kidney conserves body water during heavy exercise and in the heat by producing concentrated urine and by reabsorbing water back into the blood.

ACID-BASE BALANCE

Resting blood pH is 7.4. Blood pH varies from this norm to values as low as 7.0 (acidic) or as high as 7.8 (basic). Values beyond these points are not compatible with life. When body acidity increases, homeostasis is maintained either by adding a basic material to buffer the acid or by ridding the body of the accumulated hydrogen ions. There are three body processes that accomplish this task under nondisease conditions. The first process is the release of chemical buffers contained in blood plasma. This is a fast-reacting process that can occur within a fraction of a second. Respiratory regulation is the second process. One to 3 minutes is required for this response to occur. The third regulatory process of acid-base balance occurs in the kidney. Response of this system is much slower than the others and can take from several hours to a day or more. Exercise and sport often result in the accumulation of hydrogen ions and the reduction of blood pH. Understanding the mechanisms involved in regulating pH can help scientists protect athletes and hypothesize procedures that might minimize the debilitating effects of lowered pH.

Chemical regulation of acid-base balance

Even in the resting state the body must buffer acids created by food metabolism. By-products of oxidative metabolism are termed *volatile* acids. Carbonic acid (H_2CO_3), for example, is formed by the interaction of water and carbon dioxide during aerobic energy production. Carbonic acid dissociates to hydrogen ions (H^+) and bicarbonate ions (HCO_3^-).

$$CO_2 + H_2O \leftrightarrows H_2CO_3 \rightleftarrows H^+ + HCO_3^-$$

Nonvolatile acids in the body are produced by the breakdown of protein. These are mainly phosphoric acid and sulfuric acid.

The primary chemical buffer in body fluids is HCO_3^-. This process works as follows:

$$HCO_3^- + H^+ \leftrightarrows H_2CO_3 \rightleftarrows CO_2 + H_2O$$

The strong acid HCO_3^- forms a weak acid, H_2CO_3. To understand this buffering mechanism, it is necessary to be familiar with the Henderson-Hasselbalch equation:

$$pH = pK + \log\left(\frac{Base}{Acid}\right)$$

Bicarbonate ions (HCO_3^-) represent the base in the equation, and carbonic acid (H_2CO_3) represents the acid. When acid and base are in equilibrium in body fluids, pH is 7.4. The term *pK* is a constant related to the dissociation of acid in a buffer and is 6.1 in blood plasma. In other words, the pH of body fluids can be calculated if bicarbonate ion and carbonic acid concentrations are measured. Therefore, if the bicarbonate ion concentration is 24 mM per liter and carbonic acid concentration is 1.2 mM per liter, the pH is calculated as follows[31]:

$$pH = 6.1 + \log \frac{24 \text{ mM}}{1.2 \text{ mM}} = 7.4$$

Phosphates and proteins also buffer acids in body fluids. Hemoglobin is the most important buffer in the blood.

Respiratory regulation of acid-base balance

This mechanism is discussed in Chapter 7 in relation to respiratory acidosis and alkalosis. To reiterate, respiration controls the accumulation of carbon dioxide in body fluids. If carbon dioxide builds up, arterial partial pressure of carbon dioxide rises,

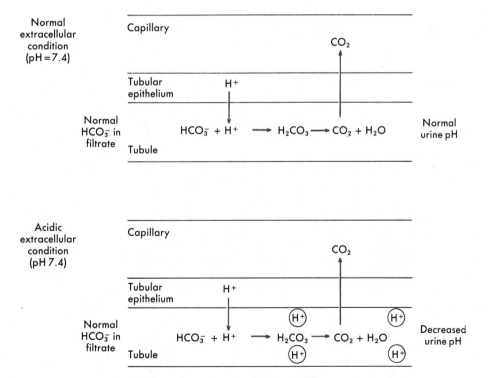

FIG. 8-13 **Mechanism by which acid-base balance is regulated by the kidney. Under normal conditions HCO$_3^-$ in filtrate is balanced by H$^+$ ions secreted by tubular epithelium. When the extracellular fluid is acidic, HCO$_3^-$ is low in the filtrate, thus all the secreted H$^+$ ions cannot be buffered. Excess H$^+$ ions are eliminated in the urine.**

resulting in decreased pH. The decrease in pH is detected by the respiratory center, which causes increased ventilation and elimination of carbon dioxide. The opposite occurs with respiratory alkalosis.

Kidney regulation of acid-base balance

The kidneys regulate acid-base balance by excreting acid urine when hydrogen ion concentration in extracellular fluid is too high, and secreting bicarbonate ions when the extracellular fluid is too basic. Acid-base regulation in the kidneys occurs primarily in the distal tubules. The process is complicated and is thus treated briefly here. Figure 8-13 indicates that under normal conditions the amount of hydrogen ion secreted by the tubular epithelium equals the amount of tubular bicarbonate. Hydrogen ions combine with bicarbonate ions to form carbonic acid, which dissociates to carbon dioxide and water. The carbon dioxide passes into capillaries and travels to the lungs to be exchanged. Under acidic conditions, smaller amounts of bicarbonate ions are filtered by the glomerulus, leaving an excess of hydrogen ions in the tubular fluid. This excess in hydrogen ions is excreted in the urine.

pH as a limiting factor during exercise

During exercise with a high anaerobic component, lactic acid is produced in quantities greater than the body's ability to buffer it. It seems reasonable to assume that the lowered pH produced in such situations might be a limiting factor for further exercise. To test this hypothesis 10 normal males were tested before and after 400 meter runs under two conditions.[22] One condition was a normal control, and in the other test subjects received an infusion of bicarbonate buffer before the run. Run time and maximum lactic acid accumulation were unchanged even though blood pH level was raised from 7.1 to 7.2 when the bicarbonate buffer infusion was given. The investigators questioned the importance of pH as a limiting factor. Similar results have been found by others.[4] However, neither study used a placebo (a similar but inert control substance) or double-blind (neither subject nor experimenter knows what substance is being received) procedures.

To resolve the experimental deficiencies of previous studies, a group of investigators administered substances to subjects that produced acidosis (NH_4Cl) and alkalosis ($NaHCO_3$), as well as substances that had no effect (placebo) during exercise at three intensity levels (33%, 66%, and 95% $\dot{V}O_2$ max).[19] During the 95% level exercise, endurance time was significantly longer with alkalosis and significantly shorter with acidosis. Lactic acid accumulation occurred in the same manner; that is, it was significantly higher with alkalosis. These researchers concluded that acidosis is an important factor in endurance performance. In other words, acidosis appears to be a limiting factor in high-intensity, primarily anaerobic events.

SUMMARY

The kidney plays an important role in maintaining body fluid balance and homeostasis. Body fluids are contained in two compartments: the intracellular compartment, which accounts for 30% to 40% of total body weight, and the extracellular compartment, which accounts for 20% of total body weight. The fluid volume of each compartment depends on the osmolality of the fluid, that is, the number of particles (solute) contained in the solution. When the osmolality of body fluids exceeds normal levels, the kidney excretes high-osmolality urine and conserves water. When body fluid osmolality is low the reverse occurs. In persons at rest daily water loss comes mostly from kidney urine production. However, during prolonged exercise most water is lost through sweating.

The basic anatomical unit of the kidney, of which there are 1,200,000, is the nephron. A nephron can be anatomically separated into the glomerulus and the tubular system. Blood entering the glomerulus is filtered through the glomerular membrane. The filtrate enters Bowman's capsule and then passes through the tubular system (proximal tubules, loop of Henle, distal tubules, and collecting tubules) where most of the water and some solutes are reabsorbed into the peritubular capillaries. Water and solutes not reabsorbed are excreted into the bladder as urine.

Renal blood flow is a function of arterial pressure and of resistance in the renal arterioles. Because renal arterioles constrict during exercise, renal blood flow decreases as exercise intensities increase. Glomerular filtration rate also decreases with exercise but less markedly than does renal blood flow.

Urine output varies directly with renal blood flow. Since renal blood flow is decreased during exercise, so is urinary output. This decrease is also related to reduction in glomerular filtration rate.

The osmolality of urine also changes with exercise. Sodium excretion during exercise is reduced by 50%. Reabsorption of water and solutes occurs along the whole tubular system. Tubules also secrete certain substances, namely, creatinine, potassium, and hydrogen ions. Proteinuria (protein in urine) has been found among athletes and thus been termed *athletic pseudonephritis*. The cause of this increase in urinary protein is unknown, but the condition is transient, and studies show that it occurs in both contact and noncontact sport athletes, increases with exercise intensities, and can be reduced with training.

The kidney's ability to concentrate urine, and so to maintain body fluid balance, is related to the permeability of the pores in the collecting tubules. This permeability can be altered by the release of antidiuretic hormone (ADH). When osmolality of extracellular fluid increases, antidiuretic hormone causes water to be reabsorbed by the kidney and results in excretion of concentrated urine.

Three processes regulate acid-base balance. First, acid can be reduced by chemical regulation. The primary chemical buffer in body fluids is bicarbonate. In this process a strong acid (HCO_3^-) combines with hydrogen ions to form a weak acid, carbonic acid, which dissociates to carbon dioxide and water. The second acid-base regulating process involves respiratory regulation. Blood pH can decrease because of accumulation of carbon dioxide. The decrease in pH is detected by the respiratory center, which causes increased ventilation and elimination of carbon dioxide. Kidney regulation is the third acid-base regulatory process. The kidneys excrete acid urine when the hydrogen ion concentration in extracellular fluid is too high and alkaline urine when the bicarbonate ion concentration in extracellular fluid is too high. Although the literature is inconsistent, it appears that acidosis is a limiting factor in high-intensity, primarily anaerobic events.

KEY TERMS

athletic pseudonephritis a transient condition found in athletes following exercise and marked by the increased excretion of protein, cells, and other substances. This condition mimics a kidney disease known as glomerular nephritis.

electrolytes ions, primarily sodium, potassium, and chloride, that play an important role in water balance.

exercise proteinuria excess protein in the urine following exercise.

glomerular filtration rate (GFR) the rate at which blood entering the kidney is filtered through the glomerulus.

osmolality a measure of the number of particles contained in a solution.

plasma clearance the extent to which the kidney excretes unwanted substances.

reabsorption the process by which the kidney returns usable substances to the blood.

renal blood flow (RBF) the rate at which blood enters the kidney (glomerulus) through the afferent arteriole.

REVIEW QUESTIONS

1. How much body water is found in the average male? How does this figure compare with the figure for females?

2. List the major anatomical units of the kidney. Briefly describe the function of each.

3. Describe the processes through which electrolytes are regulated.

4. Describe blood flow to the kidney during exercise. What are the consequences of this response?

5. Why do endurance athletes need to pay attention to electrolyte loss, especially during conditions of high temperature?

6. Is exercise proteinuria related to sports trauma (contact)? Explain.

7. How does the kidney function to conserve water during conditions of high temperature?

8. Explain the relationship between acidosis and performance in anaerobic sports.

REFERENCES

1. Alyea, E.P., and Parish, H.H.: Renal response to exercise: urinary findings, JAMA **167**:807, 1958.

2. American College of Sports Medicine: Position statement on prevention of heat injuries during distance running, Med. Sci. Sports **7**:vii, 1975.

3. Andersen, K.L.: The cardiovascular system in exercise. In Falls, H.B., editor: Exercise physiology, New York, 1968, Academic Press, Inc.

4. Asmussen, E., VonDobeln, W., and Nielsen, M.: Blood lactate and oxygen debt after exhaustive work at different oxygen tensions, Acta Physiol. Scand. **15:**57, 1948.

5. Cantone, A., and Cerretelli, P.: Effect of training on proteinuria following muscular exercise, Int. Z. Angew. Physiol. **18:**324, 1960.

6. Castenfors, J.: Renal function during exercise with special reference to exercise proteinuria and the release of renin, Acta Physiol. Scand. **70**(Suppl. 293):7, 1967.

7. Castenfors, J.: Renal clearances and urinary sodium and potassium excretion during supine exercise in normal subjects, Acta Physiol. Scand. **70:**207, 1967.

8. Castenfors, J.: Renal function during prolonged exercise, Ann. N.Y. Acad. Sci. **301:**151, 1977.

9. Castenfors, J., Mossfeldt, F., and Piscator, M.: Effect of prolonged heavy exercise on renal function and urinary protein excretion, Acta Physiol. Scand. **70:**194, 1967.

10. Costill, D.L., Branam, G., Fink, W., and others: Exercise induced sodium conservation: changes in plasma renin and aldosterone, Med. Sci. Sports **8:**209, 1976.

11. Dill, D.B.: The Harvard Fatigue Laboratory: its development, contributions and demise, Circ. Res. **20** and **21:**161, 1967.

12. Gardner, K.D.: "Athletic pseudonephritis"—alteration of urine sediment by athletic competition, JAMA **161:**1613, 1956.

13. Gottschalk, C.W., and Lassiter, W.E.: Mechanisms of urine formation. In Mountcastle, V.B., editor: Medical physiology, ed. 14, vol. 2, St. Louis, 1980, The C.V. Mosby Co.

14. Grimby, G.: Renal clearances during prolonged supine exercise at different loads, J. Appl. Physiol. **20:**1294, 1965.

15. Guyton, A.C.: Textbook of medical physiology, ed. 6, Philadelphia, 1981, W.B. Saunders Co.

16. Guyton, A.C.: Physiology of the human body, Philadelphia, ed. 6, 1984, Saunders College.

17. Howenstine, J.A.: Exertion-induced myoglobinuria and hemoglobinuria: simulation of acute glomerulonephritis, JAMA **173:**493, 1960.

18. Javitt, N.B., and Miller, A.T.: Mechanism of exercise proteinuria, J. Appl. Physiol. **4:**834, 1952.

19. Jones, N.S., Sutton, J.R., Taylor, R., and others: Effect of pH on cardiorespiratory and metabolic responses to exercise, J. Appl. Physiol. **43:**959, 1977.

20. Kachadorian, W.A., and Johnson, R.E.: Renal responses to various rates of exercise, J. Appl. Physiol. **28:**748, 1970.

21. Kachadorian, W.A., and Johnson, R.E.: The effect of exercise on some clinical measures of renal function, Am. Heart J. **82:**278, 1971.

22. Kindermann, W., Keul, J., and Huber, G.: Physical exercise after induced alkalosis (bicarbonate or tris buffer), Eur. J. Applied Physiol. **37:**197, 1977.

23. Kotchen, T.A., Hartley, L.H., Rice, T.W., and others: Renin, norepinephrine, and epinephrine responses to graded exercise, J. Appl. Physiol. **31:**178, 1971.

24. Leube, W.: Ueber Ausscheidung von Eiweiss im Harn des gesunden Menschen, Virchows Arch. **72:**145, 1878.

25. Maher, J.T., Jones, L.G., Hartley, L.H., and others: Aldosterone dynamics during graded exercise at sea level and high altitude, J. Appl. Physiol. **39**:18, 1975.

26. Marshall, E.K., and Vickers, J.L.: The mechanism of the elimination of phenolsulphonphthalein by the kidney: a proof of secretion by the convoluted tubules, Bull. Johns Hopkins Hosp. **34**:1, 1923.

27. Pappenheimer, J.R.: Passage of molecules through capillary walls, Physiol. Rev. **33**:387, 1953.

28. Perlman, L.V., Cunningham, D., Montoye, H., and others: Exercise proteinuria, Med. Sci. Sports **2**:20, 1970.

29. Poortmans, J.R.: Exercise and renal function. In Hutton, R.S., editor: Exercise and sport sciences reviews, vol. 5, Santa Barbara, 1977, Journal Publishing Affiliates.

30. Randall, H.T.: Fluid, electrolyte, and acid-base balance, Surg. Clin. North Am. **56**:1019, 1976.

31. Schultze, R.G.: Physiology of the kidney. In Ross, G., editor: Essentials of human physiology, Chicago, 1978, Year Book Medical Publishers, Inc.

32. Smith, J.H., Robinson, S., and Pearcy, M.: Renal responses to exercise, heat and dehydration, J. Appl. Physiol. **4**:659, 1952.

33. Wesson, L.G.: Kidney function in exercise. In Johnson, W.R., editor: Science and medicine of exercise and sports, New York, 1960, Harper & Brothers, Publishers.

SUGGESTED READINGS

Castenfors, J.: Renal function during exercise with special reference to exercise proteinuria and the release of renin, Acta Physiol. Scand. **70**(Suppl. 293):7, 1967.

Gottschalk, C.W., and Lassiter, W.E.: Mechanisms of urine formation. In Mountcastle, V.B., editor: Medical physiology, ed. 14, vol. 2, St. Louis, 1980, The C.V. Mosby Co.

Poortmans, J.R.: Exercise and renal function. In Hutton, R.S., editor: Exercise and sport sciences reviews, vol. 5, Santa Barbara, 1977, Journal Publishing Affiliates.

Randall, H.T.: Fluid, electrolyte, and acid-base balance, Surg. Clin. North Am. **56**:1019, 1976.

Schultze, R.G.: Physiology of the kidney. In Ross, G., editor: Essentials of human physiology, Chicago, 1978, Year Book Medical Publishers, Inc.

Wesson, L.G.: Kidney function in exercise. In Johnson, W.R., editor: Science and medicine of exercise and sports, New York, 1960, Harper & Brothers, Publishers.

CASE STUDY

A marathon (26.2 miles) race director called the other day.

DIRECTOR: I know I'm supposed to provide water and electrolyte solutions to runners during marathons, but I'm not sure how much to give them. I'm also curious about the physiological needs for taking water and electrolyte solutions during marathons.

PROFESSOR: First, the amounts of water and electrolyte solutions you should provide can be found in the American College of Sports Medicine's "Position Statement on Prevention of Heat Injuries During Distance Running."[2] The statement is based on research involving long-distance runners. The specific items that will answer your questions are as follows:

3. It is the responsibility of the race sponsors to provide fluids which contain small amounts of sugar (less than 2.5 g glucose · 100 ml^{-1} of water) and electrolytes (less than 10 mEq sodium and 5 mEq potassium per liter of solution).

4. Runners should be encouraged to frequently ingest fluids during competition and to consume 400-500 ml (12-17 oz) of fluid 10-15 minutes before competition.

The electrolyte concentrations of commercial electrolyte solutions should be provided on the labels.

DIRECTOR: OK, but exactly how will this supplementation actually work?

PROFESSOR: To begin with, prevention of heat injuries is related to the maintenance of water balance. As the body heats up, both from environmental heat and from metabolic heat, the body sweats to dissipate the heat. For example, the average marathoner has a body surface area of 1.5 m^2 (height, 68 inches and weight, 135 pounds). With a sweat rate of 1.0 L/m^2 · hr^{-1}, a 3-hour marathoner can lose about 4.5 liters of water. This loss represents roughly 7% of the body weight. Such a severe water loss would lead to significant hyperthermia if replacement fluids were not given.

DIRECTOR: So fluid ingestion replenishes the loss and prevents heat stroke.

PROFESSOR: Exactly. It keeps the internal body temperature down within acceptable physiological limits. It's important to remember that runners' natural instincts to drink are not strong enough to cause them to drink enough to maintain normal hydration. Therefore, they have to be encouraged to drink during the race.

DIRECTOR: Now, how about the electrolytes. What do they do?

PROFESSOR: Let's start with the end of a race. What would the runner's urine look like? You would expect it to be very concentrated, since the kidney does everything possible to keep water from leaving the body. Normal urine has a specific gravity, which is a measure of its concentration, of 1.010. So you could expect the specific gravity of a dehydrated runner's urine to be 1.020 or higher.

DIRECTOR: That means the body is excreting more electrolytes?

PROFESSOR: It is more likely that the body is excreting less water, and thus the fluid is more concentrated. In fact, fewer electrolytes are excreted in urine during and following exercise.

Continued.

DIRECTOR: Why?

PROFESSOR: When water is lost in sweat, electrolytes are also lost. Principally, sodium and chloride are the electrolytes lost from extracellular fluid. The kidney reacts to this electrolyte loss by conserving sodium and chloride. Severe electrolyte loss can lead to muscle cramping and significant water imbalances.

DIRECTOR: So to protect against extreme electrolyte loss we must provide marathon runners with electrolyte solutions.

PROFESSOR: Right. Good luck!

HISTORY OF EXERCISE PHYSIOLOGY

The name Henderson (Henderson-Hasselbalch equation) is often associated with the beginning of the study of exercise physiology in the United States. L.J. Henderson (1878-1942) was a physical chemist at Harvard University who was famous for his research on the physiochemical properties of blood. (One of his awards was from the French Legion of Honor.) In 1913, Henderson wrote *The Fitness of the Environment: An Inquiry into the Biological Significance of the Properties of Matter*. Every future physiologist should read this classic book. Henderson was a remarkable scientist, far ahead of his time.

D.B. Dill[11] claims that Henderson conceived the Harvard Fatigue Laboratory in 1926. He proposed the establishment of a laboratory of human physiology and received grants of $25,000 for equipment and $500,000 for 10 year's operating expenses from the Rockefeller Foundation. Research in the laboratory began in the fall of 1927. The laboratory's first treadmill operated with a motor from a streetcar. The motor was capable of four speeds forward (2.33, 3.5, 5.8, and 7.0 mph) and reverse. The usual treadmill grade (before modern treadmills, which came equipped with grade adjustments) reported in the early literature, 8.6%, was the result of the use of a streetcar jack, which could be raised no further. The 20 years of its existence (the laboratory was dissolved in 1946) were marked by research that laid the foundation for future study of human physiological response to exercise.

The scientists who worked at the Harvard Fatigue Laboratory came from all over the world to work and study there. As they left (Ancel Keys to Minnesota; R.E. Johnson to Illinois; Sid Robinson to Indiana; ''Woody'' Belding to Pittsburgh; Steve Horvath to California; E.H. Christensen to Sweden; Erling Asmussen to Denmark; Rodolfo Margaria to Italy, to name just a few), they became the pioneers of the study of exercise physiology. Most exercise physiologists today can directly or indirectly trace their scientific genealogies back to those who worked at the Harvard Fatigue Laboratory.

Foremost among the protégés of L.J. Henderson was D.B. Dill, who taught at Indiana University during the early 1960s. Still active at well past 90 years of age, Bruce Dill is considered to be the father of exercise physiology in the United States. If Dill is the father, certainly L.J. Henderson was the grandfather.

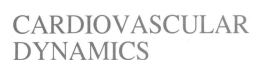

chapter 9

CARDIOVASCULAR DYNAMICS

MAJOR LEARNING OBJECTIVE
Cardiac output is the product of stroke volume and heart rate. Cardiac function can be measured invasively through cardiac catheterization and noninvasively through electrocardiography and echocardiography.

APPLICATIONS
Many physical education programs are conducted with people having cardiac abnormalities or at risk for heart disease. It is necessary to know when the heart is adapting positively to exercise.
■ Before engaging in an exercise program, persons with heart disease, or those at risk for heart disease, should be required to undergo a graded exercise test with electrocardiographic monitoring. Such a test can be used to safely and effectively prescribe an exercise program.

THE evaluation of either health- or performance-related physical fitness requires an understanding of the interaction between muscular contraction and the cardiovascular system. It is understood that muscular contraction requires the nutrients carried in the blood. To reach muscle, blood requires a pump and a series of conduits for transportation. The efficiency of this system determines the capacity for performing work or, in other words, cardiovascular fitness. This chapter addresses the very complex matter of the coupling of the cardiovascular system with muscular contraction.

GENERAL DESCRIPTION OF THE CARDIOVASCULAR SYSTEM

Reference to *the* pump is a misnomer, because in fact, the heart consists of two pumps, the right and left ventricles. The right ventricle pumps blood into the lungs, creating *pulmonary circulation*. The left ventricle pumps blood to all other body systems, creating *systemic circulation*. Figure 9-1 describes the cardiovascular system. The two pumps must work in unison; otherwise unequal volumes would result in pooling of blood on either the pulmonary or systemic side.

The systemic circulation consists of an arterial and a venous side. Successive decrements in arterial diameter occur from the *aorta* to the *arterioles* and ultimately to the *capillaries*. The diameter increases on the venous side beginning with the *venules* and progressing until the *venae cavae* are reached just before entering the heart. A continuous pressure drop of approximately 84 mm Hg (90 mm Hg in the aorta vs 6 mm Hg in the venae cavae) exists between the aorta and the venae cavae and is caused by the resistance offered by smaller diameter vessels. Blood flow can be described by the following equation:

$$\text{Blood flow} = \frac{\text{Pressure difference}}{\text{Resistance}}$$

Therefore, the greater the pressure difference, the greater is the flow, but the greater the resistance, the smaller is the flow.

Resistance can be altered to regulate blood flow, which occurs primarily in the arterioles. For example, blood flow to working skeletal muscle increases during light exercise. This increase is mostly the result of vasodilation of arterioles, which decreases resistance. Increased blood pressure during exercise is another contributing factor.

It is crucial that the heart is able to vary its output; otherwise adaptation to a stress such as exercise would be impossible. *Cardiac output* can be expressed as follows:

$$\text{Cardiac output } (\dot{Q}) = \text{Stroke volume (SV)} \times \text{Heart rate (HR)}$$

An increase in either stroke volume or heart rate can increase cardiac output. During intense exercise, for example, cardiac output can increase fivefold or sixfold (from 5 L/min at rest to 25 or 30 L/min).

Oxygen consumption $(\dot{V}_{O_2})$ by working muscles is partly a function of cardiac output

(SV × HR) and partly results from the ability of the muscle tissue to extract oxygen from the arterial blood, called the arterial-venous oxygen difference (A-V O$_2$ difference). $\dot{V}_{O_2}$ can be expressed by the following equation:

$$\dot{V}_{O_2} = SV \times HR \times \text{A-V O}_2 \text{ difference}$$

Veins are low-pressure, low-resistance vessels responsible for returning blood back to the heart *(venous return)*. Venous return is an important element in the maintenance of stroke volume and therefore the output of the heart. However, veins are able to distend greatly and hold large quantities of blood. For this reason they are referred to as *capacitance* vessels. For example, when a person rises from a lying to a standing position, veins can hold much more blood. Such a movement reduces venous return, which ultimately can cause dizziness. Reduced venous return decreases cardiac output and blood pressure, thus decreasing blood flow to the brain. Because veins are located close to muscles and because of their distensibility, contraction of muscle acts to squeeze blood through the veins, aiding venous return. Since veins contain valves that prevent backflow, muscular contraction pushes blood toward the heart.

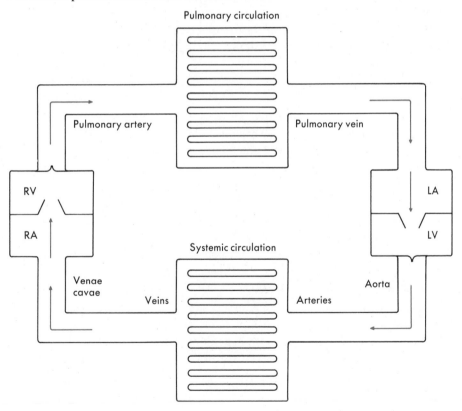

FIG. 9-1   **The cardiovascular system consisting of the heart, pulmonary circulation, and systemic circulation.**

A general description of the cardiovascular system would not be complete without a discussion of blood pressure. As mentioned previously, pressure drops between the left and right sides of the heart. The pressure that can be measured in a doctor's office is peripheral arterial pressure, as contrasted with central pressure, which would require placing a catheter through an artery up to the heart. Peripheral arterial pressure, usually measured over the upper arm, is a measurement of two separate components, *systolic* and *diastolic*. The systolic component reflects the pressure associated with the expulsion of blood from the heart, which in a normal, young adult is approximately 120 mm Hg. The diastolic component reflects the arterial pressure during the relaxation phase of the heart cycle, which is the pressure necessary to hold the arteries open.

MEASUREMENT OF CARDIAC FUNCTION

The exercise physiologist has several tools for measuring cardiac function, ranging from the *invasive* (requiring measurement under the skin) to the *noninvasive* (measurement outside the skin). Invasive techniques are more direct measurements, but noninvasive techniques are more practical. Therefore, human subject experiments use noninvasive procedures except in cases where the risk of invasive techniques is justified. For instance, people with suspected heart disease or left ventricular abnormalities are often subjected to cardiac catheterization to confirm a diagnosis. Only in rare cases are normal athletes investigated in this way.

Electrocardiography

Perhaps the most common noninvasive technique for examining cardiac function is *electrocardiography*. By placing electrodes on the limbs and chest, it is possible to record the passage of the cardiac impulse throughout the chambers of the heart. The impulse that begins the heart cycle originates in the heart itself, the sinoatrial (SA) node. Leaving the SA node, the impulse spreads across the atrial chambers to the atrioventricular (AV) node. From the AV node, the impulses pass through the AV bundle and then separate to travel along the right and left bundle branches, located on either side of the interventricular septum. Reaching the apex of the heart, cardiac innervation continues through each ventricle via Purkinje fibers. It is this impulse transport that can be seen in the electrocardiogram (ECG). Normal electrical function tells a great deal about cardiac function. Therefore, the ECG has been the most widely used cardiac diagnostic tool in the first half of the twentieth century. Figure 9-2 illustrates the normal ECG. The P wave of the ECG represents depolarization of the atria. (You remember that as an impulse passes along a membrane, the polarity changes from a resting state, where the outside is electropositive, to an electronegative state.) When the impulse passes, the polarity returns to resting conditions (repolarization) (see Chapter 2). The QRS complex depicts depolarization of the ventricles. This complex overrides atrial repolarization, making it impossible to observe. The T wave illustrates ventricular repolarization.

In ischemic heart disease patients, where the heart tissue is not receiving enough blood through the coronary arteries, changes can occur in the ECG. For example, a depressed

S-T segment can be observed (see Figure 9-2). Although it has been claimed that certain changes occur in the ECG that distinguish between the hearts of trained and untrained people, it is generally agreed that other measurements are more useful in determining degrees of normality.[9]

Echocardiography

Echocardiography is a noninvasive technique using the principle of reflected ultrasound. In this technique, a transducer is held on the subject's chest in the third or fourth intercostal space, adjacent to the sternum. Sound waves are directed at different areas of

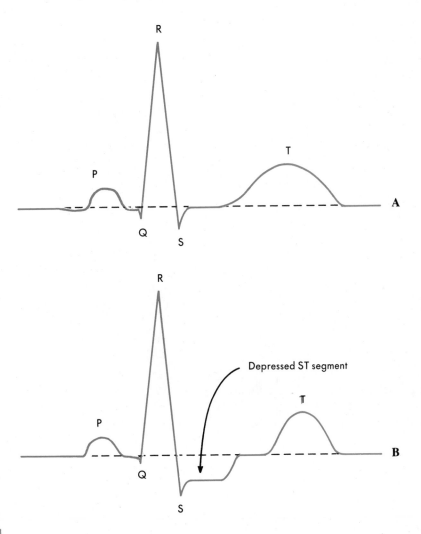

FIG. 9-2   The electrocardiogram illustrating, *A*, a normal wave pattern and, *B*, one type of cardiac abnormality, that is, depressed ST segment (ischemia).

the heart, reflected by its structures, and transmitted back through the transducer. A tracing is recorded as shown in Figure 9-3. Left ventricular size and performance can be evaluated at rest, before exercise, and following exercise. Typical measurements include end-diastolic dimension (Dd); end-systolic dimension (Ds); percent left ventricular dimension shortening ($\% \Delta D = \dfrac{Dd - Ds}{Dd} \times 100$); and posterior left ventricular wall thickness at end-diastolic dimension (PWd). The record can also be used to estimate stroke volume, ejection fraction (percentage of blood in ventricle ejected per stroke), and cardiac output.

Cardiac catheterization

Cardiac output and other measurements of cardiac function can be measured invasively by *cardiac catheterization*. This procedure involves passing a flexible catheter, either through the brachial or femoral vein, into the heart. For example, the catheter can be attached to a pressure transducer to determine pressure differences at various points in response to the dynamics of the cardiac cycle. Blood samples can be withdrawn to determine the oxygen content. Opaque substances can be injected to follow the flow of blood through the heart by x-ray. This last technique is used as a diagnostic procedure in

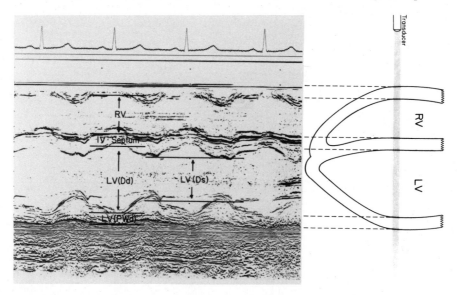

FIG. 9-3   Illustration of an echocardiographic record with special reference to the determination of left ventricular wall dimensions. The ultrasound reflection records the right ventricular cavity (RV), intraventricular (IV) septum thickness, left ventricular (LV) cavity dimension at end diastole (Dd), left ventricular cavity dimension at end systole (Ds), and left ventricular posterior wall dimension at end diastole (PWd). (This recording was provided by Dr. William Gualtierre, Cardiometrics Inc., New York.)

the detection of coronary artery disease. Occluded arteries can be identified and a decision made regarding future surgical or medical therapy (see Figure 9-4).

Catheterization, using the *Fick principle,* can directly evaluate cardiac output. A blood sample is taken from the pulmonary artery (mixed venous blood) through a catheter inserted in the brachial vein. Another sample is drawn from an artery located, for example, in the arm. These two samples allow the measurement of the oxygen content of the arterial and mixed venous blood and, thus, the A-V O_2 difference. The Fick principle states that the amount of blood flow through an organ, in this case the lung, is related to the ratio of total oxygen consumption to A-V O_2 difference.

$$\text{Cardiac output} = \frac{\text{Total } O_2 \text{ consumption (ml/min)}}{\text{A-V } O_2 \text{ difference (ml)}} \times 100$$

To compute cardiac output, the determination of total oxygen consumption is also required. In a resting condition, a subject would recline, attached to a collecting chamber by a breathing valve. If the subject consumes 300 ml of oxygen per minute, and the oxygen

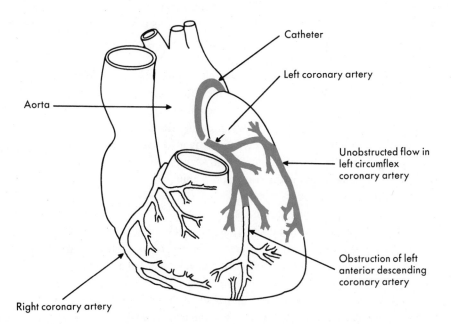

Aorta

Catheter

Left coronary artery

Unobstructed flow in left circumflex coronary artery

Obstruction of left anterior descending coronary artery

Right coronary artery

FIG. 9-4   Cardiac catheterization. One purpose of this procedure is to determine the blood flow characteristics of the coronary arteries. In this illustration, a catheter has been placed in a peripheral artery and passed upward through the aorta until its tip reaches the left coronary artery. Contrast material has been injected and can be seen passing through the left circumflex coronary artery unobstructed. However, an obstruction can be seen in the left anterior descending coronary artery, with no blood flow reaching the lower anterior surface of the heart.

content of arterial and mixed venous blood is 20 and 14 ml/100 ml of blood, respectively, the cardiac output would be 5 liters.

$$\frac{300 \text{ ml} \cdot \text{min}}{(20 - 14 \text{ ml}) \cdot 100 \text{ ml}} \times 100 = 5,000 \text{ ml} \cdot \text{min}^{-1}$$

REGULATION OF CARDIAC OUTPUT

Since cardiac output varies according to body size, it is often expressed as Cardiac index ($\dot{Q} \cdot m^2$ of body surface area). Cardiac index averages 3 L $\cdot$ m^2 in males and is about 7% to 10% lower in females. To understand how cardiac output is regulated, we must look at the control of its basic components, heart rate and stroke volume.

Control of heart rate

During exercise, heart rate is the most important mechanism for increasing cardiac output. Heart rate is directly related to cardiac output throughout the physiological range. Regulation is under the control of the autonomic nervous system. At rest, the parasympathetic branch dominates, and during exercise, the sympathetic branch dominates. In addition, adrenal hormones, epinephrine and norepinephrine, influence heart rate.

Control of stroke volume

In the most simplistic terms, the output of the pump per stroke is dependent on its input. This relationship is explained by the *Frank-Starling mechanism,* that is, the relationship between end-diastolic volume (venous inflow) and stroke volume. The mechanism states that as more blood flows in during diastole, the cardiac muscle fibers will stretch more. Diastolic filling is determined by effective filling pressure and resistance to distention offered by the ventricular wall. Increased stretch causes more cross-bridge linkages and a more powerful contraction, thus, the stroke volume is greater. Under certain controlled conditions, this mechanism is a complete explanation of stroke volume. However, recent work indicates that stroke volume is not solely explained by changes in ventricular dimensions. Additionally, it has been shown that myocardial contractility contributes to increasing stroke volume.[46] *Contractility* refers to many factors involved with rate, amount, and duration of tension development and shortening and relaxation of the myocardia.[39]

The heart contracts as a single unit without the possibility of recruiting more motor units. Thus, during exercise when stroke volume is increasing with no increase in diastolic filling, the only mechanism available is increased contractility.

Figure 9-5 describes the interrelationship between cardiac output and its two major determinants, heart rate and stroke volume. The figure depicts these variables as a function of percent of maximal oxygen consumption to show their response to increasing levels of work. It can be seen that at up to approximately one-third of maximal exercise, both heart rate and stroke volume contribute to the increase in cardiac output. However, after that point, the major contributor to increasing cardiac output is cardiac frequency.

Cardiac output remains stable during prolonged exercise; however, heart rate increases and stroke volume decreases reciprocally.[21] The decreased stroke volume is associated with a decrease in venous return, which is related to the increased heart rate. The increased heart rate is related to an increased $\dot{V}O_2$ and body temperature that occur over time.

CARDIOVASCULAR RESPONSE TO EXERCISE

Thus far, our discussion has been devoted to a general description of the cardiovascular system, the variables that describe it, and how it is measured and regulated. Much of this material has been a review of basic physiology deemed necessary so that the student could review material pertinent to the present section. This section details more specifically the coupling process between the cardiovascular system and muscular contraction. In other words, how does the body adjust its blood flow to meet exercise requirements?

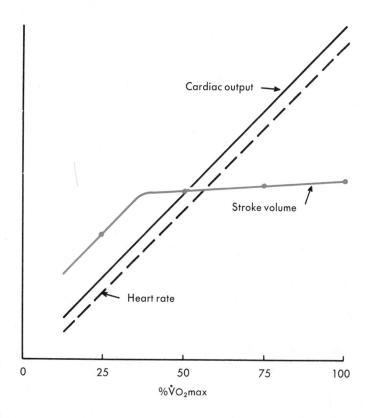

FIG. 9-5   This figure illustrates the growth of cardiac output, stroke volume, and heart rate as a function of increasing exercise intensity (% $\dot{V}O_2$ max). Stroke volume increases only to about one third of $\dot{V}O_2$ max; however, cardiac output continues to grow linearly throughout the full range. This is accomplished by the linear increase in heart rate throughout.

Response to dynamic exercise

Resting cardiac output averages approximately 5 L/min. During maximal exercise in highly trained athletes, it is common to observe a fivefold or sixfold increase. Resting blood flow distribution has been described as follows[7]:

Brain 15%

Liver 15%

Kidney 25%

Muscle 15%

Coronary 10%

Skin 10%

Other viscera 10%

During maximal exercise muscle blood flow in working skeletal muscle could be expected to be at the 85% or 90% level, thus, drastic adjustments have been made.

Increased heart rate contributes to the increased cardiac output. This response largely results from the removal of *parasympathetic* dominance, which was characteristic of the resting state. In fact, increases in cardiac output are almost exclusively caused by increased heart rate,[45] as stroke volume plays only a small role.

When exercise is performed dynamically in the supine position, stroke volume does not increase, since the postural position promotes adequate venous return. Resting stroke volume in the sitting position is lower than supine values because the blood pools in the veins. Exercise in the sitting position, however, results in some increase in stroke volume as a result of the actions of the *muscle pump,* that is, the contraction of muscle around the veins causes blood to be moved toward the heart. Stroke volume does not exceed supine values, and further increases in exercise intensity beyond about 33% of maximum do not stimulate additional stroke volume.

Increased vascular resistance, from peripheral vasoconstriction, results in decreased blood flow to such regions as the kidney and the abdomen. Conversely, vascular resistance decreases in exercising muscle. During exercise, coronary blood flow increases in direct proportion to the cardiac oxygen demand.

Practical summary. Blood flow is redistributed during exercise from areas where demand is least to those where demand is greatest, that is, working muscles.

Response to static (isometric) exercise

The term *static* refers to a condition in which local blood vessels are compressed during exercise. As mentioned, this occurs at the same time that muscle blood flow is being stimulated by vasodilation of local vessels. Therefore, continuation of static exercise depends on the balance achieved between these two opposing forces. Investigators have observed that vessels were not completely occluded until the load exceeded 70% of a maximal voluntary contraction (MVC).[23] Before this point, increasing blood pressure acts to overcome the muscular pressure by keeping vessels open. After 70% MVC, this is no longer possible.

Cardiac output response to dynamic exercise

Change in cardiac function with increasing exercise intensity has been examined using echocardiographic estimates.[34] Figure 9-6 illustrates the linear relationship between cardiac output and exercise intensity in groups of trained and untrained subjects.

As the metabolic needs of muscle tissue rise with increasing exercise intensity, the heart responds by increasing its output of blood. It is interesting to remember here that stroke volume responds nonlinearly with increasing intensity. Heart rate increases facilitate the need by muscle for greater cardiac output. However, during the recovery period following exercise (when there is a continuously falling heart rate), stroke volume increases above that observed during exercise. Recovery stroke volume has been found to remain greater than the final exercise stroke volume even after approximately 3.5 minutes.[17] Increasing stroke volume above exercise values many times during interval training periods (repeated bouts of exercise interspersed with periods of rest) is an important stimulus for cardiovascular improvement.

Cardiac output is related to the amount of muscle mass used in a given exercise. For example, cardiac output is significantly increased when one-arm or one-leg exercise is

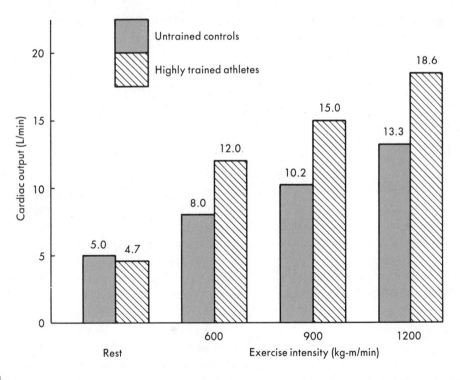

FIG. 9-6   Cardiac output of untrained subjects at rest and at three levels of exercise intensity (600, 900, and 1200 kg-m/min). (From Meerson, F.Z., Mukharlyamou, N.M., Belenkov, Y.N., and others: Effect of adaptation to physical exertion on contraction and relaxation on the weight of the left ventricle, Fiziologiya Cheloveka 5(4):650, 1977.)

compared with two-arm or two-leg exercise at the same intensity.[47] During submaximal exercise, cardiac output is higher when the exercise involves a smaller muscle mass, that is, more $\dot{Q}$ is required when exercising with one limb when the load is equal. Smaller muscle mass involvement is also characteristic of bicycle exercise as compared to tread-mill exercise. This difference is related to the supportive posture of the bicycle. Maximal cardiac output is significantly higher on the treadmill compared to the bicycle in both trained and untrained subjects.[35] A similar result has been observed at an exercise intensity of 50% $\dot{V}O_2$ max in untrained males.[11]

It was implied, but not explicitly stated, in Figure 9-6 that cardiac output during maximal exercise would be significantly greater in the highly trained athlete. To directly study this question, 33 male runners were compared with 34 sedentary males.[53] The hypothesis was confirmed, as cardiac outputs of 26.3 and 21.4 L/min, respectively, were observed.

A sex difference in cardiac output has also been observed,[15] after matching males and females on $\dot{V}O_2$ max, height, HR max, and maximal work capacity. Males showed significantly lower cardiac output and stroke volume values and significantly higher A-V O_2 difference at 35% $\dot{V}O_2$ max. These differences can be explained by the greater hemoglobin and muscle mass of the males. Males display higher cardiac outputs (23.5 vs 18.4 L/min^2) during maximal exercise as well.

Practical summary. Training cardiac output is partly a function of the degree to which stroke volume can be raised during exercise. Interval training is a valuable tool in this regard. Exercise cardiac output is related to the amount of muscle mass used in the effort.

Left ventricular response to dynamic exercise

Heart size and its relationship to sports performance have interested exercise scientists for many years. It has been known for some time, through x-ray evidence, that the gross dimensions of the heart can increase with training. Echocardiography has provided a simple noninvasive procedure for further study of this phenomenon. For example, left ventricular mass has been shown to be increased in male long-distance runners.[37,41] Similar changes have been observed in female field hockey players.[54]

To examine whether these observations are genetic or environmental, several studies have evaluated left ventricular dimensions before and after training. In all cases cardiac hypertrophy was observed.[10,14,36] The striking feature of these findings was the relatively short training duration necessary for the change to occur. Previously, it was thought that such results required many months or even years of training. Twenty-six normal men and women were studied before and after a 4-days per week walk and jog program.[10] An increase in posterior wall dimension was found after 11 weeks. Similar results were observed in only 5 weeks of using a 2-hour swimming program 6 days per week.[14] Of equal interest is the apparent transience of the effect following training. Three months after training, cross-country runners showed significantly decreased left ventricular end-diastolic diameter.[14]

Different athletic groups have been shown to display *hypertrophic specificity*. Isometrically trained athletes, with the cardiac stimulus related to increased blood pressure, display increases in wall dimensions. Conversely, isotonically trained athletes, with increased stroke volume serving as the stimulus, show a dilation of the left ventricle.[36] The first result was confirmed in a study of 13 nationally ranked weight lifters.[33] Echocardiographic recordings revealed hypertrophy of the ventricular septum and a normal sized left ventricular cavity. Although this pattern mimics abnormal cardiac responses, it is possible to diagnostically determine the underlying normality.

End-diastolic volume (EDV) and stroke volume do not change during isometric exercise, and both increase during isotonic upright exercise.[39] Heart rate increases in both cases, resulting in increases in cardiac output. Thirteen middle-aged males were studied during static handgrip (30% MVC) and dynamic bicycle exercise (85% predicted HR max).[24] Cardiac output, stroke volume, and end-diastolic volume were all significantly lower during static exercise. Dynamic exercise promotes increased cardiac contractility, decreased peripheral resistance, and increased venous return.

Cardiovascular response to isometric exercise (25% MVC) has also been examined in adolescents (age 14-16 yr).[25] As would be expected, stroke volume did not change but the cardiac index (cardiac output/m^2) increased significantly because of increased heart rate. These data indicate that adolescents respond in the same way as adults to isometric exercise.

Practical summary. Physical training results in ventricular enlargement specific to the type of training.

Muscle blood flow during dynamic exercise

Muscle blood flow increases with increasing work intensity, certainly up to 70% $\dot{V}O_2$ max,[50] and most likely up to 100% $\dot{V}O_2$ max.[19] One puzzling aspect of the study of muscle blood flow is the lack of difference between the trained and untrained subjects when values are presented per unit of muscle tissue.[19] These data are presented in Figure 9-7. It would normally be hypothesized that trained subjects would have greater muscle blood flow to support the extraction of oxygen; however, this does not seem to be the case. It seems that the larger total muscle mass of the trained subjects is not accompanied by larger blood flow. An 18% decline in muscle blood flow following 6 weeks of physical training was observed. A significant increase in succinic dehydrogenase (SDH), a Krebs cycle enzyme, was observed after training. This result indicates that an increase in oxygen extraction may be occurring without increases in blood flow. In such a situation, less blood flow would be required.

Practical summary. Training results in a lower demand for local muscular blood flow.

TABLE 9-1 ▦ REVIEW OF LITERATURE CONCERNING HEART RATE RESPONSE TO VARIOUS COMPETITIVE SPORTS

Authors	Activity	Type of subject	Number	Age	Sex	Results
Paterson	Ice hockey	Competitive players				Mean ice HR / Peak ice HR / Mean off-ice HR
			34	10.7	M	181 / 189 / 136
			33	12.2	M	187 / 189 / 148
			23	14.4	M	194 / 204 / 153
			10	21.0	M	173 / — / 120
Blanskby and others	Squash					HR mean during squash
		Sedentary	25	42.4	M	Approx. 170, −97.2% HR max at peak
		Active	25	43.9	M	Approx. 150, −85.5% HR max at peak
		A grade	25	25.6	M	Approx. 160, −83.6% HR max at peak
Corbin and others	Basketball	College				Mean rest HR / Mean game HR / Mean play HR
		Player	1	—	M	58 / 126 / 169
		Coach	1	—	M	78 / 101 / —
		Fan	1	—	M	60 / 66 / —
Magel and others	Swimming	College swimmers	7	20.1	M	Peak HR: 50 yd 172 / 100 yd 174 / 200 yd 180 / 500 yd 181 / 1000 yd 180
McArdle and others	Running	College track team				Rest HR / Anticipatory HR / Exercise HR
		60 yd	5	19.0	M	67 / 148 / 177
		220 yd	5	—		67 / 130 / 191
		440 yd	4	—		63 / 129 / 187
		880 yd	4	—		62 / 122 / 186
		1 mile	4	—		58 / 118 / 195
		2 mile	4	—		59 / 180 / 206

Heart rate response to various activities

Heart rate has been used as a general indicator of the cardiovascular stimulus provided by a given activity. Table 9-1 reviews several investigations that have examined exercise heart rate.[5,8,30,31,38] All the investigations used telemetry for recording data during competition. Although such studies can be challenged relative to sample size or representativeness of one competitive event, they do provide a guide for the practitioner.

Practical summary. Peak competitive HRs are relatively high; off-game and anticipatory HRs are well above rest; and peak HRs are highest during the longer competitive distances for both swimming and running.

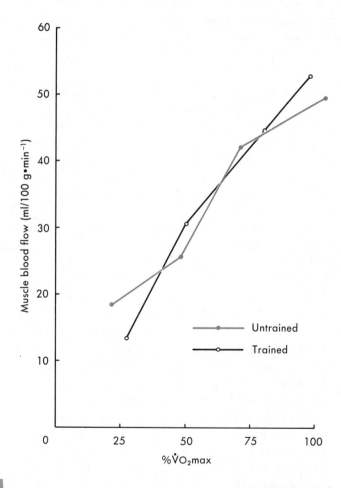

FIG. 9-7   **Comparison of muscle blood flow between trained and untrained subjects at various exercise intensities (% $\dot{V}O_2$ max). No significant differences were observed between groups. (From Grimby, G., Häggendal, E., and Saltin, B.: Local xenon 133 clearance from the quadriceps muscles during exercise in man, J. Appl. Physiol. *22:*305, 1966.)**

SUMMARY

The cardiovascular system consists of two pumps—the right and left ventricles—and the pulmonary and systemic circulations. The systemic circulation includes the arterial and venous sides. To adapt to the stress of exercise, the heart must be able to vary its output of blood. Variations in blood output can be accomplished by changes in heart rate, stroke volume, or both.

Cardiac function can be measured invasively (under the skin) or noninvasively (outside the skin). The most common noninvasive technique employs the electrocardiograph (ECG). The ECG records the movement of the electrical impulse through the heart during the heart cycle. Echocardiography uses the principle of reflected ultrasound to evaluate various structures in the heart. The record can also be used to estimate stroke volume, ejection fraction, and cardiac output. Cardiac catheterization has become a common procedure to invasively evaluate cardiac function. A catheter threaded through a vein and placed at various points in the heart is used to examine coronary blood flow and cardiac output.

Heart rate, one of the two important factors contributing to cardiac output, is regulated by the sympathetic nervous system during exercise. The other factor, stroke volume, under certain specified conditions, can be explained by the Frank-Starling mechanism. This mechanism relates cardiac muscle fiber stretch to diastolic filling. Recent evidence indicates that increased myocardial contractility, through stimulation from the sympathetic nervous system, is the best explanation for increased stroke volume during exercise.

While only 15% of resting blood flow is distributed to skeletal muscle, maximal dynamic exercise blood flow can reach 85% to 90% of total blood volume. Cardiac output changes during dynamic exercise are primarily accounted for by increased heart rate, with stroke volume playing a lesser role. In fact, stroke volume does not contribute to further increases in cardiac output beyond 33% of maximal dynamic exercise.

During static exercise, blood flow to muscles is limited by the compression force of the contracted muscle on local blood vessels. Total occlusion does not occur, however, until the load exceeds 70% MVC. As intensity increases during dynamic exercise, a linear increase occurs in cardiac output. Highly trained athletes display significantly higher cardiac outputs than untrained counterparts. During recovery, stroke volume increases beyond that observed during peak exercise. The level of the cardiac output is dependent on the muscle mass involvement.

Maximal cardiac output is significantly higher in highly trained groups. Males have significantly lower cardiac outputs during submaximal exercise and significantly higher maximal cardiac outputs compared to females. Cardiac output remains stable during prolonged exercise when increasing heart rate and declining stroke volume are present.

Left ventricular dimensions increase with training, and, contrary to past theory, these changes occur within a relatively short time, that is, 5 to 11 weeks. Left ventricular dimensions have decreased significantly in cross-country runners after 4 days, following 3 months of training. Isometrically trained athletes show increased ventricular wall dimensions, and isotonically trained athletes show a dilation of the left ventricle.

KEY TERMS

blood pressure the pressure measured in the vascular system that is associated with cardiac contraction (systolic) and relaxation (diastolic).

cardiac catheterization a technique that measures heart function in which a catheter is passed through a vein into the heart.

cardiac output the amount of blood pumped from the heart each minute.

dynamic exercise exercise marked by a change in joint angle, sometimes referred to as isotonic exercise.

echocardiography a technique that measures heart function in which sound waves are reflected from heart structures.

electrocardiography a technique that measures electrical changes during the cardiac cycle.

heart rate the number of times the heart beats each minute.

isometric exercise exercise in which tension is produced without changing the joint angle, also referred to as static exercise.

left ventricular hypertrophy increasing the cross section of the heart's left ventricle.

oxygen consumption the amount of oxygen that the body consumes each minute.

stroke volume the amount of blood pumped from the heart with each beat.

REVIEW QUESTIONS

1. Describe the anatomical components of the cardiovascular system.

2. Describe the function of the veins.

3. Compare the electrocardiograph to the echocardiograph in terms of recording method. What type of data does each record?

4. How can the heart contract more vigorously during exercise, when the heart muscle conforms to the all-or-none principle?

5. How does stroke volume change as a function of postural change?

6. Why is continued performance difficult when isometric contractions exceed 70% of maximal voluntary contraction?

7. Explain the relationship between cardiac output and muscle mass involvement.

8. How do left ventricular dimensions differ between sprinters and endurance athletes?

REFERENCES

1. Alam, M., and Smirk, F.H.: Observations in man on a pulse accelerating reflex from the voluntary muscles of the legs, J. Appl. Physiol. **92:**167, 1937.

2. Åstrand, P.O., Cuddy, T.E., Saltin, B., and others: Cardiac output during submaximal and maximal work, J. Appl. Physiol. **19:**268, 1964.

3. Beekman, R.H., Katch, V., Marks, C., and others: Validity of CO_2-rebreathing cardiac output during rest and exercise in young adults, Med. Sci. Sports Exerc. **16:**306, 1984.

4. Behr, M.J., Leong, K.-H., and Jones, R.H.: Acute effects of cigarette smoking on left ventricular function at rest and exercise, Med. Sci. Sports Exerc. **13:**176, 1981.

5. Blanksby, B.A., Elliott, B.C., and Bloomfield, J.: Telemetered heart rate responses of middle-aged sedentary males, middle-aged active males and "A" grade male squash players, Med. J. Aust. **2**:477, 1973.

6. Buck, J.A., Amundsen, L.R., and Nielsen, D.H.: Systolic blood pressure responses during isometric contractions of large and small muscle groups, Med. Sci. Sports Exerc. **12**:145, 1980.

7. Burton, A.C.: Physiology and biophysics of the circulation, Chicago, 1972, Year Book Medical Publishers, Inc.

8. Corbin, C.B., Tolson, H., Fletcher, R., and others: Heart rate variations during a basketball game, Coach Athl. **33**(2):18, 1970.

9. Cureton, T.K.: Physical fitness of champion athletes, Urbana, Ill., 1951, University of Illinois Press.

10. DeMaria, A.N., Neumann, A., Lee, G., and others: Alterations in ventricular mass and performance induced by exercise training in man evaluated by echocardiography, Circulation **57**:237, 1978.

11. Deutsch, D.T., and Knowlton, R.G.: Circulorespiratory responses to prolonged treadmill and bicycle exercise, Arch. Phys. Med. Rehabil. **61**:298, 1980.

12. Donald, K.W., Lind, A.R., McNicol, G.W., and others: Cardiovascular responses to sustained (static) contractions. In Chapman, C.B., editor: Physiology of muscular exercise, New York, 1967, American Heart Association, Inc.

13. Reference deleted in proofs.

14. Ehansi, A.A., Hagberg, J.M., and Hickson, R.C.: Rapid changes in left ventricular dimensions and mass in response to physical conditioning and deconditioning, Am. J. Cardiol. **42**:52, 1978.

15. Freedson, P., Katch, V.L., Sady, S., and others: Cardiac output differences in males and females during mild cycle ergometer exercise, Med. Sci. Sports **11**:16, 1979.

16. Gettman, L.R., Ayres, J.J., Polluck, M.L., and others: The effect of circuit weight training on strength, cardiorespiratory function, and body composition of adult men, Med. Sci. Sports **10**:171, 1978.

17. Goldberg, D.I., and Shephard, R.J.: Stroke volume during recovery from upright bicycle exercise, J. Appl. Physiol. Respir. Environ. Exerc. Physiol. **48**(5):833, 1980.

18. Green, J.F., and Jackman, A.P.: Peripheral limitations to exercise Med. Sci. Sports Exerc. **16**:299, 1984.

19. Grimby, G., Häggendal, E., and Saltin, B.: Local xenon 133 clearance from the quadriceps muscles during exercise in man, J. Appl. Physiol. **22**:305, 1966.

20. Hanne-Paparv, N., and Kellermann, J.J.: Long-term Holter ECG monitoring of athletes, Med. Sci. Sports Exerc. **13**:294, 1981.

21. Hartley, L.H., and Saltin, B.: Reduction of stroke volume and increase in heart rate after a previous heavier submaximal work load, Scand. J. Clin. Lab. Invest. **22**:217, 1968.

22. Hickson, R.C., Kanakis, C., Davis, J.R., and others: Reduced training duration effects on aerobic power, endurance, and cardiac growth, J. Appl. Physiol. Respir. Environ. Exerc. Physiol. **53**:225, 1982.

23. Humphreys, P.W., and Lind, A.R.: Blood flow through active and inactive muscles of the forearm during sustained hand-grip contractions, J. Physiol. **166**:120, 1963.

24. Korhonen, U.R., Koskinen, M., Linnaluoto, M., and others: Left ventricular response to dynamic and static exercise: evaluation by radiocardiography in healthy men, Ann. Clin. Res. **11**:189, 1979.

25. Laird, W.P., Fixler, D.E., and Huffines, F.D.: Cardiovascular response to isometric exercise in normal adolescents, Circulation **59**(4):651, 1979.

26. Lamont, L.S.: Echocardiographic findings in athletes: a review, Am. Correct. Ther. J. **34**(2): 46, 1980.

27. Lind, A.R., and McNicol, G.W.: Cardiovascular responses to static and dynamic exercise, Ergonomics **8**:379, 1965.

28. Longhurst, J.C., Kelly, A.R., Gonyea, W.J., and others: Cardiovascular responses to static exercise in distance runners and weight lifters, J. Appl. Physiol. Respir. Environ. Exerc. Physiol. **49**(4):676, 1980.

29. MacDougall, J.D., Sale, D.G., Moroz, J.R., and others: Mitochondrial volume density in human skeletal muscle following heavy resistance training, Med. Sci. Sports **11**:164, 1979.

30. Magel, J.R., McArdle, W.D., and Glaser, R.M.: Telemetered heart rate response to selected competitive swimming events, J. Appl. Physiol. **26**:764, 1969.

31. McArdle, W.D., Foglia, G.F., and Patti, A.V.: Telemetered cardiac response to selected running events, J. Appl. Physiol. **23**:566, 1967.

32. McCloskey, D.I., and Streatfield, K.A.: Muscular reflex stimuli to the cardiovascular system during isometric contractions of muscle groups of different mass, J. Physiol. **250**(2):431, 1975.

33. Menapace, F.J., Hammer, W.J., Ritzer, T.F., and others: Left ventricular size in competitive weight lifters: an echocardiographic study, Med. Sci. Sports Exerc. **14**:72, 1982.

34. Meerson, F.Z., Mukharlyamov, N.M., Belenkov, Y.N., and others: Effect of adaptation to physical exertion on contraction and relaxation on the weight of the left ventricle, Fiziologiya Cheloveka **5**(4):650, 1977.

35. Miyamura, M., Kitamura, K., Yamada, A., and others: Cardiorespiratory responses to maximal treadmill and bicycle exercise in trained and untrained subjects, J. Sports Med. **18**:25, 1978.

36. Morganroth, J., Maron, B.J., Henry, W.L., and others: Comparative left ventricular dimensions in trained athletes, Ann. Intern. Med. **82**:521, 1975.

37. Parker, B.M., Londeree, B.R., Cupp, G.V., and others: The non-invasive cardiac evaluation of long-distance runners, Chest **73**(3):376, 1978.

38. Paterson, D.H.: Respiratory and cardiovascular aspects of intermittent exercise with regard to ice hockey, Can. J. Appl. Sport Sci. **4**(1):22, 1979.

39. Paulsen, W.J., Boughner, D.R., Friesen, A., and others: Ventricular response to isometric and isotonic exercise: echocardiographic assessment, Br. Heart J. **45**:521, 1979.

40. Powles, A.C.P.: The effect of drugs on the cardiovascular response to exercise, Med. Sci. Sports Exerc. **13**:294, 1981.

41. Rashoff, W.J., Goldman, W., and Cohn, K.: The "athletic heart" prevalence and physiological significance of left ventricular enlargement in distance runners, JAMA **236**:158, 1976.

42. Reilly, T., Robinson, G., and Minors, D.S.: Some circulatory responses to exercise at different times of day, Med. Sci. Sports Exerc. **16**:477, 1984.

43. Ricci, G., Lajoie, D., Petitclerc, R., and others: Left ventricular size following endurance, sprint and strength training, Med. Sci. Sports Exerc. **14**:344, 1982.

44. Rubal, B.J., Rosentswieg, J., and Hamerly, B.: Echocardiographic examination of women collegiate softball champions, Med. Sci. Sports Exerc. **13:**176, 1981.

45. Rushmer, R.F.: Cardiovascular dynamics, ed. 4, Philadelphia, 1976, W.B. Saunders Co.

46. Sarnoff, S.J., and Mitchell, J.H.: The control of the function of the heart. In Hamilton, W.H., and Dow, P., editors: Handbook of physiology, section 2, circulation, vol. I, Washington, D.C., 1962, American Physiological Society.

47. Sechar, N.H., Clausen, J.P., Klausen, K., and others: Central and regional circulatory effects of adding arm exercise to leg exercise, Acta Physiol. Scand. **100:**288, 1977.

48. Snoeckx, L.H.E.H., Abeling, H.F.M., Lambregts, J.A.C., and others: Echocardiographic dimensions in athletes in relation to their training programs, Med. Sci. Sports Exerc. **14:**428, 1982.

49. Thompson, P.D., Lewis, S., Varady, A., and others: Cardiac dimensions and performance after either arm or leg endurance training, Med. Sci. Sports Exerc. **13:**303, 1981.

50. Tonnesen, U.H.: Blood flow through muscle during rhythmic contraction measured by 133 xenon, Scand. J. Clin. Lab. Invest. **16:**646, 1964.

51. Varnauskas, E., Björntop, P., Fahlén, M., and others: Effects of physical training on exercise blood flow and enzymatic activity in skeletal muscle, Cardiovasc. Res. **4:**418, 1970.

52. Wilmore, J.H., Parr, R.B., Girandola, R.W., and others: Physiological alterations consequent to circuit weight training, Med. Sci. Sports **10:**79, 1978.

53. Yamaji, K., and Miyashita, M.: Differences in cardio-respiratory responses to exhaustive exercise between athletes and non-athletes, Eur. J. Appl. Physiol. **38:**233, 1978.

54. Zeldis, S.M., Morganroth, J., and Rubler, S.: Cardiac hypertrophy in response to dynamic conditioning in female athletes, J. Appl. Physiol. **44:**849, 1978.

SUGGESTED READINGS

Carlsten, A., and Grimby, G.: The circulatory response to muscular exercise in man, Springfield, Ill., 1966, Charles C Thomas, Publisher.

Chapman, C.C.: Physiology of muscular exercise, New York, 1967, American Heart Association, Inc.

Marshall, J.M.: The heart. In Mountcastle, V.B., editor: Medical physiology, ed. 14, vol. 2, St. Louis, 1980, The C.V. Mosby Co.

Ross, G.: Cardiovascular system. In Ross, G., editor: Essentials of human physiology, Chicago, 1978, Year Book Medical Publishers, Inc.

Rowell, L.B.: Human cardiovascular adjustments to exercise and thermal stress, Physiol. Rev. **54:**75, 1974.

Rowell, L.B.: What signals govern the cardiovascular responses to exercise? Med. Sci. Sports **12:**307, 1980.

Rushmer, R.F.: Cardiovascular dynamics, ed. 14, Philadelphia, 1976, W.B. Saunders Co.

CASE STUDY 1

The importance of strength in many sports is undeniable. It is so important that many university and professional teams now hire a specialized coach who attends only to the development of strength in athletes. It is interesting to note that no such specialist is hired to attend to the other components of physical fitness.

We have yet to see a cardiovascular coach hired by universities or professional teams. This situation raises the question of the relative importance of each of these two components, strength and cardiovascular training, to the other. Does the strength coach develop the cardiovascular system by prescribing a program to hypertrophy muscle?

It is theoretically possible to design a weight program in which the resistance is so low and the repetitions so numerous that it mimics a running program. Therefore, if you view weights as a medium to apply overload, you can imagine a continuum of programs that emphasize cardiovascular benefits on the one extreme and strength on the other. The practical truth of the matter is that most coaches are primarily concerned with pure strength. Therefore, the athlete has to work on the end of the weight-overload continuum that promotes little, if any, cardiovascular benefit. In fact, one study[29] has found that a high-intensity strength program reduced mitochondrial density per unit of muscle. The athletes increased muscle mass, so they did not eliminate mitochondria presumably, but the fact remains that their oxidative capacity was not promoted. Oxidative capacity would usually improve in programs that stressed cardiovascular conditioning.

Let's review for a moment the physiological response to an acute session of weight lifting. This response gives us insight about any mechanism that might improve cardiovascular variables. Blood flow to muscle is completely occluded with contractions that exceed 70% MVC. In an attempt to overcome this muscular pressure on the vessels, systemic blood pressure is increased to high levels. One study,[36] discussed earlier in this chapter, demonstrates that the result of a pressure-overloaded heart is an increase in cardiac wall thickness, not internal chamber dimensions. It seems clear that ischemic exercise (>70% MVC) would not promote stroke volume and, therefore, cardiac output. The only other mechanism capable of increasing aerobic capacity, a value we use to estimate cardiovascular function, would be oxygen extraction. It has already been pointed out that neither increased blood flow nor increased mitochondrial density (both indicators of oxygen extraction) occur with training. In fact, Gettman and others[16] and Wilmore and others[52] have shown that aerobic capacity does not change with circuit weight training in males. Circuit weight training did cause a 10% increase in aerobic capacity in females.[52] This apparent sex difference may reflect the law of initial values, since the females showed initial $\dot{V}O_2$ max values 34.4% below the males, that is, the possibility of change is related to the initial level of cardiovascular condition.

Obviously, there is nothing wrong with training athletes to gain strength, but in most programs cardiovascular improvements are not made. Therefore, for athletes who require both strength and cardiovascular conditioning, both aspects must be trained independently.

CASE STUDY 2

Because of its close association with the public schools, the field of health and physical education is sometimes limited to an age range from 5 to 22 years. The vast majority of the population exceeds these boundaries. Perhaps the greatest challenge to this field lies in the people who are not of school age. Every person, from the fetus that bobs through a prenatal exercise class to our oldest senior citizen exercising in a nursing home, deserves attention.

One group that has received considerable attention within health and physical education in recent years is cardiac patients. Since the early 1960s when Dr. Herman Hellerstein pioneered the use of exercise for cardiac patients at the Cleveland Clinic, there has been a need for skilled cardiac exercise leaders and exercise stress test technicians, personnel trained in health and physical education. As the involvement of such personnel has increased in the rehabilitation process, the demand for greater knowledge of cardiovascular function has also increased. It is common, for example, for an exercise leader to receive a physician's report that includes detailed information about diagnostic tests. This information provides essential background data regarding the nature of the patient's disease and also data necessary for the development of an exercise prescription, which is the topic of a subsequent chapter. Following are typical measurements that an exercise leader might find in a physician's report. To be conversant with physicians and to be able to give the best possible care to patients, these measurements should be understood.

Patient: __John Doe__   Date: __August 6, 1982__

Age: __52__   Reason for exercise test: __Family history of heart disease__

Cholesterol: __264__   Triglycerides: __304__   Blood pressure: __108/70__

Test protocol: __Bruce__   Maximal predicted HR: __173__

	HR	BP	ECG Changes
Stage 1 (1.7 mph/10%)	112	120/80	1 mm ST depression
Stage 2 (2.5 mph/12%)	135	145/80	1 to 1.5 mm ST depression
Stage 3 (3.4 mph/14%)	170	164/80	1.5 to 2 mm ST depression

Medical impression: Positive treadmill test for ischemic heart disease.

Subsequent diagnostic evaluation: Patient John Doe was evaluated by echocardiography and found to have a 25% left ventricular ejection fraction. Cardiac catheterization revealed an 85% obstruction of the left anterior descending coronary artery and 70% obstruction of the left circumflex coronary artery.

Surgery: Patient John Doe underwent coronary bypass surgery to correct obstructions in the two left coronary arteries.

This information represents only a brief medical report but it is sufficient to illustrate a number of cardiovascular measurements that the cardiac exercise leader must understand. First, it is clear that the patient was at risk for heart disease because of his family history, and abnormally high cholesterol (>250 mg %) and triglyceride (>200 mg %) levels. Second, the patient was tested to a heart rate very close to maximum, demonstrating a normal blood pressure response but an abnormal depression (>1 mm) of the ST segment of the electrocardiogram. Therefore, the test was judged to be positive. It was the physician's decision to further evaluate the patient, first with noninvasive technology (echocardiography) and next with an invasive procedure (cardiac catheterization). Since the ''echo'' indicated that left ventricular function was abnormal, that is, low ejection fraction, further evaluation was warranted. The cardiac catheterization revealed serious obstruction of the two left coronary arteries. These obstructions were surgically corrected. Following bypass surgery, this patient was given another exercise test. Results indicated no cardiac ischemia, and an exercise prescription was prepared based on the test heart rate data. To this date, this patient is exercising successfully in a closely monitored cardiac exercise program.

PART THREE

EXERCISE PRESCRIPTION, TRAINING TECHNIQUES, AND PHYSIOLOGICAL EFFECTS

chapter 10

GRADED EXERCISE TESTING

MAJOR LEARNING OBJECTIVE
Objectives of graded exercise testing are determination of functional capacity, diagnosis of heart disease, development of an individualized exercise prescription, and evaluation of prescription effectiveness.

APPLICATION
Graded exercise testing results consist of calculation of aerobic power and electrocardiographic and blood pressure responses, and prescription of a target heart rate range.

229

$\mathbf{I}$N recent years those who study the fields of health and physical education have explored new, nontraditional options for undergraduate majors. Perhaps the most promising occupations to pursue have been in the areas of commercial fitness and cardiac rehabilitation programming. The burgeoning interest of Americans in the use of exercise as a disease prevention mechanism and of physicians in the provision of expanded rehabilitative services has created a growing job market for well-trained exercise specialists. Many preventive exercise programs and virtually all cardiac exercise programs require preentry graded exercise testing. In response to the need for highly trained exercise personnel, the American College of Sports Medicine (ACSM) has developed a certification process for four categories of exercise program employees: exercise program director, exercise specialist, fitness instructor, and exercise test technologist.[1] This last category is concerned solely with testing, but it is also essential for the exercise leader (specialist and instructor) and administrator (program director) to be knowledgeable about both the testing process and the interpretation of tests. This chapter introduces the student who may be interested in nonteaching options in health or physical education to the body of knowledge about graded exercise testing. Since emphasis in this chapter will be placed on the use of exercise testing for the diagnosis of heart disease and the prescription of preventive exercise programs, the reader should be acquainted with the definition of coronary heart disease and those factors that are known to place a person at risk for this disease.

CORONARY HEART DISEASE

For the purposes of this chapter, coronary heart disease (CHD) is defined as partial or total closure of the coronary arteries resulting in symptoms or signs of reduced or occluded coronary blood flow. The direct diagnosis of CHD is accomplished through the use of coronary catheterization (angiography), whereby a catheter is passed into the coronary arteries, dye is injected, and the dye flow is filmed by x-ray film to determine the patency (openness) of the arteries.

Risk factors

The American Heart Association[3] has identified a number of factors that increase the risk of heart attack (referred to as myocardial infarction, or MI). The three principal risk factors are hypertension (high blood pressure), smoking, and high blood cholesterol levels.[1] Individuals with one risk factor approximately double the risk of a cardiac event; two and three risk factors increase the risk at least 3 times and 10 times, respectively. Because of their increased risk for coronary disease, it is suggested that heart disease–prone individuals alter their life-styles to eliminate negative factors. If exercise is proposed for such individuals, graded exercise testing is an absolute necessity. In an attempt to categorize various patient groups differentially, the ACSM[1] developed the classification system shown in Table 10-1.

The categories in Table 10-1 can be generalized into two categories of individuals who present themselves for testing. First, there is the apparently healthy population of potential exercisers who want primarily to determine their tolerance for exercise and who seek prescriptive advice. This category spans the continuum from healthy but very unfit persons to highly trained competitive athletes (categories A to C). Second, individuals at risk for disease, specifically heart disease, and patients who have already experienced an MI (categories D-I) may request testing. The testing principles are basically the same for both groups with differences primarily noted in the performance limitations of the patients and the need to pay special attention to cardiac monitoring.

OBJECTIVES OF GRADED EXERCISE TESTING

The objectives of the graded exercise test are the following:

1. To determine the functional capacity of the individual: in other words, the exercise intensity at which it is necessary to terminate exercise because of fatigue and the symptoms and signs that contraindicate continuance

TABLE 10-1 ‖‖‖ CLASSIFICATION OF POTENTIAL EXERCISE TEST SUBJECTS BY AGE AND HEALTH STATUS*

Category	Patient description
A	Asymptomatic, physically active persons of any age without CHD risk factors or disease
B	Asymptomatic, physically active persons less than 35 years of age without CHD risk factors
C	Asymptomatic, physically inactive persons 35 years and older without CHD risk factors or disease
D	Asymptomatic, physically active or inactive persons of any age with CHD risk factors but no known disease
E	Asymptomatic persons of any age with known disease
F	Symptomatic, physically active persons clinically stable for 6 months or longer
G	Symptomatic, physically inactive persons clinically stable for 6 months or longer
H	Symptomatic persons with recent onset of CHD or a change in disease status (EXAMPLE: recent myocardial infarction, unstable angina, coronary artery bypass surgery)
I	Persons for whom exercise is contraindicated

Adapted from American College of Sports Medicine: Guidelines for graded exercise testing and exercise prescription, ed. 2, Philadelphia, 1980, Lea & Febiger.
*It is recommended that a physician should be in attendance or in close proximity when subjects from categories C through I are tested.

2. To determine the presence of coronary artery disease (diagnosis)
3. To collect information necessary to develop an individualized exercise prescription
4. To evaluate the effectiveness of the exercise prescription

The graded exercise test can either be maximal or submaximal. A maximal test requires the individual to work to fatigue or until signs or symptoms contraindicate continued exercise—that is, until functional capacity is reached. Submaximal tests usually terminate at a level that is an arbitrary percentage of maximum, for instance, 85% of the age-related maximal heart rate. Test termination below 100% with or without signs or symptoms is usually inadequate for either diagnosis or functional capacity determination. Exercise intensity during any stage of a graded exercise test is often expressed in MET (3.5 ml O_2 · kg/min^{-1}). For example, if exercise is terminated at a 10 MET stage, the equivalent oxygen consumption is 35 ml O_2 · kg/min^{-1} (3.5×10).

Exercise testing athletes

When athletes are being tested, the goal is usually to ascertain performance capacity, which is an expanded version of functional capacity. In addition to physiological responses, it is important to observe psychological and environmental factors as well.[7] For example, knowledge of pain tolerance and the interaction of temperature and performance is important in predicting the performance capabilities of an athlete.

Individualized exercise testing

It is important to remember that testing, like exercise programs, should be individually designed. Again, even though general principles remain the same among various patient populations, the specialized needs of each group and, indeed, each individual must be considered. Application of standardized testing protocols is tempting because of the economy of time and effort. However, two cardiac patients—one 8 weeks after MI, unaccustomed to physical exercise, and 60 years old, and another 5 years after MI, currently exercising regularly, and 40 years old—pose quite different testing problems for the exercise test technologist. Each person should be viewed as a unique individual for whom a special testing protocol may be necessary.

History

The first known attempt to measure electrocardiographic (ECG) response to exercise was reported by Einthoven[11] in 1908. In 1918, Bousfield[6] was the first to observe the ECG during chest pain (angina pectoris). In 1928, Feil and Seigel[13] had angina pectoris patients do sit-ups until they experienced pain, noted a depression of the ST segment of the ECG, and observed a return to normality with rest and the administration of nitroglycerin. (Depression of the ST segment has been associated with myocardial ischemia and is often associated with chest pain.) Shortly thereafter, Master and Oppenheimer[19] measured heart rate and blood pressure after a step test was performed to evaluate cardiac capacity; in 1941, Master and Jaffe[18] proposed the use of the ECG after the stepping exercise to evaluate CHD.

Exercise testing for the purpose of determining the physical fitness of schoolchildren and military recruits was pioneered by scientists at the Harvard Fatigue Laboratory.[10] The Harvard step test became the standard for exercise testing in physical education for many years to come. Gradually, the step test gave way to the bicycle ergometer and treadmill because of the greater control of exercise intensity.

Risks

The incidence of mortality and morbidity (nonfatal cardiac events) in 170,000 tests has been calculated.[21] Within 1 week of testing 16 deaths were recorded, which indicates the risk of death to be 1 in 10,000 tests. The incidence of nonfatal events was 2.4 in 10,000 tests. A similar study[20] revealed mortality and morbidity figures to be 0.25 in 10,000 and 1.8 in 10,000 tests, respectively. In the largest test sample, the mortality for 700,000 tests conducted in 1375 laboratories was 0.50 in 10,000 tests.[21] Morbidity was 3.6 in 10,000 tests. The risk is small compared to the information provided, particularly CHD diagnostic information.

PRETEST PROCEDURES

Instructions

Before testing, subjects should be informed of procedures they must follow to ensure a valid exercise test. There are few things more disappointing than the need to cancel a test because of the subject's failure to comply with pretest instructions. Instructions generally fall into four categories: physical activity, nutrition, drugs, and clothing. Subjects should be told to refrain from heavy physical activity, which may limit test performance. Usually the limiting of physical exercise to normal daily activities during the day of the test is sufficient. All food intake should be suspended within 2 hours of the test. Similarly, drugs, including caffeine, nicotine, and alcohol, should be prohibited before test administration. With cardiac patients the physician must make a decision regarding suspension of therapeutic medications. In some instances, drug usage is suspended to achieve a pure diagnostic test. For the purpose of exercise prescription, in which exercise is performed by a medicated patient, the test should be given under the same conditions. Suitable clothing should be suggested. Comfortable, lightweight walking shoes are mandatory. Women should wear a blouse that opens down the front for ECG electrodes to be attached and adjusted easily; a bra is recommended to prevent excessive breast movement and electrode interference. Athletes will probably perform best with normal exercise gear.

Health history and physical examination

The purpose of the physical examination and health history is to collect information necessary to judge whether to conduct a test and, if the answer is yes, what potential problems the individual may encounter. For example, knowledge by the exercise test technologist and physician of the patient's anginal chest pain characteristics helps to guide the course of the test. In other words, knowing the typically tolerated pain from the intolerable pain is valuable when a test termination judgment is to be made. In a diagnostic test, chest pain without ECG changes is probably only chest wall syndrome, not cardiac pain and thus not cause for termination. Even when chest pain is cardiac related, a walk-through phenomenon is often observed, whereby continued exercise enables the patient to experience a lessening or disappearance of pain.

When a physician must be in attendance or in close physical proximity (categories C to I, Table 10-1), a physical examination before the exercise test is valuable. In addition to the resting ECG (both supine and standing), heart sounds, heart rate, and blood pressure should be evaluated. Many laboratories complement this preevaluation examination with one or more of the following physical measurements: body weight, body height, abdominal girth, grip strength, percentage of body fat, and selected lung volumes.[25]

It is important to collect detailed information relative to the patient's health history before arrival at the testing site. Often pretest instruction is based on this information. Many forms are available that gather personal demographic information, risk factor data, family history of disease and mortality, personal history of disease and surgery, current medical complaints (if any), and medications.

Contraindications

Not everyone is a candidate for a graded exercise test; exercise can be lethal to some individuals. Ellestad[12] suggests that exercise testing is contraindicated for the following patients:
1. Patients with acute MI
2. Patients with acute myocarditis (inflammation of the muscular walls of the heart) or pericarditis (inflammation of the membranous sac that contains the heart)
3. Patients with unstable angina pectoris, that is, a changing pain pattern
4. Patients with rapid ventricular or atrial arrhythmias
5. Patients with second- or third-degree heart block
6. Patients with congestive heart failure
7. Acutely ill patients such as those with infections or hyperthyroidism
8. Patients with acute aortic stenosis
9. Patients with significant obstruction of the left main coronary artery or 90% occlusion of the left anterior descending and circumflex arteries

The guidelines of the ACSM[1] would add to this list the following patients:
1. Patients with a history suggesting medication effects; for example, those who take digitalis have a falsely lowered ST segment on their ECGs, suggesting myocardial ischemia
2. Patients with severe ideopathic, hypertrophic, subaortic stenosis (IHSS)
3. Patients with a suspected or known dissecting aneurysm (dilation of the arterial wall, in which blood is forced between the layers of the artery)
4. Patients with suspected or known thrombophlebitis (inflammation of the vein wall and formation of thrombi)
5. Patients with a recent systemic or pulmonary embolism

6. Patients who have taken high doses of phenothiazine agents (tranquilizers, which may cause a false positive test)

Patient safety practices begin before the graded exercise test and often may include eliminating the testing procedure altogether.

Informed consent

The provision of medical services is accompanied by the possibility of malpractice suits being brought against physicians, technologists, university or hospital adminis-trators, and/or the institution itself through its governing body (the board of directors). Patients cannot sign away their right to examination by competent personnel and properly operating equipment. Negligence by test personnel, if proven, can result in costly court litigation and payment for harm, even when the most elaborate precautions have been taken. Still, it is the obligation of every testing unit to develop a consent form for each patient to read and sign. The form usually contains an explanation of the test, a description of possible risks and discomforts, a description of expected benefits, assurance that all questions will be answered, and a declaration by the patient that he freely consents to undergo the test. Such a form should be read to or by the patient before the performance of any procedure.

Persons involved with graded exercise testing should be sure that the institution for whom they work carries liability insurance, that they personally purchase a malpractice policy, or preferably both. Most health insurance carriers provide policies for paramedical personnel.

PERSONNEL

It is advisable that each testing facility be supervised by a physician who is experi-enced in exercise testing procedures, a program director certified by the ACSM, or someone with equivalent competence. ACSM guidelines[1] spell out the requirements for program director certification: *knowledge* in functional anatomy, exercise physiology, pathophysiology, electrocardiography, human behavior and psychology, and gerontol-ogy; *functional capability* in exercise testing, emergency procedures, exercise prescrip-tion, exercise leadership, and program administration; and a 1-year *internship* involving approximately 1,600 hours. Certification is gained by successfully passing both a written knowledge test and a practical application test. The public requires and should, in fact, demand a very high standard of practice. ACSM certification is one way of achieving this objective.

Exercise testing for emergency and functional purposes requires a minimum of two persons, with a third person often being very useful. The physician or program director is responsible for monitoring the ECG oscilloscope and printouts and possibly manipulating the controls that adjust exercise intensity. When a diagnostic test is administered or a cardiac patient is tested, it is advisable for the physician to be solely responsible for monitoring the ECG and the patient's symptoms and signs. The exercise test technologist can be responsible for preparing the patient for the test, recording exercise blood pressure, and generally attending to the needs of the patient. Like the program director, the exercise test technologist is certifiable by ACSM, and must also pass both written and practical tests. The exercise test technologist is responsible for knowledge in all the areas listed for the program director and has functional capabilities in exercise testing and emergency procedures. No internship is required for certification, but practical experience is highly desirable.

A third person, if thought to be necessary, can be drawn from a pool of interested students in a university setting or from paramedical personnel in a hospital or commercial environment. An RN as the third person is very useful in emergency situations—particularly nurses with coronary care unit experience, in which defibrillating, starting IVs, and administering emergency medications are commonplace.

EQUIPMENT

A survey of 14,000 laboratories concerning exercise test procedures found that 72% were using treadmills, 17% bicycle ergometers, and only 11% step tests.[24] This section discusses these three major testing modes and the reasons why one may be favored over the others. Arm ergometry is being used increasingly in exercise testing laboratories. This instrumentation is valuable for patients with lower limb disabilities and as a supplement to the primary lower limb testing. Many programs include upper body routines; therefore collection of data specifically related to such activity can be very beneficial. Further discussion is offered in various other sources.

Step test

As mentioned earlier, the step test was the original mode of testing both patients and normal populations. The procedure is inexpensive, and the calculation of work output is relatively simple. For instance, if a 150-pound person steps to the top of a step, 1 foot in height, the person has performed 150 foot-pounds of physical work. If the same individual continues stepping for 1 minute and makes 30 excursions, the work performed is 150 foot-pounds × 30, or 4,500 foot-pounds/min. (Actually, since this calculation is work per unit time, it is a calculation of *power*.) The metric equivalent of this power output is 622 kg-m/min. Table 10-2 shows the MET equivalents of various stepping rates and bench heights. For example, with a 32-centimeter bench and a 30 steps/minute stepping rate, the MET value is 9.6, or just under 10 times the resting metabolic rate.

The inability of the test administrator to adjust the exercise intensity easily and the impracticality of the exercise mode are the major liabilities of this test procedure. It is difficult to control the height of the subject's center of gravity, particularly at high stepping rates; in other words, it is very easy for the subject to make an incomplete excursion while stepping. Also, since the work performed depends on the stepping rate, control of exercise intensity is affected by the subject's ability to stay with the beat of a metronome.[7] To reach $\dot{V}O_2$ max while stepping, the rate must be increased to a level that would make it biomechanically very difficult, if not impossible.

Bicycle ergometer

The bicycle ergometer offers a testing mode most typically in the sitting position, at which the subject does not have to move body mass. Two subjects performing the same exercise intensity would therefore have equivalent oxygen consumptions ($L \cdot min^{-1}$), but if body weights are different, they would show different capacities relative to body weight ($ml \cdot kg/min^{-1}$). The supported position on a bicycle makes recording of various physiological variables much easier. Specifically, it is much easier to record blood pressure because of the stable, upright position. The sitting posture also facilitates safety for the subject.

Two engineering designs are available. The most commonly used is the mechanically braked ergometer. This design is very easy to calibrate but requires the subject to maintain a constant pace, usually with a metronome. Typically these bicycles are calibrated with weights (resistance) suspended from a belt that surrounds the bicycle flywheel. These weights allow calibration of the resistance scale, usually measured in kiloponds. The length of the flywheel belt is normally 6 meters. To determine the power output of a bicycle ergometer of this type, the following formula should be used: Kiloponds × Length of flywheel belt × rpm. For example, a resistance of 1 kilopond and an rpm value of 50 would result in a power output of 300 kilopond meters per minute (1 × 6 × 50). The other design offers an electrically braked system, the great advantage of which is that the exercise intensity does not require subject-controlled pace. Resistance on the pedals is adjusted upward and downward as the pedal rate decreases and increases, respectively.

TABLE 10-2 |||||| ENERGY EXPENDITURE IN MET DURING STEPPING, WITH DIFFERENT RATES AND STEP HEIGHTS

Step height		Steps/min			
cm	inches	12	18	24	30
0	0	1.2	1.8	2.4	3.0
4	1.6	1.5	2.3	3.1	3.8
8	3.2	1.9	2.8	3.7	4.6
12	4.7	2.2	3.3	4.4	5.5
16	6.3	2.5	3.8	5.0	6.3
20	7.9	2.8	4.3	5.7	7.1
24	9.4	3.2	4.8	6.3	7.9
28	11.0	3.5	5.2	7.0	8.7
32	12.6	3.8	5.7	7.7	9.6
36	14.2	4.1	6.2	8.3	10.4
40	15.8	4.5	6.7	9.0	11.2

Adapted from American College of Sports Medicine: Guidelines for graded exercise testing and exercise prescription, ed. 2, Philadelphia, 1980, Lea & Febiger.

The major liability of the bicycle ergometer, and perhaps the reason for its less prevalent use, involves the nature of the movement. Bicycle activity is not a common mode of movement for most individuals. Walking is a far more common activity, so testing is predominantly accomplished on treadmills.

Treadmill

Walking is the most common mode of movement; the treadmill, however, is by far the most expensive type of testing equipment. Another advantage lost with the gain in movement practicality is that of efficient measurement. Measurement of blood pressure and oxygen consumption is more difficult because of upper body instability and total body movement (the forward and backward movement on the motorized belt).

Measurement of the oxygen requirement for treadmill walking, in contrast to that for bicycle exercise, is unrelated to body weight. Two persons of differing body weights walking at the same rate show unequal total oxygen consumption (L/min) but equal oxygen consumption relative to body weight (ml/kg · min^{-1}). The calculation can be made as follows:

$$\dot{V}_{O_2} \text{ (ml} \cdot \text{kg/min}^{-1}) = \text{Speed (m/min)} \times$$
$$0.1 \text{ (ml } O_2 \cdot \text{kg/min per m/min)} + 3.5 \text{ (ml } O_2 \cdot \text{kg/min}^{-1})$$

For a walking speed of 3 mph (80 m/min), the $\dot{V}_{O_2}$ is 11.5 ml · kg/min^{-1}.[1] To determine the MET equivalent of this $\dot{V}_{O_2}$, the value is divided by 3.5 (11.5 ÷ 3.5 = 3.3 MET). The reader should be reminded that the calculations are different for uphill walking, running, and outdoor exercise.

Other equipment

Many excellent direct writing ECGs are available on the market. Electronic specifications required of such instrumentation are discussed in detail elsewhere.[4] Other measurement devices required during exercise stress testing and discussed in this book are oscilloscopes, blood pressure sphygmomanometers, and emergency equipment such as defibrillators.

GRADED EXERCISE TESTING PRINCIPLES

Decisions regarding the structure of an exercise test are guided by certain principles. The first, mentioned earlier, emphasizes the need to tailor a test to the individual needs of the subject. Tests are not for the convenience of the administrator; maximal valid information about the subject is the goal.

General principles

Some authors suggest that the exercise test should be equally suitable for the trained and untrained[12] or for persons of various ages and health status.[7] This is a perfectly logical suggestion relative to the general structure of the test but should not specifically pinpoint attributes, such as work loads. All the necessary test interpretations and subsequent prescriptions can be made with the test work loads allowed to vary with individual needs. The test should not require any special skill by the subject, since mechanical efficiency would mask the true results of the test. The testing instrument should evaluate the large muscle groups of the body (as should all three instruments previously discussed), and the test data should be reproducible. Norms are very helpful to the interpretation of the test. Although the test is not a competition among subjects, a knowledge of the average response helps in making judgments regarding future behavior, such as on the need for an exercise program. Norms are guidelines—not absolute demarcations. It should be obvious that a test should maximize safety for the subject and minimize discomfort.

Measurement principles

Exercise tests for persons in categories C to I in Table 10-1 should comprise, as a minimum, instrumentation to record the ECG and blood pressure (sphygmomanometer). The ECG and blood pressure should be measured at rest before exercise, during exercise, and in recovery after exercise. Since both measurements are recorded for the upright position during exercise and in the supine position during recovery, both variables must be measured in these two postural positions at rest, that is, supine and standing. It is recommended that all 12 leads of the ECG should be used during an exercise test. Such a multiple-lead system allows a complete examination of possible myocardial ischemia during exercise. If a single-lead system must be used, the exploring electrode should be placed in the V_5 position (the fifth intercostal space at the anterior edge of the axilla). This is the position most sensitive to myocardial ischemia.[23] Heart rate is another variable that should be recorded during an exercise test; however, it is automatically displayed in many ECG instruments or can be easily calculated by measurement of the distance between R waves.

The student is referred to Figure 9-2, which shows the normal ECG pattern. With the patient at rest the test technician should be able to identify evidence of a previous MI: an exaggerated Q wave and elevated T wave in certain leads. During exercise the pattern should remain approximately the same, except that the increased heart rate compresses the waves. Also, it is important to monitor the ECG during exercise for signs of ischemia (lack of coronary blood flow and oxygen supply) and rhythm disturbances. Both of these signs contraindicate further testing. Ischemia most often takes the form of a displaced ST segment (horizontal or downsloping below the baseline) or an inverted T wave. ST segment displacement signals an abnormality in the ratio of myocardial oxygen supply and demand: the demand is greater than the supply. Rhythm disturbances, also called "skipped beats," can take many forms and indicate an interruption of the normal conduction of the cardiac impulse. For example, sometimes the ventricles are stimulated to contract prematurely (premature ventricular contraction, or PVC). When this occurs, the heart contracts before the chambers fill properly, thus decreasing the stroke volume. An occasional beat of this type is usually harmless, but its occurrence in rapid succession during exercise places the patient in great danger.

Principles regarding selection of exercise intensities

The following principles are useful for establishing the structure of an exercise test:

1. The entire protocol should be structured to maximize generation of the necessary information but should be short enough to be practical. The test's duration should exceed 6 minutes but be no longer than approximately 15 minutes.

2. The test's protocol should incorporate a warm-up period. A judicious method is to use the early minutes of the test—at 0 resistance on the bike or 0 grade and low speed on the treadmill—as the warm-up; that is, to include the warm-up as the first stage in the protocol.

3. The initial exercise intensity should be at a level below the estimated point of impairment in the case of a patient[3] and below the estimated maximal capacity ($\dot{V}_{O_2}$ max) in other cases.

4. The test should involve variable loads instead of a single continuous protocol (see Figure 13-1). This technique allows observation of an individual within a variety of exercise intensities, representing the possible daily range of physical activity.

5. The test protocol should be arranged in stages, with each stage progressively increasing in intensity until the termination criteria is reached. The stages' durations should ensure attainment of steady-state conditions for heart rate and oxygen consumption. Durations between 3 and 6 minutes meet this requirement. Practicality dictates a progressive test protocol; on the other hand, most physical occupations involve intermittent activity with periodic rest periods.[5] The latter procedure would also facilitate measurement of research data[22] but again would be costly in duration.

Sample test protocols

Figure 10-1 illustrates the several patterns possible when an exercise test is developed. For further elucidation, this sections attempts to show how protocols can be developed for the bicycle and treadmill, utilizing the principles previously discussed (Tables 10-3 and 10-4). The duration of the intermittent bicycle ergometer protocol is longer, but data acquisition is facilitated. Stage I, selected because of its low MET level (2.3), serves as a warm-up stage. The second stage is a mild increment (1.4 MET), and the following stages require energy increments of approximately 2.5 MET. Such a protocol is usually not appropriate for a person with very low fitness, because of the relatively high energy requirement increments from stage to stage. It should be remembered that the terminal load varies between subjects and may be higher than the highest load shown in Table 10-3. Variations in exercise intensity values and identification of higher intensities than those appearing in Table 10-3 can be found elsewhere.[1]

Table 10-4 shows a progressive walking protocol on the treadmill. This pattern illustrates one of many that can be designed for a cardiac patient or someone whose exercise capacity is severely limited. Like the previous example, this protocol utilizes the first stage as warm-up at a low MET level (2.3). Subsequent stages increase the energy

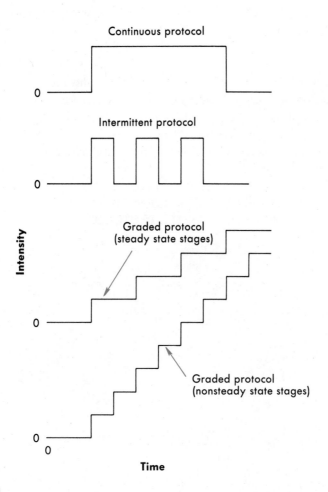

FIG. 10-1 Four typical exercise test intensity patterns. The intensity of the test stages is illustrated as a function of time. A continuous protocol illustrates a single intensity pattern which might be used to evaluate physiological response to long-term exercise. Intermittent protocols intersperse periods of exercise with periods of rest. Utilizing this protocol to test functional capacity would necessitate increasing intensity with each exercise stage. Two graded protocols are shown, one utilizing short duration, non-steady state stages and the other comprises longer duration, steady state stages. If the test administrator is desirous of utilizing stage data for prescribing exercise, for example, steady state values would be mandatory.

increment by approximately 1 MET. Many cardiac patients entering phase II (up to 12 weeks after MI) and phase III (more than 12 weeks after MI) exercise programs have functional capacities below 5 MET. If this exercise protocol is followed, additional stages can be added if necessary.[1]

Test termination criteria

Whether the test is administered to a high-risk patient or to a highly trained athlete, the result is the determination of functional capacity, that is, the physical load (or energy equivalent) at which termination occurs. In the former case, termination may occur because of the appearance of abnormal signs on the ECG or abnormal symptoms (angina). In the latter case, termination usually occurs because of physical exhaustion. In both cases

TABLE 10-3 ‖‖‖ SAMPLE OF AN INTERMITTENT, PROGRESSIVE BICYCLE ERGOMETER PROTOCOL

Stage	Time (min)	Exercise intensity (kg-m · min^{-1})	MET
I	0-5	0*	2.3
Rest	5-10	0	1.0†
II	10-15	300	3.7
Rest	15-20	0	1.0
III	20-25	600	6.1
Rest	25-30	0	1.0
IV	30-35	900	8.6
Rest	35-40	0	1.0
V	40-45	1200	11.0

*Pedaling without flywheel resistance
†MET value after metabolism returns to resting state

TABLE 10-4 ‖‖‖ SAMPLE OF A CONTINUOUS, PROGRESSIVE TREADMILL WALKING PROTOCOL

Stage	Time (min)	Speed (mph)	Grade (%)	MET
I	0-3	1.7	0	2.3
II	3-6	1.7	5.0	3.5
III	6-9	1.7	10.0	4.6
IV	9-12	2.5	7.5	5.6
V	12-15	3.0	7.5	6.4

the test can be terminated when the physician judges the work to be maximal or intolerable. An alternative to continuation until exhaustion is the use of an arbitrary endpoint, such as a percentage of maximal heart rate. Some argue that a submaximal test that automatically terminates when 85% of maximal heart rate is attained should be sufficient for evaluation of exercise tolerance in most exercise situations. Others argue that the test is not valid unless individuals reach symptoms (symptom-limited test) or maximal heart rate and/or oxygen consumption. Figure 10-2 illustrates the decline of maximal heart rate with age, which can be used to assign arbitrary test termination points; for example, the test is terminated automatically when a 45-year-old subject's heart rate reaches 175. Most exercise tests in the 1980s continue to maximal heart rate if other termination criteria have not been met by then. If $\dot{V}O_2$ max is the criterion, the test is terminated when increases in exercise intensity fail to produce increases in $\dot{V}O_2$.

The signs and symptoms that serve as criteria for terminating a test[1,12] are the following:

1. Premature ventricular contractions (PVCs) appearing in pairs, continuous bigeminy (PVC every other beat) or trigeminy (PVC every third beat), or with ventricular tachycardia (run of three or more PVCs)
2. Atrial tachycardia or fibrillation

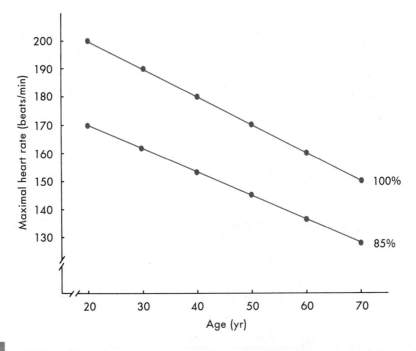

FIG. 10-2   Age-related maximal heart rate as well as 85% of maximum. It can be seen that values decline predictably with increasing age. This graph was developed utilizing the predictive formula: Maximum heart rate = 200 − Age (years).

3. Second- and third-degree heart block and sudden left bundle branch block
4. Progressive intensity of anginal pain
5. ST depression of 2 mm
6. Decrease in heart rate and systolic blood pressure (SBP) with increasing exercise intensity
7. Dyspnea, nausea, fatigue, or faintness
8. Severe musculoskeletal pain
9. Patient appears vasoconstricted (pale and clammy)
10. Exaggerated increase in SBP (>250 mm Hg), increase in diastolic blood pressure (DBP) more than 20 mm Hg, or increase above 110 to 120 mm Hg
11. Malfunctioning equipment

Medications and exercise test response

Most cardiac patients and many patients who need preventive measures require medications. When the physician elects to test these patients without withdrawing medications, the exercise test technologist must be aware of the possibility of interpretation difficulties with certain common cardiac drugs. Table 10-5 summarizes the possible interfering effects of selected cardiac drugs.[1] These drugs should probably be removed temporarily in the case of a diagnostic test.

Emergency procedures and equipment

All personnel involved with exercise testing should be trained in cardiopulmonary resuscitation (CPR)—basic life support. At least one of the testing team should addition-

TABLE 10-5 |||||| SUMMARY OF THE POSSIBLE EFFECTS OF CARDIAC MEDICATIONS ON THE INTERPRETATION OF EXERCISE TESTS

Drug type	Possible effect	
	May delay onset of ischemia	May cause false positive
Antianginal	X	
Beta blocker	X	
Antihypertensive		X
Digitalis		X
Antiarrhythmic	X	X
	(Quinidine, propranolol)	(Digoxin)
Tranquilizers		X

Adapted from American College of Sports Medicine: Guidelines for graded exercise testing and exercise prescription, ed. 2, Philadelphia, 1980, Lea & Febiger.

ally be trained in advanced cardiac life support. The testing area should contain a defibrillator, devices to maintain airways, a suction apparatus, and oxygen with an Ambu bag system. Also, emergency drugs should be available.[1] Emergency telephone numbers should be posted and emergency procedures and evacuation plans practiced periodically.[1]

PHYSIOLOGY OF THE GRADED EXERCISE TEST

It was mentioned earlier that the minimum of exercise test instrumentation would include a sphygmomanometer (blood pressure) and electrocardiogram (electrical activity plus heart rate). Figure 10-3 illustrates two important points relative to heart rate response. First, it can be seen that stage duration plays an important role in the identification of the

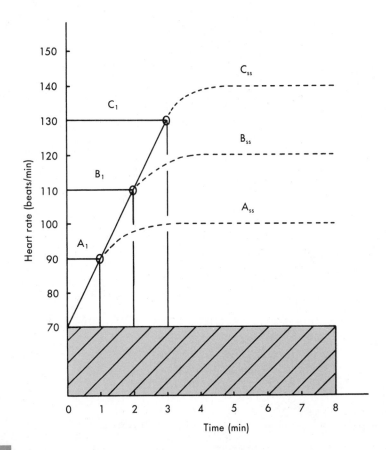

FIG. 10-3   Heart rate response to increasing exercise intensity in an exercise test. This figure illustrates the effect of using short duration (1 min) non-steady-state stages compared to longer (3 min), steady state stages. The 1 min heart rate values for the 3 stages (A_1, B_1, C_1) are 90, 110, and 130, respectively. If these stages would be extended to 3 min (approximating steady state conditions $[SS]$) the values change to 100, 120, and 140, respectively.

steady-state response. Stages with a short duration (1 minute) fail to provide steady state responses. Second, heart rate increases with each stage of the test. The magnitude of the increase is related to age, physical fitness, environmental factors, and health status. Figure 10-4 displays the plot of heart rate as a function of oxygen consumption in three groups: cardiac patients, untrained normals, and trained normals.[23] All three groups show a linear increase in heart rate as $\dot{V}_{O_2}$ increases. However, the slope of the line for patients is significantly higher than that for both trained and untrained normals.

Expected systolic blood pressure response during exercise is 7 to 10 mm Hg per

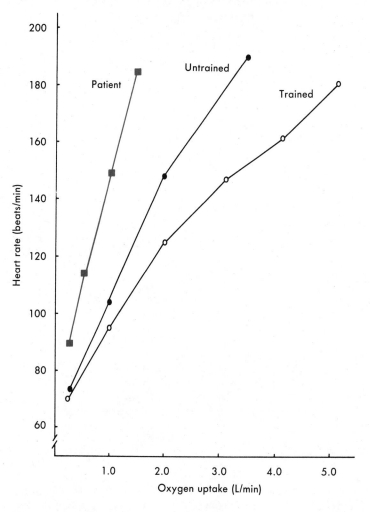

FIG. 10-4   **Comparison of the heart rate response to an exercise test protocol in cardiac patients and normal untrained and untrained subjects. Patients terminate the test at a lower oxygen uptake level and show a steeper heart rate slope throughout. (Adapted from Spiro, S.G.: Exercise testing in clinical medicine, Br. J. Dis. Chest *71*:145, 1977.)**

MET.[3] The normal ECG shows shortened PR and QT intervals and a displaced J-point. (The J-point is the point of inflection as the S wave returns to the baseline and becomes the T wave.) Normal subjects do not show anginal pain, claudication pain (legs), or intolerable dyspnea even during maximal exercise.[3]

POSTTEST PROCEDURES

As soon as the test termination criteria has been met, the exercise intensity should be reduced to a minimum. It is not advisable for the patient to stop immediately, since it is common for some patients to become hypotensive and faint when stopped abruptly after strenuous exercise. Therefore 1 or 2 minutes of easy pedaling or flat walking is a prudent procedure. Following this brief posttest activity, the patient should be placed in the supine position for the remainder of the recovery period. Usually a symptom-free recovery period lasts 6 to 8 minutes.[25] It should not be assumed that a test is normal just because no abnormal responses were observed during the exercise phase of the test. It is not uncommon to observe abnormal responses only in the recovery period after cessation of the exercise.[14] Sometimes coronary artery ischemia can be masked by exercise-induced arterial dilation. The absolute duration of the recovery period is determined by the normalization of the abnormal response.[3]

TEST INTERPRETATION
Functional capacity tests

Astrand[5] has cautioned exercise physiologists to be wary of data collected from a single test when evaluating the physical condition of an individual. He refers to the interpretation of $\dot{V}O_2$ max. Low values, could mean the presence of a disease process, low genetic endowment, or low physical condition. The presence of a disease process can be readily determined by supplementary testing. Determination of whether a low $\dot{V}O_2$ max should be interpreted as a low condition or a low genetic endowment is much more difficult. The only adequate discrimination is through a training program, which defeats the purpose of a predictive test to evaluate physical condition.

The units of expression for $\dot{V}O_2$ max should depend on the goal. For instance, when subjects increase body composition concomitantly with $\dot{V}O_2$ max—such as during the training of postpubescent girls, or any training that combines a cardiovascular stimulus with muscular hypertrophy—ml/kg should not be utilized. Expressing $\dot{V}O_2$ max per unit of body mass masks the $\dot{V}O_2$ changes.[5] Another example involves the use of ml/kg when evaluating athletes who do not have to move their body mass directly, for instance, swimmers and rowers. This expression is appropriate for runners, since the activity directly involves lifting body mass against gravity.[5]

Each stage of the exercise test should have an identified oxygen requirement. In this way, functional capacity can be expressed in oxygen consumption or MET terms. If the test protocol in Table 10-3 is used as an example, a subject who completes the third stage of the test before fatigue would be said to have a functional capacity of 6.1 MET, or 21.4 ml · kg/min^{-1} (MET value × 3.5). Most subjects like to know how such values compare with others of similar characteristics. It is often difficult to locate standards that have been determined from a large enough sample displaying the necessary demographic characteristics. One of the best fitness classifications grids appears in Table 10-6. Carrying the previous example another step, if our subject was a 45-year-old woman, the test interpretation would place the subject in the "fair" fitness classification (between 17 and 23 ml · kg/min^{-1}).

Diagnostic tests

Tests conducted for the purpose of evaluating the presence or absence of ischemic heart disease (IHD) represent a different interpretive problem. Here, a judgment is being made about a disease process. An incorrect judgment can be devastating to the patient. If the test results are interpreted to indicate the presence of IHD, but the patient does not in fact have IHD (false positive), the patient will begin a life of limitation and fear, which is not appropriate. On the other hand, if the patient has IHD that the test data do not confirm (false negative) the patient will continue normal life routines (which may be dangerous) or, at the least, omit possible therapeutic remedies. These questions are addressed in medicine by evaluating the results of a predictive test against those of a direct determination of the disease process. In this case, the exercise test results are compared with the results of coronary angiography. Angiographic evidence is said to be positive when a coronary artery is obstructed by at least 50%. Most studies have determined that IHD has to be well advanced (50% to 75% occlusion) before symptoms or ECG changes

TABLE 10-6 |||||| CARDIORESPIRATORY FITNESS CLASSIFICATION SYSTEM DEVELOPED BY THE PREVENTIVE MEDICINE CENTER IN PALO ALTO, CALIFORNIA

Women Age (yrs)	Maximal oxygen uptake (ml · kg/min^{-1})				
	Low	Fair	Average	Good	High
20-29	<24	24-30	31-37	38-48	>48
30-39	<20	20-27	28-33	34-44	>44
40-49	<17	17-23	24-30	31-41	>41
50-59	<15	15-20	21-27	28-37	>37
60-69	<13	13-17	18-23	24-34	>34
Men					
20-29	<25	25-33	34-42	43-52	>52
30-39	<23	23-30	31-38	39-48	>48
40-49	<20	20-26	27-35	36-44	>44
50-59	<18	18-24	25-33	34-42	>42
60-69	<16	16-22	23-30	31-40	>40

occur.[9,17] Because interindividual differences exist regarding the degree of coronary artery occlusion and production of symptoms or ECG changes during exercise tests, some error in prediction can be expected. The key to diagnostic test development is to keep the error at a minimum. Another way of stating the challenge is that the test must demonstrate both high *sensitivity* and high *specificity*. Simply stated, this means that false-positive and false-negative results (sensitivity and specificity, respectively) are minimized. More exactly, sensitivity and specificity are calculated as follows[12]:

$$\text{Sensitivity} = \frac{\text{Patients with positive exercise tests and positive angiograms}}{\text{All patients with positive angiograms}} \times 100$$

$$\text{Specificity} = \frac{\text{Patients with negative exercise tests and negative angiograms}}{\text{All patients with negative angiograms}} \times 100$$

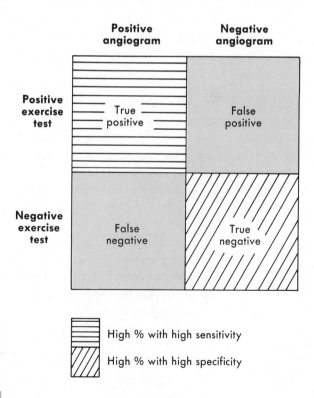

FIG. 10-5   The relationship between angiographic tests, directly examining the degree of ischemia in the coronary arteries, and exercise tests, which indirectly predict the presence of ischemia in the coronary arteries. If the two tests produce confirming results a high percentage of the time the predictive test is said to be sensitive (true positives) or specific (true negatives).

For a test to be highly sensitive, most patients with positive angiograms also must have positive exercise tests (few false positives). A highly specific test produces few false negatives. Figure 10-5 illustrates the relationship of exercise tests and angiographic tests to sensitivity and specificity.

More false positives are observed in populations showing a low disease prevalence (one-vessel disease) compared to populations with a high prevalence (three-vessel disease).[25] In other words, when the disease is not as well developed, it is more difficult to detect with exercise testing. Those with minimal and obscure signs and symptoms are therefore difficult to diagnose. The chance of a positive exercise test increases with the number of vessels occluded (40%, 65%, and 78% with 1-, 2-, and 3-vessel disease, respectively). In addition, the predictive value of the exercise test improves with the depth of the ST depression.[12] Although a 1.0 mm ST depression resulted in positive angiography 90% of the time, a 2.0 mm ST depression proved to be correct 98% of the time.

Test termination criteria and angiographic criteria play a major role in correct predictions. The degree of closure used to judge the presence of IHD is critical.[7] A 70% arterial closure criterion is more rigorous and perhaps more correct than 50% closure. It has also been found that maximal exercise tests reveal more correct positive responses than near-maximal tests.[16]

SUMMARY

The student who may be interested in a nonteaching career in health or physical education should know about graded exercise testing. Testing principles are basically the same for apparently healthy populations, those having heart disease, and those limited by a high risk of it. With patients who have the disease, more emphasis is placed on cardiac monitoring.

The objectives of graded exercise testing are the determination of functional capacity, diagnosis of heart disease, development of an individualized exercise prescription, and evaluation of that prescription's effectiveness.

Before testing, subjects should be instructed to follow selected procedures, which help to produce a more valid test result. These instructions involve physical activity, nutrition, drugs, and clothing. A comprehensive health history recorded just before testing provides valuable information, which has a bearing on decisions to be made during the test and on subsequent test interpretation. Similarly, a physical examination by a physician may reveal conditions that contraindicate testing; for example, patients with acute heart disease or unstable chest pain (angina pectoris) should not be tested. To protect the patient and the test administrator, informed consent documents must be explained and signed. The individual, however, cannot sign away the right to competent and prudent performance by the testing personnel.

Testing equipment options include the step bench, bicycle ergometer, and the treadmill. Although the step bench has historically been the device of choice, most test administrators currently use either a bicycle (17%) or a treadmill (72%). The bicycle offers several advantages, among which are that the subject does not have to move body weight because of the supported position, and exercise intensity can be easily and reliably adjusted. The major liability of this instrument is the fact that the form of movement is not common for a high percentage of the population. Treadmill testing has become popular because it tests a very common mode of movement, walking, and exercise intensity can be varied, like the bicycle, with ease and reliability.

Minimum instrumentation to conduct a valid test consists of an ECG, which also measures heart rate, and a sphygmomanometer for blood pressure measurements. Development of the test protocol should take into consideration duration (6 to 15 minutes), use of the early minutes of the test as a warm-up, beginning at an exercise intensity below the estimated point of impairment or maximal capacity ($\dot{V}O_2$ max), utilization of multiple loads, and progressive increments in load.

Exercise tests are terminated because of the appearance of abnormal signs (ECG or blood pressure) or symptoms (angina pectoris) or because of exhaustion. Usually tests are conducted with age-related maximal heart rate (100%) as an arbitrary termination point. Mandatory termination criteria include cardiac arrhythmias, decrease in the heart rate, decrease or exaggerated increase in the blood pressure, ischemic changes in the ECG, and malfunctioning equipment.

Abnormal physiological responses to the exercise test are decreased heart rate and blood pressure, increase in SBP above 250 mm Hg, ST segment depression (≥ 1 mm), certain cardiac arrhythmias (such as, continuously occurring PVCs), angina pain, claudication, severe dyspnea, and faintness.

It is difficult to determine whether a low $\dot{V}O_2$ max is a sign of poor physical condition or low genetic endowment. Units for expressing $\dot{V}O_2$ max (ml/kg or L/min) should be based on the test application. The functional capacity, ml $\cdot$ kg/min^{-1} or MET, can be estimated from the terminal stage of the exercise test.

The predictive value of a diagnostic test depends on calculated test sensitivity and specificity. Sensitivity measures the degree to which positive exercise tests agree with direct measurement of coronary artery occlusion (angiography). The more false-positive exercise tests, the lower the sensitivity. A highly specific test produces few false negatives. The predictive value of an exercise test improves both with the depth of the ST segment depression accepted for test termination and with the test extended to maximal fatigue levels, compared to near-maximal levels.

KEY TERMS

angina pectoris the pain associated with coronary artery ischemia that is usually manifested in the left side of the chest and in the left arm, but can also be sensed in the right arm, back, neck, and head.

angiography (coronary catheterization) a technique in which a catheter is inserted into the coronary arteries to determine the presence of arterial occlusion.

cardiac exercise program a supervised exercise program for cardiac patients conducted in the hospital during the acute stage (phase I), up to 12 weeks after a myocardial infarction (phase II), and 12 weeks after a myocardial infarction (phase III).

coronary heart disease (CHD) risk factors factors that when associated with a person's life-style or physiological make-up place a person at risk for coronary heart disease.

functional capacity the highest exercise intensity or physiological response attained during a graded exercise test, usually described in terms of MET or $\dot{V}O_2$ max.

ischemic heart disease (IHD) is used interchangeably with CHD and refers to decreased blood flow associated with coronary artery occlusion.

maximal test an exercise test that is terminated at subject exhaustion or when physiological variables reach maximal values.

MET a multiple of resting metabolic rate.

MI myocardial infarction (heart attack).

morbidity a nonfatal event.

mortality a fatal event.

preventive exercise program a supervised exercise program for individuals with and without CHD risk factors.

sensitivity the characteristic of a diagnostic exercise test in which false positives are minimized, that is, a positive exercise test and a negative angiogram.

specificity the characteristics of a diagnostic exercise test in which false negatives are minimized, that is, a negative exercise test and a positive angiogram.

submaximal test an exercise test that is terminated at an exercise intensity before subject exhaustion or the attainment of maximal physiological variables.

REVIEW QUESTIONS

1. Name the three primary risk factors for coronary heart disease and indicate the degree of risk with one, two, and three factors present.

2. If a patient exercises to exhaustion at the 7 MET level on a graded exercise test, what would be the estimated maximal oxygen consumption? Would this value be equivalent to functional capacity? Define functional capacity.

3. What is the range of both mortality and morbidity risk during graded exercise testing?

4. Discuss the value of obtaining a health history and physical examination before a graded exercise test.

5. Discuss the advantages and disadvantages of using a step bench, bicycle ergometer, or treadmill for a graded exercise test.

6. What are the possible criteria for terminating a graded exercise test? What is ST depression and what does it indicate?

7. Why does Astrand advise caution in interpreting functional capacity tests?

8. Define test sensitivity and specificity. How would you know that a graded exercise test was false positive?

REFERENCES

1. American College of Sports Medicine: Guidelines for graded exercise testing and exercise prescription, Philadelphia, 1980, ed. 2, Lea & Febiger.

2. American Heart Association: Exercise testing and training of apparently healthy individuals: a handbook for physicians, Dallas, 1972, American Heart Association.

3. American Heart Association: Exercise testing and training of individuals with heart disease or at high risk for its development: a handbook for physicians, Dallas, 1975, American Heart Association.

4. American Heart Association: The exercise standards book, Dallas, 1979, American Heart Association.

5. Astrand, P.O.: Quantification of exercise capability and evaluation of physical capacity in man. In Sonnenblick, E.H., and Lesch, M., editors: Exercise and heart disease, New York, 1977, Grune & Stratton.

6. Bousfield, G.: Angina pectoris: variations in electrocardiograms during paroxysm, Lancet **2:**457, 1918.

7. Cardus, D.: Exercise testing: methods and uses. In Hutton, R.S., editor: Exercise and sport sciences reviews, Philadelphia, 1978, Franklin Institute Press.

8. Costill, D.L., and Winrow, E.: Maximum oxygen intake among marathon runners, Arch. Phys. Med. Rehabil. **51:**317, 1970.

9. Diethrich, E.B., Liddicoat, J.E., Kinard, S.A., and others: Surgical significance of angiographic patterns in coronary arterial disease, Circulation **36:**155, 1967.

10. Dill, D.B.: The Harvard Fatigue Laboratory: its development, contributions and demise. In Chapman, C.B., editor: Physiology of muscular exercise, New York, 1967, American Heart Association.

11. Einthoven, W.: Weiteres uber das Elektrokardiogramm, Arch. Physiologie **122:**517, 1908.

12. Ellestad, M.H.: Stress testing: principles and practices, ed. 2, Philadelphia, 1980, F.A. Davis Co.

12a. Fairshter, R.D., Walters, J., Salness, K., and others: A comparison of incremental exercise tests during cycle and treadmill ergometry, Med. Sci. Sports Exerc. **15:**549, 1983.

13. Feil, H., and Siegel, M.L.: Electrocardiographic changes during attacks of angina, Am. J. Med. Sci. **175:**255, 1928.

14. Froelicher, V.F., and others: Value of exercise testing for screening asymptomatic men for latent coronary artery disease, Prog. Cardiovasc. Dis. **43:**265, 1976.

15. Karlsson, J.: The physiology of alpine skiing, Park City, Utah, 1978, United States Ski Coaches Association.

16. Lester, R.M., Sheffield, L.T., and Reeves, T.J.: Electrocardiographic changes in clinically normal older men following near-maximal and maximal exercise, Circulation **36:**5, 1967.

17. Mason, R.E., Likar, I., Biern, R.O., and others: Multiple-lead exercise electrocardiography, Circulation **36:**517, 1967.

18. Master, A.M., and Jaffe, H.L.: The electrocardiographic changes after exercise in angina pectoris, J. Mt. Sinai Hosp. **7:**629, 1941.

19. Master, A.M., and Oppenheimer, E.J.: A simple exercise tolerance test for circulatory efficiency with standard tables for normal individuals, Am. J. Med. Sci. **177:**223, 1929.

20. McHenry, P.L., and Morris, S.N.: Exercise electrocardiography: current state of the art. In Schlant, R., and Hurst, W., editors: Advances in electrocardiography, New York, 1976, Grune & Stratton.

21. Rochnis, P., and Blackburn, H.: Exercise tests: a survey of procedures, safety and litigation expenses in approximately 170,000 tests, JAMA **217**:1061, 1971.

22. Sheffield, L.T., and Roitman, D.: Stress testing methodology. In Sonnenblick, E.H., and Lesch, M., editors: Exercise and heart disease, New York, 1977, Grune & Stratton.

23. Spiro, S.G.: Exercise testing in clinical medicine, Br. J. Dis. Chest **71**:145, 1977.

24. Stuart, R.J., Jr.: National survey of stress-testing facilities. In Ellestad, M.H., Allen, W.H., and Stuart, R.J., Jr., editors: New developments in stress testing, Long Beach, Calif., 1977, Long Beach Memorial Hospital.

24a. Weltman, A., and Regan, J.: A reliable method for the measurement of constant load maximal endurance performance on the bicycle ergometer, Res. Q. Exerc. Sport **53**:176, 1982.

25. Wilson, P.K., Fardy, P.S., and Froelicher, V.F.: Cardiac rehabilitation, adult fitness, and exercise testing, Philadelphia, 1981, Lea & Febiger.

26. Wolfe, L.A., Cunningham, D.A., Paulseth, J.E., and others: The value of combining non-invasive techniques in exercise testing, Med. Sci. Sports Exerc. **12**:200, 1980.

SUGGESTED READINGS

Blackburn, H., editor: Measurement in exercise electrocardiography, Springfield, Ill., 1969, Charles C Thomas, Publishers.

Fardy, P.S., Bennett, J.L., Reitz, N.L., and others: Cardiac rehabilitation: implications for the nurse and other allied health professionals, St. Louis, 1980, The C.V. Mosby Co.

Pollock, M.L., and Schmidt, D.H., editors: Heart disease and rehabilitation, Boston, 1979, Houghton Mifflin.

Sonnenblick, E.H., and Lesch, M., editors: Exercise and heart disease, New York, 1977, Grune & Stratton.

CASE STUDY 1

A high school alpine ski coach called recently to discuss a young male skier formerly on his team.

COACH: My skier had an excellent high school record and should make a very good college skier. He and his parents had been invited by the U.S. Olympic ski coaches, who wanted to assess his future potential, to train with the team. This means delaying his college education by 1 or 2 years and making a certain monetary investment by the parents. His parents want to know if the young man has the potential for international competition.

PROFESSOR: I would be happy to help if everyone understands that what we study is physiological potential, not necessarily the potential for skiing per se. The whole of skiing is greater than the sum of the physiological parts. Skiing involves motor skill and certain psychological characteristics that we cannot assess.

With all this understood, a time was scheduled to assess both the aerobic and anaerobic capacities (including strength) of the skier. Karlsson[15] found that relatively high blood lactic acid levels after alpine skiing indicate a high anaerobic component as well as an aerobic component. The nature of the motor skill indicates the need for high muscular strength. Only the aerobic functional capacity ($\dot{V}O_2$ max) test results were considered.

To obtain the most valid data, it was decided to measure the $\dot{V}O_2$ directly instead of making an estimation based on physical load. It is difficult to achieve aerobic specificity with skiers, since none of the testing instruments adequately simulate the activity. However, since many international alpine skiers have been tested on the treadmill, this instrument was selected. An adaptation of the Costill test protocol[8] was chosen because it contained all the elements necessary for testing the functional capacity of a potential international athlete. Six minutes of low-intensity exercise (3.0, 4.5, and 6.0 mph) was administered to allow for warm-up. Warm-up was followed by 3-minute stages at 9.0 mph beginning at 0% grade and increasing to 4% at the second stage, with 2% increments in each succeeding stage. The following are the results:

Stage	Speed (mph)	Grade (%)	MET	Time (min)	$\dot{V}O_2$ (L/min^{-1})	$\dot{V}O_2$ (ml · kg/min^{-1})
I	3.0	0	3.3	0-2	1.18	16.7
II	4.5	0	7.9	2-4	1.54	21.8
III	6.0	0	10.2	4-6	2.38	33.7
IV	9.0	0	14.8	6-9	3.58	50.7
V	9.0	4	17.3	9-12	4.09	57.9
VI	9.0	6	18.5	12-15	4.35	61.5
VII	9.0	8	19.7	15-16*	4.33	61.3

*Subject voluntarily stopped after 1 minute of stage VII.

It is important to note that the attainment of a stage requiring close to 20 times the resting metabolic rate is an outstanding achievement in itself. The fact that a plateau in $\dot{V}O_2$ was achieved in the final 2 stages validates the maximal value. Functional capacity ($\dot{V}O_2$ max) was established at 61.5 ml · kg/min^{-1} (4.35 L/min^{-1}). Corrected for altitude (+7%), equivalent sea level $\dot{V}O_2$ max would be approximately 66.0 ml · kg/min^{-1}. (NOTE: STPD correction adjusts pulmonary ventilation, not oxygen consumption per se.) Astrand[5] reported an average value for the Swedish National Alpine Ski Team of 67 ml · kg/min^{-1} (a range of 53 to 77).

The aerobic functional capacity of this skier was judged to be high enough to compete at an international level. Again, caution should be used in making performance predictions from one physiological variable without considering motor skill and psychological factors.

CASE STUDY 2

A police officer was tested in the Human Energy Research Laboratory at the University of Wyoming; an exercise test is part of the annual physical examination administered to each officer. The subject was a 33-year-old asymptomatic man with an elevated resting blood pressure (148/94) but no other risk factors. He ran regularly, usually covering 4 miles at a pace of 8:00 min/mile. During the administration of a recent departmental physical fitness battery, the subject completed 1.5 miles in 12 minutes in the Cooper test. A Bruce protocol was administered with the following results (the age-related maximal heart rate was 185):

Stage	Speed (mph)	Grade (%)	MET	Heart rate (beats/min)	Blood pressure (mm Hg)
I	1.7	10	4.6	110	162/90
II	2.5	12	7.0	130	170/88
III	3.4	14	10.2	162	182/70
IV	4.2	16	12.1	180	—

The subject remained asymptomatic throughout the entire test. During stage II, an equivocal ST depression was observed. During stage III, a clear 3 mm ST depression appeared. The subject was taken to stage IV to see if symptomatology could be produced. No angina pain occurred, but the ST segment dropped to 5 mm. The test was terminated immediately. Recovery was unremarkable, with a rapid return of the ST segment to baseline. Further questioning revealed that the subject had previously experienced some chest tightness while jogging. Coronary angiography was recommended and resulted in the diagnosis of three-vessel disease. Subsequently, the subject received three bypasses in open heart surgery. The pretest signs were very misleading in this case. The previous exercise habits of the patient prompted continuation of a test that normally would have been terminated much sooner.

These cases are not common, but they occur often enough to encourage utmost caution with every person tested. Even a young, physically active person may exhibit coronary artery disease. Fortunately, in this case the problem was identified early before a more serious cardiac event occurred.

chapter 11

INDIVIDUALIZED EXERCISE PRESCRIPTION

MAJOR LEARNING OBJECTIVE
Prescription consists of assimilation of knowledge from the literature, dosage assignments (type, frequency, duration, and intensity), and unit conversion (converting test data to a unit useful in controlling exercise in a practical setting).

APPLICATIONS
Minimum exercise dosages for making positive physiological gains are 3 days per week, 30 minutes per day, and 70% of functional capacity.
■ Frequency and duration recommendations are derived from previous research. Intensity data are derived from a graded exercise test, usually involving heart rate. The heart rate must be monitored in the practical setting to ensure compliance with intensity recommendations.

257

$\mathbf{A}$ **LONG**-term objective of exercise physiology is the establishment of a pharmacopeia of exercise. A pharmacopeia is an authoritative book containing information on medicinal drugs. Exercise can and should be viewed as a therapeutic agent that must be thoughtfully administered, as with any drug. In the fields of health and physical education, a pharmacopeia would relate the physiological benefits of exercise to the physical properties of exercise (type, frequency, duration, and intensity). In other words, it would determine the dose-response relationship and, if a certain response is desired, the physical properties of the dose. Implicit in the development of the pharmacopeia would be the recognition that the prescribed dose for one may not be adequate for another; individualization is mandatory.

To date, not enough research has been completed to warrant an entire book devoted to dose-response relationships in exercise. However, the past 20 years have provided enough data to enable practitioners to make intelligent decisions about individualized exercise prescriptions. Exercise prescription today is possible because of research that has linked three factors: benefits, physical properties of exercise, and personal characteristics of the exerciser. The greatest portion of the research has related physical properties to cardiorespiratory benefits and has used aerobic capacity ($\dot{V}_{O_2}$ max) as the unit of measurement to describe those benefits. Physical properties, as just mentioned, include type, frequency, duration, and intensity of exercise. Personal characteristics that may modify the prescription are age, sex, and physical condition. This chapter addresses the interaction of benefits, physical properties of exercise, and personal characteristics in the development of the exercise prescription.

Figure 11-1 shows a general model that describes the prescribing of exercise. Prescription development necessitates the *assimilation* of information from the body of knowledge as well as from the exercise test. Type, frequency, duration, and intensity recommendations are provided from research that has examined the interaction of these variables with the production of benefits. Intensity recommendations are personalized through data directly generated in the exercise test. *Dosage assignment* usually takes the following form: type (aerobic or anaerobic as well as mode: walking, jogging, swimming, cycling, and so on); frequency (days/week); duration (time of the session, usually excluding warm-up and cool-down); and intensity (commonly expressed in MET). The final stage of the prescription process is the conversion of the data collected in the exercise test to intensity units usable at the exercise site *(unit conversion)*.

EXERCISE TEST AND PRESCRIPTION

At the time of the exercise test or before the development of the exercise prescription, background information should be sought from the potential exerciser. This information is separate but related to the health history and physical fitness evaluation connected to the exercise test per se. For example, prior and current exercise habits are relevant to the assignment both of the initial exercise level and of the most enjoyable type of exercise. (Compliance in exercise programs is related to enjoyment.[10]) Personal objectives of the exerciser are also relevant to the setting of the prescription. The young athlete preparing for the Junior Olympics is directed toward exercise training quite different from that of a middle-aged adult interested only in achieving optimal cardiorespiratory benefits. It has been suggested that setting short- and long-term exercise goals with the exerciser is a fruitful preliminary activity.[18]

Exercise test variables

Certain variables measured during the exercise test are very useful in developing the exercise intensity prescription. These variables are heart rate (HR), oxygen consumption ($\dot{V}O_2$), MET, electrocardiogram (ECG), blood pressure (BP), rate of perceived exertion (RPE), and double product (DP, or systolic blood pressure $\times$ heart rate). Usually the intensity component of the exercise prescription is based on the establishment of func-

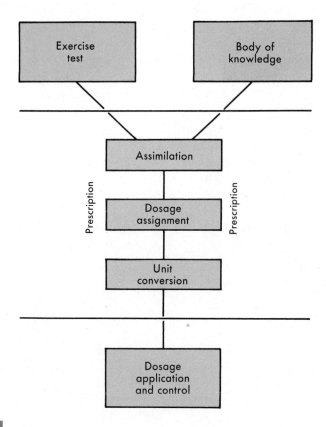

FIG. 11-1   **Steps in the development of the exercise prescription.**

tional capacity (FC) in the exercise test. The FC is expressed as a percentage of one of the units just listed, most often $\dot{V}O_2$, HR, MET, or symptoms and signs. Table 11-1 shows the most typical FC units and the translation of those units into useful values for prescribing exercise intensity. It should be noted that a field test could be devised that would estimate FC in healthy young individuals, for instance, a measurement of HR during exercise on a bicycle ergometer or step test. See Figure 11-4 for an illustration of how exercise HR might be prescribed.

Establishment of exercise intensity prescription from functional capacity determination

After the FC has been determined in the exercise test, the next question is what intensity level is most appropriate for the needs and objectives of the exerciser? A competitive athlete requires intensity levels much higher than the levels a cardiac patient requires, even though the prescriptive process is about the same. For example, a competitive cross-country skier requires intensity levels that push the upper levels of tolerance. The cardiac patient, on the other hand, needs only to be in a zone that ensures an optimal cardiorespiratory stimulus. The exact intensity levels required to provide a stimulus are discussed in detail later. For now, the figures of 70% and 90% of functional capacity will be used as values for the setting of the intensity prescription.

It should be pointed out that the prescriptive unit must be capable of being monitored or controlled during exercise. It might be quite logical and useful to prescribe exercise on the basis of lactate accumulation in the exercise test. However, the monitoring methods are not very practical or comfortable for most exercise programs. Figure 11-2 illustrates a method by which exercise intensity can be prescribed. This hypothetical patient complet-

TABLE 11-1 ‖‖‖ DESCRIPTIVE UNITS USED TO OBJECTIFY THE POINT AT WHICH AN EXERCISE TEST IS TERMINATED AND THE PRESCRIPTIVE UNIT USED TO SET EXERCISE INTENSITY ASSOCIATED WITH EACH

Test termination descriptive unit	Exercise intensity prescriptive unit
$\dot{V}O_2$	Percentage of $\dot{V}O_2$ max
MET	Percentage of MET max
HR	Percentage of HR max (preferably set as percentage of HR range)
ECG changes (such as ST depression)	Percentage of $\dot{V}O_2$, HR, or MET at which changes occur
Symptoms (such as angina pectoris)	Percentage of $\dot{V}O_2$, HR, or MET at which symptoms occur
BP (such as systolic rate $>$ 250 mm Hg)	Percentage of $\dot{V}O_2$, HR, or MET at which abnormal BP occurred
RPE	RPE associated with percentage of $\dot{V}O_2$, HR, or MET at test termination

ed three stages of the Bruce protocol with HRs of 135, 153, and 171, respectively. The reason for test termination was fatigue. FC was set at the MET equivalent of the final stage, 10 MET. Vertical lines are drawn from the 90% and 70% MET values, 9 and 7 MET, to the HR regression line. Horizontal lines drawn from the HR/MET regression line to the HR axis reveal the rates associated with the two prescribed MET levels: 165 and 153. It should be clear that although MET prescriptions cannot be directly monitored, HR equivalents can. The monitoring process is discussed later in this chapter.

Home exercise programs are occasionally prescribed directly from the MET values calculated from the exercise test. Table 11-2 provides a few examples of the MET values associated with certain modes of exercise. For example, a patient with an FC of 6 METs is allowed to play golf and tennis (doubles) but not basketball and handball. This method is deficient for most patients because there is no easy way to determine whether the prescription is maintained unless the HR is monitored periodically. Even HR monitoring may be erroneous because most sporting activity involves bursts of high energy output inter-

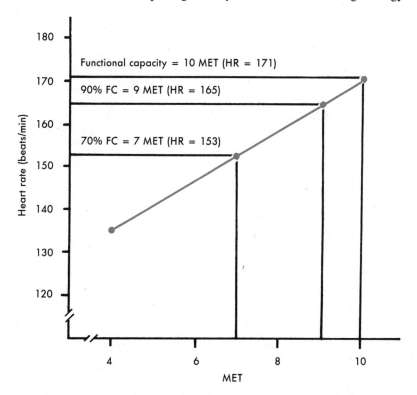

FIG. 11-2 Prescription of exercise intensity from stress test data. Functional capacity is set at the MET level of the final exercise stage. Average prescribed exercise intensity is 70% of functional capacity. This value is 7 MET in this hypothetical case and is equivalent to a heart rate of 153, the so-called target heart rate. Maximum exercise intensity for this case is 9 MET (or HR = 165).

spersed with periods of lower expenditure. Thus the table values are averages, and the absolute energy expenditure depends on the motivation of the participant. MET prescriptions are more accurate when the energy expenditure is maintained at a steady level, as in walking. MET prescriptions below 4 MET are considered low intensity; 4 to 9 MET, moderate; 8 to 12 MET, moderate to high; and greater than 12 MET, high intensity.[18]

Another common prescription method involves the calculation of the heart rate range (HRR). Called the Karvonen method after its developer, it assumes that the effective heart rate range for physical activity exists between the resting HR and the maximal HR. The maximal HR can either be predicted from tables showing the rate as a function of age or determined by direct measurement during an exercise test. If the maximal HR is the functional maximal HR, the rate achieved during the final stage of the exercise test,

TABLE 11-2 ‖‖‖‖ SAMPLE OF A MET TABLE USED TO PRESCRIBE EXERCISE FROM THE IDENTIFIED MET FUNCTIONAL CAPACITY

MET range	Exercise mode
3-4	Walking (3 mph)
	Cycling (6 mph)
	Golf (pulling cart)
4-5	Walking (3.5 mph)
	Cycling (8 mph)
	Tennis (doubles)
5-6	Canoeing (4 mph)
	Roller skating (9 mph)
6-7	Tennis (singles)
	Cross-country skiing (2.5 mph)
7-8	Jogging (5 mph)
	Basketball (recreational)
	Mountain climbing
	Ice hockey
8-9	Basketball (vigorous)
	Cycling (13 mph)
	Cross-country skiing (4 mph)
	Handball (social)
>9	Running (6 mph and above)
	Cross-country skiing (>4 mph)
	Handball (competitive)

it can be presumed that the individual is safe to exercise within the HRR. Figure 11-3 illustrates the calculation of prescribed HR with this method. The resting HR is subtracted from the maximal HR to establish the HRR. Target exercise rates are determined by multiplying the desired intensity percentage by the HRR and adding this figure to the resting HR.

PRESCRIPTION OF PHYSICAL PROPERTIES OF EXERCISE
Intensity

Of the four physical properties (intensity, duration, frequency, and type) involved in setting an exercise prescription, only intensity is developed from the exercise test. As mentioned previously, FC as determined in the exercise test is used to express prescribed exercise intensity. A percentage of FC is converted to a form usable during exercise, such as the percentage of HRR.

Intensity has been called the most important of the prescriptive components.[28] It is also the most difficult because of the necessity to bring it under control; that is, intensity is expressed in terms that are not stable, such as HR, so attention must be paid to the

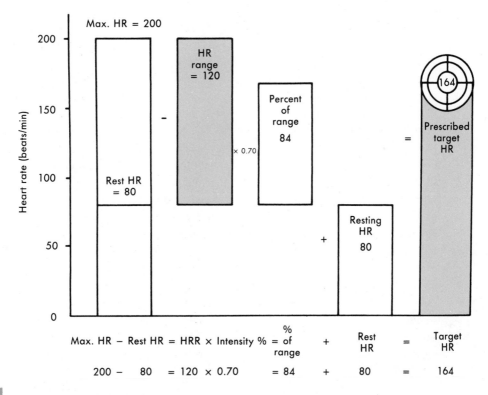

FIG. 11-3   Karvonen method of determining prescribed target heart rate (HR) as a percentage of the heart rate range (HRR). Any percentage can be used.

conditions that create stability and the methods that monitor change. This problem is discussed in more detail later.

Neither intensity nor the other components are pure factors independent of the others. For example, intensity is said to interact with duration. Beginners in cardiorespiratory exercise are said to do better with lower intensity and longer sessions.[18,19] With obese individuals and severely limited cardiac patients, the best results can be obtained by using the interactive qualities of frequency and duration. In these cases, a shorter exercise with more frequent daily sessions is recommended.

Cardiorespiratory improvement has been shown to be directly related to exercise intensity.[23] When three groups of subjects walked 3 days per week on a treadmill at HRs averaging 120, 150, and 180 beats/min, performance improvements (maximal treadmill time) were related to the stepwise increase in intensity.

Most people who have been exposed to competitive athletics have known coaches who espoused the ''no pain—no gain'' principle of training. Translated, this principle mandates maximal or near-maximal efforts during training sessions. The negative result of this principle is that many former athletes are unprepared to exercise as adults without great pain, grunting, and physical misery. In fact, research data are clear that adults interested in acquiring health benefits from exercise can gain those benefits without 100% intensity. The data have identified a variable intensity threshold for making improvements. The threshold is variable because the absolute magnitude of the threshold changes, depending on initial fitness,[7] age,[5,24] duration,[1] and disease.[2]

The concept of an intensity threshold does not negate the validity of the ''no pain—no gain'' principle for athletes. As barbaric as it may sound, elite athletes must train at high-intensity levels, which can be uncomfortably intense, to remain competitive. Greater improvement requires greater intensities. The problem with the ''no pain—no gain'' principle results from the athlete learning it exclusively.

Most of the early research concerned with the intensity factor used absolute physiological levels as a means of defining magnitude. An example of this technique was referred to earlier in the research that compared absolute HR levels: 120, 150, 180.[28] One of the first attempts to express exercise intensity on a relative basis was accomplished by Hollman and Venrath,[11] who showed that subjects made significant improvements when the training HR was approximately 60% of the HRR. Most current research reports evidence of intensity thresholds in relative terms. Subjects with varying capacities are thereby compared at equivalent exercise loads.

Table 11-3 summarizes current research on the intensity threshold level necessary to stimulate cardiorespiratory improvement. Because an exact 1:1 relationship does not exist between HR and $\dot{V}o_2$, it can be noted that the thresholds are lower when they are expressed in terms of $\dot{V}o_2$ max than when expressed in terms of HR max. Generally, the threshold for $\dot{V}o_2$ max is 50% to 80%, and for HR max it is 60% to 90%.[3,15,20,27]

Although two groups of investigators[4,19] could find no evidence of a threshold below 50%, some exceptions do exist. For instance, changes in 60- to 79-year-old men were noted at intensities between 35% and 60% of the HRR.[5] Similarly, changes were noted at

TABLE 11-3 ||||| SUMMARY OF RESEARCH CONDUCTED
TO DETERMINE OPTIMAL EXERCISE INTENSITY TO
ACHIEVE CARDIORESPIRATORY BENEFITS, WITH BOTH
$\dot{V}O_2$ MAX AND HR MAX USED AS THE BASIS FOR THE
PERCENTAGE PRESCRIPTION

$\dot{V}O_2$ max		HR max	
Percentage	**Reference**	**Percentage**	**Reference**
50	Astrand[3]	60-90	Pollock[15]
50-80	Pollock[15]	70-85	Taylor and others[27]
60-80	Roskamm[20]		

an intensity as low as 39% in older subjects.[24] Again, the intensity threshold may vary, depending on the characteristics of the group studied. It should be noted that in practice the term *intensity threshold* is sometimes interchanged with *target intensity*. However, the research goal in studies of exercise prescription has been to identify the level required for the achievement of benefit, so *threshold* is used here.

Duration

It should be repeated that the duration component is not independent of intensity; the two components are interactive. The American College of Sports Medicine[1] recommends an effective duration range of 15 to 60 minutes. Specific duration prescriptions depend on the intensity used. Cardiorespiratory changes can be made with 15-minute durations as long as the intensity is high. Adults who exercise with a health motive respond well to low to moderate intensities and longer programs.[1] However, greater improvements were observed with longer training when 20-, 40-, and 60-minute sessions were compared (with the intensity held constant).[14] It has been argued that the interaction of duration and intensity is a function of the lack of control over total work.[22] In other words, the important variable is the total work performed in training, independent of either intensity or duration.

As with intensity, some variability has been observed regarding the minimal duration threshold for improvement. English[6] and Canadian[24] scientists have both observed improvement with durations as low as 5 minutes. On the other hand, when 5-, 15-, and 25-minute durations were directly compared, no cardiorespiratory improvement could be found in the 5-minute group. Certainly the duration that provides a sufficient training stimulus is a function of initial physical fitness and disease state.[2]

Frequency

Frequency is thought to be the least important of the prescriptive components. The threshold for cardiovascular improvement appears to be 2 or 3 exercise sessions per week.

Both 2 and 4 sessions per week were found to stimulate significantly higher improvements than 1 per week.[25] Others have observed significant improvements with a frequency of 2 sessions per week.[16] Most authorities recommend a frequency of 3 to 5 sessions per week to make optimal improvements[1,28] and 2 to 3 per week for a maintenance program after initial gains have been made.[28]

As mentioned previously with regard to duration, total work performed each week, not frequency alone, may be the important factor. When total work was equated in an investigation—four sessions were compared to two and three sessions compared to five— no significant differences in improvement were observed.[25] In another confirming study, when variable frequencies of training were contrasted, with exercise intensity and weeks of training held constant, improvement was greatest with the highest frequency. In such an experimental paradigm, total work increases with the number of weeks of training. Total work, not frequency, can therefore be said to be responsible for the training improvements. However, one long workout would not be enough to achieve beneficial effects.

Type of exercise

The type of exercise does not appear to be critical to cardiovascular improvement when intensity, duration, and frequency are adequate. For example, when running, walking, and cycling were compared, with the intermode prescriptive components held constant (30 min, 3 days/wk, 85% to 95% HR max), results were approximately equal.[17]

Enjoyment is an important factor in the selection of exercise,[28] since exercise program compliance is not high when enjoyment is missing.[10] Other factors to consider are goals, available facilities, time, and physical fitness.[1] When the potential exerciser has very low fitness, the initial concern must be the development of the cardiorespiratory system to serve as a foundation for further, more specific conditioning.[19]

Cardiac patients present a special set of problems for the exercise specialist or technologist prescribing exercise. First, the exercise's intensity should be easily controlled. Games, for instance, have such a variable intensity that it is difficult to maintain exercise at a safe and beneficial level. Walking, on the other hand, can be easily controlled. Cardiorespiratory (continuous, large-muscle, aerobic) activity, such as walking and jogging, is best as the initial type of exercise for cardiac patients and is perhaps superior at all other times as well.[1] Game activity should be prudently recommended and never prescribed until the patient's FC reaches 5 MET.[1] Table 11-4 summarizes the literature relative to prescriptive advice for cardiac patients in phase I (in hospital), phase II (discharge to 12 weeks), and phase III (beyond 12 weeks).[18] These recommendations are variations of those made for normal exercisers.

Because many occupational and leisure-time activities involve muscular strength and endurance, it is practical to include activities that comprise both these factors in a program for low-fitness exercise participants. However, high resistance weight training, which produces strength, results in two physiological responses that are contraindicated: increase in systolic blood pressure and breath holding. Of course, breath holding results only from

TABLE 11-4 ||||| RECOMMENDED FREQUENCY, INTENSITY, DURATION, AND TYPE OF EXERCISE FOR CARDIAC PATIENTS PARTICIPATING IN A PHASE I (IN HOSPITAL), PHASE II (DISCHARGE TO 12 WEEKS), AND PHASE III (BEYOND 12 WEEKS) CARDIAC REHABILITATION PROGRAM*

Physical properties of prescription	Phase I	Phase II	Phase III
Frequency	2-3/day	1-2/day	3-5/wk
Intensity			
MI	RHR + 20	RHR + 20	70%-85% HRR
BS	RHR + 30	RHR + 30	
Duration			
MI	5-20 min	20-45 min	30-60 min
BS	5-30 min	30-60 min	
Type	ROM	ROM	Walking
	Treadmill	Treadmill	Bicycling
	Bicycling	Bicycling	Jogging
	Walking up stairs (1 flight)	Arm ergometer	Swimming
			Calisthenics
			Endurance sports

Adapted from Pollock, M.L., Ward, A., and Foster, C. In Pollock, M.L., and Schmidt, D.H., editors: Heart disease and rehabilitation, Boston, 1979, Houghton-Mifflin.
*MI = Myocardial infarction; BS = bypass surgery; RHR = resting heart rate; HRR = heart rate range; ROM = range-of-motion exercises.

poor weight training technique. Breath holding uses what is known as the Valsalva maneuver. Literally, a Valsalva maneuver involves closing the glottis against pressure. Such a maneuver interrupts venous return to the heart, which can be dangerous to the patient whose cardiovascular system is already compromised. Patients in categories D to H (see Table 10-1) should be encouraged to perform low-resistance exercises without breath holding to improve muscle tone.[1]

Summary of intensity, duration, frequency, and type

The keen observer should realize from the previous discussion that although basic minimal (threshold) prescriptive recommendations can be made, a great deal of flexibility is possible. Many different combinations of intensity, duration, frequency, and type can be created to meet the individual needs of the potential exerciser. Despite this flexibility the American College of Sports Medicine[1] indicates that improvements are unlikely if the exercise stimulus is less than 2 days/week at 50% of functional capacity and 10 min/day. It is generally recommended that healthy exercisers who desire to improve their cardiovascular system should participate in aerobic exercise (walking, jogging, running, cycling, swimming, and endurance sports) 3 to 5 days/week at an intensity of 60% to 90% of HR max for 15 to 60 min/day.[18]

FACTORS INFLUENCING PRESCRIPTION OF PHYSICAL PROPERTIES

It should not be surprising that certain factors influence the manner in which the perscription is developed. The factors of most importance are initial fitness level, age, and sex. These factors usually affect the magnitude of the intensity threshold and may require adjustment by the exercise specialist.

Initial fitness level

The law of initial values applies both to the initial assignment of the intensity prescription and to the expected improvement from cardiorespiratory exercise. In the former case, persons who have lower initial fitness levels do not require the same initial intensity stimulus as those with higher levels. Table 11-5 illustrates a sliding scale method of prescribing exercise, which allows for initial fitness. This method involves adding an amount to a baseline intensity level (60%), which is related to the FC (in METs) determined from the exercise test. In the latter case, cardiovascular improvement seems to be inversely related to the initial fitness level.[22] In other words, persons who begin with a high level of fitness are not expected to improve as much as those starting at low levels.

It has been observed that a lower intensity level throughout an entire training program can produce significant changes in unfit subjects. For example, an intensity level of 47% (HRR) was sufficient to elicit significant changes in very unfit women.[7] (Typical threshold recommendations indicate that such low levels would be ineffective.) In Figure 11-4, both training groups, 47% and 63% of HRR, improved $\dot{V}O_2$ max significantly. The 47% group significantly improved time to an HR of 180, and the other group did not. In contrast, maximal treadmill time was only significantly improved in the 63% group. One investigator observed improvement with a stimulus as low as 39%.[24] Chapter 19 offers a further discussion of aging.

Age

Higher intensities are usually required for younger exercisers.[24] Although the absolute physiological changes observed in middle-aged and older men are lower than in younger men, the relative change (%) has been found to be about the same.[21] Such changes can be achieved in older men with lower-intensity exercise levels, however. A significant increase in physical working capacity (34.5%) was found for older men (60 to 79 years), with exercise intensities between 35% and 60% of the HRR.[5]

Sex

Women respond to training as men do.[15] Principles associated with the application of intensity, duration, frequency, and type are quite appropriate for both sexes.

REGULATION OF EXERCISE INTENSITY

The most neglected area of exercise prescription concerns the method by which intensity is regulated: how can one know whether the prescribed intensity level is main-

TABLE 11-5 ||||| METHOD OF ADAPTING INITIAL EXERCISE INTENSITY
BASED ON THE FITNESS LEVEL (FC) OF THE PATIENT

Functional capacity (MET)	Adjusted prescriptive intensity (basic % + FC)	Training intensity (API % × FC)
3	60 + 3 = 63%	1.90
5	60 + 5 = 65%	3.25
10	60 + 10 = 70%	7.00
15	60 + 15 = 75%	11.25
20	60 + 20 = 80%	16.00

Adapted from American College of Sports Medicine: Guidelines for graded exercise testing and exercise prescription, ed. 2, Philadelphia, 1980, Lea & Febiger.

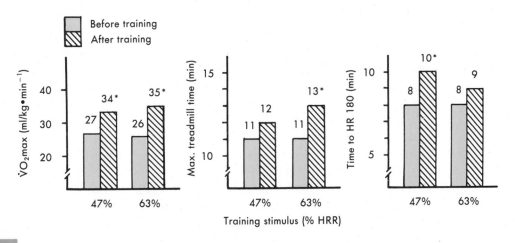

FIG. 11-4 Comparison of two unfit female groups who trained at intensities of 47% and 63%, respectively. The training stimulus was a percentage of the heart rate range (HRR). Note the significant change between before and after training ($p < .05$). (Drawn from the data of Edwards, M.A.: The effects of training at predetermined heart rate levels for sedentary college women, Med. Sci. Sports Exerc. *6*:14, 1974.)

tained? This is a very simple process if exercise is prescribed as a MET value, since a table can be consulted to determine which activities fall within an individual's FC. This assumes that the energy cost (MET) of an activity is the same for all people and under all conditions. It is difficult to accept this assumption except in the broadest sense because of the variability in activity/energy cost. Control of exercise intensity in cardiac patients, for whom strict adherence to the prescription is critical for safety, is absolutely essential. The safest method of control involves constant monitoring of the ECG and/or HR. This method provides maximal control but is very costly, and in the case of hard-wire monitoring (as opposed to radio telemetry), flexibility of movement is inhibited.

The challenge for the exercise practitioner is to find a method that effectively controls intensity and is not costly. Many programs throughout the United States incorporate speed of movement, HR, RPE, or some combination of these variables to control exercise intensity. Each is relatively inexpensive and, with some limitations, has proven to be effective. Since HR is directly related to speed of movement while walking, jogging, cycling, and stepping, this variable (speed of movement) is most often utilized as a means of control.[1] It is not advisable for any variable-speed activity (most sports) but is good for group aerobic programs. Another disadvantage of utilizing speed of movement to control exercise intensity involves complications brought about by certain environmental factors.[1] For example, if speed of movement is used to control prescribed HR at a specific percentage of FC, that control depends on HR response at a particular temperature. If a patient exercises at the same speed under higher temperatures, the HR is higher—perhaps dangerously so.

Despite these disadvantages, speed of movement has proven to be an effective control of exercise intensity. The following method has proven effective in titrating speed of movement to a prescribed HR in a walk/jog program.

1. Ask the patient to walk at a natural walking pace over a measured course so that total time exceeds 3 minutes (to achieve steady state). It is important that patients maintain a constant pace.
2. At the end of the first walk stage, record the exact time (so that speed in ft/sec can be calculated), the 10-second postwalk HR (count × 6 = beats/min), and the rate of perceived exertion (RPE).
3. If the first walk's speed produced a HR below that prescribed, ask the patient to repeat step 1 at a slightly accelerated pace. Then repeat step 2.
4. Repeat steps 1 and 2 until at least one produced HR falls above and one falls below the prescribed HR.
5. The prescribed speed of movement is calculated as shown in Figure 11-5: briefly, a horizontal line is drawn from the prescribed HR to the produced HR/speed line. From this point, a vertical line is dropped to the speed axis.
6. Next, speed must be converted to lap time, so that the speed can be controlled by a large lap clock. Table 11-6 illustrates how lap time can be converted from the prescribed speed in gyms of various sizes.

TABLE 11-6 ‖‖‖‖‖ DETERMINATION OF INDIVIDUAL LAP TIMES FROM
PRESCRIBED MOVEMENT SPEED AND GYMNASIUM OR TRACK SIZE*

Movement speed (mph)	Gymnasium or track size		
	4 laps/mile (min/lap)	8 laps/mile (min/lap)	12 laps/mile (min/lap)
2.0	7:30	3:45	2:30
2.5	6:00	3:00	2:00
3.0	5:00	2:30	1:40
3.5	4:17	2:09	1:26
4.0	3:45	1:53	1:15
4.5	3:20	1:40	1:07
5.0	3:00	1:30	1:00

*This table can also be used to determine movement speed from known lap times.

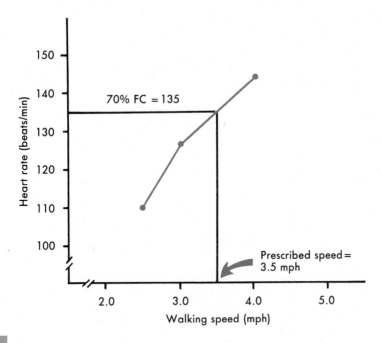

FIG. 11-5 Titration method of determining the walking speed necessary to elicit the prescribed target
HR (70% of functional capacity). Self-selected and paced walking trials are given for a
minimum of 3 min until a HR/speed point is established on either side of the prescribed
HR. Interpolation is used to establish the prescribed speed.

7. Finally, the patient is instructed to produce the control pace at the calculated lap time (>3 minutes), and the HR is checked. After the patient learns to control pace naturally, usually after 2 or 3 trials, the HR can be effectively and safely controlled. (Recording RPE during this procedure provides an opportunity to assess the individual's subjective evaluation of "feeling." These values can be used by the practitioner to monitor the subjective dimension during exercise and aids in the control of exercise intensity.)

This method does not imply that speed of movement is the only unit of control. On the contrary, it is a guide to help the patient achieve the prescribed HR and RPE. Speed of movement should be used in concert with HR and RPE for most effective control.

Another method of controlling intensity simply involves control of the prescribed HR level. Since speed ultimately must be manipulated to control HR, this variable is merely the flip side of the previous variable. As the exerciser becomes more fit, the same speed elicits a lower HR. Thus monitoring HR automatically controls speed of movement. HR, measured by palpation of the radial or carotid artery and periodically counted for 10 seconds, is an effective method of control. To be most effective, the testing mode should be similar to the intended exercise mode, for example a walking test for the walking exercise; it would be inappropriate to test on a bicycle ergometer and expect the HR to apply directly to a walking exercise program. Biomechanical differences between treadmill walking and normal locomotion also make the use of treadmill walking in assigning HR dosage only a rough approximation.

It has been suggested that cardiac patients use their own sense of discomfort as a guide to intensity dosage control.[2] Studies using the Borg scale of perceived exertion (see Chapter 19) indicate RPE to be both a promising measure[8] and a valid one.[26] In a review of clinical applications of perceived exertion,[13] I warned both scientists and clinicians that the use of RPE—collected by *estimating* the subjective intensity of exercise test loads on a treadmill—to control exercise intensity in an exercise program in which patients are asked to *produce* a specific subjective level may be an unfair test of this theoretically attractive procedure. Patients might effectively control exercise if a simple biofeedback procedure is initiated before the exercise program. For example, the titration procedure already discussed is an excellent method for teaching the patient to assess changes in feeling and thus to manipulate speed of movement in response to subjective feeling. It might be instructive to distinguish between *estimating* and *producing* a subjective level. In the former the technician provides the exercise stimulus, and the patient estimates the level. In the latter the technician provides the subjective level (for instance, the target RPE), and the patient provides the exercise output. Estimation and production require two quite different behaviors.

APPLICATION OF EXERCISE STIMULUS

Each exercise session is subdivided into a warm-up phase, exercise stimulus period, and cool-down phase. This pattern is illustrated in Figure 11-6. HR is used to demonstrate the principle of the three phases. The warm-up phase is used to raise the HR gradually to the prescribed range. During the stimulus period the HR remains at an average of 70% and should not exceed 90% of the HRR.[1] After the stimulus period the HR is allowed to return to near-resting conditions. It should be remembered that both the duration and the intensity should be adjusted initially to allow for the subject's fitness, age, and possible disease characteristics.

Progression of the exercise stimulus begins with a modification of the prescription, referred to as the *starter* stage.[18] By decreasing the prescribed intensity by 1 MET and utilizing a beginning duration of 12 minutes, muscle soreness can be kept to a minimum. This stage lasts 4 to 6 weeks. After the individual has made the initial adaptation to exercise, the *conditioning stage* begins. During this stage, the full-intensity prescription is followed. As fitness improves, it becomes necessary to increase movement speed so that the prescribed percentage is achieved. This stage usually continues for approximately 6 months. After the conditioning stage the individual should be sufficiently improved to

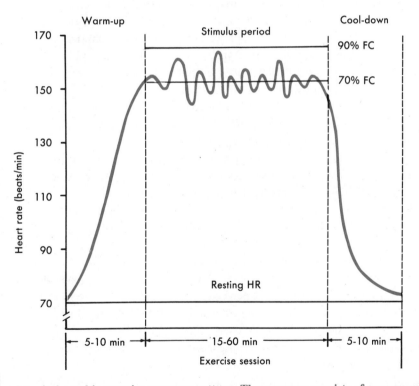

FIG. 11-6   A typical aerobic exercise program pattern. The sequence consists of a warm-up period, an exercise stimulus period (duration varies according to characteristics of the exerciser), and a cool-down period. HR is raised during the warm-up to, or close to, the target HR (70% FC). In this case the HR should average 153 during the stimulus period but not exceed 165 (see Figure 11-2). During the cool-down the HR is allowed to return toward the resting value.

allow entrance into the *maintenance stage,* in which intensity progession is no longer necessary and more enjoyable activities, such as games, can be added.[1]

With cardiac patients the graded exercise test should be repeated approximately every 6 weeks. Such a procedure aids in the medical follow-up examinations of the patient and allows fine-tuning of the exercise prescription.[2] Normal exercisers do not require such frequent testing but should be retested periodically.

Individualized prescription of exercise does not preclude group exercise, in which many persons exercise at approximately the same rate, which promotes socialization. In a large group, even with a large variability in prescribed rates, a great deal of social interaction is possible.

SUMMARY

Prescription of exercise is accomplished through the process of *assimilation, dosage assignment,* and *unit conversion.* Assimilation involves the use of knowledge accumulated in the literature concerning type, frequency, duration, and intensity of exercise combined with graded exercise test data that aid in the identification of exercise intensity. Dosage assignment is the process of explicitly stating the physical properties of the individualized exercise prescription (type, frequency, duration, and intensity). Unit conversion involves changing the intensity prescription (such as MET) to a form that can be controlled during exercise (such as HR or movement speed).

The exercise intensity prescription is based on the determination of functional capacity (FC). FC is usually expressed as the $\dot{V}O_2$, HR, or MET level at which the exercise test was terminated. Exercise is prescribed as a percentage of these units. The preferred method of prescribing exercise utilizes HR as the unit of description, since it is easy to monitor during exercise. This method prescribes exercise intensity as a percentage of the HR range (HRR; maximal HR minus resting HR).

Developing an exercise prescription involves consideration of four physical properties: intensity, duration, frequency, and type. Intensity has been called the most important of the prescriptive components and it is difficult to control during exercise. Cardiorespiratory improvement has been shown to be directly related to exercise intensity. Although elite athletes often must train at intensities at or near 100%, research indicates that optimal improvements can be achieved at percentages well below this level. The threshold for change to occur when HR max is the criterion is 60% to 90% (50% to 80% for $\dot{V}O_2$ max). Older individuals may have thresholds as low as 35%.

All physical properties of the exercise prescription are probably interactive, that is, not independent. For example, duration of exercise is thought to depend on the intensity. Cardiorespiratory changes can be made with 15-minute durations as long as the intensity is high. Some research indicates that changes can be made with durations as low as 5 minutes. Usually 15 to 60 minutes is recommended.

The least important of the prescriptive components is frequency. Most authorities recommend a frequency of 3 to 5 sessions per week to make optimal improvements and 2 to 3 per week for a maintenance program. Some research indicates that total work, not frequency, is the critical variable for change to occur.

When the prescriptive components are equated, most aerobic types of exercise produce about the same results. Aerobic exercise is the best initial form of exercise for cardiac patients and is perhaps superior at all other times as well. Cardiac patients should be cautioned to refrain from any exercise that involves a Valsalva maneuver (closing the glottis against pressure) because of the danger of provoking abnormal responses in an already compromised cardiovascular system.

Factors such as initial fitness level, age, and sex may affect the magnitude of the intensity threshold. It has been observed that very unfit and older people can improve at intensities below 50%. Gender, however, does not seem to be an important factor, since both men and women respond about equally when the prescriptive components have been equated.

The most neglected area of exercise prescription concerns the methods by which intensity is regulated. The safest but most costly method is continuous monitoring of the ECG and/or HR. Less costly and perhaps equally safe methods incorporate speed of movement, HR, and RPE to control exercise intensity. Although each can be used alone, the most preferable method involves the use of all three units in concert.

Each exercise session is subdivided into a warm-up phase, exercise stimulus period, and cool-down phase. During the stimulus period the HR remains at an average of 70% and should not exceed 90% of HRR. A starter stage is recommended for the first 4 to 6 weeks so that muscle soreness can be prevented. The conditioning stage usually lasts 6 months and is followed by the maintenance stage.

KEY TERMS

assimilation the process of merging distinct factors, for example, in exercise prescription these factors are intensity, frequency, duration, and type of exercise.

dosage assignment specification of an exercise prescription in terms of intensity, frequency, duration, and type of exercise.

double product multiplication of heart rate and systolic blood pressure used as an estimate of myocardial (heart) oxygen consumption.

functional capacity the highest exercise intensity or physiological response attained during a graded exercise test, usually described in terms of MET, HR, or $\dot{V}O_2$ max.

heart rate range maximal heart rate minus resting heart rate.

intensity threshold the minimal exercise intensity for attainment of cardiovascular benefits.

Karvonen method method of prescribing exercise target intensity using a percentage of the heart rate range.

MET a multiple of resting metabolic rate.

perceived exertion a subjective rating of the level of experienced effort during exercise.

pharmacopoeia an authoritative book containing information on medicinal drugs.

unit conversion changing physiological units derived from the graded exercise test to those that can be used at the exercise site.

REVIEW QUESTIONS

1. Describe the exercise prescription model, making sure to define assimilation, dosage assignment, and unit conversion.

2. Name three methods of prescribing exercise intensity, and contrast the relative merits of each.

3. What is the ''no pain—no gain'' principle of exercise prescription? Why is it effective for young, healthy athletes and unnecessary for middle-aged adults?

4. Define intensity threshold. Why have improvements been observed at intensities as low as 40% while some experiments have not observed improvements until 70% of functional capacity?

5. Why are intensity and duration interactive when prescribing exercise? Also, why is frequency the least important factor?

6. What is the relationship between cardiovascular improvement and initial fitness level? Explain the reason for this relationship.

7. Describe three methods of regulating exercise intensity. What are the merits of each method? Are the methods mutually exclusive?

8. Defend the use of a starter stage in exercise programs for adults.

REFERENCES

1. American College of Sports Medicine: Guidelines for graded exercise testing and exercise prescription, ed. 2, Philadelphia, 1980, Lea & Febiger.

2. American Heart Association: Exercise testing and training of individuals with heart disease or at high risk for its development: a handbook for physicians, Dallas, 1975, American Heart Association.

3. Astrand, I.: Aerobic work capacity in men and women with reference to age, Acta Physiol. Scand. **49**(Suppl. 169):45, 1960.

4. Davies, C.T.M., and Knibbs, A.V.: The training stimulus: the effects of intensity, duration, and frequency of effort on maximum aerobic power output, Int. Z. Angew. Physiol. **29**:299, 1971.

5. DeVries, H.A.: Exercise intensity threshold for improvement of cardiovascular-respiratory function in older men, Geriatrics **26**:94, 1971.

6. Durnin, J.V.G.A., Brockway, J.M., and Whitcher, H.W.: Effects of a short period of training of varying severity on some measurements of physical fitness, J. Appl. Physiol. **15**:161, 1960.

7. Edwards, M.A.: The effects of training at predetermined heart rate levels for sedentary college women, Med. Sci. Sports Exerc. **6**:14, 1974.

8. Gutmann, M.C., Squires, R.W., Pollock, M.L., and others: Perceived exertion–heart rate relationship during exercise testing and training in cardiac patients, J. Cardiac Rehabil. **1:**52, 1981.

9. Hartung, G.H., Smolensky, M.H., Harrist, R.B., and others: Effects of varied durations of training on improvement in cardiorespiratory endurance, J. Hum. Ergol. (Tokyo) **6:**61, 1977.

10. Heinzelman, F., and Bagley, R.W.: Response to physical activity programs and their effects on health behavior, Public Health Rep. **85:**905, 1970.

10a. Hickson, R.C., and Rosenkoetter, M.A.: Reduced training frequencies and maintenance of increased aerobic power, Med. Sci. Sports Exerc. **13:**13, 1981.

11. Hollman, W., and Venrath, H.: Experimentelle untersuchungen zur Bedeutung aines trainings Unterhalb und Oberhalb der Dauerbeltz Stungsgranze. In Korts, editor: Carl Diem Festschrift, W. u.a. Frankfort/Wein, 1962.

12. Karvonen, M., Kentala, K., and Muslala, O.: The effects of training heart rate: a longitudinal study, Ann. Med. Exptl. Biol. Fenn. **35:**307, 1957.

13. Noble, B.J.: Clinical applications of perceived exertion, Med. Sci. Sports Exerc. **14:**406, 1982.

14. Olree, H.D., Corbin, B., Penrod, J., and others: Methods of achieving and maintaining physical fitness for prolonged space flight, Final Progress Report to NASA (Grant no. NGR-04-002-004), 1969.

15. Pollock, M.L.: Quantification of endurance training programs. In Wilmore, J.H., editor: Exercise and sports sciences reviews, New York, 1973, Academic Press, Inc.

16. Pollock, M.L., Cureton, T.K., and Greninger, L.: Effects of frequency of training on working capacity, cardiovascular function and body composition of adult men, Med. Sci. Sports Exerc. **1:**70, 1969.

17. Pollock, M.L., Dimmick, J., Millers, H.S., and others: Effects of mode of training on cardiovascular function and body composition of adult men, Med. Sci. Sports Exerc. **2:**139, 1975.

18. Pollock, M.L., Ward, A., and Foster, C.: Exercise prescription for rehabilitation of the cardiac patient. In Pollock, M.L., and Schmidt, D.H., editors: Heart disease and rehabilitation, Boston, 1979, Houghton-Mifflin.

19. Pollock, M.L., Wilmore, J.H., and Fox, S.M.: Health and fitness through physical activity, New York, 1978, John Wiley & Sons, Inc.

20. Roskamm, H.: Optimum patterns of exercise for healthy adults, Can. Med. Assoc. J. **96:**895, 1967.

21. Saltin, B., Hartley, L., Kilbom, A., and others: Physical training in sedentary middle-aged and older men. II. Oxygen uptake, heart rate and blood lactate concentration at submaximal and maximal exercise, Scand. J. Clin. Lab. Invest. **24:**323, 1969.

22. Sharkey, B.J.: Intensity and duration of training and the development of cardiorespiratory endurance, Med. Sci. Sports Exerc. **2:**197, 1970.

23. Sharkey, B.J., and Holleman, J.P.: Cardiorespiratory adaptations to training at specified intensities, Res. Q. **41:**44, 1970.

24. Shephard, R.J.: Intensity, duration and frequency of exercise as determinants of the response to a training regimen, Int. Z. Angew. Physiol. **26:**272, 1968.

25. Sidney, K.H., Eynon, R.B., and Cunningham, D.A.: The effects of frequency of exercise upon physical work performance and selected variables representative of cardiorespiratory fitness. In Taylor, A.W., editor: Training: scientific basis and application, Springfield, Ill., 1972, Charles C Thomas, Publisher.

26. Smutok, M.A., Skrinar, G.S., and Pandolf, K.B.: Exercise intensity: subjective regulation by perceived exertion, Arch. Phys. Med. Rehabil. **61:**569, 1980.

27. Taylor, H.L., Haskell, W., Fox, S.M., and others: Exercise tests: a summary of procedures and concepts of stress testing for cardiovascular diagnosis and function evaluation. In Blackburn, H., editor: Measurement in exercise electrocardiography, Springfield, Ill., 1969, Charles C Thomas, Publisher.

28. Wilson, P.K., Fardy, P.S., and Froelicher, V.F.: Cardiac rehabilitation: adult fitness and exercise training, Philadelphia, 1981, Lea & Febiger.

SUGGESTED READINGS

American College of Sports Medicine: Guidelines for graded exercise testing and exercise prescription, ed. 2, Philadelphia, 1980, Lea & Febiger.

Amsterdam, E.A., Wilmore, J.H., and DeMaria, A.N.: Exercise in cardiovascular health and disease, New York, 1977, Yorke Medical Books.

Fardy, P.S., Bennett, J.L., Reitz, N.L., and others: Cardiac rehabilitation: implications for the nurse and other health professionals, St. Louis, 1980, The C.V. Mosby Co.

Pollock, M.L.: Quantification of endurance training programs. In Wilmore, J.H., editor: Exercise and sports sciences reviews, New York, 1973, Academic Press.

Pollock, M.L., and Schmidt, D.H.: Heart disease and rehabilitation, Boston, 1978, Houghton-Mifflin.

Pollock, M.L., Wilmore, J.H., and Fox, S.M.: Health and fitness through physical activity, New York, 1978, John Wiley & Sons, Inc.

Wilson, P.K., Fardy, P.S., and Froelicher, V.F.: Cardiac rehabilitation, adult fitness and exercise testing, Philadelphia, 1981, Lea & Febiger.

CASE STUDY 1

A 32-year-old unfit woman appeared at an exercise site for the first day of exercise. She had a functional capacity of 6.4 MET. The treadmill test was terminated, with the HR at 128 beats/min, because of dyspnea and leg fatigue. Exercise intensity was prescribed at 4.5 (70%) and 5.8 (90%) MET. Since this was a starter program, the average intensity was reduced to 60% (3.5 MET). The suggested HR for 3.5 MET was 105.

The titration test, described earlier in this chapter, was used to determine the speed of walking that would simulate the prescribed walking and to control the intensity at a stable level. Figure 11-7 shows the data collected from the test.

Continued.

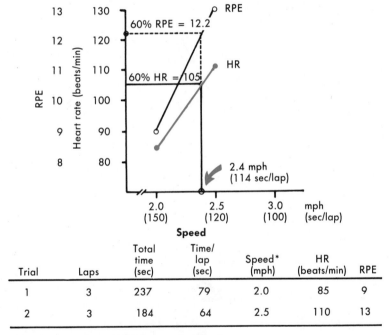

Trial	Laps	Total time (sec)	Time/ lap (sec)	Speed* (mph)	HR (beats/min)	RPE
1	3	237	79	2.0	85	9
2	3	184	64	2.5	110	13

*Based on gym size with 12 laps to the mile.

FIG. 11-7 Illustration of the determination of the movement speed and rating of perceived exertion (RPE) associated with the prescribed target HR. The titration method is used (Figure 14-5) and in this hypothetical case study a movement speed and RPE of 2.4 mph (114 sec/lap) and 12.2 mph are established. These are the initial values used by the exercise specialist to control exercise intensity at 60% FC.

The exercise specialist began exercising the patient at a lap rate of 67 seconds. Adjustments were made as necessary. So that the patient's perceptions could be correctly anchored she was told that when she exercised at the correct HR her perceived exertion should be about 12. She was advised to concentrate on her subjective feelings while exercising at the prescribed rate, so that deviations could be easily detected: tidal volume, respiratory frequency, and muscle discomfort were described as cues that could be effective. In this way, the speed of movement (lap time), HR, and RPE could be utilized in concert to regulate exercise intensity.

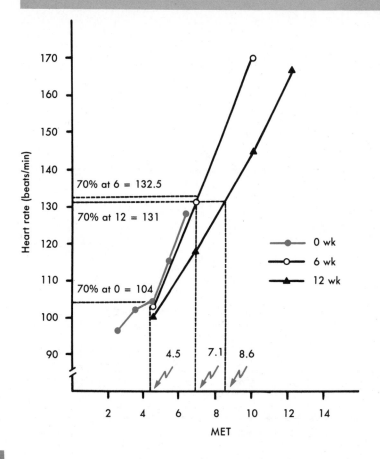

FIG. 11-8   Illustration of the change in prescribed target HR and movement speed as a function of 0, 6, and 12 weeks of training in a phase II cardiac exercise program. FC improvement can be observed by the increase in the MET value at test termination (6.4, 10.2, and 12.3). Target HR increases significantly between 0 and 6 weeks and remains essentially the same at 12 weeks. However, the training MET value (4.5, 7.1, and 8.6), or the energy level necessary to achieve target HR, increases progressively.

CASE STUDY 2

A 39-year-old male airline pilot entered a phase II exercise program after an uncomplicated hospital recovery from an acute inferior MI. Coronary catheterization revealed total occlusion of the right coronary artery and normal left coronary arteries. The right coronary artery was catheterized for percutaneous transluminal coronary angioplasty (PTCA). This technique involves expanding a balloon attached to the end of the catheter to reduce the size of the occlusion. After PTCA, the right coronary artery remained 60% to 80% occluded. The patient was given a graded exercise test on hospital discharge and again 6 weeks and 12 weeks after initiation of phase II exercise. The test data are plotted in Figure 11-8.

It was easy to observe improvement resulting from the program. The 0 test was terminated because of patient leg fatigue at an HR of 128. After 6 weeks of training the same test was terminated because of ECG changes at an HR of 170 in the 10.2 MET stage. The final phase II test (at 12 weeks) was terminated at about the same HR (167) but at a higher exercise intensity (12.3). The prescribed exercise HRs are notable. For the first 6 weeks the 70% level was set at 104 (4.5 MET). The 70% level at 6 and 12 weeks was approximately the same (132.5 and 131, respectively). An important difference can be seen, however; it takes more work to produce the 131 at 12 weeks (8.6 MET) than the 132.5 at 6 weeks (7.1 MET). This is evidence of a training effect, since the HR/MET line has shifted to the right. The plot in Figure 11-8 is not significant only for identifying the prescribed HR but also for helping the patient and exercise specialist to observe training changes.

The pilot has made a remarkable recovery with a very good FC. The Civil Aeronautics Board still will not allow him to fly. This is reassuring for us white-knuckle passengers but not so good for a young, vigorous postcoronary patient who wants to practice his profession.

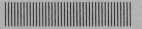

chapter 12

TRAINING TECHNIQUES

MAJOR LEARNING OBJECTIVE
Physiological training theory assumes that functional knowledge of the physiological system being trained is directly related to making correct training decisions.

APPLICATIONS
First, the physiological system to be trained is identified. This involves integrating the physical dimensions of the exercise with knowledge of the metabolic systems. Next, physiological training principles are integrated with the identified metabolic system(s). In so doing, the training dimensions are established.
■ The exercise specialist must examine the exercise closely in terms of type, frequency, duration, and intensity of the component parts. Training decisions should be as specific as possible.

$\mathbf{T}$**HIS** chapter and the one that follows contain a great deal of overlapping material, that of training techniques and training effects. It is difficult to discuss a technique without also discussing the effect it produces, and conversely, it is difficult to discuss the effects without reference to training technique. It is impossible to remove all this overlap and, in many ways, undesirable. This chapter concentrates on a description of the physical dimensions of training and how those dimensions might stimulate change. Change, as such, is discussed in the next chapter.

Physiology is not the only science that is required for an understanding of training for sport and exercise. Sport and exercise are not only physiological entities; they also involve an understanding of the psychology of learning (motor learning) and the physics of human movement (biomechanics). Questions dealing with how to train athletes relative to motor skill, or what is the most mechanically efficient technique of executing a particular skill, must be addressed by other disciplines. The material in this chapter is focused on the training of physiological systems alone. Admittedly, this is a segmented approach but, thus far, it is necessary because of the complexity of taking a wholistic approach.

PHYSIOLOGICAL TRAINING THEORY

Knowledge of physiology plays a paramount role as the teacher, coach, or exercise specialist makes training decisions for those seeking physical activity. The basis of this process might be called physiological training theory. This theory assumes that functional knowledge of the physiological system being trained is directly related to making correct training decisions. Figure 12-1 illustrates this theory. Development of the correct training program requires the integration of knowledge about physiological systems and the principles and physical dimensions of training with analysis of the physical dimensions of the activity.

What physiological system should be trained?

Answering this question requires serious examination of the demands involved in the activity under consideration. Sometimes we take this question for granted, that is, we allow biases of previous observation or word-of-mouth tradition to dictate our answer. Usually, physical educators look at sport with an orientation toward skill or strategy. It is necessary to train yourself to approach an activity relative to the stress it places on human physiology. One method for doing this involves using the prescriptive dimensions discussed in Chapter 11 as a guide. We must examine the type, frequency, duration, and intensity of exercise displayed during various components of the activity. For example, we can look at the game of basketball. The type of activity can be identified as relatively continuous movement interspersed with intervals of high-intensity exercise. Frequency refers to the frequency of essential components within the game or practice. Since basketball games are heavily oriented to repeated submaximal excursions of the court, training should attempt to duplicate this frequency pattern as closely as possible. Additionally, the frequency of short, high-intensity movement must be considered (less than 10 to 30 seconds). Game duration, depending on the competitive level, lasts 30 to 40 minutes. Intensity during play ranges from momentary standing to maximal intensity running. Of course, because of time-outs and free throws, there are many periods of rest. In summary, basketball can be described as a combination of continuous and interval activity with many repetitions within a game, 30 to 40 minutes of playing duration, and variable intensity. The components of basketball are highly anaerobic and require anaerobic training for effective performance. However, an aerobic base is essential for the basketball player to adapt to the total context of the game.

Knowledge of these dimensions must now be integrated with knowledge of the physi-

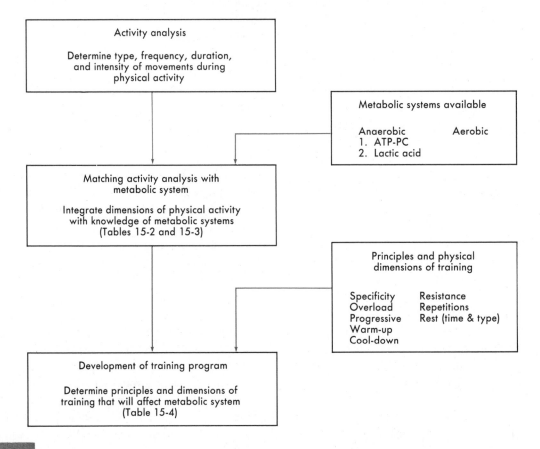

FIG. 12-1   **Physiological training theory. To determine which metabolic system to train, results of the activity analysis are integrated with a knowledge of the characteristics of the system. Then training principles and dimensions that affect the metabolic system(s) are used to develop the training program.**

ological systems. The most common approach is to concentrate on metabolic systems, since the dominant concern in training is with energy production in support of muscular contraction. Thus, we now come back to the discussions of metabolic systems in Chapter 3. Broadly speaking, metabolism during physical activity can be broken down into two categories: aerobic and anaerobic. Anaerobic can be further subdivided into ATP-PC and lactic acid systems. The problem for the coach, or exercise specialist, is to identify what system(s) need to be trained to effectively perform a particular activity. To do this, we must know how frequency, duration, and intensity interact with the metabolic systems. Table 12-1 provides a simplistic model for making this integration.* Using the previously identified characteristics of basketball, it can be seen that this sport uses all three metabolic systems. It is necessary to decide on the relative contributions of each system so that each can be appropriately trained. This decision depends a great deal on the style of play. Table 12-2 offers further guidance in this area.[14]

Principles and physical dimensions of training

After the metabolic system(s) to be trained has been identified, attention can be turned to how that system(s) is changed. It should now be clear that training theory incorporates the principle of *specificity*. This principle has been discussed in earlier chapters but usually with reference to testing or body part training (for example, arm vs leg training).

In this context, the theory proposes that a specific metabolic system needs to be

---

*This table shows the dimensions of physical activity on the vertical axis and the three metabolic systems on the horizontal axis. By determining the frequency, duration, and intensity dimensions, it should be possible to identify the dominant metabolic system in use. For example, if an activity involves maximal repetitions with durations less than 10 seconds, the system that should be trained would be ATP-PC. The integration is not always that simple, however.

TABLE 12-1 ‖‖‖ METHOD TO DETERMINE WHICH METABOLIC SYSTEM TO TRAIN

Physical dimensions*	Metabolic systems		Aerobic
	Anaerobic		
	ATP-PC	Lactic acid	
Frequency	Repeated repetitions	Repeated repetitions	Continuous movement
Duration	<10-15 sec	<2-5 min	>5 min
Intensity	Maximal	Maximal or near maximal	Submaximal

*Refers to the nature of the activity itself rather than the training dimensions.

TABLE 12-2 ||||| PERCENTAGE OF VARIOUS SPORTS DEVOTED TO VARIOUS METABOLIC SYSTEMS

Sports or sport activity	% Emphasis according to energy systems		
	ATP-PC and lactic acid	LA − O_2	O_2
Baseball	80	20	—
Basketball	85	15	—
Fencing	90	10	—
Field hockey	60	20	20
Football	90	10	—
Golf	95	5	—
Gymnastics	90	10	—
Ice hockey			
Forwards, defense	80	20	—
Goalie	95	5	—
Lacrosse			
Goalie, defense, attack men	80	20	—
Midfielders, man-down	60	20	20
Rowing	20	30	50
Skiing			
Slalom, jumping, downhill	80	20	—
Cross-country	—	5	95
Pleasure skiing	34	33	33
Soccer			
Goalie, wings, strikers	80	20	—
Halfbacks, or link men	60	20	20
Swimming and diving			
50 yd, diving	98	2	—
100 yd	80	15	5
200 yd	30	65	5
400, 500 yd	20	40	40
1500, 1650 yd	10	20	70
Tennis	70	20	10
Track and field			
100, 200 yd	98	2	—
Field events	90	10	—
440 yd	80	15	5
880 yd	30	65	5
1 mile	20	55	25
2 miles	20	40	40
3 miles	10	20	70
6 miles (cross-country)	5	15	80
Marathon	—	5	95
Volleyball	90	10	—
Wrestling	90	10	—

From Fox, E.L., and Mathews, D.: Interval training: conditioning for sports and general fitness, Philadelphia, 1974, W.B. Saunders Co.

trained. In addition, the *overload principle* must be applied to the metabolic system to stimulate change. The homeostatic predisposition of a metabolic system is to remain stable when it is under stable environmental conditions. For the system to change, the stable environmental conditions have to change. Therefore, the metabolic system must be stressed beyond that which is normal or usual. During aerobic training, for example, some combination of exercise frequency, duration, or intensity must be altered to change the load (overload) on the system. To be optimally effective, overload must be applied with *progressive resistance*. This principle acknowledges the fact that a metabolic system adapts to an overload so that the load no longer represents a stimulus for change. There-fore, in a progressive manner, the load (resistance) needs to be increased so that the system continues to be overloaded.

Of course, the assumption must be made that continued change is desired. At some point, the participant will undoubtedly be satisfied with a maintenance program in which the load conditions, and therefore the stimulus to the system, remain stable.

The final principles involve *warm-up* and *cool-down*. Gradual preparation of muscles and the cardiorespiratory system (warm-up) helps to prevent injury and promotes meta-bolic efficiency. Cool-down allows the metabolic system to decrease intensity to resting conditions in a deliberate manner. Technically, warm-up and cool-down are workout components, not training principles. However, without their inclusion, the principles of specificity overload and progressive resistance, and the physiological responses that they represent, are greatly modified.

Figure 12-2 illustrates the physical dimensions that can be applied to most physiologi-cal training programs. Overload is applied by manipulation of resistance, repetitions, and rest periods. For example, during strength training, a selected resistance is raised a certain number of repetitions. If the repetitions are ordered into sets, as usual, then the variable of rest duration between sets must be considered. Shorter rest intervals intensify the work-out, and longer intervals reduce the intensity. In the case of isometric training, a single repetition consists of force applied against an immovable load with resistance defined by the effort expended (for example, 50% of maximal voluntary contraction). At the other end of the continuum, it is possible to imagine an extremely light load that can be repeatedly lifted for an indefinite period of time (muscular endurance training).

During aerobic training, the resistance is determined by the distance traveled and the time taken to complete the distance (speed). During interval training, rest periods occur between the repetitions. But, like strength training, the repetitions can be organized into sets, in which case, time between sets can also be manipulated to alter the training stimulus. The term *exercise/rest ratio* refers to the time of the exercise bout relative to the time of rest. These two line components are interactive and require careful manipulation. A 1:2 ratio indicates that the rest period is twice as long as the exercise period.

Development of the training program

Table 12-3 illustrates how the physical dimensions of training are related to various metabolic systems. For example, many recreational long-distance runners use long, slow,

A

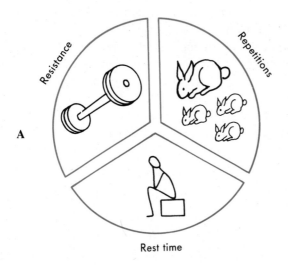

Rest time

B

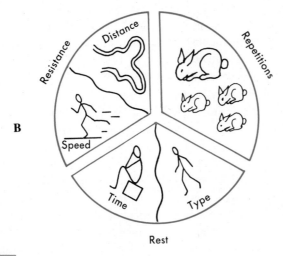

Rest

FIG. 12-2 The physical dimensions of (A) strength and (B) metabolic training.

TABLE 12-3 ▌▌▌▌ INTEGRATION OF METABOLIC SYSTEMS WITH VARIOUS TYPES OF TRAINING AND THEIR PHYSICAL DIMENSIONS*

Metabolic system	Type of training	Resistance Distance	Speed	Repetitions	Rest time	Sport application examples
Aerobic	Continuous, long, slow	Longer	Slower	0	0	Recreational jogger or recovery day for runner
Aerobic	Continuous, long, fast	Less	Faster	0	0	Quality workout for cross-country runner
ATP-PC	Interval,† short	<220 yd	1-5 sec < max	1.5-2 miles per day	1:3	Baseball, basketball, football soccer, and swimming
ATP-PC/LA	Interval, moderate	440-660 yd	1-4 sec < max	1.5-2 miles per day	1:2	Quarter mile run, soccer, swimming
LA/O₂	Interval, long	<880 yd	3-4 sec < max	1.5-2 miles per day	1:1	Mile run, soccer, swimming
ATP-PC	Sprint	50-55 yd	Max	Until fatigue	Full recovery	Baseball, basketball, football, swimming (sprint)
Aerobic/ anaerobic	Fartlek	2-3 miles	Slow and fast	0	0	All combined aerobic/anaerobic sports

*This table can be entered with a metabolic system to be trained or a sport application. In either case, an example is given of a type of training possible and its physical dimensions. Other training methods are possible.
†Interval training, particularly with extended rest periods, is known to also improve aerobic power.

distance training (a form of continuous training). As implied from the term, the distance is long and the speed is submaximal. The actual distance and speed depend on the caliber of the runner and the purpose of the training run. There are no repetitions in continuous training, since it consists of a single, continuous bout and requires no rest periods. Fartlek (Swedish speed play) training is merely a variation of continuous training that provides an anaerobic stress within the context of continuous, aerobic exercise. In this type of training, constant pace periods are interspersed with short periods of increased speed, but it is continuous movement without rest periods.

Another example found in Table 12-3 involves interval training. Baseball, for example, requires relatively short, high-speed sprints. The major system requiring attention is the ATP-PC system. Therefore, repeated short intervals with a 1:3 exercise/rest ratio would be employed. The speed would be 1 to 5 seconds slower than the maximal speed for the prescribed distance (approximately 50 yards could be used for baseball) and repeated until 1.5 to 2 miles are covered during the workout. Such a workout should be arranged so that approximately 10 repetitions would be completed during each of 5 sets. Baseball players could also use sprint training in which maximal speed sprints between 50 to 100 yards would be used. Rest periods during interval training are set with consideration for duration and intensity of exercise, that is, short, highly intense intervals (ATP-PC training) use 1:3 ratios; longer, less intense exercise intervals use 1:1 ratios.[14] Most training techniques used by coaches fit the dimensions shown in Figure 12-2 and Table 12-3. Distances for swimming need to be reduced to 25% of those used for running.

AEROBIC-ANAEROBIC TRAINING

Rather arbitrarily, strength training is discussed in a separate section of this chapter. There seems to be obvious differences between strength and aerobic-anaerobic training but there are similarities as well. Muscle hypertrophy change is the emphasis in strength training and cardiorespiratory/metabolic change is the focus of aerobic-anaerobic training. Knowledge that hypertrophy is a dominant goal, however, certainly should not discount the link between change in muscle cross section and the metabolic milieu during training, for example, anaerobic. Figure 12-3 proposes a wholistic theory in which training might be described on a continuum that considers both the metabolic system involvement and the physical dimensions of the training. On the anaerobic/strength end of the continuum, training is marked by high resistance, low repetitions, and shorter duration exercise. Perhaps the extreme here would be isometric training, in which maximal resistance and one repetition would define the exercise. Short-duration interval training would also fit on this extreme.

The aerobic/muscular endurance end of the continuum is distinguished by low resistance, high repetitions, and longer duration exercise. Training for marathons would be an example of a method on the aerobic end of the continuum, that is, continuous training using many repetitions (lifts of the center of gravity) and low resistance (body weight).

Circuit weight training is an example of a training method that is planned to achieve muscle hypertrophy, as well as improvement in aerobic capacity even though improvement in the latter is minimal. Therefore, lifting weights is performed by moving continuously between several stations (minimal rest) with high-repetition, low-resistance lifting at each station. The variables included in the model (Figure 12-3) are very sensitive, with manipulation of only one causing a shift in position on the continuum.

Continuous and interval training

Continuous training, with literally no repetitions, is submaximal by its nature. This type of training becomes more suitable the more completely an activity can be considered aerobic. Before World War II, most training for the mile run was continuous long-distance training referred to, at that time, as overdistance training. Changes in world records in this event, beginning with Roger Banister's breaking of the 4-minute barrier, have been largely the result of the use of interval training methods.

Interval training uses distance repetitions that are shorter than total race distance; however, a more highly intense workout is possible because of the rest periods. Figure 12-4 illustrates a comparison of interval and continuous training over a 30-minute period. For the purposes of the illustration, it is assumed that a runner is training for a mile run and that the current best race time is 4 minutes. The interval training workout uses 2 sets of 3 repetitions. Each repetition is 1,320 yards (¾ mile) and is followed by a rest period.

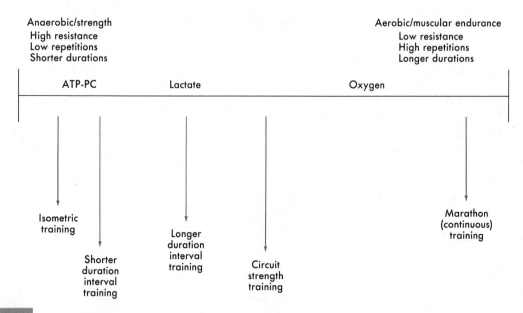

FIG. 12-3 Wholistic theory of athletic training. The training continuum considers both metabolic system involvement and the physical dimensions of training. Selection of a training technique depends on the metabolic system requiring change. Different metabolic systems require variable manipulation of the physical dimensions.

Exercise intensity is determined by adding 4 seconds to the average race pace speed (1 minute/440 yards). The intensity represents 98% of maximal mile time. With the use of this longer duration repetition, an exercise/rest ratio of 1:0.5 is selected (3:04 exercise to 1:32 rest).

In contrast, if the same runner would train with continuous training over the same time duration, the intensity would have to be less than 98%. The intensity possible would depend on the individual's anaerobic threshold, most likely 85% or less. (See Chapter 5 for a more complete discussion of the "anaerobic threshold" or more correctly termed

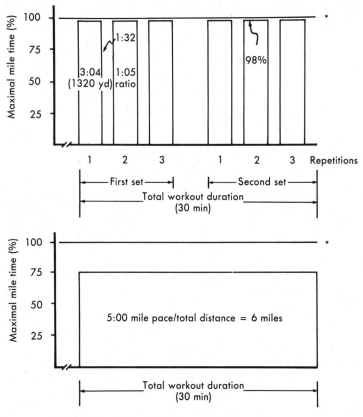

*100% is based on 4:00 mile race time.

FIG. 12-4   Illustration of a typical pattern for interval and continuous training. Training duration was intentionally equalized to contrast the two techniques. Interval training intensity is based on the addition of 4 seconds to the average race time (3:00) for the training distance (¾ mile; 1,320 yards). Training intervals were arbitrarily arranged in two sets of three to meet the total workout duration requirements. The continuous training intensity percentage (75%) was arbitrarily selected to illustrate the contrast.

OBLA—onset of blood lactate accumulation.) A more realistic training example is a single bout of continuous running at 75% of maximal mile time (5:00 minutes). It is easy to see that interval training provides the higher intensity stimulus but continuous training provides a relatively high stimulus over a longer actual exercise duration. Both are known to improve aerobic capacity, and the improvement is about equal when total training distance is equated between these methods.[23,40] Since aerobic capacity improvement is known to be a function of cardiac output changes as well as tissue level changes,[26] both continuous and interval methods must provide a stimulus for one or both of these changes. Our knowledge of the exact mechanism for change is still unfolding. It is important to note that the mile run is both aerobic and anaerobic. The anaerobic component contributes much more than scientists realized before World War II. Undoubtedly, the high anaerobic involvement in the interval training concept has aided improvement of world records in this event.

The stimulus for improvement that is provided by dynamic exercise has been called *volume stress*.[37] Volume refers to stroke volume and its contribution to the central (cardiac output) mechanism for improving aerobic capacity. It is thought that placing stress on this mechanism by increasing its magnitude over time promotes improvement of stroke volume and, therefore, cardiac output. During continuous training at intensity levels beyond 50% $\dot{V}O_2$ max, the stroke volume would attain its maximal exercise level. An interesting response occurs during interval training, illustrated in Figure 12-5, in which stroke index, cardiac output, and heart rate are followed periodically for 216 seconds following exercise.[20] The stroke index (volume) increases following the end of exercise (F) and remains elevated throughout the 216-second recording period. This occurs as heart rate is continuously decreasing. Despite the drop in heart rate, cardiac output increases during the first recovery segment (38.4 seconds) because of the proportionally larger increase in stroke index. Therefore, when exercise is intermittently stopped, an even larger stimulus can be provided to stroke volume. This change is hypothesized to explain the advantage of interval training for performance and the mechanism for change in aerobic capacity.

Manipulation of exercise and rest time has a significant effect on the intensity of the training stimulus and on the metabolic system trained. Figure 12-6 shows the results of an investigation[3] in which 4 exercise/rest combinations were compared during heavy exercise: 0.5/0.5, 1/1, 2/2, and 3/3 minutes (NOTE: The exercise/rest ratio is always 1:1). Total work performed, over 1 hour, was equated among the combinations. It can be seen that as time increased during interval training on a bicycle, both heart rate and lactic acid concentration increased linearly. The lactate system is stimulated most by the longer exercise intervals (2 and 3 minutes). The shorter exercise combinations involved the same amount of work over a 1-hour training session but produced much less physiological strain (increases in heart rate and lactic acid).

One investigation is instructive relative to the possible contribution of short and long exercise intervals to aerobic capacity.[31] Three groups of Army recruits were trained over a 2-month period according to the following schedule: Group I trained 3 days per week for 2 months using 15 seconds of exercise and 15 seconds of rest. Group II was exposed to the same total exercise time during each session, except 3-minute exercise and rest intervals were used. Group III used the same program as Group II, except they trained during the second month only. All groups improved $\dot{V}_{O_2}$ max significantly. The 3-minute interval groups seemed to improve aerobic capacity somewhat more effectively than the 15-second group (26% and 23% vs 16%).

The genius of coaching, with regard to the physiological preparation of athletes, involves the correct selection of the physical dimensions that promote the metabolic priority of the sport. When in doubt, the coach should plan training that is as specific as possible to the movements of the sport. Both continuous and interval training improve aerobic capacity. Interval training is the preferred mode for training the anaerobic meta-

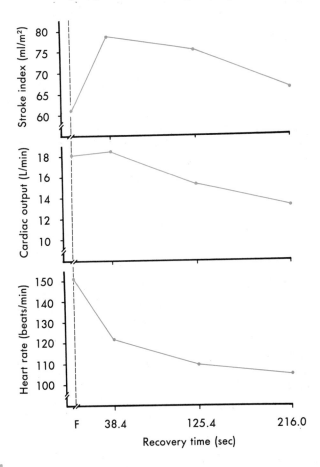

FIG. 12-5 Recovery stroke index, cardiac output, and heart rate following the final (F) exercise time point. The highest stroke volume (index) is obtained following exercise. (Adapted from Goldberg, D.I., and Shephard, R.J.: Stroke volume during recovery from upright bicycle exercise, J. Appl. Physiol. *48*:833, 1980.)

bolic systems. Subtle differences in results seem to be possible depending on manipulation of the physical dimensions of training.

Training for racing

Following is a summary of 10 principles that should be incorporated in a training program before a race.[36]

1. Gradually increase training pace up to race pace using one-half to three-quarters of the race distance.
2. Spend time on proper style at the desired race pace. When the runner becomes fatigued it is very important to concentrate on the maintenance of style.
3. Train on the same type of terrain as will be used in the race.
4. Run the race distance at a pace less than race pace.
5. Use the progressive overload principle by beginning at a pace less than race pace, gradually increase the distance from one-half to three-quarters of the race distance, and finally increase pace and decrease distance.
6. Train in racing shoes.
7. Train in the same type of clothing to be worn in the race.
8. Drink water as you intend to drink in the race.

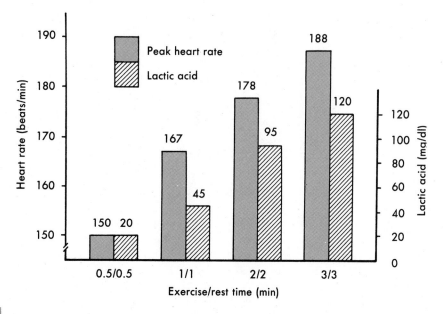

FIG. 12-6   Illustration of the peak heart rate and lactic acid response to various exercise/rest times. Both variables increase directly with the increase in time. Note that the exercise/rest ratios are the same for each example (1:1). (Adapted from Astrand, I., Astrand, P.O., Christenson, E.H., and others: Intermittent muscular work, Acta Physiol. Scand. *48:*448, 1960.)

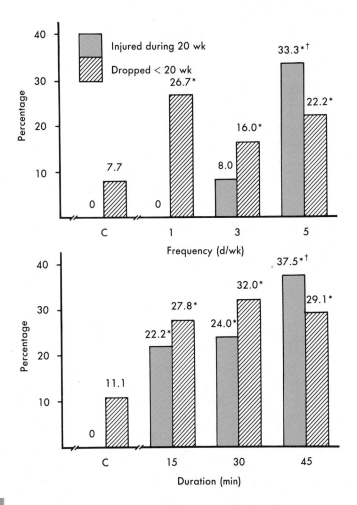

Injury and dropout percentages in a study that compared various training frequencies (1, 3, and 5 days/week, $p < .05$ compared to C) and another that compared various training durations (15, 30, and 45 minutes/session, $p < .05$ compared to 15 and 30 minutes). The experiments lasted 20 weeks. Injury columns reflect those injured but who did not drop out. Dropout columns reflect injuries and a variety of other reasons. (Adapted from Pollock, M.L.: The quantification of endurance training programs. In Wilmore, J.H., editor: Exercise and sport sciences reviews, New York, 1973, Academic Press, Inc.)

9. Train under similar environmental conditions as those expected for the race.
10. Alternate hard training days with easy days.

Injury and dropout

Even though a program may be most effective for improving a certain metabolic system, if it produces a high incidence of injury or its intensity is so stressful that participants drop out because of lack of enjoyment, it may prove to be counterproductive. Several investigators compared groups running, walking, and playing volleyball with those biking and swimming.[44] Seventy-five percent of the injuries occurred in the former groups. Intensity of training is important to both injury prevention and adherence to programs. A 15% injury rate was observed in a moderate intensity program,[52] while a moderate to high intensity program showed a 40% injury rate.[50]

Perhaps the most instructive investigation dealing with injury and dropout was conducted at two prison facilities.[51] One group (n = 87) was subdivided to study the effects of exercise duration (15, 30, and 45 minutes, 3 days per week for 20 weeks). The other group exercised at various frequencies (1, 3, and 5 days per week for 20 weeks). The overall attrition rate was 21.4% for the frequency study and 29.9% for the duration study. Injuries were highest among 5-day-per-week exercisers (39%) and the 45-minute duration exercisers (54%). Injury and dropout data are shown in Figure 12-7.

Both injury and dropout percentages were significantly higher for all experimental groups compared to the control group. The 45-minute duration and 5-day groups suffered injuries significantly more than the 15- and 30-minute duration groups and the 1- and 3-day frequency groups, respectively. Data analysis revealed that both duration and frequency have a significant effect on injury.

These data support the prescriptive recommendation of 30 minutes, 3 days per week for those seeking health benefits from exercise. In relation to dropout data, this phenomenon has been shown to be higher in interval training programs compared to continuous training.[49] In addition, coaches who need to train athletes at increased durations, frequencies, and intensities should monitor them very closely to determine when the training load might be counterproductive because of increased injury rates. It should also be remembered that injury may not be caused by duration, frequency, and intensity, as such. Often injury is caused by not paying careful attention to the rate at which these dimensions are increased. For example, increasing intensity too quickly implicates that progression may be the cause, not necessarily intensity itself.

Maintenance

Sooner or later the athlete or exerciser asks, ''How long do I have to keep increasing the resistance?'' or ''Now that I've attained my goal, what do I need to do to keep it?'' In other words, how is it possible to maintain? Most coaches provide athletes with offseason and preseason conditioning programs. Training during the season is usually placed in a maintenance mode with emphasis concentrated on competition. Some exceptions to this rule are notable. For example, swimming is a sport in which continued improvement in physiological function is essential. Cross-country (Nordic) skiing is another example. The U.S. Nordic Ski Team was studied in October (before ski training), in January (before competition), and in April (following competition).[24] A training response noted in October and January was not found in April. Although variables did not increase significantly between January and April, they did not decrease either. April was the month of the national championships, a time when physiological condition should be maximally developed. Lack of improvement in April was thought to be a negative response relative to competitive performance. The researchers faulted lack of time for training and travel requirements for this phenomenon.

Ice hockey players have also been studied over a season of play.[22] In ice hockey, game competition predominates over practice sessions during the season. Although some variables increased, they did not compare with the improvements observed in many training studies. It does not appear that participation in a sport over a season provides a sufficient stimulus for improvement. The lowered stimulus due to concentration on the game results

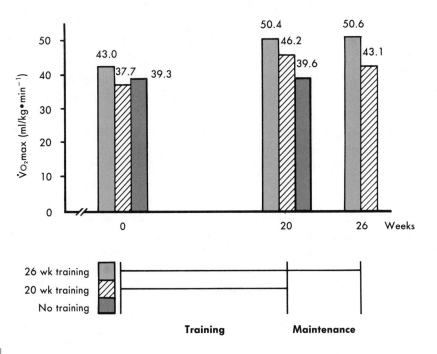

FIG. 12-8 Illustration of a maintenance experiment in which one group trained for 20 weeks at 94% of maximal heart rate followed by 6 additional weeks of training at a lowered intensity (84%). Another group trained the first 20 weeks only, while a third group did not train. The maintenance group maintained initial gains during the final 6 weeks, and the other training group decreased $\dot{V}O_2$ max significantly. (Adapted from Pollock, M.L., Gettman, L.R., Milesis, C.A., and others: Effects of frequency and duration of training on attrition and incidence of injury, Med. Sci. Sports *9*:31, 1977.)

in minimal improvement compared to preseason training, however.

Maintenance of physiological gains has been studied in sedentary men[52] (see Figure 12-8). One group (n = 9) trained for 26 weeks. During the first 20 weeks, this group trained for 30 minutes per session at 94% of maximal heart rate. In the final 6 weeks, maintenance was attempted by 32-minute sessions at 84% of maximal heart rate. A second group (n = 5) trained the same as the first for 20 weeks, but did not train the final 6 weeks. Six subjects served as a control group and did not train. Both training groups made significant physiological changes over the first 20 weeks. During the final 6 weeks the maintenance group did not change; however, the discontinued training group showed significant losses. The control group did not change. This experiment demonstrated that physiological gains can be maintained by a regimen in which training intensity is decreased. It seems reasonable that other manipulations of the exercise prescription are possible if maintenance is desired, that is, other than 32-minute sessions and 84% of maximal heart rate. It can be seen that aerobic fitness gains are easily compromised by discontinuance of training.

Another important concept to be noted is *detraining*. This concept asks the question, "If I discontinue training, how long will it take to lose what I have gained?" Studies in this area have been rather sparse. It is apparent, however, that gains begin to deteriorate rather quickly. It appears that strength gains are rather more stable than cardiovascular gains. Studies have shown that *some* strength gains remain for 6 months to 1 year after stopping training. This should obviously not be viewed as a method of training. Cardiovascular gains, on the other hand, are quite transient and can disappear within a few weeks or months. One study showed that the gains made in $\dot{V}O_2$ max over 7 weeks of training returned to pretraining levels after 8 weeks of inactivity.[34]

The antithesis of detraining is *overtraining*. Most of us have heard of athletes who "leave their game on the practice court." Typically, overtraining refers to fatigue accumulated over many and/or too intense practice periods that is not compensated for before competition. A less critical example, but nonetheless problematic, is the athlete who cannot continue training at necessary levels because of doing too much, or too much too soon. Orthopedic surgeons have been deluged in recent years by athletes, young and old, Olympic and recreational, who complain of *overuse syndrome*. These patients complain of sore muscles and joints or perhaps a general run-down condition, and typically overtraining is the source of the complaint. The best cure for such a condition is rest. Such a recommendation is not looked on with favor by the athlete when an important competition is approaching. The smart athlete and coach know that judicious use of rest may be as important as an intensive workout in the preparation for championship form.

Additional training modes

Many exercisers prefer training modes that do not easily fit into the model discussed previously in this chapter. For example, a sport like tennis is controlled by the skill of the players and the nature of the game. Intensity, frequency, and duration are dictated by the game. A match that meets the stimulus characteristics for producing both aerobic and anaerobic changes is conceivable. On the other hand, the converse may be true as well. Investigators compared a group training with tennis to two groups training on a bicycle and by jogging.[59] All groups trained 30 minutes per day, 3 days per week, for 20 weeks. Heart rate was monitored periodically and indicated that the tennis, bicycle, and jogging groups averaged 65%, 83%, and 85% of maximal heart rate, respectively. The tennis group made modest improvements in endurance capacity but only the bike and jogging groups significantly increased aerobic power. It was pointed out by the investigators that the duration of the tennis training was only 30% to 50% of the typical outing. In addition, even though the tennis intensity was about at the acceptable training threshold, it was well below that of the other two groups. Although games like tennis are probably capable of improving cardiorespiratory fitness, the unpredictability of the game intensity interferes with maximal productivity.

Rope skipping has been proposed in recent years to be an effective mode of cardio-respiratory training. Rope skipping has been studied to determine whether this activity is suitable for a graded exercise program, that is, when the rate of skipping is increased, does the energy cost rise proportionately?[58] Results showed that the stress (energy cost) was the same no matter what rate of skipping was engaged. Therefore, even though it may be possible to improve cardiorespiratory fitness with rope skipping, it is not possible to apply the stimulus in a graded fashion.

Most exercises discussed thus far have involved leg movements to apply stress to the metabolic systems. However, some recreational activities, like canoeing, involve the arms primarily. Arm exercise is the only possible mode for many handicapped persons. Arm cranking was studied over 10 weeks of training.[55] Aerobic capacity was increased by 19%, applying the usual prescription procedures. Since the muscle mass involvement is far less than for leg exercise, we would not expect improvement to be comparable to leg exercise. A group of disabled subjects was trained with arm exercise 30 minutes per day, 3 days per week, for 20 weeks.[51] As would be predicted from the previous study, the disabled subjects improved $\dot{V}O_2$ max significantly. It appears that the prescriptive principles developed for leg exercise apply to arm exercise as well.

STRENGTH TRAINING

We direct our attention back to Figure 12-3, which hypothesizes a model that has natural validity. It seems reasonable that the body reads movement stimuli as all part of a single system. Of course, there are many combinations of factors that can be manipulated to provide the stress. In addition, the body mass can be used as a resistance as well as other artificial weights or occupational loads. Still these manipulations only represent points on a continuum. Scientists fragment systems for the purpose of closer examination, but in the natural environment the systems operate as a whole. Isometric contraction is only one part of a whole system that also contains marathon running. Strength training has been arbitrarily separated here because of the differences inherent in the application of the stimulus, not because it is not part of the whole system discussed earlier.

Isotonic training

Isotonic training consists of movements that contain both concentric and eccentric contractions. Training with barbells, for example, is both concentric and eccentric. Lifting the resistance is concentric and lowering the resistance is eccentric. The earliest studies of tonic contractions, to determine how the training dimensions should be applied, were completed by DeLorme and Watkins.[12] They found that strength would increase if resistance and repetitions were manipulated in 3 sets of 10 repetitions. Each set increased resistance beginning with one-half of 10 RM* and then moving to three-fourths and on to full 10 RM.

Recent research by Anderson and Kearney lends general support to the DeLorme and Watkins[12] data as well as the model presented in Figure 12-3. These investigators compared three training regimens: high resistance–low repetition; medium resistance–medium repetition; and low resistance–high repetition. Strength and endurance changes were 20.22%, 8.22%, and 4.92% and 23.58%, 39.23%, and 41.30%, respectively. Although between-group differences were not found for either strength or endurance, trends do support training specificity depending on the end of the training continuum employed. It should be noted, however, that if either component is selected for training, the other untrained component receives benefits.

The DeLorme and Watkins hypothesis was tested to determine the optimal RM for strength training: 2, 4, 6, 8, 10, and 12 RM were compared—1 set, 3 days per week, for 12 weeks.[4] Groups using the 4, 6, and 8 RM programs significantly improved strength. It was concluded that the optimal RM stimulus was between 3 and 9. In another investigation,[5] combinations of sets (1, 2, and 3) and RM (2, 6, and 10) stimuli were studied. The best combination was 3 sets and 6 RM. However, no difference was found among 2 RM for 6 sets vs 6 RM for 3 sets vs 10 RM for 3 sets.[6] All improved strength significantly.

The stimulus for strength gain using isotonic training seems to require a 3-set program with the RM requirement, at the minimum, about 3, and, at the maximum, about 10. Therefore, a stimulus range is indicated that implicates a threshold for change and an optimal point beyond which further stimulus does not produce further gains. Currently, we know very little about the physiological mechanism that links strength gain to these training dimensions. However, muscle growth would seem to comply with simple natural laws about growth, that is, thresholds for appearance and extinction are present—too little fertilizer has no effect on the lawn and too much will begin to burn it out.

Mechanism for isotonic improvement

What is the physiological explanation for improved muscle strength? First, return to the continuum presented in Figure 12-3. High-repetition, low-resistance training with

---

*The term *RM* refers to repetitions maximum. RM literally means the maximal resistance that can be lifted a certain number of repetitions. In the DeLorme and Watkins example, 10 RM refers to the maximal weight that can be lifted 10 times. DeLorme and Watkins[12] believed strength and endurance to be specific.

weights can be thought of in the same category as running. Specific strength improvement, however, is not the primary goal during running. The goal is to make aerobic change, and that change seems to result from *volume stress*.[37] Overload provided by the body weight in running does increase muscular endurance in the legs, but strength is improved only minimally.

High strength gains are made on the other end of the continuum, with high-resistance, low-repetition exercise. The anaerobic metabolic system is certainly affected here, but there is no evidence that this system is connected to increased strength and/or muscle hypertrophy. Common sense would certainly support this connection as a viable hypothesis. Strength training alters various hemodynamic properties that undoubtedly change the metabolic milieu of muscle. For example, isometric tension, the far extreme of the continuum, is known to provide a *pressure stress* on cardiac muscle.[35,39] Increases in blood pressure occur as a result of the physical closure of vessels during intense contractions and reflexes in contracting muscles as well as in central control mechanisms. Blood flow is thought to be adequate below 15% MVC and inadequate above 15% MVC.[34] Muscle contraction begins to occlude blood vessels at resistances greater than 15% MVC.

When strength increases are coupled with hypertrophy, the result is an increase in muscle volume caused by increased muscle protein, connective tissue, etc. Protein gain is accounted for primarily by sarcoplasmic protein from a combination of increased protein synthesis and decreased protein breakdown. The stimulus for hypertrophy apparently rests with increased tension development.[21] Strength, however, is known to increase without changes in muscle volume. Such a change is said to be a function of "neural factors" rather than tension development.[41] (Additional discussion of this topic can be found in the discussion of isometric training.)

Eccentric training

Isotonic training, about which we have been speaking, contains both concentric and eccentric components. Only with physical assistance can these components be isolated in most strength training. With barbells, the weight can be removed following the lifting phase to isolate the concentric component. Conversely, the weight can be put in place for the weight trainer to make the return phase only, the eccentric component. It has been confirmed through electromyographic (EMG) analysis that more fibers are recruited (submaximal load) during concentric contractions than during eccentric contractions.[2] Thus, it was hypothesized that since eccentric contractions use fewer fibers at the same load,[45] it may be possible to train at heavier loads and make greater gains. An experiment was structured in which the right arm and leg were trained eccentrically at 120% of 1 RM (2 sets, 6 repetitions). The left arm and leg were trained concentrically at 80% of 1 RM (2 sets, 10 repetitions). Although the gains were generally greater with eccentric training, there were no significant differences. Subjects perceive eccentric exercise to be easier. Additionally, eccentric exercise may provide a protection against injury to joint ligaments and cartilage.[29] The potential of eccentric training for sport performance has not been fully explored. Certainly, eccentric movements are part of sport, but we usually pay more attention to the concentric component. One negative factor associated with eccentric training is the production of muscle soreness. This type of training produces much more soreness than does concentric training. Resulting local inflammation of muscle and connective tissue is related to edema (swollen peripheral tissue caused by the loss of fluid from tissue) in the overused area.

Strength training dilemma

The great popularity of strength training for athletes has shifted in recent years from a barbell emphasis to the use of self-contained equipment. One author indicates that as many as 60 weight training companies are marketing their version of the overload principle.[32] This equipment is largely of the variable resistance type in which resistance can be altered with the quick change of a holding pin rather than adding additional free weights. These systems provide added safety and, if used correctly, can better isolate a muscle group, but they are essentially isotonic training methods. A few exceptions are the isokinetic machines, a concept that is discussed later. Aside from the advantages just cited for variable resistance equipment, the same basic strength is being produced as with barbells. The most important question is whether the type of strength produced in any program is the type necessary for sport performances. Many sport activities are power (force times acceleration) oriented. Strength training emphasizes the force component but largely ignores the acceleration component. Steinhaus[57] made this point in 1963; however, the inertia of strength training was moving too quickly to listen to his wisdom. Weight training has been criticized because it ignores the trunk rotation strength that is needed in all sports except Olympic lifting and straight-ahead running.[28] Steinhaus recommends strengthening rotational muscles of the abdomen and lower back for more sport specificity. The whole question of strength training for sport needs to be reexamined.

Isometric training

Interest in the potential for isometric training began in 1953 following the publication of the research of Hettinger and Muller.[25] They found that strength improved at an average rate of 5% per week with the use of a single 1-second isometric contraction (5 days per week) held at two-thirds MVC. Later, after considerable scientific discussion of this work, it was determined that the best results are achieved with the use of maximal contractions repeated 5 to 10 times per day.[42] Because of the nature of the isometric process, strength improvement often occurs at only one angle. Since sport requires the production of force from many positions of the joints, this technique has not been popular. For example, groups training at 115, 135, and 155 degrees did not gain strength at any other angle.[16]

The process by which strength gains occur during isometric exercise is as obscure as with other forms of strength training. It was originally hypothesized that isometric gains may be attributed to the ischemia produced by the occlusion of vessels during isometric contraction.[25] However, an investigation failed to find strength gains by occlusion of the vessel alone without tension. If ischemia is a factor, as hypothesized,[25] it must interact with tension, or other processes that stimulate tension, to produce increased force and/or hypertrophy. Further investigation with ischemia, as a stimulant to strength improvement, should incorporate tension, perhaps with external stimulation. Tension alone, without the influence of blood flow or nervous system interaction, has been shown to account for muscle hypertrophy.[54]

Circuit strength training

One of the most interesting scientific and practical training problems involves the question of whether strength programs can be designed to develop aerobic power in addition to strength. Given the continuum described in Figure 12-3, this question appears academic. It seems logical that if the resistance is adjusted to allow repeated contractions, or the rest periods incorporate aerobic activity, then both results can be achieved simultaneously. Still, this natural hypothesis requires scientific validation. Aerobic capacity has been shown to increase with running training by 15% to 20%.[47] However, circuit strength training (CST), planned with an aerobic component, has only improved aerobic capacity by 3.5%[18] in a 10-week program and 6%[60] in a 20-week program.

One group of researchers was interested in whether combining an initial 8 weeks of CST with a subsequent 8 weeks of jogging would improve the aerobic yield.[17] Following are the components of the circuit:

1. Cycling at 900 kg-m/min for 2 minutes
2. Bench press/pull down
3. Knee extension/flexion
4. Biceps curl/pull down
5. Leg press
6. Sit-ups
7. Shoulder press/pull down
8. Rowing; push forward/pull back

$\dot{V}_{O_2}$ max improved 3% during the initial CST and an additional 8% following the jogging phase. Although aerobic changes were lower than running studies, the results were comparable. In addition, the CST training showed significant changes in treadmill time, body fat, isotonic strength, and isokinetic strength. It should be noted that items 1 and 8 are traditional aerobic exercises.

In another study, CST was integrated with running during rest periods (30 seconds between stations) and compared to CST with complete rest intervals.[19] Both programs significantly improved $\dot{V}_{O_2}$ max (17% and 12%, respectively) and were not significantly different from each other. Both programs used 3 circuits of 10 exercises each, with each exercise repeated 12 to 15 times at 40% 1 RM. Emphasis on lower resistance and moderate repetitions seems to promote aerobic power. Adding running to rest periods further enhances this process.

Isokinetic training

Isokinetic contractions involve the development of maximal tension as the muscle shortens at a constant speed through a full range of motion. In other words, it can be said that isokinetic training is isotonic training with speed of movement under control. Such training requires specialized equipment, often at a prohibitive cost for wide use. The great advantage of isokinetic training, however, is the possibility to develop strength at speeds that approximate athletic motions.[32] As mentioned earlier, strength as such should not be the preferential goal for improvement of human performance.

Although "Nautilus" type equipment has sometimes been associated with the term *isokinetic,* in fact these machines are of the variable resistance type and basically employ isotonic principles. In contrast to some variable resistance machines, Nautilus type equipment provides a system of cams so that resistance is applied according to human strength curves. These curves show that force application of muscle depends on joint angle. Variable resistance machines assume that force is the same at all joint angles. This is not the case. For example, with a biceps curl, the force production possible at a joint angle of 180° (full extension) is less than the force capability at other joint angles. In other words, Nautilus type equipment attempts to apply resistance in concert with the muscle's capability of applying force.

Isokinetic training was compared to isotonic and isometric training.[57] Gains in total work performed were 35%, 27.5%, and 9.4%, respectively. Lesmes and others[33] found that isokinetic training increased maximal muscle torque (angular force production) without increasing muscle mass. Training consisted of maximal knee extensions and flexions at a velocity of 180 degrees/second either for 6 seconds (one leg) or 30 seconds (other leg). Total work was equated between legs. The authors suggest that the gains made in this type of training may be explained by a change in the recruitment pattern of muscle fibers. Improvements were not observed at high contractile velocities, that is, above the training velocity. These results suggest that isokinetic training is specific to velocity. Therefore, athletes should train at velocities that are close to typical sport movements if isokinetic training is to be incorporated. Sports movements that require high velocities may be best suited for athletes with high percentages of FT fibers. Predominantly FT fiber subjects have been shown to generate higher isokinetic peak torques than predominantly ST fiber subjects, and the difference increased as movement velocity increased from 115 to 400 degrees/second.

Comparison of weight training programs

Comparative research of various weight training programs has been reviewed by Fleck and Schutt (see Suggested Readings). Isokinetic training increases both isokinetic and isotonic strength more than isotonic training does. In addition, isokinetic training appears to cause less muscle soreness. Isokinetic training has also been found to be superior to isometric training when evaluated either by isokinetic strength gains or isometric testing. It should be noted again that some equipment advertised as isokinetic is really variable resistance equipment. If isokinetic strength procedures are thought to be desirable, the teacher or coach should be sure that the equipment is truly isokinetic, that is, constant velocity with no resistance setting.

Comparisons of isotonic training programs with either isometric or variable resistance programs present a confusing picture. Part of the contoversy involves the type of testing equipment used in the experiment. For example, isometric testing shows isometric training to be better and isotonic testing, using the same subjects, shows isotonic training to be superior. Therefore, a specificity problem arises. Another factor in the controversy involves variable results. In one study isotonic training proved to be better than variable resistance, and in another, the reverse was found. It seems that any of these techniques could be used beneficially for strength training. Remember, however, that isometric strength gains are limited to the joint angle used during training.

Development of weight training programs for athletes

Before beginning advanced weight training, athletes should undertake a *base program* of 4 to 6 weeks. This is particularly important for novice weight trainers, but it is also applicable to the more experienced who have not been training recently. The base program allows for initial adaptation before progressing to high-intensity training. The base program is designed to exercise each part of the body. Rest periods, lasting 3 to 4 minutes, should be interspersed between exercises. Multiple sets are recommended, that is, perform all sets of one exercise before moving to a new exercise. Because this procedure can be stressful, the beginner is advised to perform only one set at first and progress to 2 or 3 sets as tolerance improves. The repetition maximum (RM) system is recommended for arriving at appropriate resistances. This program should be conducted 3 days per week with 1 day of rest between sessions.

Following is a sample base program for use with athletes:

	Set 1	Set 2	Set 3
Warm-up	—	—	—
Bench press	10-12	10-12	10-12
Leg press	10-12	10-12	10-12
Sit-ups (bent leg)	10	10	10
Military press	10	10	10
Single leg extensions	10	10	10
Lat pull down	10-12	10-12	10-12
Single leg flexions	10	10	10
Arm curls	10	10	10
Calf raisers	15	15	15

Advanced programs for athletes should be designed with event specificity in mind. A program suitable for a football player is usually not suitable for a volleyball player or wrestler. Following are examples of programs designed for and successfully used by volleyball players and wrestlers. The sport of volleyball requires great jumping ability along with strength to perform specific tasks like "bumps," "digs," and "spikes." Many of these tasks are performed over a single supporting leg. Therefore, when possible, exercises should include this postural consideration. Each of the following exercises should be performed in multiple sets with 3 to 4 minutes of rest between exercises. The advanced program should be conducted 4 days per week (MT ThF).

	Set 1	Set 2	Set 3	Set 4
Warm-up	—	—	—	—
Split squats	10	8	8	—
Sit-ups (bent leg)	20	20	20	—
Lat pull down	10	10	10	—
Squats/leg press	5	5	5	5
Single arm front and lateral raises	10	10	10	—
Two arm pull overs	8	8	8	—
Side squats	10	8	8	—
Two arm "bump" front raises	10	8	8	—
Bench press	5	5	5	5
Plyometric drills (box jumping)	—	—	—	—

Wrestling requires the athlete to exhibit great power and strength. In addition, wrestlers must be able to tolerate lactic acid. A weight training program for wrestlers should address these specific needs. A structural strength and power program (MWF) should be interspersed with a local muscular endurance program (TTh). The strength and power program uses a multiple set order with 3 to 4 minutes of rest between exercises.

	Set 1	Set 2	Set 3	Set 4	Set 5
Warm-up	—	—	—	—	—
Power clean	5	5	5	5	5
Squats	5	5	5	5	5
Sit-ups (bent leg)	25	25	—	—	—
Push presses	8	8	8	8	—
Hang cleans	5	5	5	5	5
Dead lifts	7	7	7	7	7
Optional lift	—	—	—	—	—

The local muscular endurance program is performed in circuit order (1 set per exercise before proceeding to the next set) with a 2- to 4-minute rest between sets.

	Set 1	Set 2	Set 3 (optional)
Warm-up	—	—	—
Bench press	10	10	10
Double leg extensions	10	10	10
Military press	10	10	10
Leg press	10	10	10
Curls	10	10	10
Calf raisers	10	10	10
Upright rows	10	10	10
Double leg curls	10	10	10
Lat pull downs	10	10	10

These programs were designed by Captain William Kraemer, Ph.D., exercise physiologist, U.S. Army Institute of Environmental Medicine, Natick, Massachusetts.

Maintenance of strength gains

Muscular strength and endurance do not seem to be easily compromised by stopping training. Strength gains were not significantly reduced after 6 weeks without isotonic training,[7] and subjects still retained 45% of the gains after 1 year.[38] Endurance was not significantly reduced after 4 weeks[10] and after 65 days.[27] Strength can be maintained, following attainment of an optimal level, by as few as one training session per month.[53]

SUMMARY

This chapter presented various techniques of training by concentrating on the physical dimensions of training and how those dimensions might stimulate change. A physiological training theory was discussed that has been proposed to help the teacher and coach make training decisions. Decisions are based on the integration of knowledge about physiological systems and the principles and physical dimensions of training, with an analysis of the physical dimensions of the activity.

The first step is to identify the physiological system used in the physical activity. This involves the determination of the type, frequency, duration, and intensity of its various components. Next, these dimensions must be integrated with knowledge of metabolic systems. In so doing, the coach or teacher determines the system(s) to be changed (oxygen, ATP-PC, lactate) and the proportion of time to be devoted to each. Metabolic systems are changed by applying the principles of specificity, overload, and progressive resistance and incorporating time for warm-up and cool-down. Resistance, repetitions, and rest time are manipulated to adapt training to the metabolic system and the needs of the activity.

All training can be represented on a continuum with high-resistance/low-repetition/short-duration methods on one extreme (for example, isometric) and low-resistance/high-repetition/long-duration methods at the other (for example, marathon). Continuous training falls on the latter end of the continuum and interval training on the first. Both types of training are known to improve aerobic capacity; however, one major advantage of interval training is the high-intensity stimulus provided in a short period of time.

Volume stress has been hypothesized as the stimulus for improvement during aerobic exercise. By providing training dimensions that increase stroke volume, the mechanisms responsible for improving systemic blood flow are enhanced. Interval training is thought to be particularly beneficial in this regard, since stroke volume rises above peak exercise values during the rest interval between exercise bouts.

Manipulation of training dimensions can result in subtle differences regarding the effect on metabolic systems. For example, 3-minute exercise intervals were found to be more effective than 15-second intervals for improvement in aerobic capacity. Likewise, the lactate system is more effectively stimulated with longer intervals, 2 to 3 minutes, than shorter intervals, 0.5 to 1 minute.

Dropout rate has been shown to be higher in interval programs compared to continuous programs. Both duration and frequency have a significant effect on injury. Groups training with 15- and 30-minute exercise durations had significantly fewer injuries than a group using 45-minute sessions. Moderate to high intensity training resulted in a 40% injury rate compared to 15% for a moderate intensity program.

Aerobic fitness gains are easily compromised by the discontinuance of training. In one study, significant losses were observed after 6 weeks; however, continued training at a lower intensity was able to maintain previous gains. A competitive season may be able to maintain previous gains, but it is unlikely that additional improvements will be observed.

When training dimensions are equated between various modes of training (jogging and cycling), approximately the same aerobic gains can be expected. Games like tennis most likely achieve the same results; however, the nature of the game and the skill of the opponent govern the playing intensity and, in a competitive situation, the duration. Rope skipping is not a preferred training mode because the exercise cannot be graded. Energy cost remains constant across a wide range of skipping rates. Arm cranking can improve aerobic capacity, although results are not as great as with leg training, since the muscle mass involvement is much less.

Isotonic strength training consists of movements that contain both concentric (shortening) and eccentric (lengthening) contractions. Early research by DeLorme and Watkins[12] found that strength could be improved by using 3 sets of 10 repetitions (one-half, three-fourths, and full 10 RM). The term *RM* refers to the maximal resistance that can be lifted for a certain number of repetitions. Later work confirmed these results, but suggested the optimal RM range was between 3 and 9.[4] Strength appears to enhance endurance and vice versa, but there is a tendency for high-resistance, low-repetition programs to produce strength and for low-resistance, high-repetition programs to produce endurance. The mechanism responsible for improved isotonic strength and muscle hypertrophy is unclear.

At equal submaximal loads, more fibers are recruited during eccentric training. Subjects perceive eccentric training to be less stressful.

Strength training emphasizes the force component of sport but not the acceleration component. More attention should be given to the production of force at velocities that mimic sport movements. Most barbell and variable resistance equipment fails to consider this point. In addition, this equipment does not promote trunk rotation strength, which is needed in most sports.

Isometric contractions are known to increase muscle strength. However, the gains are made only at the joint angle trained.

Circuit strength training has been promoted as a method to enhance both strength and aerobic capacity. Research indicates that aerobic capacity can be improved by this method, although often at a lower level than running.

Isokinetic contractions involve the development of maximal tension as the muscle shortens at a constant speed through a full range of motion. This type of training offers the possibility that strength could be developed at speeds that approximate athletic motions. Isokinetic training may be specific to the training velocity.

Maintenance of strength and endurance appears to be less fragile than maintenance of cardiorespiratory fitness. Cessation of training for 4 and 6 weeks does not significantly reduce strength and endurance, respectively.

KEY TERMS

concentric contraction force created by shortening of muscle, as in the up portion of a push-up; sometimes referred to as positive exercise.

contraction since this term usually implies change in length of muscle, generally shortening, and we know that other length changes are possible (lengthening), contraction should be defined as the "attempt to shorten."

eccentric contraction force created by lengthening of muscle, as in the down portion of a push-up; sometimes referred to as negative exercise.

isokinetic contraction dynamic contraction in which the speed of movement is constant throughout a range of movement.

isometric contraction muscular force resulting in no change in muscle length or movement of the skeleton.

power performance of work with time as a consideration ($P = W \times T^{-1}$). Power is measured in watts.

work when muscular contraction results in shortening (concentric) of muscle, the resulting body movement is considered work ($W = f \times d$). Work is also performed when muscles lengthen (eccentric), in which case, muscles are said to be worked on. Since work does not involve time, which is usually the case in sport and exercise, and can be accomplished when no movement occurs ($d = 0$), such as with isometric force, "exercise" is the preferred term to use as an encompassing term for force created by muscular contraction within the context of sport and exercise.

REVIEW QUESTIONS

1. Briefly discuss the physiological training theory.

2. What metabolic system would you train to prepare yourself for racquetball? What variables did you use to arrive at your decision?

3. Briefly describe why interval training would be a preferred approach for a miler.

4. What is thought to be the stimulus for improvement during interval training? Explain.

5. How would you prescribe exercise duration, frequency, and intensity if you were concerned with both cardiorespiratory improvement and injury prevention?

6. Briefly discuss the mechanism for improvement during isotonic weight training.

7. Define eccentric training. In what context might such training be useful? Name one positive and one negative argument regarding the use of eccentric training.

8. Can weight training provide aerobic benefits? How?

9. How is Nautilus type equipment different from most variable resistance systems?

REFERENCES

1. Anderson, T., and Kearney, J.T.: Effects of three resistance training programs on muscular strength and absolute and relative endurance, Res. Q. Exerc. Sport **53**:1, 1982.

2. Asmussen, E.: Positive and negative work, Acta Physiol. Scand. **28**:364, 1963.

3. Astrand, I., Astrand, P.O., Christensen, E.H., and others: Intermittent muscular work, Acta Physiol. Scand. **48**:448, 1960.

4. Berger, R.A.: Effect of varied weight training programs on strength, Res. Q. **33**:168, 1962.

5. Berger, R.A.: Optimum repetitions for the development of strength, Res. Q. **33**:334, 1962.

6. Berger, R.A.: Comparative effects of three weight training programs, Res. Q. **33**:396, 1963.

7. Berger, R.A.: Comparison of the effect of various weight training loads on health, Res. Q. **36**:141, 1965.

8. Capra, F.: The turning point, New York, 1982, Simon & Schuster.

9. Clarke, D.H., and Stull, G.A.: Endurance training as a determinant of strength and fatigability, Res. Q. **41**:19, 1970.

10. Clarke, H.H., Shay, C.T., and Mathews, D.K.: Strength decrement of elbow flexor muscles following exhaustive exercise, Arch. Phys. Med. Rehabil. **8**:184, 1954.

11. Coyle, E.F., Costill, D.L., and Lesmes, G.R.: Leg extension power and muscle fiber composition, Med. Sci. Sports **11**:12, 1979.

11a. Coyle, E.F., Feiring, D.C., Rotkis, T.C., and others: Specificity of power improvements through slow and fast isokinetic training, J. Appl. Physiol. **51**:1437, 1981.

12. DeLorme, T.H., and Watkins, A.L.: Techniques of progressive resistance exercise, Arch. Phys. Med. Rehabil. **29**:263, 1948.

13. Dressendorfer, R.H.: Endurance training of recreationally active men, Physic. Sports Med. **6**:122, 1978.

14. Fox, E.L., and Mathews, D.: Interval training: conditioning for sports and general fitness, Philadelphia, 1974, W.B. Saunders Co.

15. Fox, E.L., and Mathews, D.K.: The physiological basis of physical education and athletics, ed. 3, Philadelphia, 1981, Saunders College Publishing.

16. Gardner, G.W.: Specificity of strength changes of the exercised and nonexercised limb following isometric training, Res. Q. **34**:98, 1963.

17. Gettman, L.R., Ayres, J.J., Pollock, M.L., and others: Physiological effects on adult men of circuit strength training and jogging, Arch. Phys. Med. Rehabil. **60**:115, 1979.

18. Gettman, L.R., Ayres, J.J., Pollock, M.L., and others: The effect of circuit weight training on work capacity, cardiorespiratory function, and body composition of adult men, Med. Sci. Sports **10**:171, 1978.

19. Gettman, L.R., Ward, P., and Hagan, R.D.: A comparison of combined running and weight training with circuit weight training, Med. Sci. Sports Exerc. **14**:229, 1982.

20. Goldberg, D.I., and Shephard, R.J.: Stroke volume during recovery from upright bicycle exercise, J. Appl. Physiol. **48**:833, 1980.

21. Goldberg, A.L., Etlinger, J.D., Goldspink, D.F., and others: Mechanism of work-induced hypertrophy of skeletal muscle, Med. Sci. Sports **7**:248, 1975.

22. Green, J.J., and Houston, M.E.: Effect of a season of ice hockey on energy capacities and associated functions, Med. Sci. Sports **7**:299, 1975.

23. Gregory, L.W.: The development of aerobic capacity: a comparison of continuous and interval training, Res. Q. **50:**199, 1979.

24. Hanson, J.S.: Decline of physiological training effects during the competitive season in members of the U.S. Nordic ski team, Med. Sci. Sports **7:**213, 1975.

25. Hettinger, T., and Muller, E.A.: Muskelleistung und Muskeltraining, Arbeitsphysiologie **5:** 111, 1953.

26. Holloszy, J.O.: Biochemical adaptations to exercise: aerobic metabolism. Exerc. Sport Sci. Rev. **1:**46, 1973.

27. Houtz, S.J., Parrish, A.M., and Hellebrandt, F.A.: The influence of heavy resistance exercise on strength, Physiother. Rev. **26:**299, 1946.

28. Jesse, J.P.: Misuse of strength development training programs in athletic training, Physic. Sports Med. **7:**46, 1979.

29. Johnson, B.L., Adamczyk, J.W., Tennoe, K.O., and others: A comparison of concentric and eccentric muscle training, Med. Sci. Sports **8:**35, 1976.

29a. Kakkihen, K., and Komi, P.V.: Electromyographic changes during strength training and detraining, Med. Sci. Sports Exerc. **15:**455, 1983.

30. Knuttgen, H.G.: Force, work, power, and exercise, Med. Sci. Sports **10:**227, 1978.

31. Knuttgen, H.G., Nordesjo, L.O., Ollander, B., and others: Physical conditioning through interval training with young male adults, Med. Sci. Sports **5:**220, 1973.

32. Kraemer, W.J.: Weight training: what you don't know will hurt you, Wy. J. Health, Phys. Ed. Recr. Dance **5:**8, 1982.

33. Lesmes, G.R., Costill, D.L., Coyle, E.F., and others: Muscle strength and power changes during maximal isokinetic training, Med. Sci. Sports **10:**226, 1978.

34. Lind, A.R., and McNicol, G.W.: Cardiovascular responses to static and dynamic exercise, Ergonomics **8:**379, 1965.

35. Lind, A.R., McNicol, G.W., and Donald, K.W.: Circulatory adjustments to sustained (static) muscular activity. In Evang, K., and Andersen, K.L., editors: Proceedings of the International Symposium of Physical Activity in Health and Disease, Norway, 1966, Universitelesforlaget.

36. Londeree, B.: How to customize workouts, Run. World **13:**172, 1978.

37. McCloskey, D.I.: Isometric exercise and cardiovascular stress, Aust. N.Z. J. Med. **6:**15, 1976.

38. McMorris, J.D., and Elkins, E.C.: A study of production and evaluation of muscular hypertrophy, Arch. Phys. Med. Rehabil. **35:**420, 1954.

39. Mitchell, J.H., and Wildenthal, K.: Static (isometric) exercise and the heart, Annu. Rev. Med. **25:**369, 1974.

40. Moffatt, R.J., Stamford, B.A., Weltman, A., and others: Effects of high intensity aerobic training on maximal oxygen uptake capacity and field test performance, J. Sports Med. **17:**351, 1977.

41. Moritani, T., and DeVries, H.A.: Neural factors versus hypertrophy in the time course of muscle strength gain, Am. J. Phys. Med. **58:**115, 1979.

42. Muller, E.A., and Rohmert, W.: Die Geschwindigkeit des Muskelkraftzunahme bei isometrischem Training, Int. Z. Physiol. enischl. Arbeits-physiol. **19:**403, 1963.

43. Noble, B.J.: The effect of two-thirds maximal static contractions on the rate of improvement in static strength. Unpublished master's thesis, Michigan State University, 1957.

44. Oja, P., Teraslinna, P., Partanen, T., and others: Feasibility of an 18 months' physical training program for middle-aged men and its effect on physical fitness, Am. J. Public Health **6:**459, 1975.

45. Orlander, J., Kiessling, K-H., Karlsson, J., and others: Low intensity training, inactivity and resumed training in sedentary men, Acta Physiol. Scand. **101:**351, 1977.

46. Petrofsky, J.S., and Lind, A.R.: Comparison of metabolic and ventilatory responses of men to various lifting tasks and bicycle ergometry, J. Appl. Physiol. **45:**60, 1978.

47. Pollock, M.L.: The quantification of endurance training programs, Exerc. Sport Sci. Rev. **1:**155, 1973.

48. Pollock, M.L.: How much is enough? Physic. Sports Med. **6:**50, 1978.

49. Pollock, M.L., Broida, J., Kendrick, Z., and others: Effects of training two days per week at different intensities on middle-aged men, Med. Sci. Sports **4:**192, 1972.

50. Pollock, M.L., Gettman, L.R., Milesis, C.A., and others: Effects of frequency and duration of training on attrition and incidence of injury, Med. Sci. Sports **9:**31, 1977.

51. Pollock, M.L., Miller, H., Janeway, R., and others: Effects of walking on body composition and cardiovascular function of middle-aged men, J. Appl. Physiol. **30:**126, 1971.

52. Pollock, M.L., Miller, H.S., Linnerud, A.C., and others: Arm pedaling as an endurance training regimen for the disabled, Arch. Phys. Med. Rehabil. **55:**418, 1974.

53. Pollock, M.L., Ward, A., and Ayres, J.J.: Cardiorespiratory fitness: response to differing intensities and durations of training, Arch. Phys. Med. Rehabil. **58:**467, 1977.

54. Rose, D.L., Radzyminski, S.F., and Beatty, R.R.: Effect of brief maximal exercise on the strength of the quadriceps femoris, Arch. Phys. Med. Rehabil. **38:**157, 1957.

55. Schiaffino, S., and Hanzlikova, V.: On the mechanism of compensatory hypertrophy in skeletal muscles, Experientia **26:**152, 1970.

56. Stamford, B.A., Cuddihee, R.W., Moffatt, R.J., and others: Task specific changes in maximal oxygen uptake resulting from arm versus leg training, Ergonomics **21:**1, 1978.

57. Steinhaus, A.H.: Toward an understanding of health and physical education, Dubuque, Iowa, 1963, William C. Brown Co.

58. Thistle, H.G., Hislop, H.J., Moffroid, M., and others: Isokinetic contraction: a new concept of resistive exercise, Arch. Phys. Med. Rehabil. **48:**279, 1967.

59. Town, G.P., Sol, N., and Sinning, W.E.: The effect of rope skipping rate on energy expenditure of males and females, Med. Sci. Sports Exerc. **12:**295, 1980.

60. Wilmore, J.H., Davis, J.A., O'Brien, R.S., and others: Physiological alterations consequent to 20-week conditioning programs of bicycling, tennis, and jogging, Med. Sci. Sports Exerc. **12:**1, 1980.

61. Wilmore, J.H., Parr, R.B., Vodak, P.A., and others: Strength, endurance, BMR, and body composition changes with circuit training, Med. Sci. Sports (Abstract) **8:**59, 1976.

SUGGESTED READINGS

Clarke, D.H.: Adaptations in strength and muscular endurance resulting from exercise, Exerc. Sport Sci. Rev. **1:**74, 1973.

Fleck, S.J., and Schutt, R.C.: Types of strength training, Orthop. Clin. North Am. **4:**449, 1983.

Fox, E.L., and Mathews, D.: Interval training: conditioning for sports and general fitness, Philadelphia, 1974, W.B. Saunders Co.

Gettman, L.R., and Pollock, M.L.: Circuit weight training: a critical review of its physiological benefits, Physic. Sports Med. **9**:44, 1981.

Goldberg, A.L., Etlinger, J.D., Goldspink, D.D., and others: Mechanism of work-induced hypertrophy of skeletal muscle, Med. Sci. Sports **7**:248, 1975.

Jesse, J.P.: Misuse of strength development training programs in athletic training, Physic. Sportsmed. **7**:46, 1979.

McDonagh, M.J.N., and Davies, C.T.M.: Adaptive response of mammalian skeletal muscle to exercise with high loads, Eur. J. Appl. Physiol. **52**:139, 1984.

Pollock, M.L.: How much is enough? Physic. Sports Med. **6**:50, 1978.

Stull, G.A., and Clarke, D.H.: Muscular strength testing and training. In Leon, A.S., and Amundson, G.J., editors: Proceeding of the First International Conference on Lifestyle and Health, Minneapolis, 1978, The University of Minnesota.

CASE STUDY 1

The following conversation took place after a recent lecture about training techniques.

STUDENT: Remember what you said at the beginning of class about exercise physiology not being able to explain all factors involved with human performance? When does it all get put back together? I mean, the mind and the body get dissected many times in my classes.

PROFESSOR: I'm afraid that health, physical education, recreation, and dance have been significantly affected by the scientific revolution. We have often been accused of selling ourselves out to arts and sciences to obtain respectability. The problem is probably much more complex than that. Capra[8] has written about the pervasive nature of Cartesian thought (Descartes is thought to be the father of the scientific revolution) on all elements of Western culture. Interest has been oriented toward segmenting structures, including the human structure, into subunits that can be more easily analyzed. The theory is that the sum of the parts is equal to the whole. However, some people argue that the whole is greater than the sum of the parts. Anyway, the so-called movement sciences have merely followed a pattern similar to other sciences. In addition to exercise physiology, we have biomechanics, motor learning, sport psychology, sport sociology, etc. I agree with your point that after you take all these courses, no attempt is made to put the knowledge back together.

STUDENT: I'm not sure that I understand all that, but I'm glad you see there's a need to pull it back together. It can be overwhelming.

PROFESSOR: It's overwhelming to faculty members as well, so overwhelming that we don't talk about it much. We live in a time when wholism is a key concept, but we can't deal with it within HPERD as a whole or movement science, specifically. We have not been trained as generalists. Momentum leads us to further fragmentation and less wholistic conceptualization.

STUDENT: Are you saying that we need to stop our scientific efforts and try to put it all together as a whole?

PROFESSOR: I don't think we could or should stop our scientific thrust. The problem has been one of imbalance. Almost all our effort has been directed toward scientific output. What we need now is a concerted, creative effort directed toward wholism, which runs parallel to science.

STUDENT: So, I'm left out!

PROFESSOR: In one sense, yes. However, in another sense, you are the beginning of efforts to lift us out. The main responsibility will be placed on your generation.

CASE STUDY 2

A tennis coach recently asked me to assist her in developing a preseason training program for her team. Our initial conversations were centered on a physical description of the game. Tennis has an aerobic component in that points, games, and entire matches *can* consist of low-resistance/high-repetition/long-duration play. Therefore, some aerobic improvement is desirable. However, court dimensions, as well as many strategic styles, would point to a predominance of short bursts of high-intensity movements lasting only a few seconds. Anaerobic training would also be required, perhaps predominately. Training should be individualized to the player's court style. It would seem that the aerobic-anaerobic nature of tennis would make interval training an efficient technique. Such a technique would provide an overload that enhances both metabolic systems. For specificity, ATP-PC training that comprises short-duration (1 to 5 seconds), straight-ahead, and diagonal movements mimicking court actions should be used. Moderate intervals, between 440 and 660 yards, would promote the lactate system necessary for longer, high-intensity points.

A good, solid base of continuous training before preseason (2 to 4 miles, 3 to 5 times per week) would provide a preparation for the rigors of hard practices and make a significant contribution to the aerobic requirements of tennis. A less frequent use of continuous training (1 to 2 per week) could be included in preseason practice. However, aerobic benefits will also be achieved from the interval training.

Strength training should also be included in the physiological preparation of tennis players. Training should be specific to typical movement velocities and the movements of tennis as such. If isokinetic training of the upper body is possible, it should be included. Movements that mimic the stroking motions are necessary. For example, pulley weights are easily adapted to the various strokes. High muscle bulk and force are not required of tennis players. Circuit training, which uses tennis movements, tennis velocities, and low-resistance, high-repetition dimensions, would be very effective. Adding jogging to the interstation rest periods would add to the aerobic contribution.

Establishing a training program for any sport requires seeking answers to the following questions:

1. What physiological system is involved?
2. How does that system change?
3. What physical dimensions of training are related to the change?

chapter 13

BODY COMPOSITION AND WEIGHT CONTROL

MAJOR LEARNING OBJECTIVE

Obesity is a function of both the number and size of fat cells. The number of fat cells can continue to increase until maturity but increases especially quickly during preadolescence.

APPLICATIONS

Adult obesity can be a function of childhood fat accumulation and fat cell proliferation.

■ Elementary school children should be encouraged to exercise as much as possible to prevent a positive caloric balance, which can add to the number of fat cells.

317

Body composition is usually described as having two components: fat tissue and lean tissue (Figure 13-1). Lean tissue consists of muscle, bone, and other organic factors. Since bone and other tissue that make up lean mass are relatively stable, change in lean mass is usually a function of changes in the muscle component. Although body weight is the most common body composition measurement, we shall see that it is also the least specific. We should be interested in whether we have too much fat or too little muscle rather than body weight as such. Figure 13-2 illustrates the goals we typically have regarding change in body composition. Positive body composition changes involve a desire to increase either fat or lean tissue. Seldom do we strive to lose muscle tissue but most individuals, at one time or another, attempt to lose some accumulated fat (negative change). For our purpose, positive and negative refer to direction, not value.

Sport application

Most athletes want to increase muscle tissue. For example, weight lifters and football players seek increased muscle mass to improve their ability to apply force. Occasionally athletes are desirous of increasing fat tissue. The channel swimmer needs fat for purposes of insulation, for instance. Also the heavyweight wrestler may want to add fat to increase total body bulk. A classic example of the athlete striving to lose fat is the wrestler, particularly in the lower weight classes. Several other athletic groups, such as long-distance runners, try to keep their fat weight as low as possible.

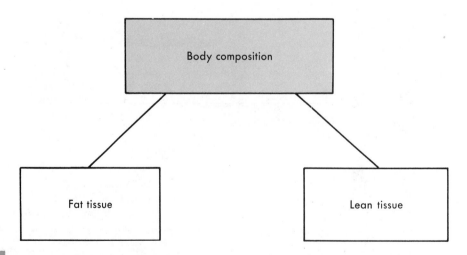

FIG. 13-1   The components of body composition.

General application

Most individuals in our culture want to decrease fat, sometimes fanatically so. Some very thin persons want to increase either fat or muscle to improve appearance or functional capabilities. Muscle tissue increase is a dream of most people in the Western world. We spend a great deal of time and money in the United States thinking, or attempting to do something, about our body composition. The growth of the commerical fitness industry is to no small extent a function of the American compulsion with body composition (decreasing fat and increasing lean tissue). Improving our health and making our body proportions more acceptable can both be achieved by paying attention to the elimination of fat tissue and the addition of lean tissue. Therefore, knowledge of body composition and weight control is absolutely essential for the exercise specialist.

Purpose

This chapter has three basic goals, which are reflected in its three major headings:
1. To describe the physiology of body composition and its control
2. To discuss how body composition is measured
3. To answer the question: How can body composition be changed? (Weight control)

PHYSIOLOGY

Since the growth and development of muscle, a principal component of lean body mass, has been dealt with in previous chapters, concentration in this chapter will be placed on fat tissue development. Fat tissue can be subdivided into essential and storage fat. Essential fat is located in bone marrow, nerve tissue, and various organs. Storage fat, as its name implies, is stored as an energy reserve in adipose tissue. Essentially, the amount of storage fat does not differ between the sexes; however, essential fat is four times greater

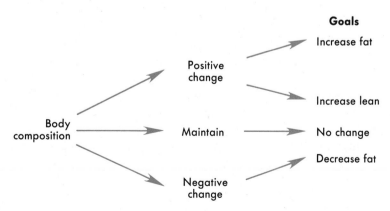

FIG. 13-2 Typical body composition goals.

TABLE 13-1 ||||| BODY COMPOSITION OF
THE ''REFERENCE'' PERSON

	Reference man	Reference woman
Age (yr)	20-24	20-24
Height (in)	68.5	64.5
Weight (lb)	154	125
Total fat (lb)	23.1	33.8
(%)	15.0	27.0
Storage fat (lb)	18.5	18.8
(%)	12.0	15.0
Essential fat (lb)	4.6	15.0
(%)	3.0	12.0
Muscle (lb)	69	45
(%)	44.8	36.0
Bone (lb)	23	15
(%)	14.9	12.0
Remainder (lb)	38.9	31.2
(%)	25.3	25.0
Lean body weight (lb)	136	107

Modified from McArdle, W.D., Katch, F.I., and Katch, V.L.: Exercise physiology: energy, nutrition, and human performance, Philadelphia, 1981, Lea & Febiger.

in females. The higher percentage of essential fat in females is related to the protection of reproductive organs. Therefore the percentage of total body fat for a reference man and woman is 15% and 27%, respectively[39] (Table 13-1).

Storage fat can be further categorized as brown and white adipose tissue. Both tissues use the same metabolic pathways (for example, for fatty acid storage and release) and are histologically similar in the newborn infant.[31] The difference in these tissues concerns function. Brown tissue is used for the generation of heat (thermogenesis) while white adipose tissue serves as a substrate for energy metabolism. In man, until 10 years of age, brown adipose tissue is widely distributed throughout the body.[31] In subsequent years brown tissue disappears, presumably taking on the morphological characteristics of white tissue.

Obesity, defined as adipose tissue 15% in excess of normal, is a definite cultural problem. In 1975, more than half of American males and 40% of females were obese.[36] Metropolitan Life Insurance data have been analyzed to determine the effects of being obese on the life span.[57] The following equation provides a ratio that indicates the risk of an obese condition:

$$\text{Risk} = \frac{\text{Expected age at death}}{\text{Actual age at death}} \times 100$$

TABLE 13-2 ||||| MORTALITY RISK AND REDUCTION IN MORTALITY RISK FOR VARIOUS DEGREES OF OVERWEIGHT*

Age (yr)	% > Average weight		
	10	**20**	**30**
Males			
15-39	110	124	142
40-69	116	126	142
Females			
15-39	107	115	122
40-69	111	125	136

	Moderate overweight		Marked overweight	
	Original	**After weight loss**	**Original**	**After weight loss**
Males	142	113	179	109
Females	142	90	161	135

(Modified from Schlenker, E.D.: Obesity and the lifespan. In Schemmel, R., editor: Nutrition, physiology, and obesity, Boca Raton, Florida, 1980, CRC Press, Inc.)
*Standard risk of mortality equals 100; numbers less than 100 indicate a reduced risk.

For example, a ratio greater than 100 (standard risk) indicates a higher than normal risk for early death. Data for males and females of various ages are shown in Table 13-2. It indicates that as the percentage of overweight increases, so does the risk of early death.

It is important to realize the fallacy of using excess body weight as a criterion for obesity. As mentioned previously, body composition is made up of lean and fat weight. A condition of overweight can result from an excess of either component. During World War II a number of muscular football players were rejected by the Draft Board for being overweight based on standard height-weight tables. These men were not overweight based on excess fat but on higher than average muscular development. Height-weight tables that do not account for various body structures can be misleading. In fact, body weight as such is such a broad description of body composition it is a wonder that some dynamic entrepreneur has not replaced the bathroom scale with a fat caliper. It would make millions of dollars and, unlike many gadgets sold on the market, would make a significant contribution to evaluation of health status.

Theories describing the development of obesity stress the involvement of hereditary, environmental, or a combination of hereditary and environmental factors. Observations have been made concerning genetic influences (Table 13-3).[35] Two "slender" parents are not likely to produce an "obese" child, whereas two "obese" parents will most likely produce "obese" children. Thus our genetic inheritance can place us at risk for obesity.

One can speak of the "push" theory of obesity (for example, obesity arising from nonphysiological reasons). If persons are excluded who become obese because of inherited tendencies, metabolic abnormalities, or brain damage, mechanisms such as stress-related overeating can be hypothesized. Another environmental but physiologically based mechanism would be sedentary living (reduced energy output).

Figure 13-3 illustrates a genetic/environmental interaction model for obesity.[12] Although basic tendencies for leanness and fatness are inherited, they can be modified by diet. This model provides an answer to the age-old question: How can two people eat the same diet and one can maintain normal body composition while the other becomes obese? It seems plausible that genetic and environmental factors, not to mention traumatic (brain damage) or metabolic pathologic conditions (endocrine abnormality), are all important to our understanding of obesity.

TABLE 13-3 |||||| DAVENPORT'S GENETIC OBSERVATIONS

Parent		Children
Slender × slender	→	Slender (very few obese)
Obese × obese	→	Obese (a few medium or slender)
Slender × fleshy	→	Majority obese

Adapted from Mayer.

Diet

	Scanty	Normal	Abundant
Leanness	Skinny	Normal	Obese
Fatness	Normal	Obese	Very obese

Genes

FIG. 13-3   Genetic and environmental interaction with regard to the accumulation of excess body fat. (Modified from Dobzhansky, T.: Mankind evolving, New Haven, Conn., 1962, Yale University Press.)

Adipocyte hypertrophy and hyperplasia

Obesity can develop from enlargement of existing adipocytes (hypertrophy), the increase of adipocytes (hyperplasia), or a combination of both.[19] Needle aspiration of human fat tissue indicates that nonobese people have 25 to 30 $\times$ 10^9 adipocytes. It is commonly believed that obesity occurs more rapidly and easily with those who have more adipocytes.

Recently adipose tissue hypertrophy and hyperplasia have been observed after birth. In fact, cell size and number can increase fourfold to fivefold in humans from birth to adulthood.[19] Studies in animals indicate that the period during childhood, before adolescence, is the most critical.[48] Therefore eating and exercise habits during childhood are important to the development of adult obesity. Cell number remains stable in adulthood. The mechanism for adult obesity is adipocyte hypertrophy. It appears to be advantageous to do anything possible to prevent hyperplasia before physiological maturation.

One study examined young, growing animals paired for body weight and divided into an exercise group, a sedentary, food-restricted group, and a sedentary, free-eating control group.[47] Both the exercised and food-restricted animals had significantly lighter fat pads as adults. In a subsequent study[48] the role of early exercise on adult body weight was investigated. The exercising animals participated in a 28-week swimming program followed by 34 weeks of restricted activity. Compared with free-eating sedentary control animals, exercising animals had significantly lower body weight at 64 weeks. To the extent that we can make extrapolations from animals to humans, we might suggest that childhood dietary precautions and physical activity may prevent or inhibit adult obesity by decreasing adipocyte hyperplasia.

Appetite and obesity

Exercise suppresses the appetite in male animals, and the degree of suppression is related to exercise intensity.[45] Animals who participated in a high-intensity, short-term program consumed fewer calories than did nonexercising control animals. Confirmation of these data in humans is difficult given the problems with assessment of calorie intake and expenditure.[74] However, it has been observed that appetite and food intake are related in active people but not in inactive persons. For example, inactive people do not consume calories in direct response to physical activity,[36] but rather they eat more calories than their activity levels require. Also, a decrease in activity does not always result in a decrease in appetite.[38] This means that active people must be careful during inactive periods because their appetite will not necessarily adapt to the decrease in energy expenditure with a decrease in intake. Those with muscular body types (mesomorphs) need to exercise more than do those with thin body types (ectomorphs) for the appetite to adjust food intake correctly.[36]

Contrary to popular belief, obese people do not necessarily have a high caloric intake. Table 13-4 illustrates the results of a survey of obese and nonobese high school girls.[24] The mean daily caloric intake was 741 kcal lower in obese compared with nonobese girls. The

TABLE 13-4 ||||| MEAN CALORIC INTAKE PER DAY IN OBESE AND
NONOBESE GIRLS

| | | Caloric intake per day | | | | |
	No.	>2,500	2,500-2,000	<2,000	Mean	SD
Obese	28	3	6	19	1,965	453
Nonobese	28	15	10	3	2,706	633

(Modified from Johnson, M.L., Burke, B.S., and Mayer, J.: Relative importance of inactivity and overeating in energy balance of high school girls, Am. J. Clin. Nutr. **4:**37, 1956.)
NOTE: Nonobese girls consumed an average of 741 more calories per day compared with obese girls.

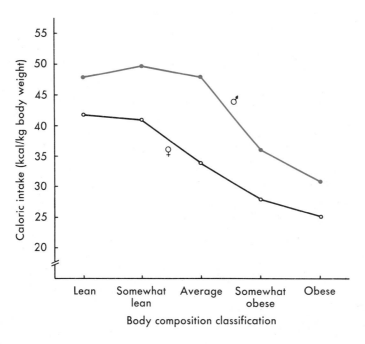

FIG. 13-4   Caloric intake corrected for body weight (BW) of boys and girls plotted as a function of body composition classification. Both boys and girls in the "somewhat obese" and "obese" categories consume fewer calories. (Modified from Heald, F.P., Dangela, M., and Brunschuyler, P.: Physiology of adolescence, N. Engl. J. Med. *268:*243, 1963.)

relative importance of an inactive life-style rather than dietary intake was noted. Further evidence of this phenomenon is offered in Figure 13-4. Both boys and girls show a decreased caloric intake as the body fat continuum moves from lean to obese. Obesity is more a function of inactivity than of food intake. Lean children tend to be more active.

Setpoint theory

The so-called setpoint theory has been proposed in recent years to explain why obese people often eat less than do lean people. Why does the appetite fail to adapt to changes in physical activity and vice versa? Also, why does metabolism fail to change in response to changes in appetite or physical activity to maintain a stable body composition? Setpoint theory hypothesizes that the body contains a hypothalamic ''thermostat'' that attempts to maintain body fat at a predetermined ''set'' level.[4] If each individual were left to his or her own devices, body fat would seek this level and remain stable. Attempts to increase and decrease body fat can be accomplished only by resisting this ''natural'' setpoint. Human will can attempt to overpower the setpoint, for example, by dieting, but sooner or later the will exhausts itself and body weight returns. This observation is confirmed by the thousands, if not millions, of people each year who lose weight by dieting only to gain it back. If the setpoint could be lowered, perhaps this futile repetition would not occur. Physical activity is said to lower the setpoint.[4] It has been speculated that setpoint alterations may be regulated by changes in metabolic rate mediated by hormonal or neural signals. Confirmation of setpoint theory, as well as the role of exercise in this theory, requires further investigation.

BODY COMPOSITION MEASUREMENT

If we are to assess body composition, reliable and valid measures of body fat and lean are needed. It is obviously not possible to assess these components directly in the intact human. Therefore measurement possibilities are indirect estimates. However, a few direct determinations have been made with human cadavers. In the twentieth century, only seven human cadavers have been dissected and analyzed for this purpose.[56] Many more small animals have been dissected, but whether these data can be translated for the assessment of human body composition is not known.[3]

Techniques

Below is a list of techniques used to evaluate body composition indirectly.

1. *Hydrometry*. Because body water is indirectly related to body fat, measurement of total body water can be used to predict body fat. This technique requires the injection of a radioactive tracer, which limits its usefulness with normal human subjects.
2. *Potassium-40*. Lean tissue naturally emits ^{40}K. Scintillation counters are used to count the ^{40}K emission. The counts are calibrated according to the quantity of lean tissue. This equipment has been used extensively in animal science for the evalua-

tion of various feeding protocols. Extensive use of ^{40}K counting in exercise physiology is limited by its expense.

3. *Computerized tomography (CT scan).* X-rays are passed through a single cross-sectional plane of the body at different angles. The absorption or deflections of the x-rays can be recorded, amplified, digitized, stored, and transformed into an image. The image can be photographed for measurement. The technique involves the intravenous injection of a contrast agent.[1] Human thigh muscles have been photographed and their areas measured with a planimeter[21] (Figure 13-5). This technique shows promise for research in body composition.

4. *Volume displacement.* Volume displacement is used to determine the body density by submerging the body in a tank and measuring the water displaced (by collecting overflow water passing through a cannula at the initial water level and into a burette). The volume of the water displaced is related to body volume and density by the formula: Body density = Body mass + Body volume. In turn, body density is related to body fat.

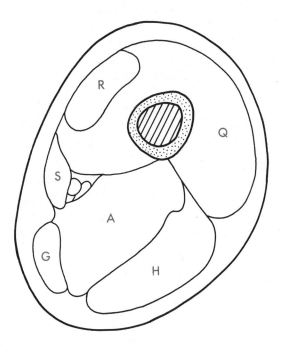

FIG. 13-5   Diagram showing the image produced with computerized tomography. The diagram illustrates a cross section of the thigh with: R-rectus femoris, Q-quadriceps femoris, A-adductors, G-gracilis, S-sartorius, H-hamstrings. Using planimetry the area of each muscle can be calculated. (Modified from Ingemann-Hansen, T., and Halkjaer-Kristensen, J.: Computerized tomographic determination of human thigh components, Scand. J. Rehabil. Med. *12:*27, 1980.)

5. *Underwater weighing*. By measuring the loss of weight in water, body volume can be determined. Body volume can be converted to body density and body fat as described earlier and subsequently in greater detail. A significant difference has been reported between the percentage of fat calculated from underwater weighing (20.1%) and volume displacement (19.4%).[68] This difference may not be physiologically significant, however.

6. *Anthropometric measurement*. With underwater weighing used as a validity criterion, various anthropometric girths and diameters have been used to estimate body density and body fat.

7. *Skinfold measurement*. Several fat pad sites have been measured for skinfold thickness, again with underwater weighing used as a validity criterion, with these measurements serving as estimates of body density and body fat.

8. *Anthropometric and skinfold measurement*. Some equations have used a combination of measurements to estimate body density and body fat.

With the exception of [40]K counting and CT, body fat is measured or estimated and lean mass is computed by subtraction. For example, if a 150-pound person is found to have 15% fat, the fat weight would be 22½ pounds, and by subtraction lean weight would be 127½ pounds (150 − 22½ pounds).

Anthropometric estimation of body density

It seems logical that measurement of the external dimensions of the body (girths and diameters) might provide valuable information about body composition and body type. Early in this century, Sheldon[58] introduced the concept of somatotype in an attempt to classify what he thought to be basic types of body structure. He hypothesized that human bodies could be grouped by a predominance of one of three characteristic components: ectomorphy (linear), mesomorphy (muscular), and endomorphy (fleshy). For example, one could be described as a mesomorph. In cases in which two components were high, one could be described as an ectomesomorph. Each component was placed on a 7-point scale, with 7 indicating a maximum and 1 a minimum of the component. A system of subjectively rating somatotypes was developed in which a person was classified by three numbers associated with the degree of each component present (for example, 3-5-1 [endomorphy, mesomorphy, and ectomorphy, respectively]). However, the system was highly subjective. Heath and Carter[18] later developed a more objective system of arriving at the somatotype numbers by using a number of body girths, diameters, skinfold measurements, and the ponderal index. In a later section of this chapter, examples will be given of typical somatotypes observed in various athletic groups.

Bone diameters (sliding anthropometric caliper), muscle girths (tape measure), and skinfold (fat caliper) measurements have been used successfully as predictors of body density. For example, correlations from 0.87 to 0.92 have been found between anthropometric predictions of lean body weight and underwater weighing.[74] In 1969 and 1970, the following results were reported in prediction experiments with college-age men (R^2 = 0.867)[76] and women (R^2 = 0.755).[77]

Density, g/ml (males) = 1.05721 − 0.00052 (abdominal fat, mm) + 0.00168 (biiliac diameter, cm) + 0.00014 (neck circumference, cm) + 0.00048 (chest circumference, cm) − 0.00145 (abdominal circumference, cm)

Density, g/ml (females) = 1.07685 − 0.00063 (scapular fat, mm) − 0.00336 (knee diameter, cm) + 0.00227 (neck circumference, cm) − 0.00049 (minimal abdominal circumference, cm) − 0.00043 (maximal abdominal circumference)

These authors are quick to caution that such equations have highest predictive accuracy when the test sample is similar to the original sample, that is, college age men and women. The validity of equations has been shown to depend on the age and fitness of the population studied.[14]

Recently an attempt has been made to develop generalized equations for males[22] and females[23] that are thought to be valid across a wide spectrum of age and physical conditions. The following are examples of equations that used the sum of seven skinfolds; however, equations are available for the sum of four and three skinfolds as well. The multiple correlations of these two equations are 0.917 and 0.867, respectively.

Density, g/ml (males) = 1.17615 − 0.2394 (log of the sum of chest, axilla, triceps, subscapula, abdomen, suprailium, and front thigh skinfolds) − 0.00022 (age) − 0.0070 (waist circumference, cm) + 0.02120 (forearm circumference, cm)

Density, g/ml (females) = 1.25186 − 0.03048 (log sum of 7 skinfolds above) − 0.00011 (age) − 0.00064 (gluteal circumference, cm)

Several problems have been identified when body composition is estimated from anthropometric measures.[61]

1. Accuracy of body composition depends on the correct use of anthropometric equipment.
2. If generalized equations are correct, they can be used with accuracy. If other nongeneralized equations are used, it is essential to select an equation that has been developed with subjects similar to the investigator's target population.
3. Equations are based on group data. These equations may be inappropriate for individuals.
4. Equations may not be sensitive to the changes brought about by physical training.

Skinfold measurement

Measurement of skinfolds is an anthropometric determination, as are skeletal and muscle dimensions. Skinfold measurement has been separately categorized here because it has become a method of choice in field studies and large-sample research. Measurement of skinfold thickness in one or more sites can be accomplished quickly and provides a valid estimate of body density and percent body fat. The sites most often selected are illustrated in Figure 13-6. Each site is pinched up with a fold of fat encased between two thicknesses of skin. The fold must be pulled up and away from the muscle to be sure only fat is being measured. Directionality (vertical, diagonal, or horizontal) of the fold depends on the natural contour of the site. For example, midaxilla, triceps, and front thigh folds are usually vertical, while the chest, suprailiac, and subscapular sites are basically diagonal. The abdominal fold is horizontal. A constant distance should be maintained between the thumb and finger with the fold and caliper held below. Each repeat trial should involve releasing and repinching the fat fold. Multiple skinfolds should be measured on the same side of the body. Following are descriptions of anatomical landmarks used for identification of each skinfold site[3]:

1. Chest: over the lateral border of the pectoralis major muscle, just medial to the axilla.
2. Midaxilla: on the midaxillary line approximately at the level of the fifth rib.
3. Subscapular: at the inferior angle of the scapula.
4. Triceps: midway between the acromion and olecranon process on the posterior aspect of the arm, with the arm held vertically.
5. Abdomen: adjacent to the umbilicus.
6. Suprailiac: on the crest of the ilium at the midaxillary line.
7. Front thigh: on the anterior aspect of the thigh midway between the hip and knee joints.

Table 13-5 contains the percent fat computations based on the generalized regression equations (three skinfolds) for men[22] and women.[23] The tables for men use the front thigh, abdomen, and chest skinfolds. Thigh, suprailiac, and triceps skinfolds are used for

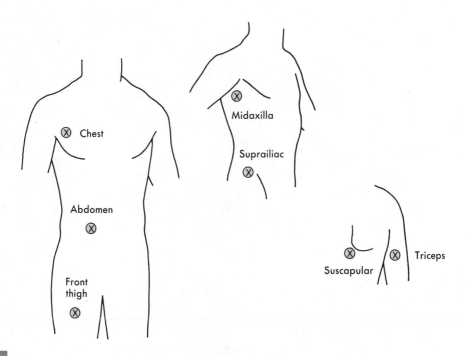

| **FIG. 13-6** | Typical sites for measurement of skinfold fat. |

TABLE 13-5 |||||| ESTIMATES OF PERCENT FAT

Sum of 3 skinfolds*	Age to the last year							
	Under 19	20-22	23-25	26-28	29-31	32-34	35-37	38-40
8-10	.9	1.3	1.6	2.0	2.3	2.7	3.0	3.3
11-13	1.9	2.3	2.6	3.0	3.3	3.7	4.0	4.3
14-16	2.9	3.3	3.6	3.9	4.3	4.6	5.0	5.3
17-19	3.9	4.2	4.6	4.9	5.3	5.6	6.0	6.3
20-22	4.8	5.2	5.5	5.9	6.2	6.6	6.9	7.3
23-25	5.8	6.2	6.5	6.8	7.2	7.5	7.9	8.2
26-28	6.8	7.1	7.5	7.8	8.1	8.5	8.8	9.2
29-31	7.7	8.0	8.4	8.7	9.1	9.4	9.8	10.1
32-34	8.6	9.0	9.3	9.7	10.0	10.4	10.7	11.1
35-37	9.5	9.9	10.2	10.6	10.9	11.3	11.6	12.0
38-40	10.5	10.8	11.2	11.5	11.8	12.2	12.5	12.9
41-43	11.4	11.7	12.1	12.4	12.7	13.1	13.4	13.8
44-46	12.2	12.6	12.9	13.3	13.6	14.0	14.3	14.7
47-49	13.1	13.5	13.8	14.2	14.5	14.9	15.2	15.5
50-52	14.0	14.3	14.7	15.0	15.4	15.7	16.1	16.4
53-55	14.8	15.2	15.5	15.9	16.2	16.6	16.9	17.3
56-58	15.7	16.0	16.4	16.7	17.1	17.4	17.8	18.1
59-61	16.5	16.9	17.2	17.6	17.9	18.3	18.6	19.0
62-64	17.4	17.7	18.1	18.4	18.8	19.1	19.4	19.8
65-67	18.2	18.5	18.9	19.2	19.6	19.9	20.3	20.6
68-70	19.0	19.3	19.7	20.0	20.4	20.7	21.1	21.4
71-73	19.8	20.1	20.5	20.8	21.2	21.5	21.9	22.2
74-76	20.6	20.9	21.3	21.6	22.0	22.3	22.7	23.0
77-79	21.4	21.7	22.1	22.4	22.8	23.1	23.4	23.8
80-82	22.1	22.5	22.8	23.2	23.5	23.9	24.2	24.6
83-85	22.9	23.2	23.6	23.9	24.3	24.6	25.0	25.3
86-88	23.6	24.0	24.3	24.7	25.0	25.4	25.7	26.1
89-91	24.4	24.7	25.1	25.4	25.8	26.1	26.5	26.8
92-94	25.1	25.5	25.8	26.2	26.5	26.9	27.2	27.5
95-97	25.8	26.2	26.5	26.9	27.2	27.6	27.9	28.3
98-100	26.6	26.9	27.3	27.6	27.9	28.3	28.6	29.0
101-103	27.3	27.6	28.0	28.3	28.6	29.0	29.3	29.7
104-106	27.9	28.3	28.6	29.0	29.3	29.7	30.0	30.4
107-109	28.6	29.0	29.3	29.7	30.0	30.4	30.7	31.1
110-112	29.3	29.6	30.0	30.3	30.7	31.0	31.4	31.7
113-115	30.0	30.3	30.7	31.0	31.3	31.7	32.0	32.4
116-118	30.6	31.0	31.3	31.6	32.0	32.3	32.7	33.0
119-121	31.3	31.6	32.0	32.3	32.6	33.0	33.3	33.7
122-124	31.9	32.2	32.6	32.9	33.3	33.6	34.0	34.3
125-127	32.5	32.9	33.2	33.5	33.9	34.2	34.6	34.9
128-130	33.1	33.5	33.8	34.2	34.5	34.9	35.7	35.5

From the Jackson and Pollock generalized equations for men under 40 years of age; men over 40 years of age; and women.
*Sum of thigh, abdomen, and chest skinfolds.

TABLE 13-5 ||||| ESTIMATES OF PERCENT FAT—cont'd

Sum of 3 skinfolds*	Age to the last year							
	41-43	44-46	47-49	50-52	53-55	56-58	59-61	Over 62
8-10	3.7	4.0	4.4	4.7	5.1	5.7	5.8	6.1
11-13	4.7	5.0	5.4	5.7	6.1	6.4	6.8	7.1
14-16	5.7	6.0	6.4	6.7	7.1	7.4	7.8	8.1
17-19	6.7	7.0	7.4	7.7	8.1	8.4	8.7	9.1
20-22	7.6	8.0	8.3	8.7	9.0	9.4	9.7	10.1
23-25	8.6	8.9	9.3	9.6	10.0	10.3	10.7	11.0
26-28	9.5	9.9	10.2	10.6	10.9	11.3	11.6	12.0
29-31	10.5	10.8	11.2	11.5	11.9	12.2	12.6	12.9
32-34	11.4	11.8	12.1	12.4	12.8	13.1	13.5	13.8
35-37	12.3	12.7	13.0	13.4	13.7	14.1	14.4	14.8
38-40	13.2	13.6	13.9	14.3	14.6	15.0	15.3	15.7
41-43	14.1	14.5	14.8	15.2	15.5	15.9	16.2	16.6
44-46	15.0	15.4	15.7	16.1	16.4	16.8	17.1	17.5
47-49	15.9	16.2	16.6	16.9	17.3	17.6	18.0	18.3
50-52	16.8	17.1	17.5	17.8	18.2	18.5	18.8	19.2
53-55	17.6	18.0	18.3	18.7	19.0	19.4	19.7	20.1
56-58	18.5	18.8	19.2	19.5	19.9	20.2	20.6	20.9
59-61	19.3	19.7	20.0	20.4	20.7	21.0	21.4	21.7
62-64	20.1	20.5	20.8	21.2	21.5	21.9	22.2	22.6
65-67	21.0	21.3	21.7	22.0	22.4	22.7	23.0	23.4
68-70	21.8	22.1	22.5	22.8	22.2	23.6	23.9	24.2
71-73	22.6	22.9	23.3	23.6	24.0	24.3	24.7	25.0
74-76	23.4	23.7	24.1	24.4	24.8	25.1	25.4	25.8
77-79	24.1	24.5	24.8	25.2	25.5	25.9	26.2	26.6
80-82	24.9	25.3	25.6	26.0	26.3	26.6	27.0	27.3
83-85	25.7	26.0	26.4	26.7	27.1	27.4	27.8	28.1
86-88	26.4	26.8	27.1	27.5	27.8	28.2	28.5	28.9
89-91	27.2	27.5	27.9	28.2	28.6	28.9	29.2	29.6
92-94	27.9	28.2	28.6	28.9	29.3	29.6	30.0	30.3
95-97	28.6	29.0	29.3	29.7	30.0	30.4	30.7	31.1
98-100	29.3	29.7	30.0	30.4	30.7	31.1	31.4	31.8
101-103	30.0	30.4	30.7	31.1	31.4	31.8	32.1	32.5
104-106	30.7	31.1	31.4	31.8	32.1	32.5	32.8	33.2
107-109	31.4	31.8	32.1	32.4	32.8	33.1	33.6	33.8
110-112	32.1	32.4	32.8	33.1	33.5	33.8	34.2	34.5
113-115	32.7	33.1	33.4	33.8	34.1	34.5	34.8	36.2
116-118	33.4	33.7	34.1	34.4	34.8	35.1	35.5	36.8
119-121	34.0	34.4	24.7	35.1	35.4	35.8	36.1	36.5
122-124	34.7	35.0	35.4	35.7	36.1	36.4	36.7	37.1
125-127	35.3	35.6	36.0	36.3	36.7	37.0	37.4	37.7
128-130	35.9	36.2	36.6	36.9	37.3	37.6	38.0	38.3

*Sum of thigh, abdomen, and chest skinfolds.

Continued.

TABLE 13-5 ||||| ESTIMATES OF PERCENT FAT—cont'd

Sum of 3 skinfolds*	Age to the last year								
	Under 22	23-27	28-32	33-37	38-42	43-47	48-52	53-57	Over 58
23-25	9.7	9.9	10.2	10.4	10.7	10.9	11.2	11.4	11.7
26-29	11.0	11.2	11.5	11.7	12.0	12.3	12.5	12.7	13.0
29-31	12.3	12.5	12.8	13.0	13.3	13.5	13.8	14.0	14.3
32-34	13.6	13.8	14.0	14.3	14.5	14.8	15.0	15.3	15.5
35-37	14.8	15.0	15.3	15.5	15.8	16.0	16.3	16.5	16.8
38-40	16.0	16.3	16.5	16.7	17.0	17.2	17.5	17.7	18.0
41-43	17.2	17.4	17.7	17.9	18.2	18.4	18.7	18.9	19.2
44-46	18.3	18.6	18.8	19.1	19.3	19.6	19.8	20.1	20.3
47-49	19.5	19.7	20.0	20.2	20.5	20.7	21.0	21.2	21.5
50-52	20.6	20.8	21.1	21.3	21.6	21.8	22.1	22.3	22.6
53-55	21.7	21.9	22.1	22.4	22.6	22.9	23.1	23.4	23.6
56-58	22.7	23.0	23.2	23.4	23.7	23.9	24.2	24.4	24.7
59-61	23.7	24.0	24.2	24.5	24.7	25.0	25.2	25.5	25.7
62-64	24.7	25.0	25.2	25.5	25.7	26.0	26.2	26.4	26.7
65-67	25.7	25.9	26.2	26.4	26.7	26.9	27.2	27.4	27.7
68-70	26.6	26.9	27.1	27.4	27.6	27.9	28.1	28.4	28.6
71-73	27.5	27.8	28.0	28.3	28.5	28.8	29.0	29.3	29.5
74-76	28.4	28.7	28.9	29.2	29.4	29.7	29.9	30.2	30.4
77-79	29.3	29.5	29.8	30.0	30.3	30.5	30.8	31.0	31.3
80-82	30.1	30.4	30.6	30.9	31.1	31.4	31.6	31.9	32.1
83-85	30.9	31.2	32.4	31.7	31.9	32.2	32.4	32.7	32.9
86-88	31.7	32.0	32.2	32.5	32.7	32.4	33.2	33.4	33.7
89-91	32.5	32.7	33.0	33.2	33.5	33.7	33.9	34.2	34.4
92-94	33.2	33.4	33.7	33.4	34.2	34.4	34.7	34.9	35.2
95-97	33.9	34.1	34.4	34.6	34.9	35.1	35.4	35.6	35.9
98-100	34.6	34.8	35.1	35.3	35.5	35.8	36.0	36.3	36.5
101-103	35.2	35.4	35.u	35.9	36.2	36.4	36.7	36.9	37.2
104-106	35.8	36.1	36.3	36.6	36.8	37.1	37.3	37.5	37.8
107-109	36.4	36.7	36.9	37.1	37.4	37.6	37.9	38.1	38.4
110-112	37.0	37.2	37.5	37.7	38.0	38.2	38.5	38.7	38.9
113-115	37.5	37.8	38.0	38.2	38.5	38.7	39.0	39.2	39.5
116-118	38.0	38.3	38.5	38.8	39.0	39.3	39.5	39.7	40.0
119-121	38.5	38.7	39.0	39.2	39.5	39.7	40.0	40.2	40.5
122-124	39.0	39.2	39.4	39.7	39.9	40.2	40.4	40.7	40.9
125-127	39.4	39.6	39.9	40.1	40.4	40.6	40.9	41.1	41.8
138-130	39.8	40.0	40.3	40.5	40.8	41.0	41.3	41.5	41.4

*Sum of thigh, suprailium, and triceps skinfolds.

women. If the sum of three skinfolds for a 44-year-old woman was added to 48, her estimated fat would be 20.7%.

There are many calipers available on the market. They range from plastic calipers without any accommodation for the amount of pressure applied to the skinfold to expensive metal calipers that apply constant pressure. Two plastic calipers, with and without pressure devices, were compared with a metal, uniform-tension caliper.[33] Results indicated that when the plastic calipers are used by inexperienced testers, reliable measurements may not be obtained. Even though calipers without constant-pressure devices are not recommended for research, after 20 minutes of training, inexperienced testers obtained satisfactory results with all three calipers. Therefore, with minimal instruction, the less expensive calipers appear to be suitable in a field situation.

Five equations have been compared to evaluate the densitometric validity of skinfold predictions.[28] Although the equations successfully ordered individuals on a continuum of leaness/fatness, validity was only moderate. Another study compared results obtained from 14 equations.[27] These authors agreed that the available equations did a "fairly good" job of ranking body composition of individuals. Equations were found to be more valid for men than for women. The equations just reported[22,23] have been shown to be valid for both male and female adolescent athletes.[68] (For females the quadratic equation was the most appropriate for predicting body density, while with males either the linear or the quadratic equation can be used.)

CHANGING BODY COMPOSITION (WEIGHT CONTROL)

Now that body composition has been defined and we know how to measure it, we can address the matter of change. Is exercise the best intervention to change body composi-

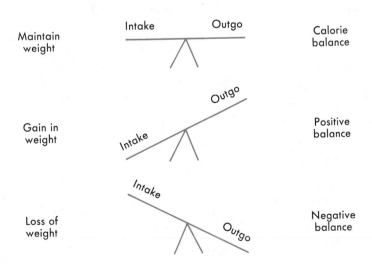

FIG. 13-7   A simplistic model illustrating the relationship of caloric balance to body weight.

tion? Diet? A combination? Certainly we would automatically turn to exercise to increase muscle mass, but the matter of fat reduction is more problematic.

A simplistic model regarding change in body weight or fat is shown in Figure 13-7. When energy input is equally compensated by output, the body is said to be in caloric balance. However, if input exceeds output, tipping the "scales" toward a positive balance, body weight will increase. This can occur from an excessive intake of calories or from a very low physical activity level (energy output). In contrast, when output exceeds input the body will lose weight and is said to be in negative balance. Again, the important

TABLE 13-6 ||||| SOMATOTYPES OF VARIOUS ELITE ATHLETES

Investigators	Sample	Sex	Endomorph	Mesomorph	Ectomorph
Wilmore	World class athletes	M			
	Sprinters		2.7	3.9	2.9
	Middle-distance runners		2.0	3.3	3.7
	Jumpers		2.2	3.3	3.7
	Throwers		5.3	5.2	1.7
	Track and field athletes ($\overline{X}$)		3.1	3.9	3.0
	Swimmers		3.4	4.0	3.0
Cureton	Olympic athletes	M			
	Swimmers		3.6	4.8	4.0
	Divers		3.0	5.0	4.4
	Track and field athletes ($\overline{X}$)		2.7	4.9	4.6
Thorland and others	Junior Olympic athletes	M			
	Sprinter and hurdle jumpers		2.3	4.5	3.4
	Middle-distance runners		2.1	3.7	4.2
	Jumpers and vaulters		2.4	4.2	4.0
	Throwers		3.9	5.8	2.1
	Track and field athletes ($\overline{X}$)		2.6	4.6	3.4
	Gymnasts and divers		2.3	5.0	3.2
	Wrestlers		2.6	5.4	2.9
Thorland and others	Junior Olympic athletes	F			
	Sprinters and hurdle jumpers		2.8	3.3	3.6
	Middle-distance runners		2.4	2.6	4.5
	Jumpers		2.8	2.3	4.6
	Throwers		4.5	4.7	2.0
	Track and field athletes ($\overline{X}$)		3.1	3.2	3.7
	Gymnasts and divers		2.7	3.8	3.3
Wilmore and others	Pro football players	M			
	Defensive backs		3.2	5.6	1.9
	Offensive backs, wide receivers		3.5	6.2	1.6
	Linebackers		4.6	6.7	1.3
	Offensive lineman, tight ends		5.5	6.7	0.9
	Defensive lineman		5.4	6.9	1.2
	Quarterbacks, kickers		5.0	5.9	1.3

question remains: Is it best to exercise to produce negative balance, to diet, or both?

Arguments have been brought forward against exercise on the grounds of the magnitude of the effort involved and the counterbalancing effects of appetite. The latter argument has been countered by studies in animals showing the suppressive effects of exercise on appetite.[45] Although the data on humans are not so impressive, several studies have shown that appetite should not be blamed for what is basically a problem of inactivity.[20]

The former argument is based on knowledge that a pound of fat contains 3,500 kcal. The argument states that it would take just too much exercise to lose weight, particularly for those whose goal is to lose 20 to 30 pounds. To be sure, exercise would provide no quick "snake medicine" cure for obesity. It would take time and effort. On the other hand, it takes time to become obese. A positive metabolic balance of 250 kcal/day, a mild imbalance, can produce a gain of 1 pound every 2 weeks. This would result in a gain of 26 pounds in 1 year. To reverse that trend would require a mild increase in exercise with little or no calorie restrictions. Indeed, it would take time to counteract previous imbalances. However, it is prudent to consider exercise in any weight control regimen.

TABLE 13-7 ‖‖‖ FAT PERCENTAGES IN VARIOUS ATHLETIC GROUPS

Athletic group	Sex	Age (yr)	% Fat	Investigators
Distance runners	M	9-16	16.5	Wilmore, Brown, and Davis
	M	17-51	16.9	
Sprint and middle-distance runners	M	9-16	10.7	
	M	17-51	11.1	
Throwers	M	—	27.0	
Swimmers				
Sprint	M	—	14.6	
Middle-distance	M	—	24.1	
Distance	M	—	17.1	
Distance runners	M	26.1	7.5	Costill, Bowers, and Kammer
Distance runners	M	40-49	11.2	Pollock and others
Distance runners	M	—	4.7	Pollock and others
Endurance runners	M	18-24	7.0	Pollock and Jackson
	M	40-50	11.0	
Sprinters	M	18-24	10.0	
Sedentary persons	M	18-28	16.0	
	M	40-50	23.0	
Basketball players	F	19.4	26.9	Conger and Macnab
Volleyball players	F	19.4	25.3	
Swimmers	F	19.4	26.3	
Runners	F	—	13.3	Novak and others
Swimmers	F	—	18.9	
Gymnasts	F	—	6.8	

The effects of exercise—descriptive studies of elite athletes

As a first approach to answering the question of the effectiveness of exercise in weight control, one can examine the body composition of elite athletes. Admittedly, such an examination involves a "chicken and egg" problem (for example, is the cause of leanness in the athlete a genetic predisposition for leanness or the result of the exercise involved in the sport?). Nevertheless, such data are valuable if only to describe the body composition requirements of various athletic events. Tables 13-6 and 13-7 illustrate examples of somatotypes and body fat percentages observed in elite athletes. Keeping in mind that variability exists within and among these athletic groups relative to somatotype and body fat, certain general observations can be made. First, the highest somatotype component among high-level male athletes is mesomorphy. Second, mesomorphy is highest among the power athletes (for example, the throwers) and lowest among distance runners. Third, endomorphy is the lowest component among male athletes, with throwers as an exception. Fourth, the highest somatotype component among female track and field Junior Olympians is ectomorphy, with the exception of throwers. Fifth, the highest somatotype component among female throwers, gymnasts, and divers competing in the Junior Olympics was mesomorphy.

Skinfold measurements were made on 456 Olympic athletes at the 1976 Montreal Games.[34] The male athletes studied represented 20 sports and 68 events. The female athletes came from 10 sports and 45 events. It was concluded that fatness "is more influenced by sport and, by inference, training." On the other hand, the patterning of the fat (anatomical distribution) was not related to sport and training. These data indicate that patterning may be genetic, but fatness is a function of physical activity. (The results of this study are related to the concept of spot reduction, which will be discussed later.)

Changes in fat that occur from an exercise program are related to the total energy expenditure of the program.[49] Longer programs, beyond 2 months, show greater fat loss. Fat loss is also related to the initial level of obesity, with the more obese losing more fat.

One investigation described the fat and somatotype characteristics of 71 female gymnasts competing in an AIAW gymnastics meet.[23] The somatotype components were not different between the placers (endomorphy, 3.06; mesomorphy, 4.04; ectomorphy, 2.61) and nonplacers (endomorphy, 2.61; mesomorphy, 4.39; ectomorphy, 2.61). However, nonplacers had significantly higher skinfold fat than had placers: 18.41% and 16.82%, respectively. The body types of these athletes were almost identical to those of Olympic-caliber gymnasts and were significantly different from those of a group of 54 nonathletes (endomorphy, 3.92; mesomorphy, 3.80; ectomorphy, 2.57). The fat percentages in this study are similar to those reported in another study of 44 female college gymnasts (15.34%).[62]

Body composition of professional football players has been described.[80] The somatotype data from this study appear in Table 13-6. The authors concluded that similarities in body type exist within the backs (offensive and defensive) and, separately, within linemen (offensive and defensive). Linebackers, quarterbacks, and kickers have somatotypes that fall between those of backs and linemen. College football players were found to be smaller and fatter than professional players.[70]

The demand for frequent and fast weight reduction in preparation for wrestling competition has been a concern of exercise physiologists for years. The practice sometimes requires wrestlers to acquire and maintain body compositions that are not natural for their body types. For example, variables of body composition were measured at the completion of a high school season and again 2 months later.[63] Lean body weight did not change during this period. However, after competitors had returned to normal diet and exercise behavior, body weight (64.1 kg vs 67.1 kg) and percent fat (9.4% vs 11.7%) increased significantly. To combat the tendency for wrestlers to go to extraordinary means to "make weight," the concept of "minimal wrestling weight" has been proposed.[65] The concept uses various anthropometric measures to predict the body weight associated with 5% fat. It is assumed that any procedure that lowers body fat below this level may be harmful to the health and performance of the wrestler. Table 13-8 describes the long form (seven items) and short form (five items) for predicting minimal weight.

TABLE 13-8 |||||| METHOD FOR CALCULATING MINIMAL WRESTLING WEIGHT

Long form

Minimal weight	=		1.84	×	Height (in)	_____
		+	3.28	×	Chest diameter (cm)	_____
		+	3.31	×	Chest depth (cm)	_____
		+	0.82	×	Biiliac diameter (cm)	_____
		+	1.69	×	Bitrochanteric diameter (cm)	_____
		+	3.56	×	Diameter of both wrists (cm)	_____
		+	2.15	×	Diameter of both ankles (cm)	_____
		−	281.72			

Short form

Minimal weight	=		2.05	×	Height (in)	_____
		+	3.65	×	Chest diameter (cm)	_____
		+	3.51	×	Chest depth (cm)	_____
		+	1.96	×	Bitrochanteric diameter (cm)	_____
		+	8.02	×	Left ankle diameter (cm)	_____
		−	282.18			

Adapted from Tcheng, T.K., and Tipton, C.: Iowa wrestling study: anthropometric measurements and the prediction of a "minimal" body weight for high school wrestlers, Med. Sci. Sports **5**:1, 1973.

The effects of exercise—experimental studies

Moving from descriptive analyses of high-level athletes, which contain a probable genetic bias, the question can be asked: What changes in body composition occur when studied in a longitudinal, experimental setting?

As a beginning, it would be fair to ask what are the physiological and performance consequences of excess weight. In an attempt to answer this question, a group of six distance runners ran a series of treadmill runs under conditions of 0%, 5%, 10%, and 15% added weight.[10] When excess weight was added, both treadmill run time and aerobic power (ml/kg · min^{-1}) were significantly reduced. Twelve-minute run distance was decreased significantly in all cases.

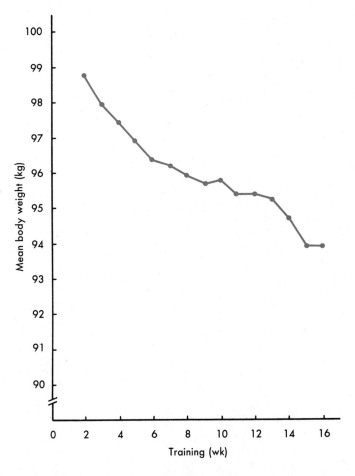

FIG. 13-8 Loss of body weight in six young males participating in a 16-week vigorous walking program. (Modified from Leon, A.S., Conrad, J., Hunningshake, D.B., and others: Effects of a vigorous walking program on body composition, and carbohydrate and lipid metabolism of obese young men, Am. J. Clin. Nutr. *32:*1776, 1979.)

Changes in body composition have been studied as a function of frequency of training (2 vs 4 days per week).[51] Changes were judged to be directly proportional to frequency. In fact, the group training 2 days per week changed percentage of fat very little, while the group training 4 days per week lowered body fat significantly (20.7% to 17.4%).

The intensity factor has also been studied.[52] With a protocol of 2 days per week, normally not an effective frequency for making changes in body composition, a significant decrease in percentage of fat (22.9% to 22.1%) was noted for a group working at 90% of maximal heart rate. No changes in body composition were observed in the group working at 80% of maximal heart rate or the control group. In another investigation, a high-intensity program (840 kg-m/min, intermittent exercise for 5 to 7.5 minutes) was compared to a low-intensity program (420 kg-m/min, continuous exercise for 10 to 15 minutes).[15] No changes in body composition were made in the high-intensity group. On the contrary, significant changes were made in the low-intensity group. The author concluded that the results supported "the contention that to reduce body fat stores an exercise program of low intensity and long duration is required." Low-intensity exercise is notable for its low respiratory exchange ratio (R), which means that fat utilization is greater.

It can be seen that changes in body fat are a function of precise manipulation of frequency, intensity, and duration. Perhaps a prudent recommendation would involve using an intensity that would allow for frequent exercise of long duration. In fact, daily exercise would be a reasonable prescription for those interested in losing weight. For example, walking 5 days per week was found to be an effective method for losing body fat.[32] Figure 13-8 illustrates the effects of a 16-week walking program on body weight.

Weight training, normally concerned with increasing lean body mass, has produced significant decreases in body fat in both men (13.24% to 11.92%) and women (24.51% to 22.65%).[72] This experiment required subjects to train 2 days per week (40 minutes per day) for 10 weeks.

To gain perspective regarding the role of exercise in weight control, 55 studies were reviewed in which protocols varying in duration from 6 to 104 weeks were used.[74] The mean loss of fat across these studies was only 1.6%. The implication of this review is that exercise, although effective, cannot be counted on for large weight reductions. Diet is a more effective method for those who need to lose a large amount of fat. However, it should be remembered that the 1.6% average reported can be misleading. Experiments that used the right combination of frequency, intensity, and duration were more effective than others.

Exercise plus diet

Many believe that the most productive procedure for losing body weight is to combine an exercise regimen with a plan to reduce caloric intake. In this way, a negative balance is produced on both the intake and the output sides. Studies in both animals and humans have confirmed that dietary restriction alone produces weight loss, with a high proportion coming from lean tissue.[46]

In a study of 25 women, interventions were compared in which one group dieted only, another exercised only, and a third group combined diet and exercise.[84] All groups decreased input, output, or input and output by 500 kcal. The three groups lost an average of 11.38 pounds with no significant differences between groups. The group that dieted only lost both fat and lean tissue. Those who exercised alone, as well as those who combined diet and exercise, increased lean weight and decreased fat weight.

OTHER CONSIDERATIONS

Spot reduction

The concept of spot reduction hypothesizes that exercise in any specific anatomical area containing excess fat will result in exclusive fat reduction in that area. Research with spot reduction has been controversial. For example, 32 subjects were trained during a 6-week period with biceps curls and triceps extensions in one arm.[44] Results indicated that a significant reduction was made in the triceps skinfold on the exercised arm, with no change in the other arm. Several other studies support this investigation.[30,40,83] Still others,[54,55] however, do not support spot reduction but propose that fat is lost in relation to the makeup of the fat pad (for example, different fat pads have different tendencies to gain and lose fat). This view is supported when localized exercise (calisthenics) is compared to generalized exercise (aerobics).[42] Each program was equated relative to frequency (3 days per week), duration (30 minutes per day), and intensity (relative to heart rate). The two programs were equally effective in altering body composition. These authors suggest that fat is lost from the "most labile" fat pads first followed by loss in the "most stable deposits." This suggestion agrees with those of others,[81] who have proposed that fat is deposited selectively rather than consistently throughout the body. Additionally, the results of an investigation of skinfold thickness in Olympians in 1976 suggest that fat patterning may be genetic.[34]

Aging

It seems reasonable to assume that the various body composition components change with age, corresponding to alterations in diet, exercise, and perhaps bone density. Fat, muscle, and muscle-free lean percentages were compared in men and women between the ages of 20 and 50 years. Results are shown here:

	Women		Men	
	20 yr	**50 yr**	**20 yr**	**50 yr**
Fat	30.7	30.0	13.6	26.5
Muscle	16.8	3.6	32.6	19.6
Muscle-free lean	53.8	58.4	53.8	53.9

Women change very little in relative fat during this 30-year period; however, muscle percentage drops drastically. During the same period, men have increases in percentage of fat and decreases in percentage of muscle. Results of the Tecumseh, Michigan, study support the hypothesis that much of this change in body composition results from changes in physical activity.[41] It should also be remembered that basal metabolic rate declines with age.

The underweight condition

Western culture has become inordinately enamored with the youthful body. Millions of dollars are spent annually to counteract the effects of aging and our excessive living habits. In and of itself, such a desire is not without many positive benefits. However, combined with the compulsive personality, such a desire can lead to a loss of fat that may place individuals in danger. Recently the problem of anorexia nervosa (compulsive loss of appetite leading to severe losses of body weight) appears to have either increased or received increased attention. This problem has been increasingly identified in recent years, especially among young women. Anorexic women can often be seen in exercise environments because of their compulsion for added calorie expenditure. A related problem concerns a recent notice of the number of hard-training women who are developing amenorrhea. Loss of the menstrual period is usually associated with large decreases in body fat, although this factor does not seem to be causative. Both anorexia nervosa and exercise-induced amenorrhea are clinically recognized by a common loss of the menstrual period. They do not have the same cause. The coach or exercise specialist may be the first professional to become aware of such conditions, and is in a good position to suggest remedial alternatives.

Whether the underweight condition results from a normal desire to lose weight, a pathological compulsion, or a genetic tendency, it represents a major problem for the exercise clinician. The psychological and medical aspects of such problems need to be handled by other health professionals.

When the underweight is genetic in origin, the condition can be problematic (for example, genetic predisposition to extreme thinness). It is interesting that women with fat weight more than 20% below the average have been shown to have a similar physique and anthropometric dimensions compared with average and obese women.[26] Weight training can be used effectively with the underweight individual but probably should be combined with an increase in caloric intake and, in some cases, a decrease in excessive exercise leading to a serious negative caloric balance.

SUMMARY

Body composition consists of fat and lean tissue. Decreasing fat and increasing lean tissue are the major concerns of both the athlete and the lay public.

Fat tissue consists of essential fat and storage fat. The former can be found in bone marrow, nerve tissue, and other organs. The latter is stored in adipose tissue. Storage fat can be further subdivided into white and brown adipose tissue.

Excess body weight has been associated with early death. However, body weight is not a good criterion of obesity, since it does not differentiate between lean and fat tissue.

Obesity can develop from an enlargement of existing adipocytes (hypertrophy), the increase of adipocytes (hyperplasia), or a combination of both. Cell size and number can increase fourfold to fivefold in humans from birth to adulthood. Cell number remains stable in adulthood, and the sole mechanism for obesity appears to be adipocyte hypertrophy.

Exercise suppresses appetite in male animals, and the degree of suppression is related to exercise intensity. Active people tend to consume calories in direct response to their physical activity, unlike inactive people. On the other hand, when active people decrease physical activity, appetite does not necessarily decline in response. Obese people are more likely to be underexercisers than overeaters.

Setpoint theory has been developed to account for the repetitive tendency of people to lose and regain body weight. The theory hypothesizes that the body contains a hypothalamic "thermostat" that attempts to maintain body fat at a predetermined "set" level. Physical activity is said to lower the setpoint.

Body composition can be estimated by the following techniques: hydrometry, ^{40}K, computerized tomography, volume displacement, underwater weighing, anthropometric measurement, skinfold measurement, and a combination of anthropometric girths and diameters and measurement of skinfold thickness.

Underwater weighing is the "gold standard" for the measurement of body density. Density is determined by dividing body mass (weight) by body volume. Volume is determined by measuring the loss of body weight in water. Several equations have been developed to compute body fat percent from body density.

Anthropometric measurement has been used to evaluate body composition and type. Sheldon[58] developed the concept of a somatotype in which individuals could be identified according to a predominance of endomorphic (fleshy), mesomorphic, (muscular), and ectomorphic (linear) components.

Skinfold prediction equations seem to order individuals correctly; however, validity, relative to underwater weighing, is only moderate and appears to be better for men than for women.

When energy input is equally compensated by output, the body is said to be in caloric balance. Positive and negative balances are created by input exceeding output or vice versa, respectively. Since a pound of fat contains 3,500 kcal, the use of exercise as a weight control mechanism has been criticized. However, given the view that weight reduction should not be undertaken rapidly, exercise is an effective addition to diet for use in weight control.

College gymnasts do not differ from Olympic gymnasts with regard to somatotype, but college competitive placers and nonplacers differ in percent fat (16.82% vs 18.41%, respectively). Professional football players show similarities in somatotype according to position: back, lineman, etc.

To combat the tendency for wrestlers to go to extraordinary means to "make weight," the concept of "minimal weight" has been proposed. Anthropometric measurements are used to predict the body weight associated with 5% body fat.

It is perhaps most prudent to combine exercise with diet when weight control is the goal. When caloric restriction alone is used, a high proportion of the weight lost comes from lean tissue.

Fat is deposited, and most likely lost, selectively. Fat is lost from certain fat pads first and others later. Failure to understand this phenomenon has caused some to suggest that spot reduction is possible.

KEY TERMS

adipose tissue hyperplasia increasing the number of adipocytes.

adipose tissue hypertrophy enlargement of existing adipocytes.

body composition division of the body into two principal tissue components— fat and lean.

densiometry measurement of body density for the purpose of determining body fat and lean proportions.

minimal weight the lowest safe weight for athletic competition, usually associated with wrestling.

obesity fat accumulation greater than 15% above normal.

skinfold measurement determination of fat-pad thickness at various anatomical sites for the purpose of predicting total body fat percentage.

somatotype determination of body structure by identifying the relative contributions of three components: endomorph (flesh), mesomorph (muscle), and ectomorph (linearity).

spot reduction the theory that exercise over a specific anatomical area (spot) will result in exclusive fat reduction in that area.

REVIEW QUESTIONS

1. What is the difference between essential fat and storage fat? Explain the sex difference in these two factors.

2. Why is "overweight" a less meaningful term than "excess fat" relative to the determination of obesity?

3. Discuss hypertrophy and hyperplasia during childhood. What recommendations would you make to parents based on current data? Is childhood obesity a function of overeating or underexercising?

4. Defend the use of one technique for the determination of body composition in a laboratory setting and another technique in a field setting.

5. Name five skinfold sites, their identifying anatomical landmarks, and the recommended directionality of the skinfold.

6. Defend the use of a combined exercise and diet approach to weight control.

7. What advantages would be provided for differences among football positions relative to somatotype? Do athletes who specialize in a particular sport tend to exhibit a more or less common somatotype?

8. What prescriptive advice (frequency, duration, and intensity) would you offer to someone who wanted to lose weight with exercise?

9. What factors might account for higher fat and lower muscle percentages among older men?

REFERENCES

1. Abrams, H.L., and McNeil, B.J.: Medical implications of computed tomography ("CAT scanning"), N. Engl. J. Med. **298:**255, 1978.

2. Behnke, A.R.: Absorption and elimination of gases from a body in relation to its fat content, Medicine **24:**359, 1945.

3. Behnke, A.R., and Wilmore, J.H.: Evaluation and regulation of body build and composition, Englewood Cliffs, N.J., 1974, Prentice-Hall Inc.

4. Bennett, W., and Gurin, J.: Do diets really work? Science **3:**42, 1982.

5. Brozek, J., Grande, F., Anderson, J.T., and others: Densitometric analysis of body composition: revision of some quantitative assumptions, Ann. N.Y. Acad. Sci. **110:**113, 1963.

5a. Bulbulian, R.: The influence of somatotype on anthropometric prediction on body composition in young women, Med. Sci. Sports Exerc. **16:**389, 1984.

5b. Buskirk, E.R., and Mendez, J.: Sports science and body composition analysis: emphasis on cell and muscle mass, Med. Sci. Sports Exerc. **16:**584, 1984.

6. Canary, J.J.: When is fat excessive? In Hafen, B.Q., editor: Weight and obesity: causes, fallacies, treatment, Provo, Utah, 1975, Brigham Young University Press.

7. Comroe, J.H., Forster, R.E., Dubois, A.B., and others: The lung, Chicago, 1962, Year Book Medical Publishers Inc.

8. Conger, P.R., and Macnab, R.B.J.: Strength, body composition, and work capacity of participants and nonparticipants in women's intercollegiate sports, Res. Q. **38:**184, 1967.

9. Costill, D.L., Bowers, R., and Kammer, W.F.: Skinfold estimates of body fat among marathon runners, Med. Sci. Sports **2:**93, 1970.

10. Cureton, K.J., Sparling, P.B., Evans, B.W., and others: Effect of experimental alterations in excess weight on aerobic capacity and distance running performance, Med. Sci. Sports **10:**194, 1976.

11. Cureton, T.K.: Physical fitness of champion athletes, Champaign, Ill., 1951, University of Illinois Press.

12. Dobzhansky, T.: Mankind evolving, New Haven, Conn., 1962, Yale University Press.

13. Falls, H.B., and Humphrey, L.D.: Body type and composition differences between placers and nonplacers in an AIAW gymnastics meet, Res. Q. **49:**38, 1978.

14. Flint, M.M., Drinkwater, B.L., Wells, C.L., and others: Validity of estimating body fat of females: effect of age and fitness, Hum. Biol. **49:**559, 1977.

15. Girandola, R.N.: Body composition changes in women: effects of high and low exercise intensity, Arch. Phys. Med. Rehabil. **57:**297, 1976.

16. Girandola, R.N., Wiswell, R.A., Mohler, J.G., and others: Effects of water immersion on lung volumes: implications for body composition analysis, J. Appl. Physiol.: Respir. Environ. Exerc. Physiol. **43:**276, 1977.

17. Heald, F.P., Dangela, M., and Brunschuyler, P.: Physiology of adolescence, N. Engl. J. Med. **268:**243, 1963.

18. Heath, B., and Carter, J.: A modified somatotype method, Am. J. Phys. Anthropol. **27:**57, 1967.

19. Hirsch, J.: Can we modify the number of adipose cells? In Hafen, B.Q., editor: Weight and obesity: causes, fallacies, treatment, Provo, Utah, 1975, Brigham Young University Press.

20. Huenemann, R.L., Hampton, M.C., Behnke, A.R., and others: Teenage nutrition and physique, Springfield, Illinois, 1974, Charles C Thomas, Publisher.

21. Ingemann-Hansen, T., and Halkjaer-Kristensen, J.: Computerized tomographic determination of human thigh components, Scand. J. Rehabil. Med. **12:**27, 1980.

22. Jackson, A.S., and Pollock, M.L.: Generalized equations for predicting body density of men, Br. J. Nutr. **40:**497, 1978.

23. Jackson, A.S., Pollock, M.L., and Ward, A.: Generalized equations for predicting body density of women, Med. Sci. Sports Exerc. **12:**175, 1980.

24. Johnson, M.L., Burke, B.S., and Mayer, J.: Relative importance of inactivity and overeating in energy balance of high school girls, Am. J. Clin. Nutr. **4:**37, 1956.

25. Katch, F.I.: Pre- and post-test changes in the factors that influence computed body density changes, Res. Q. **42:**280, 1972.

26. Katch, F.I., Katch, V.L., and Behnke, A.R.: The underweight female, Physic. Sports Med. **8:**55, 1980.

27. Katch, F.I., and McArdle, W.D.: Validity of body composition equations for college men and women, Am. J. Clin. Nutr. **28:**105, 1975.

28. Katch, F.I., and Michael, E.D.: Densitometric validation of six skinfold formulas to predict body density and percent body fat of 17-year-old boys, Res. Q. **40:**712, 1969.

29. Keys, A., and Brozek, J.: Body fat in adult man, Physiol. Rev. **33:**245, 1953.

30. Kireilis, R.W., and Cureton, T.K.: The relationship of external fat to physical education activities and fitness tests, Res. Q. **18:**123, 1947.

31. Leibel, R.L., Berry, E.M., and Hirsch, J.: Biochemistry and development of adipose tissue in man. In Kuo, and others, editors: Health and obesity, New York, 1983, Raven Press.

32. Leon, A.S., Conrad, J., Hunninghake, D.B., and others: Effects of a vigorous walking program on body composition, and carbohydrate and lipid metabolism of obese young men, Am. J. Clin. Nutr. **32:**1776, 1979.

32a. Lohman, T.G.: Research progress in validation of laboratory methods of assessing body composition, Med. Sci. Sports Exerc. **16:**596, 1984.

33. Lohman, T.G., and Pollock, M.L.: Which caliper? How much training? J. Phys. Ed. Recr. Jan.:27, 1981.

34. Malina, R.M., Mueller, W.H., Bouchard, C., and others: Fatness and fat patterning among athletes at the Montreal Olympic Games, 1976, Med. Sci. Sports Exerc. **14:**445, 1982.

35. Mayer, J.: Overweight: causes, cost, and control, Englewood Cliffs, N.J., 1968, Prentice-Hall, Inc.

36. Mayer, J.: Fat babies grow into fat people. In Hafen, B.Q., editor: Weight and obesity: causes, fallacies, treatment, Provo, Utah, 1975, Brigham Young University Press.

37. Mayer, J.: An hour of exercise vs a pound of flesh. In Hafen, B.Q., editor: Weight and obesity: causes, fallacies, treatment, Provo, Utah, 1975, Brigham Young University Press.

38. Mayer, J., Marshall, N.B., Vitale, J.J., and others: Exercise, food intake, and body weight in normal rats and genetically obese adult mice, Am. J. Physiol. **177:**544, 1954.

39. McArdle, W.D., Katch, F.I., and Katch, V.L.: Exercise physiology: energy, nutrition, and human performance, Philadelphia, 1981, Lea & Febiger.

40. Mohr, D.R.: Changes in waistline and abdominal girth and subcutaneous fat following isometric exercises, Res. Q. **36:**168, 1965.

41. Montoye, H.J.: Physical activity and health: an epidemiologic study of an entire community, Englewood Cliffs, N.J., 1975, Prentice-Hall, Inc.

42. Noland, M., and Kearney, J.T.: Anthropometric and densitometric responses of women to specific and general exercise, Res. Q. **49:**322, 1978.

43. Novak, L.P., Woodward, W.A., Bestit, C., and others: Working capacity, body composition, and anthropometry of Olympic female athletes, J. Sports Med. Phys. Fitness **17:**275, 1977.

44. Olson, A.L., and Edelstein, E.: Spot reduction of subcutaneous adipose tissue, Res. Q. **39:**647, 1968.

45. Oscai, L.B.: The role of exercise in weight control. In Wilmore, J.H., editor: Exercise and sport sciences reviews, New York, 1973, Academic Press, Inc.

46. Oscai, L.B., and Holloszy, J.O.: Effects of weight changes produced by exercise, food restriction, or overeating on body composition, J. Clin. Invest. **48:**2124, 1969.

47. Oscai, L.B., Spirakis, C.N., Wolff, C.A., and others: Effects of exercise and of food restriction on adipose tissue cellularity, J. Lipid Res. **13:**588, 1972.

48. Oscai, L.B., Babirak, S.P., McGarr, J.A., and others: Effect of exercise on adipose tissue cellularity, Fed. Proc. **33:**1956, 1974.

49. Pollock, M.L., and Jackson, A.: Body composition: measurement and changes resulting from physical training. In Burke, E.J., editor: Toward an understanding of human performance: readings in exercise physiology for the coach and athlete, Ithaca, N.Y., 1977, Mouvement Publications.

49a. Pollock, M.L., and Jackson, A.: Research progress in validation of clinical methods of assessing body composition, Med. Sci. Sports Exerc. **16:**606, 1984.

50. Pollock, M.L., Miller, H.S., and Wilmore, J.H.: Physiological characteristics of champion American track athletes 40 to 75 years of age, J. Gerontol. **29:**645, 1974.

51. Pollock, M.L., Tiffany, J., Gettman, L., and others: Effects of frequency of training of serum lipids, cardiovascular function and body composition. In Franks, B.D., editor: Exercise and fitness, 1969, Chicago, 1970, The Athletic Institute.

52. Pollock, M.L., Broida, J., Kendrick, Z., and others: Effects of training two days per week at different intensities on middle-aged men, Med. Sci. Sports **4:**192, 1972.

53. Pollock, M.L., Gettman, L.R., Jackson, A., and others: Body composition of elite class distance runners, Ann. N.Y. Acad. Sci. **301:**361, 1977.

54. Roby, F.B.: The effect of exercise on regional subcutaneous fat accumulations. Unpublished doctoral dissertation, University of Illinois, 1960.

55. Schade, M., Hellebrandt, F.A., Waterland, J.C., and others: Spot reducing in overweight college women: its influence on fat distribution as determined by photography, Res. Q. **33:**461, 1962.

56. Schemmel, R.: Assessment of obesity. In Schemmel, R., editor: Nutrition, physiology, and obesity, Boca Raton, Florida, 1980, CRC Press, Inc.

57. Schlenker, E.G.: Obesity and the lifespan. In Schemmel, R., editor: Nutrition, physiology, and obesity, Boca Raton, Florida, 1980, CRC Press, Inc.

58. Sheldon, W.: Atlas of men, New York, 1954, Harper & Brothers.

59. Sinning, W.E.: Body composition analysis by body densitometry. In Adrian, M., and Brame, J., editors: NAGWS research reports, Washington, D.C., 1977, American Alliance of Health, Physical Education, Recreation and Dance.

60. Sinning, W.E.: Anthropometric estimation of body density, fat and lean body weight in women gymnasts, Med. Sci. Sports **10**:243, 1978.

61. Sinning, W.E.: Use and misuses of anthropometric estimates of body composition, J. Phys. Ed. Recr. **51**:43, 1980.

62. Sinning, W.E., and Lindberg, G.D.: Physical characteristics of college age women gymnasts, Res. Q. **43**:226, 1972.

63. Sinning, W.E., Wilensky, N.F., and Meyers, E.J.: Post-season body composition changes and weight estimation in high-school wrestlers. In Brockhoff, J., editor: Physical education, sports and the sciences, Eugene, Oregon, 1976, Microform Publications.

64. Siri, W.E.: Body composition from fluid spaces and density, report 19. Berkeley, Calif., 1956, University of California Press.

64a. Smith, J.F., and Mansfield, E.R.: Body composition prediction in university football players, Med. Sci. Sports Exerc. **16**:398, 1984.

65. Tcheng, T.K., and Tipton, C.: Iowa wrestling study: anthropometric measurements and the prediction of a ''minimal'' body weight for high school wrestlers, Med. Sci. Sports **5**:1, 1973.

66. Thorland, W.G., Johnson, G.O., Fagot, T.G., and others: Body composition and somatotype characteristics of Junior Olympic athletes, Med. Sci. Sports Exerc. **13**:332, 1981.

67. Thorland, W.G., Johnson, G.O., Tharp, G.D., and others: Validity of anthropometric equations for the estimation of body density in adolescent athletes, Med. Sci. Sports Exerc. **16**:77, 1984.

68. Ward, A., Pollock, M.L., Jackson, A.S., and others: A comparison of body fat determined by underwater weighing and volume displacement, Am. J. Physiol. **234**:E94, 1978.

68a. Watson, A.W.S.: The physique of sportsmen: a study using factor analysis, Med. Sci. Sports Exerc. **16**:287, 1984.

69. Weredein, E.J., and Kyle, L.H.: Estimation of the constancy of the fat-free body, J. Clin. Invest. **39**:626, 1960.

70. Wickkisser, J.D., and Kelly, J.M.: The body composition of a college football team, Med. Sci. Sports **7**:199, 1975.

71. Wilmore, J.H.: The use of actual, predicted and constant residual volumes in the assessment of body composition by underwater weighing, Med. Sci. Sports **1**:87, 1969.

72. Wilmore, J.H.: Alterations in strength, body composition and anthropometric measurements consequent to a 10-week weight training program, Med. Sci. Sports **6**:133, 1974.

73. Wilmore, J.H.: Body composition and athletic performance. In Haskell, W., Scala, J., and Whittam, J., editors: Nutrition and athletic performance, Palo Alto, 1982, Bull Publishing Co.

74. Wilmore, J.H.: Appetite and body composition consequent to physical activity, Res. Q. Exerc. Sport **54**:415, 1983.

75. Wilmore, J.H., and Behnke, A.R.: Predictability of lean body weight through anthropometric assessment in college men, J. Appl. Physiol. **25**:349, 1968.

76. Wilmore, J.H., and Behnke, A.R.: An anthropometric estimation of body density and lean body weight in young men, J. Appl. Physiol. **27**:25, 1969.

77. Wilmore, J.H., and Behnke, A.R.: An anthropometric estimation of body density and lean body weight in young women, J. Appl. Physiol. **23**:267, 1970.

78. Wilmore, J.H., Brown, C.H., and Davis, J.A.: Body physique and composition of the female distance runner, Ann. N.Y. Acad. Sci. **301**:764, 1977.

79. Wilmore, J.H., Girandola, R.N., and Moody, D.L.: Validity of skinfold and girth assessment for predicting alterations in body composition, J. Appl. Physiol. **29**:313, 1970.

80. Wilmore, J.H., Parr, R.B., Haskell, W.L., and others: Football pros' strengths—and weaknesses—charted, Physic. Sports Med. **4**:45, 1976.

81. Wilmore, J.H., Royce, J., and Girandola, R.N., and others: Body composition changes with a 10-week program of jogging, Med. Sci. Sports **2**:113, 1970.

82. Wilmore, J.H., Vodak, P.A., Parr, R.B., and others: Further simplification of a method for determination of residual lung volume, Med. Sci. Sports Exerc. **12**:216, 1980.

83. Yuhasz, M.S.: The effects of sports training on body fat in man with predictions of optimal body weight. Unpublished doctoral dissertation, University of Illinois, 1962.

84. Zuti, W.B., and Golding, L.A.: Comparing diet and exercise as weight reduction tools, Physic. Sports Med. **4**:49, 1976.

SUGGESTED READINGS

Behnke, A.R., and Wilmore, J.H.: Evaluation and regulation of body build and composition, Englewood Cliffs, N.J., 1974, Prentice-Hall, Inc.

Bray, G.A.: The energetics of obesity, Med. Sci. Sports Exerc. **15**:32, 1983.

Fleck, S.J.: Body composition of elite American athletes, Am. J. Sports Med. **11**:398, 1983.

Keys, A., and Brozek, J.: Body fat in adult men, Physiol. Rev. **33**:245, 1953.

Mayer, J.: Overweight: causes, cost, and control. Englewood Cliffs, N.J., 1968, Prentice-Hall, Inc.

Oscai, L.B.: The role of exercise in weight control. In Wilmore, J.H., editor: Exercise and sport sciences reviews, New York, 1973, Academic Press, Inc.

Pollock, M.L., and Jackson, A.: Body composition: measurement and changes resulting from physical training. In Burke, E.J., editor: Toward an understanding of human performance: readings in exercise physiology for the coach and athlete, Ithaca, N.Y., 1977, Mouvement Publications.

Sinning, W.E.: Body composition analysis by body densitometry. In Adrian, M., and Brame, J., editors: NAGWS research reports, Washington, D.C., 1977, American Alliance of Health, Physical Education, Recreation and Dance.

Wilmore, J.H.: Body composition and athletic performance. In Haskell, W., Scala, J., and Whittam, J., editors: Nutrition and athletic performance, Palo Alto, 1982, Bull Publishing Co.

Wilmore, J.H.: Appetite and body composition consequent to physical activity, Res. Q. Exerc. Sport **54**:415, 1983.

LABORATORY APPLICATION: MEASUREMENT OF BODY COMPOSITION BY UNDERWATER WEIGHING
Densitometry—measurement and calculations

Underwater weighing has become the gold standard for the measurement of body density.[74] Density (D) is defined as weight (M) per unit of volume (V). Therefore

$$D = \frac{M}{V}$$

Since whole body mass (weight) is easily measured, the density can be calculated by determining body volume. Body volume is determined by measuring the loss of weight in water. Thus

$$\text{Body density} = \frac{\text{Body weight on land}}{\text{Loss of body weight in water}} \times \text{Density of water*}$$

Since some air remains in the lungs even after full exhalation (residual volume [RV]) and this air has the effect of buoying the body, making the weight seem less, a correction must be made in the equation for lung RV. A simplified version of the body density equation follows:

$$\text{Body density} = \frac{\text{Body weight on land}}{\dfrac{\text{Loss of body weight in water}}{\text{Water density}}} - RV$$

Equations to compute percent of fat have been developed by making certain assumptions about the density of human fat and lean tissue. For example,

$$\% \text{ Fat} = \left(\frac{4.950}{D} - 4.500\right) \times 100^{[64]}$$

$$\% \text{ Fat} = \left(\frac{4.570}{D} - 4.142\right) \times 100^{[5]}$$

$$\% \text{ Fat} = \left(\frac{4.201}{D} - 3.813\right) \times 100^{[29]}$$

$$\% \text{ Fat} = \left(\frac{5.053}{D} - 4.614\right) \times 100^{[2]}$$

Following are the assumptions underlying the measurement of body density[74]:
1. Density of fat and lean are known (0.90 and 1.10 g/cm^3, respectively[56]).
2. Density is relatively constant between individuals.
3. Density of bone and muscle is constant within and between individuals.
4. Individuals being measured differ from subjects, on whom the equations are based, only in the fat component.

---

*Note the addition of the water density factor in the equation. Otherwise the formula would compute specific gravity. Since the density of water changes with its temperature, water temperature must be recorded at the time of underwater weighing. Water density data are available in most collections of weights and measures.

These assumptions are basically valid but have been challenged. It seems that variations in the mineral content of bone in young and elderly subjects argues against the concept of constant bone density. Variations in bone density would lead to an invalid estimation of body fat. For example, osteoporosis leads to a decrease in bone density and an underestimation of body fat.[69] Also, body fat can be overestimated in many athletes because of their tendency to have lean tissue densities higher than assumed in the available equations.[74]

Underwater weighing procedure

The basic equipment for underwater weighing consists of the following: medical scale for land weight, water tank, hanging scale for water weight, body suspension system,

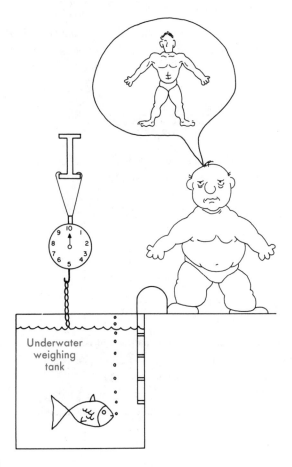

FIG. 13-9   Typical middle-aged athlete waiting to have his body volume determined by underwater weighing.

weight belt, hygrometer, and equipment (or prediction equation) for determination of RV. Figure 13-9 shows a typical middle-aged athlete waiting his turn for underwater weighing.

To avoid serious errors in measurement the following suggestions are appropriate:

1. Make sure both the land and underwater scales are calibrated.
2. The subject should be weighed early in the morning or after abstinence from drinking, eating, and exercise for 4 hours.[61]
3. Avoid weighing women 3 to 4 days before menstruation when water retention is possible.[61]
4. Weighing should be performed only when the bladder and bowels are empty.
5. A preweighing soap shower removes the tendency for bubbles to collect on the body.
6. Swim suits (two-piece suit for women) should be emptied of all trapped air after submersion.
7. RV should be measured in the tank with the subject in the approximate posture of the test.
8. A weight belt placed across the lap tends to stabilize the subject in the suspension system, resulting in smaller sweeps of the scale dial.
9. The subject should practice taking one or two deep inhalations followed by a complete exhalation. The subject must hold his or her breath during submersion and the body must be stabilized to prevent excessive variation of the scale.

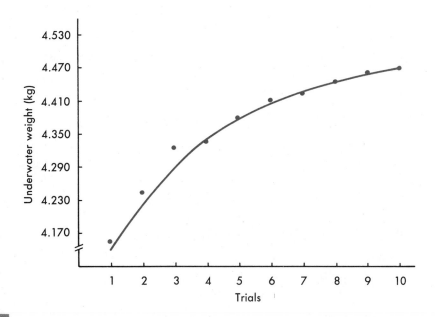

FIG. 13-10   Increase in underwater weight as a function of trials. (From the work of Katch, F.I., and McArdle, W.D.: Validity of body composition equations for college men and women, Am. J. Clin. Nutr. *28:*105, 1975.)

10. The subject repeats the submersion procedure for 10 trials. It has been shown that underwater weight measurements increase to asymptote over 10 trials (Figure 13-10).[25]

11. Since the scale dial will have some fluctuation even with the most quiescent subject, the scale should be read at the midpoint of the dial excursion.

12. The mean of the three highest weights can be used for computations of body fat.[61]

Below is a sample data collection sheet:

Water density hygrometer _____

RV _____ (L)

Weight of belt and suspension system _____ (kg)

Underwater trials:

	lb	**kg**		**lb**	**kg**
1.	_____	_____	6.	_____	_____
2.	_____	_____	7.	_____	_____
3.	_____	_____	8.	_____	_____
4.	_____	_____	9.	_____	_____
5.	_____	_____	10.	_____	_____

Three heaviest trials (kg)

1. _____
2. _____
3. _____
$\overline{X}$. _____ (Gross underwater weight)

Net underwater weight (kg) = Gross underwater weight − Weight of belt and suspension system

Calculations:

1. Body volume $= \left[\dfrac{\text{Land weight} - \text{Net underwater weight}}{\text{Water density}} \right] - RV$

2. Body density (BD) $= \dfrac{\text{Land weight}}{\text{Body volume}}$

3. % Fat $= \left(\dfrac{4.950}{\text{BD}} - 4.500 \right) \times 100$[64]

4. Fat weight (kg) $= \text{Land weight} \times \dfrac{\text{% Fat}}{100}$

5. Lean weight (kg) = Land weight − Fat weight

6. % Lean $= \dfrac{\text{Lean weight}}{\text{Land weight}} \times 100$

7. Desired weight $= \dfrac{\text{Lean weight}}{1 - \text{Desired % fat (expressed as a decimal)}}$

Measurement of RV

As mentioned previously, RV must be accounted for or the loss of weight in water will appear greater. RV can be measured, estimated from the vital capacity, or assumed to be constant for each sex according to age. These three methods were compared; however, no significant differences were found between body density, percent of fat, and lean body weight calculated by the three methods. Because of individual variation, measured RV was recommended for research in body composition. Likewise, it has been pointed out that use of constant RV values in training studies may mask changes in body composition (for example, changes in training RV mask true changes in body density.)[25]

Three methods of direct determination of RV have been reported to result in accurate measurement: nitrogen washout,[71] helium dilution,[7] and oxygen dilution.[82]

Some have argued whether RV should be measured in or out of the water. Significant differences in RV were observed between measurements made in and out of the water.[16] Other studies have shown no difference between measurements made on land or in water. Although either method may yield the same RV, it should be recorded consistently in the same medium. A good reference for those interested in a simple but accurate method of estimating RV is Wilmore and others.[82]

CASE STUDY 1

Following are data collected during an underwater weighing experiment on a 27-year-old man, including subsequent computations of body composition.

Body weight: 175   (lb)   79.55   (kg)
Water density (hygrometer):   0.995
Weight of belt and suspension system: 9.18   (kg)
Residual volume: 1.70   (L)
Underwater trials:

	lb	kg			lb	kg
1.	27.25	12.39		6.	28.00	12.73
2.	27.00	12.27		7.	27.75	12.61
3.	28.50	12.73		8.	27.75	12.61
4.	27.50	12.50		9.	28.00	12.73
5.	27.50	12.50		10.	28.00	12.73

Three heaviest trials (kg):
1.   12.73
2.   12.73
3.   12.73
$\overline{X}$.   12.73   (Gross underwater weight)

$$\text{Net underwater weight (kg)} = \frac{(12.73)}{\text{Gross underwater weight}}$$

$$- \frac{(9.18)}{\text{Weight of belt and suspension system}} = 3.55$$

Calculations:

1. Body volume $= \left[\dfrac{\overset{(79.55)}{\text{Land weight}} - \overset{(3.55)}{\text{Net underwater weight}}}{\underset{(0.995)}{\text{Water density}}} \right] - \overset{(1.70)}{\text{Residual volume}}$

$$= 76.38 - 1.70$$
$$= 74.68$$

2. Body density $= \dfrac{\overset{(79.55)}{\text{Land weight}}}{\underset{(74.68)}{\text{Body volume}}} = 1.065$

3. % Fat = $\left[\dfrac{4.950}{\dfrac{\text{Body density}}{(1.065)}}\right] - 4.500 \times 100$

$= [4.648 - 4.500] \times 100$

$= 14.80\%$

4. Fat weight (kg) = $\overset{(79.55)}{\text{Land weight}} \times \dfrac{\overset{(14.8)}{\text{\% Fat}}}{100}$

$= 11.77$ kg

5. Lean weight (kg) = $\overset{(79.55)}{\text{Land weight}} - \overset{(11.77)}{\text{Fat weight}}$

$= 67.78$ kg

6. % Lean = $\dfrac{\overset{(67.78)}{\text{Lean weight}}}{\underset{(79.55)}{\text{Land weight}}} \times 100 = 85.20\%$

CASE STUDY 2

A high school wrestling coach had two excellent heavyweight wrestlers. To capitalize on this talent, he wanted to move one of the wrestlers, currently wrestling at 225 pounds, down to the 185-pound class. He asked our advice and subsequently brought the boy in for testing. We applied the Tcheng-Tipton formula[65] for determining "minimal weight." Following are the data and resulting calculations:

Height (in)	70.00	× 1.84 =	128.80
Chest diameter (cm)	35.75	× 3.28 =	117.26
Chest depth (cm)	27.75	× 3.31 =	91.85
Biiliac diameter (cm)	30.25	× 0.82 =	24.81
Bitrochanteric diameter (cm)	35.50	× 1.69 =	60.00
Sum of wrist diameters (cm)	6 + 6 = 12	× 3.56 =	42.72
Sum of ankle diameters (cm)	7.2 + 7.3 = 14.5	× 2.15 =	31.18
			496.62
			−281.72
			214.90

It was recommended that it would be unwise to allow this wrestler to drop to the 185-pound class, since it would place him 30 pounds below "minimal weight" based on body structure.

chapter 14

PHYSIOLOGICAL EFFECTS OF TRAINING

MAJOR LEARNING OBJECTIVE

Positive gains from exercise assume that known type, frequency, duration, and intensity recommendations have been followed.

APPLICATIONS

The exercise specialist can almost exactly specify the gains possible from a particular type of training.

■ Teachers and coaches should be capable of explaining, in both scientific and lay terms, the effects of exercise. For example, aerobic programs should produce increases in maximal oxygen consumption, stroke volume, cardiac output, and muscle and blood lactate levels.

SCIENTISTS in many biological disciplines are concerned with the so-called nature-nurture question. They ask whether observed changes are due to nature (genetics) or nurture (training). This question is a scientific variant of the practical question of whether an athlete is "born or made." A famous Swedish physiologist is fond of saying that the best way to ensure athletic success is to choose your parents properly. This tongue-in-cheek statement emphasizes the importance of the genetic component. However, neither the teacher/coach nor the scientist would deny the important role of training.

Twenty-five years ago the dominant goal in physical education was to show that exercise "worked." Lay people asked, "Yes, I seem to feel better but is there objective evidence that my physiological systems have changed?" At that time, answers were laced with more hope than evidence. The picture has changed dramatically in the 1980s. There is little doubt that many important changes are made.

The purpose of this chapter is to summarize the most important of these changes. It has been unavoidable to discuss many of the changes in the previous chapters. Therefore to a large extent this chapter will be duplication. However, the topic is important enough to risk some redundancy. Teachers and coaches are often asked to defend the inclusion of exercise and sports in the school curriculum. Perhaps this chapter will provide a guide for such a defense.

It should be remembered that changes are predicated on the proper administration of the exercise stimulus. In other words, the principles of exercise prescription should be followed. With the exclusion of any one of these principles, the typical change may be either reduced or completely eliminated.

CIRCULATORY AND METABOLIC CHANGES
Bed rest

One method of discerning the value of exercise is to determine what occurs with its absence. Normal subjects given total bed rest for 21 days were found to have decreased aerobic power ($\dot{V}O_2$ max) by 28%.[36] Therefore even regular daily activity serves to maintain aerobic power. These results were confirmed in a study in which 14 days of bed rest reduced aerobic power by 12.3%.[40] In this same experiment the effects of bed rest were not eliminated by low-level reclining exercise, but they were reduced. These data reveal the value of physical therapy during prolonged medical inactivity.

Rest

The first condition from which to examine the effects of training is, of course, rest. Such an analysis asks the question: can training alter the physiological response to nonactivity, that is, rest? Several authors have observed a posttraining bradycardia (reduced heart rate) in previously sedentary subjects.[9,25,41] At the same time, an increase can be observed in resting stroke volume. This parallel response results in an unchanged resting cardiac output. The trained heart can pump the same quantity of blood per minute at rest with fewer heartbeats. Resting bradycardia has been attributed to an increased vagal tone and decreased sympathetic drive and plasma catecholamines.[8] Increased stroke volume is accounted for by increased left ventricular end-diastolic volume and the Frank-Starling mechanism.[8]

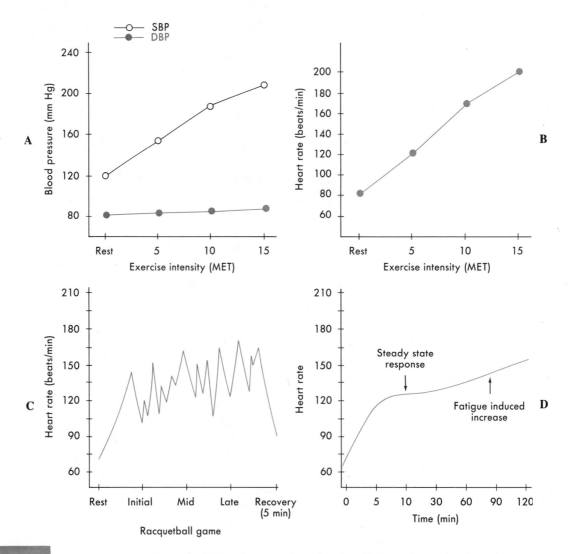

FIG. 14-1   **Illustration of heart rate and blood pressure response in relation to increasing intensity (A and B, respectively), as well as heart rate response to a hypothetical racquetball game (C) and long-duration exercise (D).**

Submaximal exercise

Since most of our active life is spent at submaximal exercise intensities, it is of interest to determine whether a training program positively affects physiological response to these intensities. Exercise administered at the same physical intensity before and after training has no apparent effect on submaximal oxygen consumption. It is presumed that the body does not change its energy requirement for the same physical challenge.

On the contrary, at the same $\dot{V}O_2$ level, the trained individual has a lower heart rate and a higher stroke volume[22] as well as a lower pulmonary ventilation.[3] Thus the physiological strain of the exercise has been reduced. Reduced muscle blood flow has been observed during submaximal exercise and appears incongruous given the lack of change in $\dot{V}O_2$. This change is explained by the increase in arteriovenous (A-V) oxygen difference, which compensates for the decreased flow.[22] Additionally, the production of muscle and blood lactate is decreased with training, as is the utilization of muscle and liver glycogen.[22] To place in perspective the effect of training on heart rate, it is important to know the acute response of heart rate to physical activity.

Figure 14-1 illustrates the submaximal heart rate response in three situations: (A) during a graded exercise test, (B) during a racquetball match, and (C) during a run of long duration (2 hours). During graded exercise, heart rate rises linearly with increasing exercise intensity. Heart rate during a game situation (for example, racquetball) will wax and wane with the intensity of the point, duration of the match, and level of competition. Heart rate shows a transient increase to steady state during 3 to 5 minutes of submaximal exercise. As long as the duration of exercise does not exceed 15 to 30 minutes, the steady-state heart rate is maintained. However, as fatigue and body temperature increase with lengthy exercise, heart rate will begin to creep upward.

Maximal exercise

Training may produce changes in maximal performance measures (speed, distance, etc.) or physiological variables. Usually changes in performance are accompanied by an increase in maximal oxygen consumption. Depending on the nature of the training conditions and the subject sample, usually an increase of 10% to 20% can be expected during a 3- to 6-month period.[19] For example, one investigator found an increase of 9% with a 24 min/week program.[47] On the other hand, an improvement of 35% has been observed in a 4 day/week program (30 minutes).[34] Using a bicycle ergometer, others[1,2] observed improvements of 16% and 18%. Using similar training programs, gains for women and men were 14% and 19%, respectively.[4] There is no doubt that women's physiological status after training changes in about the same way as that for men. Improvement in $\dot{V}O_2$ max exhibits linearity over time, with an increase of 44% in 10 weeks (Figure 14-2).[17]

In addition to the increase in $\dot{V}O_2$ max, both maximal stroke volume and maximal cardiac output increases while maximal heart rate remains unchanged or slightly lower.[22] Blood flow to the working muscles (milliliter per kilogram of muscle) is unchanged with training but, as with the submaximal response, as increase in A-V O_2 difference is observed.[22] This implies that an increase in oxygen extraction is occurring per unit of blood flow. Muscle and blood lactate increases less after training during a maximal challenge while the rate of glycogen depletion is about the same.[22]

Practical summary. The circulatory and metabolic changes achieved from training depend on the type of training (Table 14-1). Aerobic athletes, like cross-country runners and skiers, make changes that reflect the endurance nature of the training and the requirements of the competition. For example, the "volume stress" of the training increases stroke volume whether it is measured at rest, during submaximal exercise, or during maximal exercise. Thus the heart, which is needed to push large volumes of blood and oxygen to the tissues during endurance exercise, is enlarged (hypertrophy of the ventricular cavity) to facilitate this need. Anaerobic sport is a different matter. The task of the sprinter or weight lifter is to make a short-duration explosive effort. In these activities the emphasis is placed on skeletal muscle hypertrophy and training of the nervous system rather than on circulatory and metabolic changes. However, these athletes often do display a resting and submaximal exercise bradycardia (lowered heart rate) and, if interval training is structured properly, can minimally increase maximal oxygen consumption.

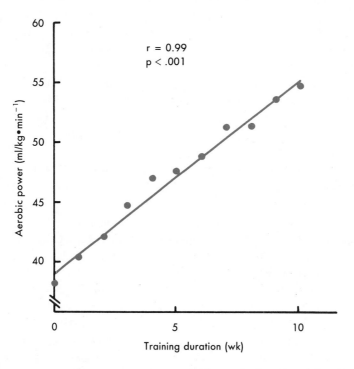

FIG. 14-2   The relationship of aerobic power (ml/kg · min⁻¹) and training duration. (Modified from Hickson, R.C., Bomze, H.A., and Holloszy, J.O.: Linear increase in aerobic power induced by a strenuous program of endurance exercise, J. Appl. Physiol. *42*:372, 1977.)

MUSCLE MORPHOLOGY
Cardiac muscle

Perhaps the most important change in cardiac muscle resulting from exercise is an increased heart weight/body weight ratio.[32] Since cardiac muscle is principally aerobic in nature, because of its continuous function, no change is observed in cardiac respiratory enzymes. The changes in heart size that have been observed are related to increases in either chamber size or wall dimensions. For example, one study examined echocardiographs of trained runners, cyclists, and weight lifters.[39] Compared with untrained control subjects, the runners and cyclists showed significantly larger left ventricular mass. This enlargement resulted from a thickening of the septum, left ventricular posterior wall, and

TABLE 14-1 ||||| THE RELATIONSHIP BETWEEN TYPE OF TRAINING (AEROBIC OR ANAEROBIC) AND THE PREDICTED CHANGE

Predicted training change	Type of training	
	Aerobic	**Anaerobic**
Rest		
Heart rate	↓	↓
Stroke volume	↑	NC
Cardiac output	NC	NC
Hypertrophy		
Cardiac muscle	↑	NC
Skeletal muscle	NC	↓
Submaximal		
Heart rate	↓	↓
Stroke volume	↑	NC
Cardiac output	↑ or NC	NC
$\dot{V}_{O_2}$	NC	NC
$\dot{V}_E$	↓	↓
Blood flow	↓	NC
HL-a	↓	↓
Maximal		
Heart rate	↓ or NC	NC
Stroke volume	↑	NC
Cardiac output	↑	NC
$\dot{V}_{O_2}$	↑	↑ or NC
$\dot{V}_E$	↑	NC
HL-a	↑	↑

NC, No change.

TABLE 14-2 ‖‖‖‖ THE RELATIONSHIP BETWEEN
TYPE OF TRAINING AND CARDIAC HYPERTROPHY

	Type of training	
Cardiac hypertrophy	**Aerobic**	**Weight training**
Ventricular mass	NC	Increased
Ventricular volume	Increased	NC
NC, No charge.		

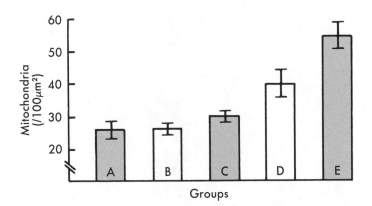

FIG. 14-3 The concentration of skeletal muscle mitochondria following various experimental manipulations. Group A consists of untrained rats sacrificed at rest. Group B was also untrained but sacrificed following exhaustive swimming. Group C was untrained sacrificed 2 hours following an exhaustive swim. Group D was trained and sacrificed immediately after running to exhaustion. Group E was a counterpart of Group D but sacrificed 24 hours following exercise. These data support the increase in mitochondria with training. (Adapted from Gollnick, P.D., and King, D.W.: Effect of exercise and training on mitochondria of rat skeletal muscle, Am. J. Physiol. *216:*1502, 1969.)

left ventricular internal diameter. Although weight lifters had increased left ventricular mass, they were not significantly different from control subjects. In a separate study, previously sedentary male subjects were evaluated before and after 6 months of jogging.[48] An 18% increase in aerobic power was accompanied by an increase in left ventricular end-diastolic dimension. Wall thickness was unchanged. Athletes involved in isometric exercise show normal left ventricular volume but increased wall thickness.[31] Although changes in weight lifters resemble those of some patients with heart disease, they have been shown to be normal variants.[28] Echocardiographic studies appear to confirm a specificity of left ventricular response depending on whether exercise is primarily aerobic or primarily of the weight-lifting type. A summary of the probable relationship between type of training and cardiac hypertrophy can be seen in Table 14-2.

Skeletal muscle

When the overload is of the aerobic type, very little hypertrophy is achieved. However, when the overload is achieved through more intense activities, such as weight lifting, greater hypertrophy is expected. This hypertrophy is primarily accounted for by an increase in protein content in muscle but also can be observed in tendons and ligaments. Also, hypertrophy found after isokinetic training was observed exclusively in fast-twitch fibers.[42]

From a metabolic point of view, a 60% increase has been observed in the protein content of skeletal muscle mitochondria after training.[18,21] This growth is attributed to both the number and the size of mitochondria.[1] Figure 14-3 displays the results of this investigation. Untrained animals show little difference in mitochondrial concentration whether they are sacrificed at rest or after exhaustive exercise. However, impressive increases are seen in trained animals. Obviously, such a change in morphology provides the opportunity for greater development of aerobic energy.

There does not seem to be evidence that would indicate a change in the number of muscle fibers. Hyperplasia has been argued as a reason for observed changes in performance after training. However, this area of research has been fraught with many technical difficulties. Therefore current evidence supports that there has been no change. For example, investigators studied 12 previously sedentary subjects who trained for 8 weeks on bicycle ergometers.[1] Significant changes were observed within the fast-twitch muscle fiber types (FOG and FG). No significant change was found in slow-twitch fiber areas and no evidence of hyperplasia was observed. Changes in fiber area are accompanied by an increase in capillary supply.[2] Increases in capillary density seem to be equally distributed to fast- and slow-twitch fiber types. The relationship of capillary density and weeks of training is shown in Figure 14-4. Although some studies do support the finding of hyperplasia, these findings are related to experimental technique (for example, evidence is found to support hyperplasia with multiple-fiber analysis, but with the more definitive single-fiber analysis the evidence becomes experimental artifact).

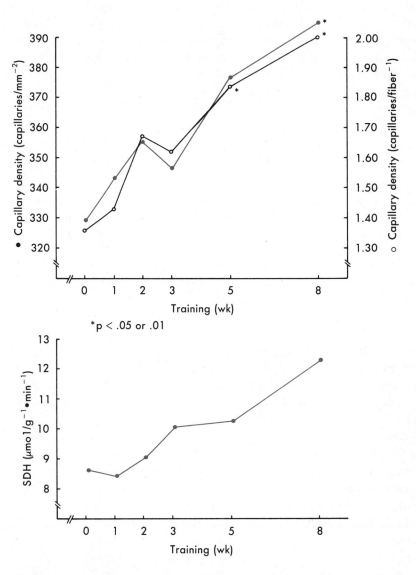

The growth of capillary density, expressed as cap/mm^{-2} and cap/fiber^{-1} (upper graph) and succinate dehydrogenase (lower graph) shown as a function of training duration. Both variables show significant increases after 8 weeks. (Adapted from Anderson, P., and Henriksson, J.: Capillary supply of the quadriceps femoris muscle of man: adaptive response to exercise, J. Physiol. *270*:677, 1977.)

Practical summary. Athletes engaged in aerobic exercise show cardiac hypertrophy through increases in ventricular cavity size. Athletes engaged in anaerobic exercise also show cardiac hypertrophy, but the change is manifested in ventricular wall size. The latter is most likely due to the maximal efforts required of these athletes whereby the heart muscle must pump against great peripheral resistances. Because of the high-resistance training often associated with anaerobic events, skeletal muscle is increased in size and production of force. On the other hand, athletes engaged in aerobic exercise usually have only minimal changes in skeletal muscle size.

MUSCLE METABOLISM

Myoglobin

Since myoglobin aids the movement of oxygen to the mitochondria, this variable has been a likely candidate for change resulting from training. In fact, an 80% increase has been observed.[33] Rats were exposed to running on a treadmill for 15 weeks. Increases in myoglobin were found in the quadriceps and hamstring muscles but not in the abdominal muscles. This result led the authors to conclude that only muscles directly involved are changed. Again, specificity of response is observed.

Respiratory enzymes

To repeat an earlier statement, no changes are observed in respiratory enzymes of cardiac muscle after training[32]; however, unlike skeletal muscle, aerobic training stimulates hypertrophy of cardiac muscle.[20] On the other hand, the less aerobic skeletal muscle does show significant alteration in respiratory enzymes. For example, a twofold increase in mitochondrial respiratory chain enzymes was found in rats.[18] Examples of these enzymes are citrate synthase and succinate dehydrogenase (SDH). Figure 14-3 demonstrates changes in SDH observed during 8 weeks of training. Likewise, significant changes have been observed in humans.[14] In addition, increases in enzymes associated with the metabolism of long chain fatty acids have been reported.[29] Fat mobilization is known to improve with training even though free fatty acid levels do not increase. Thus it can be said that aerobic training improves the capacity of skeletal muscle to oxidize both carbohydrate and fat.

Glycolytic enzymes

Another question is whether training changes are observed in the glycolytic pathway. A review of the research in this area reveals that few changes have been found in glycolytic enzymes.[10] For example, differences could not be found in a major glycolytic enzyme, phosphofructokinase (PFK), between trained and untrained males.[13] Suspecting that glycolytic changes may be a function of exercise intensity, subjects were trained for 5 months on bicycle ergometers at 75% to 90% $\dot{V}O_2$ max and PFK doubled.[14] This change occurred in fast-twitch fibers only. Small changes in phosphocreatine (PC) were not thought to functionally improve anaerobic capacity. When rats and humans were exposed to endurance training, a significant change in another glycolytic enzyme, hexokinase, was reported.[18]

Strength training is largely anaerobic. To study the glycolytic response to anaerobic strength training, five male subjects were trained for 7 weeks with isokinetic exercise.[6] Although total work was held constant, one leg was trained with 30-second exercise bouts and the other with 6-second bouts. Significant increases in PFK, muscle phosphorylase, PC, and myokinase were observed in the leg trained for 30 seconds. Biopsy specimens of the leg trained for 6 seconds revealed increases only in PFK. Changes were related to duration of exercise, but enzymatic changes were not related to either fatigue or muscle strength. These changes are obviously far more complex than can be solely accounted for by enzymatic changes.

Practical summary. As predicted from the principles of exercise prescription, the physiological system trained is specific to the type of sports training. When the overload is placed on the oxidative mechanisms (aerobic), changes are observed in mechanisms that support the oxidative process (that is, myoglobin and respiratory chain enzymes). When

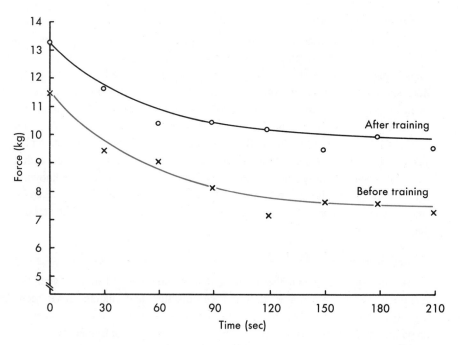

FIG. 14-5 This figure illustrates both the decline in force with a continuous hand grip task (3.5 minutes), defined as muscular endurance, and the significant increase in this variable before and following training in age group swimmers. (Modified from Clarke, D.H., and Vaccaro, P.: The effect of swimming training on muscular performance and body composition in children, Res. Q. *50:9*, 1979.)

the overload is placed on the ATP-PC and lactate systems, changes are observed in mechanisms that support anaerobic metabolism (for example, increased phosphogens and PFK). Also, anaerobic changes are made largely in fast-twitch fibers.

ADDITIONAL CHANGES

Muscular endurance

Many exercise activities involve the use of continuous contractions at submaximal intensity, that is, muscular endurance. One would hypothesize that training which involves continuous contractions should improve muscular endurance. Such a hypothesis was tested in a study of young, age-group swimmers.[5] Boys and girls were tested before and after 7 months of swimming training and compared with control subjects. Figure 14-5 shows force/time curves for the swimmers before and after training. These curves were developed from a continuous handgrip task for 3½ minutes. A decrease in force (fatigue) occurred during both tests but the curve after training was significantly displaced upward. Such a result demonstrates improvement in muscular endurance.

Strength

Previous chapters have reviewed literature related to changes resulting from various kinds of strength training. Suffice it to say that skeletal muscle increases its capacity to apply force and, in many cases, an increase in cross section is observed. Hypertrophy of skeletal muscle is less likely with predominately aerobic exercise and very likely with high overload strength training. The principle of specificity applies in that only the muscles trained improve and primarily in the fast-twitch fibers. Also, in the case of isometric exercise, the strength improvement is observed only at the angle of training.

Blood lipid levels

Epidemiological studies related to coronary heart disease have implicated physical activity as a potential preventive measure. Reports from the Framingham Heart Disease Study[24] in suburban Boston indicate that increasing levels of physical activity (physical activity index) are associated with a decreasing incidence in all deaths, deaths caused by cardiovascular disease, and deaths caused by ischemic disease (Figure 14-6). Assuming that such a relationship does exist, and there is considerable debate, the mechanism by which physical activity exerts its influence has yet to be isolated. One possibility involves circulating levels of blood lipids, for example, cholesterol and triglycerides. Therefore exercise physiologists have been interested in the link between changes in these lipids and exercise. For example, a group of scientists studied 1,000 age-matched male subjects separated into groups according to physical activity level.[30] Those classified as active in their occupational and leisure pursuits had lower serum cholesterol and triglyceride levels than those classified as moderately active and sedentary. Diet did not account for the differences, but when calculations were corrected for subject body fatness there was no relationship between activity and serum lipids. In other words, serum lipid levels tend to be higher in people who carry more body fat, irrespective of physical activity. In another study,[7] recreational runners (mean age = 38.8 years) were found to have lower serum lipids than normal control subjects. However, there was no discernable difference between three groups established by weekly running mileage (8.6, 17.7, and 36.2 miles per week).

Recent technology has made it possible to separate total blood cholesterol into its component lipoprotein fractions. These fractions include high density lipoproteins (HDL), low density lipoproteins (LDL), and very low density lipoproteins (VLDL). High quantities of HDL and low quantities of LDL have been associated with protection against coronary heart disease. Therefore, it is possible for two people to have high serum cholesterol levels, but if one level is produced by high HDL and the other by high LDL, there is a far different expectation of heart disease. The apparent explanation of this finding is that HDL breaks down cholesterol while LDL transports triglycerides in the blood, that is, high LDL levels in blood make it more available for accumulation on arterial walls. Recent research indicates that the ratio of total serum cholesterol to HDL (total cholesterol/HDL) is the best predictor of coronary heart disease. Thus, either a decrease in total cholesterol levels or an increase in HDL would decrease the risk. This

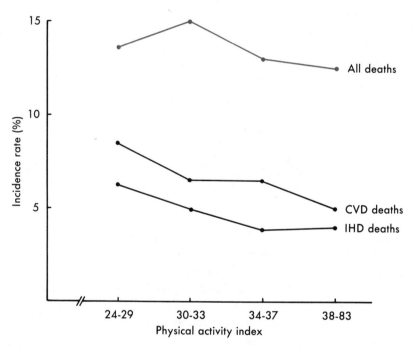

FIG. 14-6 The relationship of incidence rate for death (all, cardiovascular disease, and ischemic heart disease) and physical activity index. A higher index indicates higher physical activity levels. (Modified from Kannel, W.B., and Sorlie, P.: Some health benefits of physical activity. The Framingham study, Arch. Intern. Med. *139:*857, 1979.)

hypothesis has not been fully confirmed, but exercise physiologists have studied the relationship between exercise behavior and lipoprotein fractions. Runners who completed at least 25 km/week have been compared with age-matched control subjects.[26] HDL level was found to be significantly higher in the running group (1.77 vs 1.42 mmol/L). Another study examined 100 middle-aged men randomly assigned to exercise and control groups.[23] The exercise group trained 3 to 4 days/week for 4 months and made significant improvement in aerobic capacity. Even though no changes were observed in body weight between groups, the exercisers increased HDL levels and reduced triglyceride levels significantly. The control group had no change in their lipid levels. These results indicate that changes are not dependent on weight loss. Figure 14-7 presents the results of an interesting study that compares runners with nonrunners in both men and women.[49] In both sexes, runners showed significantly lower serum cholesterol and triglyceride concentrations. Likewise, LDL levels were significantly lower and HDL significantly higher in the runners. If the hypothesis linking serum lipid levels to coronary heart disease is confirmed, it appears that physical activity, particularly running, may have a positive influence on the prevention of the disease.

Blood pressure

Since high blood pressure (hypertension) is a known risk factor for coronary heart disease, it is of interest to note whether exercise might be a preventive intervention. Blood pressure is known to increase with emotional stress. Thus if exercise has a relaxing effect, perhaps the blood pressure may be induced to decrease. However, blood pressure is also known to increase with kidney disease and arteriosclerosis (hardening of the arteries creating increased resistance to blood flow). Exercise probably has no effect on renal hypertension, but considerable scientific interest has been shown in its effect on what has been termed *essential hypertension* (caused by arteriosclerosis). It should be pointed out that it is sometimes difficult in an experimental situation with humans to differentiate between blood pressure reduction caused by reduction in emotional stress (for example, relaxation) and mechanisms that effect arterial resistance. Most research shows aerobic exercise to cause a mild but significant decrease in systolic blood pressure. Such a reduction by no means serves to normalize the blood pressure of a serious hypertensive patient. However, hypertension is a complex disease, so any positive effect is important. More research is required in this area, since previous studies have shown methodological deficiencies.

Although acute exercise response is not the subject of this chapter, it will be helpful for the student to place training responses into perspective with an understanding of exercise-induced blood pressure response. Blood pressure rises to steady state over time and linearly with exercise intensity in a graded exercise test (Figure 14-1). An increase in systolic blood pressure during an exercise test is thought to be a positive adaptive response to the exercise. Increasing cardiac output with increasing exercise intensity is thought to promote this increase in systolic pressure. (Diastolic pressure usually increases very little with increasing exercise intensity.)

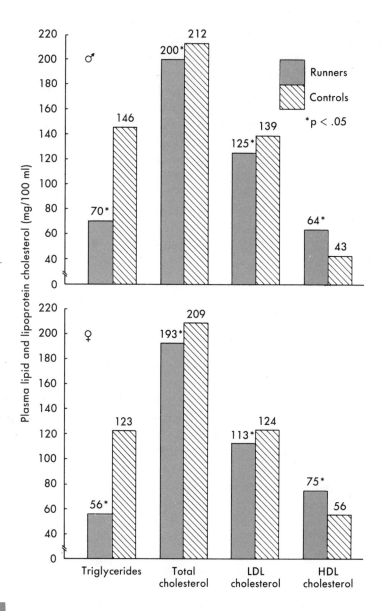

FIG. 14-7 Comparison of plasma lipids and lipoproteins between runners and control subjects. The upper panel displays the male data and the lower panel the female data. Lipoprotein fractions shown here are low-density lipoprotein (LDL) and high-density lipoprotein (HDL). In all cases, the runners respond in a manner compatible with heart disease prevention. (Modified from Wood, P.D., and Haskell, W.L.: The effect of exercise on plasma high density lipoproteins, Lipids *14:*417, 1979.)

Ligament strength

Practitioners of sports medicine have been concerned about the value of certain types of exercise in the prevention or rehabilitation of joint injury. A related interest involves the effect of immobilization (casting) of joints on subsequent ligament and tendon strength. This is a difficult area of study in the intact human. These questions have been studied with animals with casted limbs trained with sprint or endurance exercise.[43] The medial collateral ligament was tested for separation force after the experimental interventions. Force required to separate the ligament-bone junction was significantly less in the casted animals compared with controls indicating reduced ligament strength. Animals trained in endurance showed significantly greater ligament strength than did untrained animals. There was no difference between sprint-trained and untrained animals. Immobilization is contraindicated unless absolutely necessary, while endurance training appears to be a worthy protective measure. These results are shown in Figure 14-8.

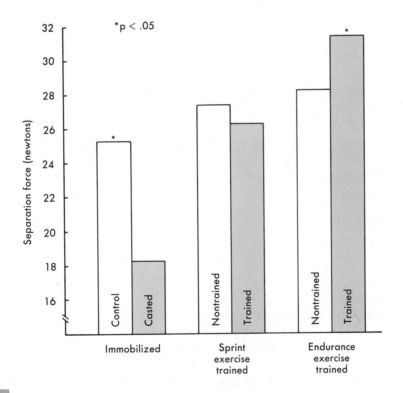

FIG. 14-8 Separation force of the medial collateral ligament in rats that were immobilized with casts, sprint trained, or endurance trained. (Modified from Tipton, C.M., Matthes, R.D., Maynard, J.A., and others: The influence of physical activity on ligaments and tendons, Med. Sci. Sports 7:165, 1975.)

TABLE 14-3 |||||| SUMMARY OF RESEARCH ON THE AEROBIC POWER
OF MALE AND FEMALE ELITE ATHLETES

Sport	Sex	$\dot{V}O_2$ max (ml/kg · min^{-1})	Authors
Distance runners	F	59.1	Wilmore and Brown[45]
Cross-country skiers	F	55.0	Hermansen and Anderson[16]
Basketball players	F	49.6	Vaccaro, Clarke, and Wrenn[44]
Basketball players	F	42.9	Sinning[37]
Olympic speed skaters	F	46.1	Maksud and others[27]
College football players	M	56.5	Smith and Byrd[38]
Pro football players	M	50.1	Wilmore and Haskell[46]
Cross-country skiers	M	75.0	Hanson[15]
Olympic speed skaters	M	56.1	Maksud and others[27]
Soccer players	M	58.4	Raven and others[35]

Elite athletes

Previous chapters have considered the physiological characteristics of various elite athletic groups. Table 14-3 presents a limited summary of the literature dealing with the aerobic power displayed in selected elite athletes. These athletes collectively show high levels of aerobic power compared with nonathletes. The question remains relevant whether these figures represent a genetic predisposition to high-caliber sport, an acquired characteristic, or both. Most likely the answer is both, with the heaviest loading on the side of the genetic component.

SUMMARY

This chapter reviews the changes that are typically observed after training conducted according to the principles of exercise prescription. At the outset, bed rest studies were examined to show the antithesis of training, that is, the effects of no activity. Complete inactivity causes a significant decline in aerobic power.

Some physiological changes produced by exercise can be observed during a state of rest. For example, a common profile would show a decreased heart rate, increased stroke volume, and no change in cardiac output. During submaximal exercise repeated after training at equal physical intensities, oxygen consumption does not change. At equivalent physiological levels ($\dot{V}O_2$), heart rate is lower and stroke volume is higher. Maximal oxygen consumption increases between 10% and 20% after appropriate aerobic training. In addition, increases are observed in maximal stroke volume, cardiac output, arteriovenous O_2 difference, muscle lactate, and blood lactate.

Cardiac muscle shows hypertrophy with training; however, respiratory enzymes do not change. The changes in heart size depend on the training stimulus. Usually aerobic training increases chamber size while anaerobic training promotes wall thickness.

On the contrary, skeletal muscle shows essentially no increase in external cross section after endurance training, but there is an increase in respiratory enzymes and muscle myoglobin. These increases parallel increases in mitochondrial size and number. Likewise, the fiber area of individual fibers grows as well as the capillary network supplying the fibers. Less dramatic changes have been observed in the glycolytic pathway. The most consistent change is in the enzyme phosphofructokinase. However, when training is predominately anaerobic (for example, isokinetic training), a number of glycolytic enzymes increased (for example, phosphorylase, PC, myokinase, phosphofructokinase).

Improvements in muscular endurance have been seen in young swimmers after intensive training. Likewise, training improves the capacity of muscle to apply force.

Epidemiological evidence has led to the hypothesis that increased physical activity decreases the rate of death from heart disease. If the hypothesis is correct, blood lipids may be linked to the relationship. Generally, more active persons have lower blood cholesterol and triglyceride levels. This change may be due to the change in body weight and fat associated with physical activity.

The separation of blood cholesterol into its lipoprotein fractions has enabled better understanding of its possible role in heart disease. High levels of HDL are associated with a lower incidence of heart disease and increase with training in both sexes.

Ligament strength increases with endurance training and decreases with immobilization. Elite athletes generally show higher aerobic capacities than do nonathletes. While some of this capacity can be produced by nurture, the highest proportion is set genetically. Detraining causes rapid decay in the aerobic power gains produced by physical training.

KEY TERMS

bradycardia a condition in which the heart rate is lower than normal.

glycolytic enzymes substances that cause or accelerate the process of anaerobic glycolysis, for example, phosphofructokinase.

high-density lipoprotein (HDL) a lipoprotein fraction of total cholesterol responsible for breaking down cholesterol, and is thought to protect against coronary artery disease.

hyperplasia change in tissue cross section caused by growth of new fibers.

low-density lipoprotein (LDL) a lipoprotein fraction of total cholesterol responsible for transporting triglycerides in the blood.

maximal exercise exercise that continues to exhaustion or until maximal physiological values are attained.

respiratory enzymes substances that cause or accelerate the process of aerobic energy production, for example, succinate dehydrogenase.

submaximal exercise exercise at an intensity below that observed for maximal exercise.

ventricular mass the size of the left ventricular walls, which may increase (hypertrophy) with certain types of training.

ventricular volume the size of the left ventricular cavity, which may increase (hypertrophy) with certain types of training.

volume stress the stimulus for the increase in cardiac stroke volume thought to be a result of training that exposes the heart to high levels of blood exchange.

$\dot{V}o_2$ **max** maximal oxygen consumption or aerobic power.

REVIEW QUESTIONS

1. Contrast the training response of heart rate, stroke volume, and cardiac output during conditions of rest, submaximal, and maximal exercise. Why doesn't cardiac output decrease during submaximal exercise following aerobic training?

2. What are the differential effects of aerobic training and weight training with regard to ventricular mass and ventricular volume? What might explain these differential effects?

3. What is the difference between muscle hypertrophy and hyperplasia? What is the state of the evidence regarding training-induced hyperplasia of skeletal muscle?

4. Briefly explain how changes in muscle metabolism might account for performance changes observed in athletes who have undertaken either aerobic or anaerobic training.

5. Discuss the relationship between training and changes in lipoprotein fractions with respect to protection against coronary artery disease.

6. What can be said relative to gender differences in $\dot{V}o_2$ max among elite athletes? What about sport type differences?

REFERENCES

1. Andersen, P., and Henriksson, J.: Capillary supply of the quadriceps femoris muscle of man: adaptive response to exercise, J. Physiol. **270:**677, 1977.

2. Andersen, P., and Henriksson, J.: Training induced changes in the subgroups of human type II skeletal muscle fibres, Acta Physiol. Scand. **99:**123, 1977.

3. Andrew, G.M., Guzman, C.A., and Becklake, M.R.: Effect of athletic training on exercise cardiac output, J. Appl. Physiol. **21:**603, 1966.

4. Burke, E.J.: Physiological effects of similar training programs in males and females, Res. Q. **48:**510, 1977.

5. Clarke, D.H., and Vaccaro, P.: The effect of swimming training on muscular performance and body composition in children, Res. Q. **50:**9, 1979.

5a. Clutch, D., Wilton, M., McGown, C., and others: The effect of depth jumps and weight training on leg strength and vertical jump, Res. Quart. Exerc. Sport **54:**5, 1983.

6. Costill, D.L., Coyle, E.F., Fink, W.F., and others: Adaptations in skeletal muscle following strength training, J. Appl. Physiol. **46:**96, 1979.

7. Dressendorfer, R.H., and Gahagen, H.: Serum lipid levels in male runners, Physic. Sportsmed. **7:**119, 1979.

7a. Fosler, C., Pollock, M., Farrell, P., and others: Training responses of speed skaters during a competitive season, Res. Quart. Exerc. Sport **53:**257, 1982.

8. Frick, M.H.: Long-term excess physical activity and central haemodynamics in man, Adv. Cardiol. **18:**136, 1976.

9. Frick, M.H., Konttinen, A., and Sarajas, H.S.S.: Effects of physical training on circulation at rest and during exercise, Am. J. Cardiol. **12:**142, 1963.

9a. George, C., Kopetzky, M.T., Hughes, M.J., and others: Changes in myocardial mass associated with age and stress: reexamination of ventricular hypertrophy, Res. Quart. Exerc. Sport **56:**25, 1985.

10. Gollnick, P.D., and Hermansen, L.: Biochemical adaptations to exercise: anaerobic metabolism. In Wilmore, J.H., editor: Exercise and sport sciences reviews, New York, 1973, Academic Press, Inc.

11. Gollnick, P.D., and King, D.W.: Effect of exercise and training on mitochondria of rat skeletal muscle, Am. J. Physiol. **216:**1502, 1969.

12. Gollnick, P.D., and King, D.W.: The immediate and chronic effect of exercise on the number an structure of skeletal muscle mitochondria, Med. Sport **3:**239, 1969.

13. Gollnick, P.D., Armstrong, R.B., Saubert, C.W., and others: Enzyme activity and fiber composition in skeletal muscle of untrained and trained men, J. Appl. Physiol. **33:**312, 1972.

14. Gollnick, P.D., Armstrong, R.B., Saltin, B., and others: Effect of training on enzyme activity and fiber composition of human skeletal muscle, J. Appl. Physiol. **34:**107, 1973.

15. Hanson, J.S.: Maximal exercise performance in members of the U.S. Nordic ski team, J. Appl. Physiol. **35:**592, 1973.

15a. Haymes, E.M., and Dickinson, A.L.: Characteristics of elite male and female ski racers, Med. Sci. Sports Exerc. **12:**153, 1980.

16. Hermansen, L., and Anderson, K.L.: Aerobic work capacity in young Norwegian men and women, J. Appl. Physiol. **20:**425, 1965.

17. Hickson, R.C., Bomze, H.A., and Holloszy, J.O.: Linear increase in aerobic power induced by a strenuous program of endurance exercise, J. Appl. Physiol. **42:**372, 1977.

18. Holloszy, J.O.: Biochemical adaptations in muscle. Effects of exercise on mitochondrial oxygen uptake and respiratory enzyme activity in skeletal muscle, J. Biol. Chem. **242:**2278, 1967.

19. Holloszy, J.O.: Biochemical adaptations to exercise: aerobic metabolism. In Wilmore, J.H., editor: Exercise and sport sciences reviews, New York, 1973, Academic Press, Inc.

20. Holloszy, J.O.: Adaptation of skeletal muscle to endurance exercise, Med. Sci. Sports **7:**155, 1975.

21. Holloszy, J.O., and Oscai, L.B.: Effect of exercise on α-glycerophosphate dehydrogenase activity in skeletal muscle, Arch. Biochem. Biophys. **130:**653, 1969.

22. Holloszy, J.O., Rennie, J.J., Hickson, R.C., and others: Physiological consequences of the biochemical adaptations to endurance exercise. In Milvy, P., editor: The marathon: physiological, medical, epidemiological and psychological studies, Ann. N.Y. Acad. Sci. **301:**440, 1977.

23. Huttunen, J.K., Lansimies, E., Voutilainen, E., and others: Effect of moderate physical exercise on serum lipoproteins. A controlled clinical trial with special reference to serum high-density lipoproteins, Circulation **60:**1220, 1979.

24. Kannel, W.B., and Sorlie, P.: Some health benefits of physical activity. The Framingham study, Arch. Intern. Med. **139:**857, 1979.

25. Knehr, C.A., Dill, D.B., and Neufeld, W.: Training and its effects on man at rest and at work, Am. J. Physiol. **136:**148, 1942.

26. Lehtonen, A., Viikari, J., and Ehnholm, C.: The effects of exercise on high density (HDL) lipoprotein apoproteins, Acta Physiol. Scand. **106:**487, 1979.

27. Maksud, M.G., Wiley, R.L., Hamilton, L.H., and others: Maximal $\dot{V}_{O_2}$, ventilation, and heart rate of Olympic speed skating candidates, J. Appl. Physiol. **29:**186, 1970.

28. Menapace, F.J., Hammer, W.J., Ritzer, T.F., and others: Left ventricular size in competitive weight lifters: an echocardiographic study, Med. Sci. Sports Exerc. **14:**72, 1982.

29. Molé, P.A., Oscai, L.B., and Holloszy, J.O.: Adaptation of muscle to exercise. Increase in levels of palmityl Coa synthetase, carnitine palmityltransferase, and palmityl Coa dehydrogenase, and in the capacity to oxidize fatty acids, J. Clin. Invest. **50:**2323, 1971.

30. Montoye, H.J., Block, W.D., Metzner, H.L., and others: Habitual physical activity and serum lipids: males aged 16-64 in a total community, J. Chronic Dis. **29:**697, 1976.

31. Morganroth, J., Maron, B.J., Henry, W.L., and others: Comparative left ventricular dimensions in trained athletes, Ann. Intern. Med. **82:**521, 1975.

32. Oscai, L.B., Molé, P.A., Brei, B., and others: Cardiac growth and respiratory enzyme levels in male rats subjected to a running program, Am. J. Physiol. **220:**1238, 1971.

33. Pattengale, P.K., and Holloszy, J.O.: Augmentation of skeletal muscle myoglobin by a program of treadmill running, Am. J. Physiol. **213:**783, 1967.

34. Pollock, M.L., Cureton, T.K., and Greninger, L.: Effects of frequency of training on working capacity, cardiovascular function and body composition of adult men, Med. Sci. Sports **1:**70, 1969.

35. Raven, P.B., Gettman, L.R., Pollock, M.L., and others: A physiological evaluation of professional soccer players, Br. J. Sports Med. **10:**209, 1976.

36. Saltin, B., Blomquist, G., Mitchell, J.H., and others: Response to exercise after bed rest and after training, Circulation **38:**1, 1968.

37. Sinning, W.E.: Body composition, cardiorespiratory function and rule changes in women's basketball, Res. Q. **44:**313, 1973.

38. Smith, D.P., and Byrd, R.J.: Body composition, pulmonary function and maximal oxygen consumption of college football players, J. Sports Med. **16:**301, 1976.

39. Snoeckx, L.H.E.H., Abeling, H.F.M., Lambregts, J.A.C., and others: Echocardiographic dimensions in athletes in relation to their training programs, Med. Sci. Sports Exerc. **14:**428, 1982.

39a. Spence, D.W., Disch, J.G., Fred, H.L., and others: Descriptive profiles of highly skilled women volleyball players, Med. Sci. Sports Exerc. **12:**299, 1980.

40. Stremel, R.W., Convertino, V.A., Bernauer, E.M., and others: Cardiorespiratory deconditioning with static and dynamic leg exercise during bed rest, J. Appl. Physiol. **41:**905, 1976.

41. Taylor, H.L., Wang, Y., Rowell, L., and others: The standardization and interpretation of submaximal and maximal tests of working capacity, Pediatrics **32:**703, 1963.

41a. Thompson, P.D., Lewis, S., Varady, A., and others: Cardiac dimensions and performance after either arm or leg endurance training, Med. Sci. Sports Exerc. **13:**303, 1981.

42. Thorstensson, A.: Observations on strength training and detraining, Acta Physiol. Scand. **100:**491, 1977.

43. Tipton, C.M., Matthes, R.D., Maynard, J.A., and others: The influence of physical activity on ligaments and tendons, Med. Sci. Sports **7:**165, 1975.

44. Vaccaro, P., Clarke, D.H., and Wrenn, J.P.: Physiological profiles of elite women basketball players, J. Sports Med. Phys. Fitness **19**:45, 1979.

45. Wilmore, J.H., and Brown, C.H.: Physiological profiles of women distance runners, Med. Sci. Sports **6**:178, 1974.

45a. Wilmore, J.H., Davis, J.A., O'Brien, R.S., and others: Physiological alterations consequent to 20-week conditioning programs of bicycling, tennis and jogging, Med. Sci. Sports Exerc. **12**:1, 1980.

46. Wilmore, J.H., and Haskell, W.L.: Body composition and endurance capacity of professional football players, J. Appl. Physiol. **33**:564, 1972.

47. Wilmore, J.H., Royce, J., Girandola, R.N., and others: Physiological alterations resulting from a 10-week program of jogging, Med. Sci. Sports **2**:7, 1970.

48. Wolfe, L.A., Cunningham, D.A., Rechnitzer, P.A., and others: Effects of endurance training on left ventricular dimensions in healthy men, J. Appl. Physiol. **47**:207, 1979.

49. Wood, P.D., and Haskell, W.L.: The effect of exercise on plasma high density lipoproteins, Lipids **14**:417, 1979.

SUGGESTED READINGS

Gollnick, P.D., and Hermansen, L.: Biochemical adaptations to exercise: anaerobic metabolism. In Wilmore, J.H., editor: Exercise and sport sciences reviews, New York, 1973, Academic Press, Inc.

Holloszy, J.O.: Biochemical adaptations to exercise: aerobic metabolism. In Wilmore, J.H., editor: Exercise and sport sciences reviews, New York, 1973, Academic Press, Inc.

Holloszy, J.O.: Adaptation of skeletal muscle to endurance exercise, Med. Sci. Sports, **7**:155, 1975.

Kannel, W.B., and Sorlie, P.: Some health benefits of physical activity. The Framingham study, Arch. Intern. Med. **139**:857, 1979.

Montoye, H.J., Block, W.D., Metzner, H.L., and others: Habitual physical activity and serum lipids: males aged 16-64 in a total community, J. Chron. Dis. **29**:697, 1976.

Saltin, B., Blomquist, G., Mitchell, J.H., and others: Response to exercise after bed rest and after training, Circulation **38**:1, 1968.

Saltin, B., and Rowell, L.B.: Functional adaptations to physical activity and inactivity, Fed. Proc. **39**:1506, 1980.

Taylor, H.L., Wang, Y., Rowell, L., and others: The standardization and interpretation of submaximal and maximal tests of working capacity, Pediatrics **32**:703, 1963.

APPLICATION: PHYSIOLOGICAL BENEFITS VERSUS HEALTH BENEFITS

The student should not assume that the known physiological benefits that can be documented to result from exercise are synonomous with evidence supporting health enhancement or disease prevention. The term *support* must be thought of as a spectrum that ranges from a position of very little supportive data to virtually unquestioned substantiation of a hypothesis. Of course, there are all levels of support in between. The question is not about the support per se but about the assumption that one kind of support translates to another. At the present time it is clear that there is considerable support regarding physiological changes, including cardiac changes, after exposure to an exercise program. Support for exercise as a preventive tool for heart disease is much less clear. Just because it is possible to show that the heart is a more efficient organ after training (for example, improved stroke volume and heart rate) does not mean that the process of heart disease has been changed. Coronary heart disease is generally a matter of closure of the coronary arteries. The process of closure with lipid material can take place over many years, perhaps from childhood. It is not clear that the process that makes the heart a better "pump," exercise, also makes an impact on the accumulation of lipids along the arterial walls. Certainly the hypothesis is intriguing and, some would say, promising. For example, some studies have shown that lipids circulating in blood are reduced by exercise. It is presumed that this may have a protective effect. However, the definitive evidence that exercise retards the development of lipids in the coronary arteries has not yet been presented.

For most professionals, the physiological change/disease prevention argument is intriguing and must be faced when facing exercise skeptics, but it does not inhibit enthusiasm for judiciously promoting exercise for health enhancement. *Health,* perhaps better termed *wellness,* is a broad concept involved with not only physical parameters but also psychological and spiritual parameters. It is impossible to see a patient with cardiac disease change dramatically in an exercise program and not say that the change is documented health enhancement whether the disease process has been changed or not.

STUDENT: You said that the effects of exercise can be attained only if the principles of exercise prescription are followed. And the principles tell us that it is necessary to exercise two, or preferably three, times per week for 30 minutes per session. From a practical point of view, how many public school physical education programs comply with that requirement?

PROFESSOR: Many don't. In many high schools, in addition to the limitation associated with time exposure, physical education is required for only 1 year. Also, it's not uncommon to see elementary physical education, when it's offered at all, scheduled only once per week.

STUDENT: But the goals of physical education are more general than just the acquisition of physical fitness.

PROFESSOR: Quite true, but your question concerns the inability to make changes in physical fitness when time is limited. Another point that can be made relates to the actual amount of exercise during a given class period. Many times when sport skills are being taught, actual movement is a matter of seconds rather than minutes.

STUDENT: But, how does a teacher deal with this problem?

PROFESSOR: I'm afraid the answer to that question depends on philosophy and not science. It depends on what you want to achieve as a teacher. The important thing to remember is that if the goal is improvement in physical fitness, that is, to change the physiology of the body, movement is required—movement that is applied with the correct principles of frequency, duration, and intensity. If you don't follow these principles, you're only kidding yourself about potential benefits of your program.

STUDENT: But if a teacher decides to emphasize physical fitness, how can it be done, considering the typical school time constraints?

PROFESSOR: I would mislead you if I indicated that there is a simple answer to your question; there isn't. Most curricular time allocations are based on either the necessity of fitting all subjects into a prescribed school day, which is a practical problem, or a certain historical precedence. Most school subjects have not been based on how long it takes to apply a certain teaching stimulus to achieve a particular learning response. For instance, the school year still clings to the cycles of an agrarian culture. We dismiss school in the summer months whether there is an agricultural purpose or not. The idea that gains in physical education, or any school subject, require a set amount of time is relatively new. At least the support of hard data is recent.

STUDENT: Are you saying there is no chance of changing the school structure?

PROFESSOR: No, but certainly the probability is not high and requires the development of a long-range strategy to educate those who make decisions.

STUDENT: What do you mean?

PROFESSOR: I mean that it will take a concerted effort on the part of teachers to present the scientific reasons why physical fitness benefits cannot be gained by short exposure to the joy of the activity. Many so-called active people in the American culture exercise only 1 day per week for maybe 1 hour at a time. Quite a few educators are among this group. They believe that they are staying fit with this activity. It will take patience and the presentation of hard data to make an impact.

PART FOUR

ENVIRONMENTAL EFFECTS
ON PHYSICAL
PERFORMANCE

chapter 15

THE EFFECT OF HEAT STRESS ON PHYSIOLOGICAL RESPONSE AND PERFORMANCE

MAJOR LEARNING OBJECTIVE
Metabolic and environmental heat loads are removed from the body by passive (radiation, convection, and conduction), as well as active (evaporation) mechanisms.

APPLICATIONS
Heat injury to people as they exercise can be prevented by being aware of effective temperature (dry- and wet-bulb temperature, globe temperature, and wind velocity).
■ Coaches and race directors in certain geographical areas who are involved with sports in which heat injury is probable should be able to determine effective temperature and limit participation accordingly.

A 150-pound runner maintaining a pace of 5:30 min/mile expends energy at a rate of approximately 20 kcal/min.[9] Since the human machine is only about 25% efficient, 75% of this energy production is released as heat. If this heat cannot be dissipated, the body temperature increases to dangerous levels (>105° F [41° C]) very quickly. Effective thermoregulation is therefore mandatory for the athlete not only for efficient performance but for survival itself.

Since athletes must occasionally perform in environments that are hot and humid, the thermoregulatory problem is compounded. The threat is not only internal, from metabolic heat production, but external, from the environment. Technically, humans are homeotherms, maintaining a relatively constant internal temperature independent of environmental temperature. However, because of man's mobility, carrying him into extreme environments and his propensity for extending the limits of human performance, homeothermic mechanisms are placed under severe strain.

The purposes of this chapter are to review the mechanisms by which the body regulates its temperature within safe limits, that is, 98.6° ± 7.0° F (37° C); to discuss the physiological responses to heat exposure; to present the means by which heat strain might be modified; and to indicate the means by which heat injuries might be prevented.

THERMOREGULATION

A number of thermosensitive zones that detect changes in body temperature have been identified in the body.[23] These receptors are located on the body surface (cutaneous), in

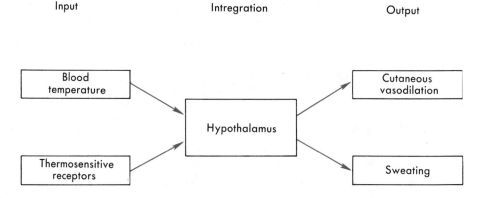

Input   Intregration   Output

FIG. 15-1   **The hypothalamus integrates temperature inputs received from thermosensitive receptors and through the blood. If the core temperature requires adjustment, cutaneous blood vessels are vasodilated and/or the sweat glands are stimulated.**

the peritoneal cavity, in the brainstem, and in the spinal cord. The area within the brainstem found to be thermally responsive is the preoptic portion of the anterior hypothalamus. Both heat- and cold-sensitive neurons are located here, but far more of the former. The hypothalamus serves as the integrating center for inputs about body temperature. Figure 15-1 illustrates the function of the hypothalamus in the regulation of body heat. Inputs to the hypothalamus arrive via the blood, which can be heated by metabolic or environmental stimuli, or via the nervous system from thermosensitive receptors (such as skin receptors); this information is integrated in the hypothalamus. The hypothalamus works like a thermostat. If the body core becomes overheated, signals are sent to cutaneous blood vessels (causing vasodilation) and/or to the sweat glands (causing sweat secretion). In the latter case, the message is delivered to the sweat glands by sympathetic motor nerves, and acetylcholine is released.

"Set point" theory of temperature regulation

Evaporation of sweat is the primary mechanism of heat loss during exercise and in a hot environment; sweating is essential to continued athletic performance. An unabated rise in core temperature leads to decreased muscular performance and can lead to heat injury (both are discussed later). It should be pointed out, however, that during exercise

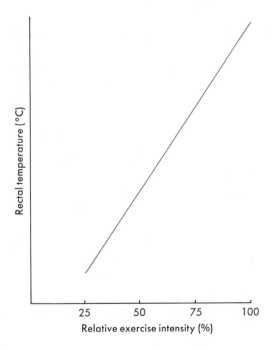

FIG. 15-2   **The linear relationship between rectal temperature and relative exercise intensity (%).**

the body functions optimally with the core temperature above resting normal (approximately 100° to 101° F [39° C]). Increased core temperature improves enzyme activity and results in more pliable connective tissue.

How is sweating controlled for maintenance of body temperature regulation? At rest, body temperature is regulated around a set point; that is, increases above a certain level result in the initiation of cooling mechanisms such as sweating. The hypothalamus regulates this set point. The mechanical analogue of the set-point theory is the operation of a thermostat. When the furnace heats the room to the set point, the furnace shuts down until the temperature changes again.

Core temperature grows linearly with relative exercise intensity (percentage of maximal exercise intensity).[64] This relationship is depicted in Figure 15-2. In turn, sweat rate increases proportionally with core temperature and skin temperature.[17,18,52] However, changes in core temperature have 10 times more effect on sweating than changes in skin temperature. Therefore control of sweating seems to be primarily related to increases in core temperature. It is said that during exercise, temperature is controlled from an ''elevated set point,'' since the optimal level of physiological function is at a point above core temperature. Thus the ''trigger'' for sweating is controlled from the elevated set point, not the resting set point.

MECHANISMS OF HEAT LOSS
Passive heat loss mechanisms

As core temperature increases during exercise in the heat, blood flow is redistributed to the periphery by vasodilation of cutaneous vessels. The blood serves as the vehicle for transporting heat to the periphery. When heat reaches the periphery it must be released from the body shell. The so-called passive heat loss mechanisms—*radiation, convection, and conduction*—contribute to this release. Figure 15-3 illustrates the use of these mechanisms when the air temperature is 75° F (24° C) and 95° F (35° C). When the air temperature is 75° F (24° C), a favorable gradient exists for heat to radiate away from the body shell. Under this condition most body heat (67%) is lost via radiation. However, when the gradient is absent (95° F [35° C]), only 4% of the heat is lost by this mechanism. Under both conditions conduction essentially does not contribute to heat loss, although theoretically it is possible. Convection, of course, depends on currents of air or water to pick up heat from the shell. This mechanism accounts for a relatively small percentage of heat loss, with air temperatures of 75° F (10%) and 95° F (6%). The convective properties of water and air have been compared in exercising subjects.[55] Both skin and core temperatures were lower (by 0.4° C) during swimming in a flume compared to pedaling a bicycle ergometer. It was concluded that exercise in water increases the body's capacity for heat dissipation because of the higher convective heat transfer from the skin to water.

Active heat loss mechanism

Evaporation is the principal active heat loss mechanism. It is active because the mechanism requires physiological changes that allow the sweat glands to secrete sweat.

Figure 15-3 illustrates the vital role of evaporation of sweat from the skin when the temperature gradient is not favorable. With the air temperature at 95° F (35° C), evaporation accounts for 90% of the heat loss.

Before discussing evaporation further, heat conduction from the core to the shell should be discussed. As mentioned earlier, when the hypothalamus detects an increase in core temperature above a certain threshold, skin vessels are stimulated to dilate. This results in an increase in blood flow to the skin. Heat from the core is thus conducted via the blood to the shell. On a hot day in the desert, to maintain a stable core temperature, the body can lose between 0.5 and 4.2 L/hr^{-1} (0.53 − 4.4 quarts · hr^{-1}) by sweating.[29] Paradoxically, as the body loses heat, it can become seriously dehydrated because of water loss.

Evaporation occurs in three forms.[29] First, water leaves the skin and lungs at all times; this is called *insensible* evaporation. Over a 24-hour period approximately 1,300 ml can be lost by this mechanism. Second, nonthermal sweating occurs during emotional stress and is termed *emotional* evaporation. The third form is *thermal* evaporation, which involves sweating through eccrine glands located on the head, face, trunk, arms, and legs.

Influence of body composition

Since heat production during exercise is nearly proportional to body weight, heavy persons must be concerned about possible heat storage. Generally, a tall and heavy or

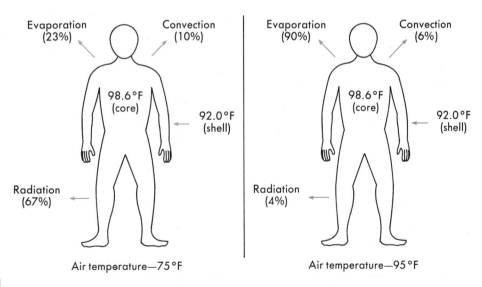

FIG. 15-3   The relative contribution of the various heat loss mechanisms in a person at rest when air temperature is 75° F (left) and 95° F (right). In each case the shell and core temperatures are identical.

short and stocky physique has greater heat storage because of greater body volume per unit of surface area. Obese people are at a disadvantage in the heat because the greater thickness of the body shell makes conductance of heat through the tissue more difficult.

CIRCULATORY AND METABOLIC RESPONSES TO HEAT STRESS
Cardiac output

As mentioned previously, it is necessary to redistribute blood flow from the central circulation to the periphery, so that heat can be dissipated. If an excess of the cardiac output is directed to the periphery, the core of the body would have to operate with deficient blood volume, which is not desirable. On the other hand, if too little is redistributed, hyperthermia is created, which is equally undesirable. The precise control of peripheral blood flow during exercise in the heat is therefore absolutely essential. This can be accomplished by increasing cardiac output, thus allowing more blood flow to be distributed to the periphery. Generally, cardiac output increases in the heat when exercise is moderately severe. During moderate to heavy exercise, cardiac output increases via increases in heart rate. Cardiac output becomes much more difficult to increase during very heavy exercise, when stroke volume and heart rate are at or close to maximum.[52]

Blood lactate levels

Several authors[19,26,41,72] have observed increases in exercise lactate in hot compared to cool environments; others[42,60] found no significant difference. It has been suggested[59] that

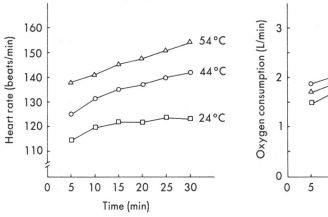
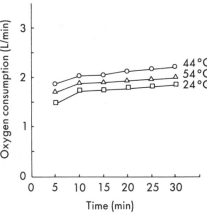

FIG. 15-4   Increasing the environmental temperature from 24° C to 44° C and 54° C results in a proportional increase in heart rate while oxygen consumption remains stable. All subjects rode the bicycle ergometer at a load that stimulated 40% $\dot{V}_{O_2}$ max during the 24° C condition. (From Pandolf, K.B., Cafarelli, E., Noble, B.J., and others: Perceptual responses during prolonged work, Percept. Mot. Skills *35:*975, 1972.)

increases in lactate were observed in some experiments because the experimental conditions resulted in decreased muscle blood flow, reduced removal of lactate by the liver, and increased muscle glycogenolysis. Lactate is most likely a factor contributing to fatigue in the heat. However, most research data indicate that thermal fatigue also appears to be related to variables other than lactate.

Oxygen consumption

Submaximal exercise oxygen consumption in cool and hot environments has been examined, and no difference was observed.[71] Generally, heat elevates heart rate but not oxygen consumption at submaximal exercise intensities. This point is illustrated in Figure 15-4. Increases in environmental temperature from 75° F (24° C) to 111° F (44° C) to 129° F (54° C) result in proportional increases in heart rate, while oxygen consumption remains stable.[56] The elevated heart rate is related to the need to increase cardiac output, whereas the oxygen consumption is responsive to the exercise intensity alone.

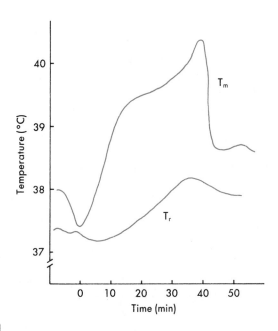

FIG. 15-5   Illustration of the increase in muscle temperature (T_m) and rectal temperature (T_r) during high-intensity exercise in a warm, humid environment. It should be noted that a favorable gradient exists for the movement of heat from muscle to the core (T_r) during exercise. Both T_m and T_r drop with cessation of exercise (40 minutes). (From Saltin, B., Giagge, A.P., and Stolwijk, J.A.S.: Body temperature and sweating during thermal transients caused by exercise, J. Appl. Physiol. *28:318*, 1970.)

Most investigators agree that maximal oxygen consumption is not affected by heat up to 122° F (50° C).[2,46,60,62] In addition, it has been shown that a group with high $\dot{V}O_2$ max (60.1 ml/kg · min^{-1}) showed a better response to submaximal work in the heat (102° F [39.4° C]) than a group with low $\dot{V}O_2$ max (35.6 ml/kg · min^{-1}).[65] This observation was based on a lower heart rate and core temperature in the high $\dot{V}O_2$ max group.

INFLUENCE OF HEAT STRESS ON MUSCLE FUNCTION

At rest, muscle temperature varies between 77° F (25° C) and 91° F (33° C), depending on environmental conditions.[25] With an average core temperature of 98.6° F (37° C), it is clear that the temperature gradient that exists favors the movement of heat from the core to muscles.

During exercise with exercise intensities greater than 25% $\dot{V}O_2$ max and in environments above 68° F (20° C), a shift in the muscle-to-core gradient occurs; that is, muscles lose heat to the core by virtue of their higher temperature. During high-intensity exercise in warm, humid environments, rectal temperature increases continuously.[63] Therefore the gradient can be interrupted, making it difficult to keep the muscle from overheating. Figure 15-5 illustrates an effective response to exercise in a warm, humid environment. A favorable gradient is maintained between the muscle and body core.

During isometric exercise, endurance decreases when muscle temperature exceeds 90° F (32° C) because of the rapid accumulation of metabolites.[11] It seems that the optimal muscle temperatures for running, cycling, and swimming are higher than for isometric exercise.[25] This temperature is approximately 104° F (40° C).[6] Aerobic exercise promotes muscle blood flow as well as peripheral blood flow; heat can thus be removed from the core of the body, preventing drastic rises in core temperature. The constrictive nature of isometric exercise with reduced or occluded blood flow probably makes it difficult to maintain a muscle/blood temperature gradient that allows efficient heat dissipation.

MODIFICATION OF PHYSIOLOGICAL RESPONSES TO HEAT STRESS
Acclimation/acclimatization

Acclimation is the artificially induced physiological adaptation to a particular temperature; acclimitization is a naturally induced adaptation.

Major changes in physiological response to heat stress begin occurring within the first 4 days of exercise in a heated environment. These changes are essentially complete within 12 to 14 days[59]; very few changes are observed with resting exposure. As mentioned previously, adaptive changes to a heated environment are referred to as either acclimation or acclimatization. The changes represent a positive adaptation to heat strain. The following changes have been observed during submaximal exercise[40]:

Decreased heart rate
Increased stroke volume
No change in cardiac output

Decreased core and skin temperature
Earlier onset of sweating
Increased sweat output
Decreased core and skin temperature at onset of sweating

Physical training and heat tolerance

A practical question for the coach, athlete, and scientist alike has been whether high physical conditions aids heat tolerance and in fact mimics acclimation/acclimatization. It is generally believed that more fit people acclimatize more quickly. Male distance runners who have trained for several years appear to have a natural acclimatization to 2 hours of mild work in dry heat.[32] Trained women acclimatize to heat in less time than their untrained counterparts.[12] The acclimatization process of women appears to be about the same as with men when exercise is expressed in relative terms (% $\dot{V}o_2$ max).[44] Acclimation/acclimatization is a transient process, which needs to be reestablished when one leaves a hot environment for as long as a month.[40]

What physiological changes consequent to physical training allow improved heat tolerance? The beneficial effects afforded to trained subjects are less heat storage, faster adjustment to a thermal steady state, and maintenance of a lower rectal temperature.[50] When untrained subjects are exposed to heat and exercise, exaggerated fluid shifts occur: more fluid is shifted from the blood plasma volume.[67] Adjustment to the heat partly depends on maintenance of cardiac output, which is related to plasma volume. Plasma volume is more stable in trained subjects. In fact, training increases plasma volume and the capacity of the sweating mechanism.[67] Several authors have confirmed an increase in sweat rate with training.[54,65]

Acclimation/acclimatization has been shown to modify the physiological response to heat. In turn, physical training appears to modify the acclimation/acclimatization process. However, even the best physical condition cannot eliminate the need for acclimation/acclimatization.[7]

Hydration and heat tolerance

Evaporation of sweat is a paradox. Without it, exercise in the heat would be impossible. But although evaporation cools the body, it can also lead to dehydration. Figure 15-6 helps to define the several terms associated with body hydration. Normal hydration is *euhydration.* Excessive water loss *(dehydration)* leads to *hypohydration,* and excessive water intake *(overhydration)* leads to *hyperhydration.* Dehydration can also mean the return to euhydration from the state of hyperhydration. Return from hypohydration to euhydration is called *rehydration.*[35]

The body can lose fluid at the rate of 1 L/hr^{-1} (1.057 qts/hr^{-1}) during hard physical training at a temperature of 90° F (32° C).[9] Core temperature rises as the body becomes hypohydrated. For example, in one experiment subjects were asked to ride a bicycle ergometer at 49% of $\dot{V}o_2$ max at a temperature of 74° F (23.6° C) and 50% relative humidity.[36] They manipulated the hydration state of the subjects in three ways: hyperhydration, hypohydration, and *ad libitum* water intake. Body weight was altered by $+1.2\%$, -5.2%, and -1.6%, respectively. The authors determined that core temperature increased $0.1°$ C for each 1% body weight (kg) loss. In other words, if a 150 lb athlete loses 5% of body weight (7.5 lb), the body temperature increases $0.5°$ C. Under certain conditions this could be equivalent to elevating temperature from a rather comfortable exercising level of $101.5°$ F to $102°$ F (approximately $39°$ C), which is on the borderline of danger. There does not appear to be a difference between static and dynamic exercise with regard to the rate of sweating or the increase in core temperature.

Football, because of the season in which practice begins, and wrestling, because of the use of dehydration techniques to ''make weight,'' are sports in which heat injury and/or performance decrements are likely. Strength and endurance have been examined in groups of subjects exposed to ad libitum water intake, water restriction, and starvation (neither food nor water). A significant reduction in both strength and endurance was observed in the water-restricted group. Greater losses were observed in the starvation group. Hypohydration is known to decrease cardiac output because of a decrease in stroke volume,[52] decreased blood plasma volume,[27] and increased heart rate during exercise.[27]

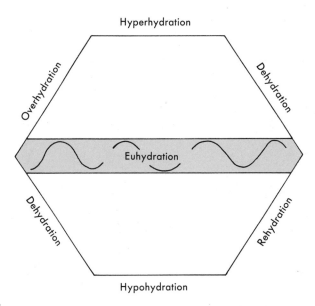

FIG. 15-6   **Illustration of the functional relationship between the various hydration terms. Normal hydration is called euhydration. (Adapted from Greenleaf, J.E.: Hyperthermia and exercise. In Robertshaw, D., editor: Environmental physiology, vol. 20, Baltimore, 1979, University Park Press.)**

Electrolyte replacement

As the body loses fluid by evaporation of sweat it also loses electrolytes, at a rate that could reach 3 g/hr[-1].[9] The main electrolytes lost in the sweat are sodium and chloride—not potassium, as has been often stated.[14] Such losses are more likely to occur with long-duration activities or with practices in the heat conducted over several days; the heat strain and exercise intensity must be heavy. When subjects are dehydrated a small amount (up to 3% of the body weight), electrolytes can be replaced naturally through the ingestion of food and drink ad libitum.[15]

When exercise continues for 2 hours or more at intensities above 50% $\dot{V}_{O_2}$ max, the replacement of fluid and electrolytes is advisable. Administration of water or a glucose-electrolyte solution periodically during a 2-hour run in the heat (98.6°F [37° C]) resulted in a reduction of heart rate to 18% below that after a run with no fluid ingestion.[27] The ingestion of an electrolyte supplement can replace 42% of the sodium lost by sweat and urine over 2 hours.[28] Water or glucose-electrolyte solutions administered during a 2-hour run caused core temperature to level off after 45 minutes, compared to a no-fluid condition in which the temperature did not level off.[16] The administration of a glucose-electrolyte solution was found to maintain serum electrolytes near preexercise levels and elevated blood pressure during the final 60 minutes of a 2-hour run.[16]

Influence of cooling

Cooling of the skin before and during exercise can modify the physiological responses to heat strain. One experiment used two cooling methods while the patient pedaled a bicycle ergometer at 105° F (41° C).[24] One method was the application of a cold towel to the head and abdomen; the second method combined the first with a 10-minute preexercise cold shower. Heart rate, rectal temperature, and sweat losses were significantly less under both conditions compared to a control condition. Head and neck cooling has also been shown to increase plasma volume during exercise in the heat.[35]

Age

Although age appears to have little effect on the rate of heat acclimation,[58] there are age-related differences in heat tolerance.[70] For example, adolescent boys and young men have better heat tolerance than boys before puberty or men 46 years or older. These results were also found in girls and women.[22,38] The increased risk of heat injury in prepubertal children and older adults seems to be related to the instability of the cardiovascular system and to lower aerobic power, respectively.[21] Age by itself is probably not related to heat tolerance. The older one becomes, the greater is the probability of lower aerobic power.[21]

Sex

Early studies reported that sweat gland density was greater in women than in men[4]; women sweat less.[39] In addition, women seem to have difficulty retaining plasma volume in the heat.[68] One would hypothesize from this information that women do not perform as well in the heat as men. In fact, when comparisons are made between men and women of equal aerobic capacities, sex differences in heat tolerance disappear.[3] Later studies indicate that men and women have the same number of sweat glands. Sweat glands are more widely distributed in men; however, women have more per unit of surface area. In dry heat there is no set difference in sweat rate. Women sweat less in wet heat, and they also maintain a lower core temperatue. Men and women have been compared at 73° F (23° C) and 102° F (39° C) (desert) at an exercise intensity of 50% $\dot{V}o_2$ max.[71] No sex differences were observed for change in $\dot{V}o_2$, heart rate, or rectal temperature. Thermoregulatory response of women to intermittent exercise in the heat has been investigated.[20] Exercise intensity was set at 75% of $\dot{V}o_2$ max. As with men, rectal temperature rose with environmental temperature, and stroke volume declined while heart rate rose. Rectal temperature does vary significantly with the day of the menstrual cycle (higher at days 14 and 20 compared to days 2, 8, and 26).[69] Time to exhaustion did not vary, however.

Adjustments to acclimation/acclimatization occur in both men and women about equally,[33] especially when exercise is expressed in relative terms.[44] Progressive reductions in thresholds for sweating and vasodilation of skin vessels are observed in both sexes.[53] Men maintain a lower absolute threshold for the onset of sweating, however.

HEAT INJURY AND EFFECTIVE TEMPERATURE

The mechanisms that cause heat injury and appropriate preventive measures have been well known for some time. Although the incidence of heat injury in athletics has declined recently, not a year goes by that death precipitated by heat stress is not recorded. This is particularly true for sports like football, conducted in hot and humid climates of the United States. If proper precautions are taken, such occurrences can be greatly minimized if not eliminated. For instance, the following factors are important to remember if one is responsible for protecting athletes against heat injury[8]:

1. The first days of exposure are the most critical.
2. Acclimation/acclimatization offers protection.
3. Obese individuals or those with a previous history of heat injury are most susceptible.
4. Individuals with infection, gastrointestinal disorders, or other conditions likely to influence temperature regulation should be closely watched.
5. Those with electrolyte imbalances or those with abnormal sweat gland function are likely candidates for heat injury.
6. Sunburn or skin lesions need to be treated immediately and not exposed to additional sunlight or heat stress.

The box on p. 395 is the position statement of the American College of Sports Medicine on prevention of heat injuries during distance running. Coaches responsible for organizing distance running competitions should be aware of these recommendations to protect athletes and decrease the possibility of being held liable for negligence.

Based on research findings and current rules governing distance running competition, it is the position of the American College of Sports Medicine that:

1. Distance races (>16 km or 10 miles) should *not* be conducted when the wet-bulb temperature–globe temperature* exceeds 28° C (82.4° F).

2. During periods of the year, when the daylight dry bulb temperature often exceeds 27° C (80° F), distance races should be conducted before 9:00 a.m. or after 4:00 p.m.

3. It is the responsibility of the race sponsors to provide fluids which contain small amounts of sugar (less than 2.5 g glucose per 100 ml of water) and electrolytes (less than 10 mEq sodium and 5 mEq potassium per liter of solution).

4. Runners should be encouraged to frequently ingest fluids during competition and to consume 400-500 ml (13-17 oz.) of fluid 10-15 minutes before competition.

5. Rules prohibiting the administration of fluids during the first 10 kilometers (6.2 miles) of a marathon race should be amended to permit fluid ingestion at frequent intervals along the race course. In light of the high sweat rates and body temperature during distance running in the heat, race sponsors should provide "water stations" at 3-4 kilometer (2-2.5 mile) intervals for all races of 16 kilometers (10 miles) or more.

6. Runners should be instructed in how to recognize the early warning symptoms that precede heat injury. Recognition of symptoms, cessation of running, and proper treatment can prevent heat injury. Early warning symptoms include the following: piloerection on chest and upper arms, chilling, throbbing pressure in the head, unsteadiness, nausea, and dry skin.

7. Race sponsors should make prior arrangements with medical personnel for the care of cases of heat injury. Responsible and informed personnel should supervise each "feeding station." Organizational personnel should reserve the right to stop runners who exhibit clear signs of heat stroke or heat exhaustion.

It is the position of the American College of Sports Medicine that policies established by local, national, and international sponsors of distance running events should adhere to these guidelines. Failure to adhere to these guidelines may jeopardize the health of competitors through heat injury.

*WBGT = 0.7 (WBT) + 0.2 (G%) + 0.1 (DBT)
Adapted from Minard, D.: Prevention of heat casualties in Marine Corps Recruits, Milit. Med. **126**:261, 1961.

This statement calls attention to the use of the *wet-bulb globe temperature (WBGT)* index[49] as a means of monitoring the risk involved under certain environmental conditions. This and other formulas are estimates of what is referred to as *effective temperature*. The lay person and the media typically monitor environmental conditions by what is called dry-bulb temperature; dry-bulb temperature, however, presents only one part of the picture relative to the possibility of heat injury. What is really necessary is an estimate of the total heat strain experienced by the body. Gagge[30] stated that a single index "must relate in some logical way to our sensory experience of warmth and cold and to our satisfaction with the thermal environment." Such an estimate must also include wet-bulb temperature, which in combination with dry-bulb temperature can be used to calculate relative humidity; black-globe temperature, which determines incident radiation; and wind velocity. Effective temperature thus evaluates how well the various heat loss mechanisms (radiation, evaporation, and convection) function. It would be prudent for every athletic program to purchase the equipment necessary for determining effective temperature.

Several rule-of-thumb estimates have been recommended, such as a rule that exercise in the heat should be curtailed when the addition of dry-bulb temperature and relative humidity results in a number greater than 150. Such estimates do not include either black-globe temperature or wind velocity, but do serve to illustrate an important point: heat injury can occur at a relatively low dry-bulb temperature if the humidity is high enough. For example, with the humidity above 80%, a dry-bulb temperature greater than 70° F (21° C) could be dangerous. The use of WBGT for football practice is illustrated in the following[57]:

1. *Application of safety index*

   Each component of the instrument is given a factor of importance, as relates to heat stress, in arriving at a safety index or scale. The index reading is obtained by adding:

   $$0.1 \times \text{the dry-bulb temperature}$$
   $$+0.2 \times \text{the black-globe temperature}$$
   $$\underline{+0.7 \times \text{the wet-bulb temperature}}$$
   $$\text{WBGT index}$$

2. *Activity adjusted accordingly during acclimatization period*

   WBGT index from 82° to 85° F (28° to 29.5° C): light exercise

   WBGT index from 85° to 88° F (29.5° to 31° C): no exercise but may give instructions in the shade

   WBGT index above 88° F (31° C): all activity discontinued

3. *After acclimatization (10 days)*

   WBGT index above 85° F (29.5° C): strenuous exercise is stopped

   WBGT index above 88° F (31° C): all exercise is stopped

4. *During and after acclimatized period*

   When the wet-bulb reading is within 3 degrees of the dry-bulb reading, all activity should be suspended.

When the wet-bulb reading is from 3 to 5 degrees below the dry-bulb reading, helmets, sweat shirts, and shoulder pads should be disgarded and activity slowed down.

Of additional interest to the teacher and coach is the effect of clothing on heat tolerance. The "clo" unit has been used to express the resistance to heat transfer with respect to convection, radiation, and evaporation. One clo "will maintain a resting-sitting person with a metabolic rate of 50 kcal · m²/hr^{-1} comfortably in an environment of 70° F (21° C) with relative humidity less than 50% and air movement of 6 m/min^{-1} (20 ft/min^{-1})."[29] If clothing fails to transfer heat away from the body properly, heat loss mechanisms will be ineffective. Beautiful uniforms might lose games if athletes become fatigued because of high heat storage. Vapor-barrier suits, which have become popular as a water loss technique or a method of acclimating athletes for competition in hot, humid environments, can place the individual at high risk for heat injury.[7]

Artificial playing surfaces, which have become popular in recent years because of the possibility of continuing activity following or during inclement weather, can have negative side effects. One side effect is that all synthetic turfs create warmer environments than grass. Not only the surface but the air directly above the surface is warmer. Coaches or field supervisors can reduce the possibility of heat injury by irrigating the surface of the artificial turf before competition.[7]

SUMMARY

Surface (cutaneous) receptors are of prime importance as sensors of body temperature. Integration of peripheral thermal cues occurs in the hypothalamus. When the body becomes overheated, as reflected by an increase in core temperature beyond a certain threshold level, the hypothalamus signals the sweat glands to secrete and the peripheral vessels to dilate. Heated blood can be directed to the skin, where it is radiated to the environment or where it can be dissipated by evaporation of sweat. Radiation, convection, and conduction are passive heat loss mechanisms. Evaporation is an active heat loss mechanism and is the most important such mechanism when the environmental temperature is greater than the skin temperature and during exercise at any temperature. Evaporation can account for a water loss of 0.5 to 4.2 L/hr. Generally, a tall, heavy or short, stocky physique stores more heat because of greater body volume per unit of surface area. Sweat rate is critical to control of body temperature, if effective adaptation to exercise in the heat is to be achieved. Sweat rate is proportional to the rise in core temperature and is controlled about an elevated set point relative to the resting state.

It is necessary to increase blood flow to the skin for the dissipation of heat. During moderate exercise in the heat, cardiac output increases to accommodate this process. However, cardiac output decreases with heavy exercise in the heat, limiting continued performance. Whether blood lactate accumulates in the heat beyond the level expected in a cool environment is unclear; investigators have observed increases as well as no change. Submaximal and maximal oxygen consumption does not change in the heat, in contrast to heart rate, which is elevated. During exercise, muscle temperature increases above core temperature, thus creating a gradient that increases body temperature. Optimal muscle temperatures are necessary for continued performance. When muscle temperature exceeds 90° F (32° C) during isometric work, or approximately 104° F (40° C) during dynamic work, performance can be impaired.

Physiological changes include decreased heart rate and increased stroke volume and sweat rate. They are essentially complete within 12 to 14 days. Physically fit people acclimatize more quickly, but people with a fit physical condition cannot do without a certain amount of acclimation/acclimatization.

Core temperature rises as the body becomes dehydrated. Temperature rises 0.1° C for each 1% of body weight loss. A significant reduction in both strength and endurance was observed when water was restricted during exercise. As the body loses fluid by evaporation, it also loses sodium chloride. During long-duration exercises, in which electrolyte losses can be high, electrolyte supplementation can maintain preexercise serum electrolyte levels.

Prepubertal children and older adults tolerate heat less well. This seems to be related to instability of the cardiovascular system and low aerobic capacity, respectively. Women sweat less in the heat and have difficulty retaining plasma volume, but they appear as well equipped to tolerate heat as men. Progressive reductions in thresholds for sweating and vasodilation of skin vessels is observed in both sexes during acclimation/acclimatization.

Effective temperature should be measured to protect athletes from heat injury. In addition to dry-bulb temperature, effective temperature considers wet-bulb temperature, black-globe temperature, and wind velocity, or factors that evaluate the effectiveness of the body's heat loss mechanisms. One formula that estimates effective temperature is the wet-bulb globe temperature (WBGT) index.

Some athletic clothing, like vapor-barrier suits, can place the body at high risk for heat injury. Artificial playing surfaces are hotter than grass.

KEY TERMS

acclimation physiological change in response to heat stress caused by artificial environments, such as saunas.

acclimatization physiological change in response to heat stress caused by natural environments, such as a visit to a hotter environment.

adaptation general term referring to the ability of organisms to adjust to their environments.

body core central portion of the body. The temperature of the core (98.6° F [37° C]) is measured in the rectum, esophagus, or tympanum.

body shell casing of the body, the skin, which is the interface between the body and the environment at which heat dissipation takes place.

conduction movement of heat from one tissue to another, caused by physical contact with a temperature gradient (high to low).

convection movement of heat from the body by circulation of air or water across its surface.

dehydration excessive water loss.

euhydration normal hydration ($\pm 1\%$ to 2%).

evaporation transfer of water to water vapor, with a resulting decrease in temperature of the object previously holding the water.

heat strain response of the body to the heat stress.

heat stress temperature stimulus acting on the body.

radiation movement of heat from one object to another without direct physical contact and in proportion to temperature difference between the objects (high to low temperature).

REVIEW QUESTIONS

1. Briefly discuss the set point theory of temperature regulation. What is controlled?

2. Why is evaporation referred to as an *active* heat loss mechanism? How does evaporation work to dissipate heat from the body?

3. Why does submaximal heart rate increase in the heat but oxygen consumption does not?

4. Briefly discuss the adaptive advantage of the temperature gradient between the core and the muscle during rest and exercise.

5. Why are increased exercise sweat rate and earlier onset of sweating advantageous acclimation/acclimatization changes?

6. What conditions prevail during physical training that allow physical fitness to mimic the effects of acclimation/acclimatization?

7. What are the performance consequences of dehydration?

8. Briefly discuss the heat tolerance of exercising women.

9. What is effective temperature, and why is it superior to dry-bulb temperature for protection against heat injury?

REFERENCES

1. American College of Sports Medicine: Prevention of heat injuries during distance running, Med. Sci. Sports Exerc. **7**:7, 1975.

2. Adams, W.C., Fos, R.H., Fry, A.J., and others: Thermoregulation during marathon running in cool, moderate, and hot environments, J. Appl. Physiol. **38**:1030, 1975.

3. Avellini, B.A., Kamon, E., and Krajewski, J.T.: Physiological responses of physically fit men and women to acclimation to humid heat, J. Appl. Physiol. **49**(2):254, 1980.

4. Bar-Or, O., Lundegren, H.M., Magnusson, L.T., and others: Distribution of heat-activated sweat glands in obese and lean men and women, Hum. Biol. **40**:235, 1968.

5. Bosco, J.S., Greenleaf, J.E., Bernauer, E.M., and others: Effects of acute dehydration and starvation on muscular strength and endurance, Acta Physiol. Pol. **25**(5):411, 1974.

6. Brooks, G.A., Hittelman, K.J., Faulkner, J.A., and others: Temperature, skeletal muscle mitochondrial functions, and oxygen debt, Am. J. Physiol. **220**:1053, 1971.

7. Buskirk, E.R.: Temperature regulation with exercise. In Hutton, R.S., editor: Exercise and sport sciences reviews, vol. 5, Santa Barbara, Calif., 1977, Journal Publishing Affiliates.

8. Buskirk, E.R., and Grasley, W.C.: Heat injury and conduct of athletics. In Johnson, W.R., and Buskirk, E.R., editors: Science and medicine in exercise and sports, New York, 1974, Harper & Row Publishers, Inc.

9. Claremont, A.D.: Coping with the weather. The basic book on marathoning, 1979, Consumers Guide.

10. Claremont, A.D., Costill, D.L., Fink, W., and others: Heat tolerance following diuretic-induced dehydration, Med. Sci. Sports Exerc. **8**(4):239, 1976.

11. Clark, R.S.J., Hellon, R.F., and Lind, A.R.: The duration of sustained contractions of the human forearm at different muscle temperatures, J. Physiol. **143**:454, 1958.

12. Cohen, J.S., and Gisolf, C.V.: Effects of interval training on work-heat tolerance of young women, Med. Sci. Sports Exerc. **14**(1):46, 1982.

13. Convertino, V.A.: Heart rate and sweat rate responses associated with exercise-induced hypervolemia, Med. Sci. Sports Exerc. **15**:77, 1983.

14. Costill, D.L.: Sweating: its composition and effect on body fluids. In Milvy, P., editor: The marathon: physiological, medical, epidemiological and psychological studies, vol. 301, New York, 1977, The New York Academy of Sciences.

15. Costill, D.L., Cole, R., Miller, E., and others: Water and electrolyte replacement during repeated days of work in the heat, Aviat. Space Environ. Med. **46**(6):795, 1975.

16. Costill, D.L., Kammer, W.F., and Fisher, A.: Fluid ingestion during distance running, Arch. Environ. Health **21**:520, 1970.

17. Costill, D.L., and Saltin, B.: Changes in ratio of venous to body hematocrit following dehydration, J. Appl. Physiol. **36**:608, 1974.

18. Damato, A.N., Lau, S.H., Stein, E., and others: Cardiovascular response to acute thermal stress (hot, dry environment) in unacclimatized normal subjects, Am. Heart J. **76**:769, 1968.

19. Dill, D.B., Yousef, M.K., and Nelson, J.D.: Response of men and women to two-hour walks in desert heat, J. Appl. Physiol. **35**:231, 1973.

20. Drinkwater, B.L., Denton, J.E., Raven, P.B., and others: Thermoregulatory response of women to intermittent work in the heat, J. Appl. Physiol. **41**(1):57, 1976.

21. Drinkwater, B.L., and Horvath, S.M.: Heat tolerance and aging, Med. Sci. Sports Exerc. **11**(1):49, 1979.

22. Drinkwater, B.L., Kupprat, I.C., Denton, J.E., and others: Response of prepubertal girls and college women to work in the heat, J. Appl. Physiol. **43**(6):1046, 1977.

23. Eisenman, J.S.: Sensory organs and thermogenesis, Isr. J. Med. Sci. **12**(9):916, 1976.

24. Falls, H.B., and Humphrey, D.: Cold water application effects on responses to heat stress during exercise, Res. Q. **42**(1):21, 1971.

25. Faulkner, J.A.: Heat and contractile properties of skeletal muscle. In Horvath, S.M., and Yousef, M.K., editors: Environmental physiology: aging, heat and altitude, Amsterdam, 1981, Elsevier/North Holland.

26. Fink, W.J., Costill, D.L., and Van Handel, P.J.: Leg metabolism during exercise in the heat and cold, Eur. J. Appl. Physiol. **34**:183, 1975.

27. Francis, K.T.: Effect of water and electrolyte replacement during exercise in the heat on biochemical indices of stress and performance, Aviat. Space Environ. Med. **50**(2):115, 1979.

28. Francis, K.T., and MacGregor, R., III.: Effect of exercise in the heat on plasma renin and aldosterone with either water or a potassium-rich electrolyte solution, Aviat. Space Environ. Med. **49**(3):461, 1978.

29. Frisancho, A.R.: Human adaptation: a functional interpretation, St. Louis, 1979, The C.V. Mosby Co.

30. Gagge, A.P.: The new effective temperature (ET): an index of human adaptation to warm environments. In Horvath, S.M., and Yousef, M.K., editors: Environmental physiology: aging, heat and altitude, Amsterdam, 1981, Elsevier/North Holland.

31. Gisolfi, C.V.: Temperature regulation during exercise: directions, Med. Sci. Sports Exerc. **15**:15, 1983.

32. Gisolfi, C.V.: Work-heat tolerance of distance runners. In Milvy, P., editor: The marathon: physiological, medical, epidemiological, and psychological studies, vol. 301, New York, 1977, The New York Academy of Sciences.

33. Gisolfi, C.V., and Cohen, J.S.: Relationships among training, heat acclimation, and heat tolerance in men and women: the controversy revisited, Med. Sci. Sports Exerc. **11**(1):56, 1979.

34. Goldman, R.F.: Clothing design for comfort and work performance in extreme thermal environments, Trans. N.Y. Acad. Sci. (Series II) **36**:531, 1974.

35. Greenleaf, J.E.: Hyperthermia and exercise. In Robertshaw, D., editor: Environmental physiology, vol. 20, Baltimore, 1979, University Park Press.

36. Greenleaf, J.E., and Castle, B.L.: Exercise temperature regulation in man during hypohydration and hyperhydration, J. Appl. Physiol. **30**(6):847, 1971.

37. Hancock, P.A.: Predictive validity of a computer model of body temperature during exercise, Med. Sci. Sports Exerc. **13**:31, 1981.

38. Haymes, E.M., Buskirk, E.R., Hodgson, J.L., and others: Heat tolerance of exercising lean and heavy prepubertal girls, J. Appl. Physiol. **36**:556, 1974.

39. Hertig, B.A., Belding, H.S., Kraning, K.K., and others: Artificial acclimatization of women to heat, J. Appl. Physiol. **18**:383, 1963.

40. Horvath, S.M.: Historical perspectives of adaptation to heat. In Horvath, S.M., and Yousef, M.K., editors: Environmental physiology: aging, heat and altitude, Amsterdam, 1981, Elsevier/North Holland.

41. Irondelle, M., and Freund, H.: Carbohydrate and fat metabolism of unacclimatized men during and after submaximal exercise in cool and hot environments, Eur. J. Appl. Physiol. **37**:27, 1977.

42. Klausen, K., Dill, D.B., Phillips, E.E., and others: Metabolic reactions to work in the heat, J. Appl. Physiol. **22**:292, 1967.

43. Kobayashi, Y., Ando, Y., Okuda, N., and others: Effects of endurance training on thermoregulation in females, Med. Sci. Sports Exerc. **12**:361, 1980.

44. Kupprat, I.C., Drinkwater, B.L., and Horvath, S.M.: Interaction of exercise and ambient environment during heat acclimatization, Hung. Rev. Sports Med. **21**:5, 1980.

45. Lemon, P.W.R.: A simple and inexpensive method for making sweat collection capsules, Res. Q. Exerc. Sports **54**:299, 1983.

46. Matsui, H., Shimaoka, K., Miyamura, M., and others: Seasonal variation of aerobic work capacity in ambient and constant temperature. In Folinsbee, L.J., and others, editors: Environmental stress, New York, 1978, Academic Press., Inc.

47. McConnell, T.R., and Sinning, W.E.: Exercise and temperature effects on human sperm production and testosterone levels, Med. Sci. Sports Exerc. **16:**51, 1984.

48. Reference deleted in proofs.

49. Minard, D.: Prevention of heat casualties in Marine Corps recruits, Milit. Med. **126:**261, 1961.

50. Nadel, E.R.: Circulatory and thermal regulations during exercise, Fed. Proc. **39**(5):1491, 1980.

51. Nadel, E.R., Cafarelli, E., Roberts, M.F., and others: Circulatory regulation during exercise in different ambient temperatures, J. Appl. Physiol. **46**(3):430, 1979.

52. Nadel, E.R., Fortney, S.M., and Wenger, C.B.: Effect of hydration state on circulatory and thermal regulations, J. Appl. Physiol. **49**(4):715, 1980.

53. Nadel, E.R., Roberts, M.F., and Wenger, C.B.: Thermoregulatory adaptations to heat and exercise: comparative responses of men and women. In Folinsbee, L.S., and others, editors: Environmental stress, New York, 1978, Academic Press, Inc.

54. Nadel, E.R., and Stolwijk, J.A.J.: Sweat gland response to the efferent thermoregulatory signal, Arch. Sci. Physiol. **27:**A67, 1973.

55. Nielsen, B., and Davies, C.T.M.: Temperature regulation during exercise in water and air, Acta Physiol. Scand. **98:**500, 1976.

56. Pandolf, K.B., Cafarelli, E., Noble, B.J., and others: Perceptual responses during prolonged work, Percept. Mot. Skills **35:**975, 1972.

57. Pearl, A.J.: Heat and physical activity, J. Fla. Med. Assoc. **67**(4):396, 1980.

58. Robinson, S., Belding, H.S., Consolazig, F.C., and others: Acclimatization of older men to work in the heat, J. Appl. Physiol. **20:**583, 1965.

59. Rowell, L.B.: Human cardiovascular adjustments to exercise and thermal stress, Physiol. Rev. **54**(1):75, 1974.

60. Rowell, L.B., Blackman, J.R., Martin, R.H., and others: Hepatic clearance of indocyane green in man under thermal and exercise stresses, J. Appl. Physiol. **20:**384, 1965.

61. Rowell, L.B., Marx, R.A., Bruce, R.D., and others: Reductions in cardiac output, central blood volume and stroke volume with thermal stress in normal man during exercise, J. Clin. Invest. **45:**1801, 1966.

62. Saltin, B., Gagge, A.P., Bergh, V., and others: Body temperature and sweating during exhaustive exercise, J. Appl. Physiol. **32:**635, 1972.

63. Saltin, B., Gagge, A.P., and Stolwijk, J.A.S.: Body temperature and sweating during thermal transients caused by exercise, J. Appl. Physiol. **28:**318, 1970.

64. Saltin, B., and Hermansen, L.: Esophageal, rectal and muscle temperature during exercise, J. Appl. Physiol. **21:**1757, 1966.

65. Shvartz, E., Magazanic, A., and Glick, Z.: Thermal responses during training in a temperate climate, J. Appl. Physiol. **36:**572, 1974.

66. Shvartz, E., Glick, Z., and Magaanik, A.: Responses to temperate, cold, and hot environments and the effect of physical training, Aviat. Space Environ. Med. **48**(3):254, 1977.

67. Senay, L.C., Jr.: Effects of exercise in the heat on body fluid distribution, Med. Sci. Sports **11**(1):42, 1979.

68. Senay, L.C., Jr.: Change in plasma volume and protein content during exposures of working man to various temperatures before and after acclimatization to heat: separation of the roles of cutaneous and skeletal muscle circulation, J. Physiol. **224**:61, 1972.

69. Stephensen, L.A., Kolka, M.A., and Wilkerson, J.E.: Metabolic and thermoregulatory responses to exercise during the human menstrual cycle, Med. Sci. Sports Exerc. **14**(4):270, 1982.

70. Wagner, J.A., Robinson, S., Tzankoff, S.P., and others: Heat tolerance and acclimatization to work in the heat in relation to age, J. Appl. Physiol. **33**:616, 1972.

71. Wells, C.L.: Responses of physically active and acclimatized men and women to exercise in a desert environment, Med. Sci. Sports Exerc. **12**(1):9, 1980.

72. Williams, C.G., Bredell, G.A.G., Wyndham, C.H., and others: Circulatory and metabolic reactions to work in heat, J. Appl. Physiol. **17**:625, 1962.

SUGGESTED READINGS

Milvy, P.: The marathon: physiological, medical, epidemiological and psychological studies, vol. 301, New York, 1977, The New York Academy of Sciences.

Horvath, S.M. and Yousef, M.K.: Environmental physiology: aging, heat and altitude, Amsterdam, 1981, Elsevier North Holland.

Folinsbee, L.J., and others: Environmental stress, New York, 1978, Academic Press.

APPLICATION: HEAT INJURY PREVENTION IN FOOTBALL

Much of the original work dealing with the prevention of heat injuries originated from interest generated by the military because of the high incidence of heat injury among recruits in basic training. The problems of military recruits are not unlike those of football players: they may be wearing clothes not conducive to heat transfer, they may be unacclimatized, they may be unfit, and water may not be readily available.

Football coaches often ask what procedures they can use in preseason practice to prevent heat injury. The following recommendations are essentially the same as those used by the U.S. Marine Corps[49]:

1. When heat stress is high, as judged by the WBGT index, activity should be curtailed. One alternative is to conduct practice early in the morning or in the evening when environmental conditions are more favorable.
2. Heavy practice should not be implemented immediately. The intensity, frequency, and duration of practices should be gradually increased over 1 or 2 weeks.
3. Players should be encouraged to arrive at preseason practice already physically fit. Acclimatization to the heat occurs more rapidly and with much less strain when players are fit.
4. Water should be always available, and an unlimited quantity should be allowed. High performance levels cannot be achieved when an athlete is hypohydrated. Research indicates that when hypohydrated individuals are provided with water ad libitum they remain hypohydrated after satisfying their thirst. Fluids should be forced rather than restricted.

5. Until players are at least partially acclimatized, full uniforms should not be required. Even the most effective material (regarding heat transfer) can prove to be harmful to unacclimatized athletes. Shorts and T-shirts can be used in drills for the first few days.

The question of salt replacement during exercise in the heat is often asked. If an athlete is receiving a normal diet, there is usually no need for supplementary salt intake. If the coach or trainer suspects that a player is not receiving an adequate diet, minimal amounts of supplementary salt may be required.

APPLICATION: DISTANCE RUNNING RECOMMENDATIONS

Thermoregulation is a popular topic among undergraduate students. The topic is straightforward and very practical for the future teacher and coach. A typical dialogue in class follows the following pattern:

> STUDENT: Are there limits to the heat loss mechanisms during distance running?
>
> PROFESSOR: Definitely! The limits depend on the physical properties of the environment.
>
> STUDENT: For example, how about radiation?

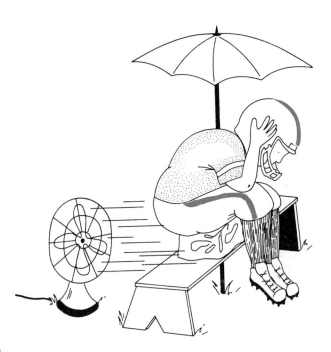

FIG. 15-7   The air-conditioned athlete.

PROFESSOR: Well, first to review. Average skin temperature is approximately 92° F (33° C). Radiation from the body shell to the environment depends on a temperature gradient with the environmental temperature below that of the shell (<92° F).

STUDENT: Then when dry-bulb temperature is above 92° F (33° C), the body begins to take on heat from the environment?

PROFESSOR: Exactly. The effect is analogous to the radiation from a wood-burning stove with a temperature much higher than the body.

STUDENT: Evaporation must depend on the relative humidity?

PROFESSOR: Right. Evaporation from the skin to the air depends on the water saturation of the air. The dryer the air, such as in a desert environment, the easier it is to evaporate and thus to lose heat. However, as the relative humidity increases so does the difficulty of evaporating.

STUDENT: With a relative humidity of close to 100%, would it be virtually impossible to evaporate water from the skin while running?

PROFESSOR: Yes.

STUDENT: How about by convection?

PROFESSOR: As you can imagine, increasing convective currents across the skin (such as wind velocity) aids the dissipation of heat. That's why we retreat to a fan on hot days.

STUDENT: It's obvious that the runner can be in a lot of trouble when dry-bulb temperature is above 92° F (33° C), relative humidity approaches 100%, and there is no wind.

PROFESSOR: The only alternative is to seek an environment that artificially conditions the air (Figure 15-7). With running, it is best to discontinue training or competition when conditions push the body's ability to adapt.

chapter 16

THE EFFECT OF COLD STRESS ON PHYSIOLOGICAL RESPONSE AND PERFORMANCE

MAJOR LEARNING OBJECTIVE
The body adapts to the cold by shivering and cutaneous vasoconstriction. Metabolic heat productivity is also an important cold adaptation mechanism.

APPLICATIONS
Hypothermia while exercising in the cold is a life-threatening condition. Summer backpacking in the mountains can result in hypothermia when lack of physical fitness and compulsive "pushing" are combined with quick changes in mountain weather that can lower body temperature. Prior planning, quick detection, and warming are essential to protect against hypothermia.

$\mathbf{I}$N the last 20 years, more and more people have begun participating in activities that take place in the winter season or that expose the body to cold stress. Skiing, both downhill and cross-country, climbing, backpacking, snowmobiling, and scuba diving all expose the body to the cold. Some of these activities, backpacking for example, can result in thermal imbalance even during the summer. Packing in the mountains, with generally cooler dry-bulb temperatures, during a summer rain shower can lead very quickly to a drop in core temperature to dangerous levels (hypothermia).

When the environmental temperature falls below a comfortable level, various mechanisms must be called into play to maintain core temperature. First, we can call on physiological thermoregulatory responses to achieve thermal balance. Second, we can alter our behavior by choosing to seek shelter, add clothing, or begin exercising.

It should be pointed out that, paradoxically, sometimes athletes can suffer from heat stress in the cold. Kaare Rodahl,[28] a famous Norwegian physiologist, states that "under

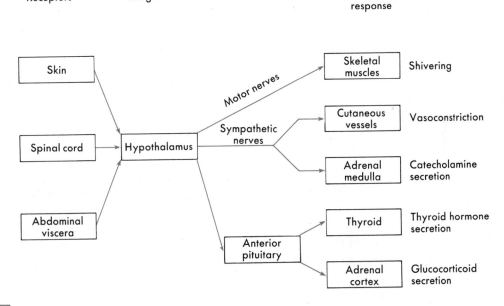

FIG. 16-1   Illustration of the mechanisms by which the body regulates its response to cold stress. A decrease in temperature is sensed by receptors and the message(s) is relayed to the hypothalamus, which integrates incoming signals. Effector organs are "instructed" to respond so that body heat is conserved (vasoconstriction) or produced (shivering and hormonal secretions).

most circumstances a man is over protected against heat loss, including most real arctic circumstances . . . .'' In other words, we underestimate the extent to which exercise creates metabolic heat, and we overdress in the cold.

This chapter discusses the ways in which the body regulates heat balance under cold stress, the effects of cold stress on performance and training practices, the process of acclimation/acclimatization in a cold environment, and ways in which we might survive a severely cold stimulus.

PHYSIOLOGICAL THERMOREGULATION IN THE COLD

The body regulates itself either by heat conservation or heat production. In the first case, the body conserves heat by *vasoconstriction* of the surface vessels and by shutting down the sweating mechanism. Heat production, increasing metabolic rate, is accomplished by *shivering* of skeletal muscles or by stimulating increased tissue oxidation by the intervention of various *hormones*.

As mentioned in Chapter 10, cold receptors are located in the skin but they are far fewer than heat receptors. When skin temperature falls below normal, signals from cold receptors increase in frequency.[31] Receptors are sensitive to both absolute temperature and the rate of change in temperature.[32] Cold receptors are also located in the spinal cord and abdominal viscera (Figure 16-1).

Signals received by the hypothalamus are integrated and directed by motor nerves to stimulate muscles to shiver; the sympathetic nervous system to cutaneous blood vessels, which vasoconstrict, and the adrenal medulla to release catecholamines (adrenalin and noradrenalin); and the anterior pituitary, which stimulates the thyroid to release hormone secretions and the adrenal cortex to release glucocorticoids (cortisol and corticosterone).[32]

MECHANISMS OF HEAT CONSERVATION AND PRODUCTION
Vasoconstriction

The major mechanism of heat conservation is vasoconstriction of cutaneous vessels. When this occurs, the flow of heat from the core to the shell is limited. This results in decreased skin temperature, which decreases the temperature gradient with the environment and thus reduces heat loss. Generally, blood pressure and heart rate are increased with vasoconstriction. When the face is exposed to cold water, an interesting response occurs. The blood pressure increases but the heart rate decreases, most likely a result of the parasympathetic (vagus nerve) influence on the heart.[10] The chest pain felt by some cardiac patients in the winter (angina pectoris) may be caused by the stress of increased blood pressure and decreased heart rate.

Muscular shivering

As mentioned earlier exercise, that is, voluntary muscular contraction, is a powerful source for heat production. When we are not exercising, involuntary muscular shivering is the main source of increased heat production. The nude body begins shivering when the environmental temperature falls below 77° F (25° C).[10] Shivering causes an increase in muscle temperature that decreases the gradient with core temperature, thus reducing muscular heat loss.

Hormonal response

It is known that several hormones are secreted during cold stress (see Figure 16-1). One class of hormones, the catecholamines, is known to increase the release of free fatty acids that increase oxidative phosphorylation, that is, increase metabolic rate.[32] Catecholamines also stimulate hyperglycemia, again producing a condition favoring tissue oxidation. Thyroxin has also been implicated in the increase in metabolic rate, particularly during cold acclimation/acclimatization.[10] Glucocorticoids, cortisol and cortisone, produced by the adrenal cortex, stimulate the formation of glucose. The availability of glucose during cold exposure may be important to increasing oxidative metabolism for cold adaptation. The secretion of catecholamines, thyroxin, and glucocorticoids all favor adaptation to cold.

Practical summary. The body is protected from the cold by reducing heat loss from the skin (vasoconstriction) and by producing heat (shivering and hormone release).

PHYSIOLOGICAL RESPONSE TO COLD STRESS
Extremities

Since the ears, feet, and fingers have very little metabolically active tissue, they depend heavily on blood supply for heat. Therefore, when skin vessels vasoconstrict, the shell temperature decreases to a point close to the environmental temperature. During this condition, very little heat is lost by convection and radiation, but the skin becomes susceptible to frostbite. A *hunter's response* has been observed in which a cold-induced vasodilation occurs, possibly protecting the skin from injury.[10] Cross-country skiers may have noticed this sensation of periodic warming and cooling of the extremities.

Oxygen consumption

Apparently $\dot{V}O_2$ max is independent of environmental temperatures.[17,19] It may be that changes in aerobic power occur only when muscle temperature falls below a certain point (100° F, 38° C).[3] Figure 16-2 illustrates the relationship between aerobic power and muscle temperature.

Research studying the response of $\dot{V}O_2$ to submaximal exercise has produced mixed results. Some studies have found increased $\dot{V}O_2$[5] and others report no differences.[9,30] This is probably because changes are not a matter of the environmental temperature as such but are changes produced in core temperature. For instance, $\dot{V}O_2$ is known to increase only after core temperature falls below 97° F (36° C).

Practical summary. Short-term exposure to cold conditions does not alter submaximal $\dot{V}O_2$ or $\dot{V}O_2$ max unless core temperature is changed.

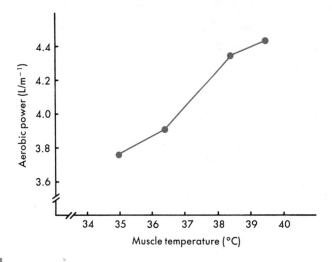

FIG. 16-2 The relationship between changes in muscle temperature and aerobic power. (Adapted from Bergh, J.: Human power at subnormal body temperatures, Acta Physiol. Scand. *478:*1, 1980.)

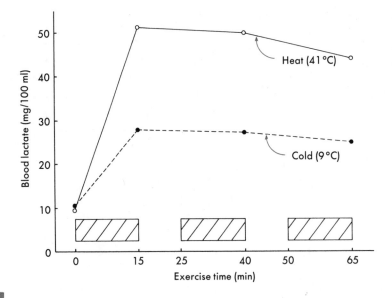

FIG. 16-3 Illustration of the blood lactate response to intermittent exercise (70% to 85% $\dot{V}O_2$ max) in the heat (106° F, 41° C) and cold (48° F, 9° C). The horizontal, hatched bars show the 15-minute exercise periods. (Adapted from Fink, W.J., Costill, D.L., and Van Handel, P.J.: Leg muscle metabolism during exercise in the heat and cold, Eur. J. Appl. Physiol. *34:*183, 1975.)

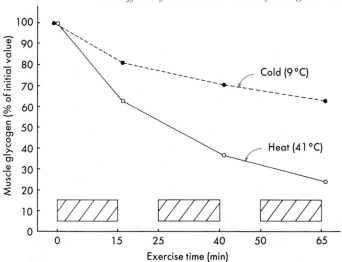

FIG. 16-4 Illustration of the muscle glycogen response to intermittent exercise (70% to 85% $\dot{V}_{O_2}$ max) in the heat (106° F, 41° C) and cold (48° F, 9° C). The horizontal, hatched bars show the 15-minute exercise periods. (Adapted from Fink, W.J., Costill, D.L., and Van Handel, P.J.: Leg muscle metabolism during exercise in the heat and cold, Eur. J. Appl. Physiol. *34:*183, 1975.)

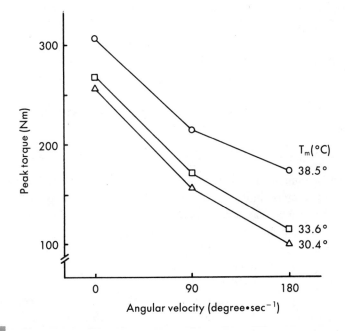

FIG. 16-5 Peak torque (Newton meters) is plotted against angular velocity of the limb (degrees · sec^{-1}) at various muscle temperatures (T_m). (Adapted from Bergh, J.: Human power at subnormal body temperatures, Acta Physiol. Scand. *478:*1, 1980.)

Blood lactate and muscle glycogen

Figures 16-3 and 16-4 illustrate the results of an experiment conducted in the heat (106° F, 41° C) and cold (48° F, 9° C).[9] Subjects exercised in three 15-minute segments (70% to 85% $\dot{V}O_2$ max) separated by 10-minute rest periods. Immediately following each exercise period, blood and muscle samples were taken. Blood lactate levels (glycolysis) were elevated in the heat compared to the cold and glycogen appears to be spared in the cold; that is, exercise is more aerobic in the cold with more reliance on fat as a fuel.

Practical summary. The physiological strain of exercise in the cold does not appear to be nearly as severe as in the heat. The athlete should be cautioned against overheating in the cold; that is, heat production may far exceed the need, given typical athletic winter dress.

STRENGTH AND ENDURANCE DURING COLD STRESS

Maximal isometric strength does not seem to be affected by the lowering of muscle temperature.[3] Figure 16-5, however, illustrates that peak torque achieved during dynamic muscular contractions, at selected angular velocities, decreases with reduced muscle temperature. Eccentric strength is increased as muscle temperature is lowered.[2] Thus, the effect of lowered muscle temperature on the development of force seems to be dependent on the type of exercise. When temperature does have an effect, it is a result of its influence on the myosin cross-bridges, that is, the rate of breaking and forming actomyosin.[2]

Muscular endurance has also been studied at various environmental temperatures: 50° F (10° C), 55° F (13° C), 65° F (18° C), and 75° F (24° C).[6] Subjects were instructed to contract maximally every 2 seconds for 6 minutes on a finger ergograph. Muscular endurance was improved by 30% in the 50° F (10° C) condition compared to 75° F (24° C).

Practical summary. Muscular strength may be improved during exposure to the cold with eccentric exercise but not with dynamic or isometric exercise.

TRAINING DURING COLD CONDITIONS

Contrary to popular opinion, it is seldom necessary to discontinue training in cold weather. As mentioned, exercise in itself is a powerful stimulus for heating the body and protecting it from hypothermia. Vasoconstriction increases the insulative capacity of the body shell and decreases the possibility of heat transfer by convection and radiation. However, fatigued or unfit individuals can run into trouble because they cannot produce enough heat to maintain thermal balance.[4]

Many people worry about possible damage to lung tissue while exercising in the cold. Environmental air, at a temperature of −25° F (−32° C), is known to be heated to 75° F (24° C) before it reaches the bronchi.[4] The respiratory discomfort sometimes associated with breathing cold air is most likely related to the fact that cold air is usually very dry. When subjects exercise at submaximal exercise intensities while breathing air cooled to

$-31°$ F $(-35°$ C), there is not only an absence of harmful tissue effects but $\dot{V}o_2$, respiratory rate, and rectal temperature are unaffected as well.[13]

Since air is such a good insulator, the athlete requires only a lightweight clothing material that is porous so that sweat can wick to the surface where it can be removed. The clo requirements of cold-resistant clothes are discussed later. However, nylon offers a good protection for the skin at a windchill equal to $-40°F$ $(-40°$ C).[4]

Practical summary. No harmful effects on lung tissue have been observed with exercise at temperatures as low as $-31°$ F $(-35°$ C).

ACCLIMATION/ACCLIMATIZATION TO COLD STRESS

Do athletes acclimatize to the cold? Does the Chicago Bears football team have an advantage over the Dallas Cowboys when playing in a cold northern stadium? Of course, psychological adaptation is important under any thermal stress. But it can be shown that a physiological adjustment has taken place that would offer an advantage to the cold-exposed player. Very few studies have probed this topic with athletes as subjects. Therefore, it is necessary to turn to other groups and animal studies to answer the question.

It has been suggested that one or more of the following criteria must be met to prove that man has acclimatized[33]:

1. Evidence of an increased metabolic rate in a thermoneutral environment, that is, neither hot nor cold.
2. Evidence of increased tissue insulation, that is, tissue characteristics that reduce heat loss, such as fat.
3. A decreased susceptibility to pain, numbness, or cold injury in the extremities.
4. A decreased cutaneous threshold for cold thermogenesis.

Subjects placed in a cold chamber begin to show acclimation effects after 1 week.[15] Acclimation is marked by an increase in metabolic rate,[15] a decrease in shivering response,[8] an increase in nonshivering thermogenesis,[8] and a decrease in skin thickness.[22] These changes are related to increased fat mobilization in the cold that reduces skinfold fat thickness.[22,23]

Practical summary. It appears that a good case can be made for acclimation (artificial) to the cold. It is necessary, however, to look for additional evidence from native populations that are naturally and habitually exposed to the cold.

Acclimatization in Eskimos and aborigines

The Eskimos are an ideal population in which to study cold acclimatization. They, particularly male hunters, spend many hours each day exposed to subzero conditions. Basal metabolic rate of Eskimos has been observed to be raised by 13% to 45% above nonnative groups.[10] One author claims that the increased specific dynamic action arising from the high-protein diet of the Eskimo accounts for this increase.[28] Others[21] have found that inland Eskimos, exposed to high cold stress, have higher metabolic rates than coastal Eskimos, who are exposed to a milder stress. This indicates that the response is environmentally induced. Genetic mediation of cold tolerance should not be discounted either. The genetic factor is evidenced by data that women and children who have less cold exposure display the same cold tolerance as males exposed to more cold.[18]

It is interesting to note that Australian aborigines, exposed to great temperature extremes on essentially nude bodies, adapt differently than Eskimos. The aborigines maintain a low metabolic rate in the cold.[10] This may be a result of their poor nutritional status compared with the Eskimos. On the other hand, the lower metabolic rate may be a consequence of genetic influences; that is, they can maintain homeostasis at a lower metabolic rate.

Acclimatization in European whites

When European whites are placed in a severely cold climate, they show an increased metabolic rate.[29] However, most whites dress and house themselves so well when exposed to a cold environment that they do not show a typical adaptive response.[10] In other words, although cold tolerance can be improved in European whites, unlike Eskimos, it is usually accomplished without a change in metabolic rate. Figure 16-6 compares the metabolic rate of Eskimos and whites at the same skin temperature and illustrates the difference in adaptive response to the cold.

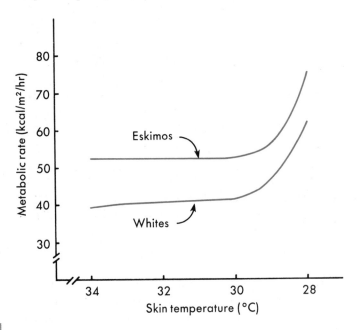

FIG. 16-6 Comparison of metabolic rate in Eskimos and Caucasians at the same skin temperatures. (Adapted from Adams, T., and Covino, B.G.: Racial variations to a standardized cold stress, J. Appl. Physiol. *12*:9, 1958.)

White workers whose occupations require exposure of specific areas of the body do show a local acclimatization. For example, fishermen display higher blood flows in the hands when exposed to cold water than nonacclimatized persons.[10] But no general acclimatization is achieved. Most likely, North American athletes do not show a physiological acclimatization to the cold because of their clothing and short exposure time.

Practical summary. Acclimatization to the cold is partly genetic and partly environmental. It is difficult to determine whether racial differences exist because whites generally protect themselves so well from the cold by their dress and housing.

SURVIVAL IN COLD AIR

Although humans, acclimatized to the cold, can adapt physiologically to abrupt cold exposure, prevention of hypothermia is not in any way ensured. When the temperature falls below −40° F (− 40° C) and clothes no longer offer a protection, thermal balance cannot be maintained at rest.[27] In remote areas, often the only alternative for survival is exercise. Rodahl[27] states, "He who can maintain a high level of physical exercise longest has the best chance of survival."

Following are seven hypothermic signs and symptoms of those exposed to severely cold conditions[26]:
1. The hands cool very rapidly and lose strength.
2. The fingers become numb and clumsy.
3. The feet and legs also become numb and clumsy.
4. Brain efficiency is impaired so that it is difficult to think clearly.
5. When the core temperature reaches 90° F (32° C), the body stops shivering and becomes rigid.
6. Gradually consciousness is lost.
7. Death from heart failure occurs when the body temperature reaches 75°F (24° C).

Factors related to cold tolerance

Age, physical fitness, body surface area, and body composition all play a role in the body's ability to acutely respond to the cold.[10] Older persons (>70 years) do not respond as well to immersion in cold water as do children and younger adults.[10] Although the research is limited, it is plausible that increased physical fitness would aid cold tolerance because of increased vascularity, muscle size, aerobic power, and the time necessary to reach fatigue.

The frequency and intensity of shivering is greater in thin people. Perhaps one of the reasons that channel swimmers survive in the cold water for long periods of time is because they ordinarily carry a large fat layer.[26] In fact, channel swimmers intentionally try to increase their body fat percentage. It is more difficult for a smaller person to survive because more heat is required to maintain a constant core temperature with a smaller surface area.

Another factor related to cold tolerance is clothing. As mentioned earlier, the unit used to evaluate the heat transfer value of clothing is called the clo. One clo ''will maintain a resting-sitting person with a metabolic rate of 50 kcal $\cdot$ m^2 $\cdot$ hr comfortably in an environment of 21° C (70° F) with relative humidity less than 50% and air movement of 6 m $\cdot$ min^{-1} (20 feet $\cdot$ min^{-1}).''[10] Naturally, in the cold it would be desirable to protect against heat transfer, that is, hold in the metabolic heat and guard the skin from cooling by the wind. At the same time, the clothing must be porous enough to allow evaporation. The recreational cross-country skier, for example, learns to use layers of clothing, that is, when the environmental temperature increases or when the work intensity increases, layers can be removed. Another common rule for the skier is to keep the intensity of the exercise and the clothing such that sweating is kept to a minimum. The clo value required in various environmental temperatures then depends on the intensity of the exercise. As the metabolic rate increases (MET value), the clo value required at any environmental temperature is reduced (Figure 16-7).[4] Therefore, when working hard even in a very cold environment, the clo requirement is quite low.

For the athlete in competition, clothing cannot be altered in response to changes in

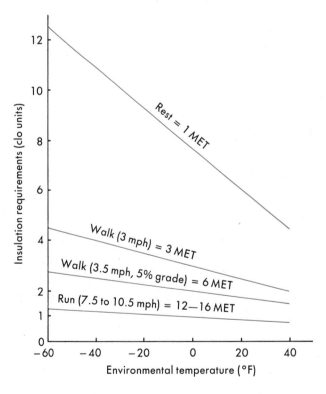

FIG. 16-7   **Illustration of the insulation requirements for clothing (clo units) at rest and at various exercise intensities when a person is exposed to a variety of environmental temperatures. One MET is defined as the energy requirement for resting metabolism. (Adapted from Claremont, A.D.: Taking winter in stride requires proper attire, Physic. Sports Med. *4:*65, 1976.)**

sweat rate. Thus, the competitive skier needs clothing to keep out the wind and protect against frostbite but that will "breathe" to allow evaporation. To study this problem eight cross-country skiers exercised for 90 minutes, at 55% to 60% $\dot{V}o_2$ max, with an environmental temperature of $-4°$ F $(-20°$ C), with and without a wind speed of 4.1 m · sec^{-1}.[14] The skiers wore regulation competitive cross-country ski uniforms that had a clo value of 1.59. Without the wind, core temperature remained relatively constant, but with the wind, it was significantly decreased, that is, they became colder. This was due to a significant increase in heat loss in the wind. A windchill chart appears in Table 16-1. The windchill concept implies that the addition of wind can make an otherwise harmless environmental temperature quite dangerous. Table 16-1 indicates that a dry-bulb temperature of 10° F $(-12°$ C) is equivalent to $-25°$ F $(-32°$ C) in a 20 mph wind. In other words, exposed skin could freeze within 1 minute.

One additional finding reported in the experiment is worthy of mention.[14] During the wind condition, the experimental group increased metabolic rate as an adaptive response. However, even though there was an increase on the average, some subjects did not increase metabolic rate. This means that these subjects did not have to increase metabolic rate to remain in thermal balance. The subjects who did not increase metabolic rate were working at an exercise intensity of 10 MET or above and the others were lower. Therefore, as mentioned, if you are working hard enough and can maintain such a level, you can tolerate the cold stress without additional physiological adaptations, that is, the exercise metabolism warms the body.

Practical summary. In a resting state in the cold, a person should dress to conserve body heat, that is, use a high clo value. When exercising, with the accompanying increase in a

TABLE 16-1 ||||| WINDCHILL CHART

Wind speed (mph)	Temperature (°F)								
	40	30	20	10	0	−10	−20	−30	−40
5	35	25	15	5	5	−15	−25	−35	−45
10	30	15	5	−10	−20	−35	−45	−60	−70
15	25	10	−5	−20	−30	−45	−60	−70	−85
20	20	5	−10	−25	−35	−50	−65	−80	−95
25	15	0	−15	−30	−45	−60	−70	−90	−105
30	10	0	−20	−30	−50	−65	−80	−95	−110
35	10	−5	−20	−35	−50	−65	−80	−100	−115
40	10	−5	−20	−35	−55	−70	−85	−100	−115
	Little danger			Danger			Great danger		

The interaction of wind speed (mph) and environmental temperature (°F), referred to as windchill, relative to the danger of freezing exposed flesh. Danger means that exposed flesh may freeze in 1 minute. Great danger means that exposed flesh may freeze in 30 seconds.

person's metabolic rate, the clo value of clothing can be reduced, that is, it is not as necessary to conserve body heat. Consequently, it is best to use a *layering* technique of dress in the cold.

SURVIVAL IN COLD WATER

Heat transfer by conduction and convection is proportional to the gradient between the skin and the environment. Because of a favorable gradient and the convective properties of water, heat is transferred 20 to 26 times faster in water than in air. Exposed to a water temperature of 32° F (0° C), thermal balance is lost in 2 minutes, and the body can become incapacitated in 15 minutes.

The Ama women of Korea represent an interesting contrast to normal response in cold water.[10] These women work by deep diving in water for plant and animal food. Diving temperatures range from 50° F (10° C) in the winter to 80.6° F (27° C) in the summer. Oral temperatures while diving drop to between 91.4° and 95.0° F (33° and 35° C). These women have a higher basal metabolic rate (35% in the winter) and a lower threshold for shivering. This is an environmentally induced acclimatization resulting from diving since an early age. Such activity would represent a severe stress for unacclimatized persons.

Aerobic power in cold water

While swimming in cold water 68° to 104° F (20° to 40° C), the temperature of a person's quadriceps muscle group has been found to vary between 100° F and 101° F (37.7° and 38.5° C).[25] $\dot{V}O_2$ max has been reported to decrease in very cold water.[25] To receive the stimulating effect of cool water but not to decrease $\dot{V}O_2$ max it has been recommended not to allow competitive pool temperatures to fall below 77° to 79° F (25° to 26° C).[7] Cardiac output has been measured during submaximal swimming at various water temperatures (64°, 77°, and 91° F; 18°, 25°, and 33° C) and was found to be constant.[20]

Survival

There is great potential for hypothermia and eventual death in cold water. Core temperature falls quickly when a person swims in water colder than 59° F (15° C). Even though heat production increases, the net loss of heat by convection is greater.[10] Remaining still in the water is the recommended survival procedure. If several persons are exposed simultaneously, they should remain still and huddled together.

In an experiment concerning survival in the cold, investigators suddenly immersed human subjects in very cold (52° F, 11° C) and less cold (82° F, 28° C) water.[11] Pulmonary ventilation was extremely high in the cold water during the first three breaths (equivalent to 94.3, 71.3, and 94.6 L · min⁻¹, respectively). The authors suggest that the high rate of ventilation increases the probability of water inspiration and may contribute to death.

Hypothermia can be counteracted by removing the wet clothing, ingesting warm liquids, providing carbohydrate supplementation, and rewarming in warm water (104° F, 40° C).[26]

The interaction of alcohol with cold exposure can potentiate the effect. An experiment was conducted in which bicycle exercise (40% $\dot{V}_{O_2}$ max) was administered under three experimental conditions: water, water and alcohol consumption, and alcohol and dextrose consumption.[12] Subjects rode intermittently for 2 hours at an environmental temperature of 23° F (−5° C). The alcohol plus water condition resulted in significant decreases in rectal temperature, skin temperature, and blood glucose levels.

Practical summary. People accidentally exposed to very cold water should not swim but remain still and huddle with a companion if available. Since alcohol potentiates the effect of cold exposure, it should not be consumed when the possibility of hypothermia is high.

SUMMARY

The zone of thermal comfort in which the body is able to maintain thermal balance (homoiothermy) is very narrow. Under cold stress, the body maintains homoiothermy either by heat conservation or heat production. Thermal balance is regulated by the hypothalamus. Cold stimulation received by receptors in the skin, spinal cord, and abdominal viscera is sent to and integrated by the hypothalamus, resulting in the stimulation of muscle shivering, cutaneous vasoconstriction, and various hormonal secretions. Vasoconstriction conserves heat by reducing blood flow to the skin. Involuntary shivering increases muscular heat production and decreases the temperature gradient between muscles and the body core. Catecholamines, thyroid hormones, and glucocorticoids are apparently involved in the stimulation of tissue oxidation, that is, increased metabolic rate.

Aerobic power (on land) has been found to be independent of environmental temperature unless conditions cause a decrease in muscle temperature, in which case aerobic power values are decreased. Variable results have been observed relative to submaximal oxygen consumption, most likely due to methodological differences between experiments and the fact that $\dot{V}_{O_2}$ varies with muscle temperature, which was not affected equally by all experimental protocols. Compared to exercise in the heat, exercise under cold conditions does not stimulate high levels of glycolysis and spares glycogen.

The effect of lowered muscle temperature on muscle strength seems to be dependent on the type of exercise. For example, isometric strength is not affected but peak torque during dynamic contractions decreases. Muscular endurance was improved by 30% at 50° F (10° C) compared to 75° F (24° C).

Exercise itself is a powerful stimulus for heating the body and acts to protect against hypothermia. There is no evidence to suggest that cold air damages lung tissue during exercise.

The question is often asked whether humans acclimate or acclimatize to cold. Human data are scarce but it appears that a good case can be made for acclimation (artificial) to the cold. Native populations such as Eskimos chronically exposed to the cold clearly display changes in metabolic rate that are indicative of acclimatization (natural). At the same skin temperatures, Eskimos show increased metabolic rates compared to European whites. Because most white populations dress and house themselves so adaptively and keep cold exposure to a minimum, acclimatization to the cold is not observed, nor is it necessary.

Cold tolerance is modified by age, physical fitness, body surface area, and body composition. Old age, low level of fitness, small body surface area, and small amounts of body fat are factors that decrease cold tolerance.

The heat transfer properties of clothing, measured by the clo unit, are important to cold tolerance. As the metabolic rate increases during exercise, the clo value required at any environmental temperature is reduced. Cross-country skiers clothed in regulation uniforms (clo = 1.59) and exercising at 55% to 60% $\dot{V}_{O_2}$ max in the wind (4.1 m $\cdot$ sec^{-1} at $-4°$ F, $-20°$ C) lose body heat during 90 minutes of exercise and decrease rectal temperature. The windchill factor must be evaluted when considering the ability of an athlete and the clothes worn to maintain thermal balance and combat hypothermia.

Heat leaves the body 20 to 26 times faster in water than air. Aerobic capacity decreases as a function of decreasing water temperature. The best competitive pool temperature is 77° to 79° F (25° to 26° C).

Swimming is not recommended during a survival situation in the water. Swimming increases the loss of temperature from the body. Increased mortality in cold water may result from inspiration of water because of increased pulmonary ventilation with sudden cold water immersion. The interaction of alcohol with cold exposure decreases survival capabilities.

KEY TERMS

acclimation physiological change in response to heat stress caused by artificial environments, such as saunas.

acclimatization physiological change in response to heat stress caused by natural environments, such as a visit to a hotter environment.

clo measurement unit used to evaluate the heat transfer value of clothing.

cold tolerance the ability of the body to adapt its physiological processes to protect against cold temperatures.

cold zone homoiothermy maintained by thermogenesis (increasing metabolic rate above normal).

cool zone heat conservation is necessary but increased heat production by increasing metabolic rate is not required.

cutaneous vasoconstriction the process by which skin blood vessels are compressed to reduce blood flow and, therefore, loss of body heat.

MET one MET is equivalent to resting metabolic rate. Thus, 5 MET would refer to a metabolic rate that is five times that of rest.

metabolic rate the rate at which the body produces energy and, therefore, heat. This variable is used as a measure of the degree to which the body adapts to the cold.

shivering involuntary muscle contraction by which the body can increase its metabolic rate and adjust to cold temperatures.

thermogenesis production of heat by physiological processes.

zone of intolerable cold maintenance of homoiothermy is impossible (core temperature falls).

zone of thermal comfort narrow thermal zone in which homoiothermy is maintained.

REVIEW QUESTIONS

1. Discuss the methods by which the body conserves and produces heat to adapt to the cold.

2. Since adaptation to the cold involves increasing metabolic rate, why does $\dot{V}O_2$ not increase with exercise in the cold?

3. What is meant by glycogen sparing and what causes it with exercise in the cold?

4. Does it seem reasonable that muscle strength would decrease in the cold? What mechanism might be responsible for such a decrease?

5. Summarize the major points illustrated in Figure 16-7 relative to the insulation requirements of clothes worn during exercise in the cold.

6. Why does the cold tolerance of Eskimo women and children demonstrate the role of genetics in acclimatization?

7. What is meant by local and general acclimatization?

8. Why does alcohol potentiate the effect of cold exposure?

REFERENCES

1. Adams, T., and Covino, B.G.: Racial variations to a standardized cold stress, J. Appl. Physiol. **12:**9, 1958.

2. Asmussen, E., Bonde-Petersen, F., and Jorgensen, K.: Mechanoelastic properties of human muscles at different temperatures, Acta Physiol. Scand. **96:**83, 1976.

3. Bergh, U.: Human power at subnormal body temperatures, Acta Physiol. Scand. (Suppl.) **478:**1, 1980.

4. Claremont, A.D.: Taking winter in stride requires proper attire, Physic. Sports Med. **4:**65, 1976.

5. Claremont, A.D., Nagle, F., Reddan, W.D., and others: Comparison of metabolic, temperature, heart rate and ventilatory responses to exercise at extreme ambient temperatures (0° and 35° C), Med. Sci. Sports **7:**150, 1975.

6. Clark, D.H., and Wojciechowicz, R.A.: The effect of low environmental temperatures on local muscular fatigue parameters, Am. Correct. Ther. J. **32:**35, 1978.

7. Costill, D.L.: Effects of water temperature on aerobic working capacity, Res. Q. **39:**67, 1967.

8. Davis, T.R.A.: Chamber cold acclimatization in man, J. Appl. Physiol. **16:**1011, 1961.

9. Fink, W.J., Costill, D.L., and Van Handel, P.J.: Leg muscle metabolism during exercise in the heat and cold, Eur. J. Appl. Physiol. **34:**183, 1975.

10. Frisancho, A.R.: Human adaptation: a functional interpretation, St. Louis, 1979, The C.V. Mosby Co.

11. Goode, R.C., Duffin, J., Miller, R., and others: Sudden cold water immersion, Respir. Physiol. **23**:301, 1975.

12. Graham, T., and Dalton, J.: Effect of alcohol on man's response to mild physical activity in a cold environment, Aviat. Space Environ. Med. **51**:793, 1980.

13. Hartung, G.H., Myhre, L.G., and Nunneley, S.A.: Physiological effects of cold air inhalation during exercise, Aviat. Space Environ. Med. **51**:591, 1980.

14. Haymes, E.M., Dickinson, A.L., Malville, N., and others: Effects of wind on the thermal and metabolic responses to exercise in the cold, Med. Sci. Sports Exerc. **14**:41, 1982.

15. Iampietro, P.F., Bass, D.E., and Buskirk, E.R.: Diurnal oxygen consumption and rectal temperature of men during cold exposure, J. Appl. Physiol. **10**:398, 1957.

16. Jaeger, J.J., Deal, E.C., Roberts, D.E., and others: Cold air inhalation and esophageal temperature in exercising humans, Med. Sci. Sports Exerc. **12**:365, 1980.

17. Kung, M., Tachmes, L., Birch, S.J., and others: Hemodynamics at rest and during exercise in comfortable, hot and cold environments. Measurement with a rebreathing technique, Bull. Eur. Physiopathol. Respir. **16**:429, 1980.

18. Le Blanc, J.: Man in the cold, Springfield, Ill., 1975, Charles C Thomas, Publisher.

19. Matsui, H., Shimaoka, K., Miyamura, M., and others: Seasonal variation of aerobic work capacity in ambient and constant temperature. In Folinsbee, L.J., and others, editors: Environmental stress, New York, 1978, Academic Press, Inc.

20. McArdle, W.D., Magel, J.R., Lesmes, G.R., and others: Metabolic and cardiovascular adjustment to work in air and water at 18, 25 and 33° C, J. Appl. Physiol. **40**:85, 1976.

21. Milan, F.A., Elsner, R.W., and Rodahl, K.: Thermal and metabolic responses of men in the Antarctic to a standard cold stress, J. Appl. Physiol. **16**:401, 1961.

22. O'Hara, W.J., Allen, C., and Shephard, R.J.: Loss of body weight and fat during exercise in a cold chamber, Eur. J. Appl. Physiol. **37**:205, 1977.

23. O'Hara, W.J., Allen, C., Shephard, R.J., and others: Fat loss in the cold—a controlled study, J. Appl. Physiol. **46**:872, 1979.

24. Patton, J.F., and Vogel, J.A.: Effects of acute cold exposure on sub-maximal endurance performance, Med. Sci. Sports Exerc. **16**:494, 1984.

25. Prinay, F., Deroanne, R., and Petit, J.M.: Influence of water temperature on thermal, circulatory and respiratory responses to muscular work, Eur. J. Appl. Physiol. **37**:129, 1977.

26. Poulton, E.C.: Environment and human efficiency, Springfield, Ill., 1972, Charles C Thomas, Publisher.

27. Rodahl, K.: Basal metabolism of the Eskimo, J. Nutr. **48**:359, 1952.

28. Rodahl, K.: Human performance in the cold. In Spector, H., Brozek, J., and Peterson, M.S., editors: Performance capacity, Washington, D.C., 1961, U.S. Department of the Army, Quartermaster Food and Container Institute.

29. Scholander, P.F., Hammel, H.T., Andersen, K.L., and others: Metabolic acclimation to cold in man, J. Appl. Physiol. **12**:1, 1958.

30. Suzuki, Y., Tsukagoshi, K., Amemiya, T., and others: Effect of alteration of peripheral blood flow on the central circulation in man during supine cycling in different ambient temperatures, Eur. J. Appl. Physiol. **45**:69, 1980.

31. Thompson, G.E.: Physiological effects of cold exposure. In Robertshaw, D., editor: Environmental physiology II, Baltimore, 1977, University Park Press.

32. Webster, A.J.F.: Physiological effects of cold exposure. In Robertshaw, D., editor: Environmental physiology I, Baltimore, 1974, University Park Press.

33. Webster, A.J.F.: Adaptation to the cold. In Robertshaw, D., editor: Envrionmental physiology I, Baltimore, 1974, University Park Press.

SUGGESTED READINGS

Bergh, U.: Human power at subnormal body temperatures, Acta Physiol. Scand. (Suppl.) **478:**1, 1980.

Frisancho, A.R.: Human adaptation: a functional interpretation, St. Louis, 1979, The C.V. Mosby Co.

Le Blanc, J.: Man in the cold, Springfield, Ill., 1975, Charles C Thomas, Publisher.

Thompson, G.E.: Physiological effects of cold exposure. In Robertshaw, D., editor: Environmental physiology II, Baltimore, 1977, University Park Press.

Webster, A.J.F.: Physiological effects of cold exposure. In Robertshaw, D., editor: Environmental physiology I, Baltimore, 1974, University Park Press.

Webster, A.J.F.: Adaptation to the cold. In Robertshaw, D., editor: Environmental physiology I, Baltimore, 1974, University Park Press.

CASE STUDY 1

I remember standing at the starting line of my first long-distance competition (5 miles) on a cold winter day (20° F, 7° C) in Pittsburgh, Pennsylvania. I was a newcomer to road racing although a middle-aged adult. My entire concentration in preparation for the race was focused on weekly mileage and completion of the race distance with a minimum of discomfort. Clothing was the least of my considerations before the race so when I awoke to an unusually cold day, I stuffed every cold weather item available in my car. Feeling the cold air on my face completely counteracted any logic that could have been expected of a person of my training. There at the starting line, with several other novices dressed like members of Admiral Byrd's Arctic Expedition, I remember looking smugly at the experienced runners and thinking "look at those macho, foolish optimists." They were standing in shorts and light shirts, some condescending to long sleeves and a wool hat.

The race started and my competitive instincts caused me to run the first mile a full minute faster than planned. That was only the beginning. It wasn't long before it was clear that I was going to have to discard some clothing. Sweating was profuse and my rectal temperature was 102° F (39° C). My only intelligent action of the day was stopping to remove all but my shorts, shoes, T-shirt, and wool cap. As I crossed the finish line I looked more like a runner and learned a valuable lesson concerning exercise in the cold, fortunately without harmful effects to myself. Military reports indicate that it is not rare to admit recruits to hospitals with heat stroke after they have been working hard in an environmental temperature of −40° F (−40° C). I was lucky.

This experience helped when I later entered a 10 km race in Cheyenne, Wyoming in which the temperature with windchill was −52° F (−47° C). At such a temperature, exposed flesh can freeze within 1 minute. The primary problem was to cover the skin to protect against frostbite and still allow for heat dissipation. I covered my face with a bandana so that, with a wool cap pulled down, only my eyes were exposed. A light nylon jacket was worn over a cotton long-sleeved shirt. The jacket protected against the wind and an open collar and waist allowed the heat to leave, similar to the effect achieved by the Eskimo parka, that is, a chimney effect. The cotton shirt provided warmth and facilitated sweat evaporation from the skin (as does wool). Cotton and wool wick sweat from the skin so that it doesn't become excessively chilled. The uniform was completed by placing nylon wind pants over regular shorts and long underwear.

I stopped at the aid stations to drink because the water loss can't be underestimated in the cold. (Also, the incidence of frostbite is increased with dehydration.) To be perfectly honest, it wasn't the most comfortable race I've been in, nor will I do it again, but I felt perfectly safe and suffered no aftereffects.

CASE STUDY 2

Mountains provide the outdoors person with many recreational possibilities —backpacking, hunting, fishing, climbing, and skiing, to name just a few. Behind the beauty and the recreational possibilities lurk a number of dangers, however. The effects of altitude are certainly significant and are discussed in the next chapter. Other dangers include polluted drinking water, solar radiation, and hypothermia. Along with an increase in altitude comes a drop in average temperature. Thus, a rather pleasant day in Denver, Colorado (elevation 5,280 feet) can become quite cool at 12,000 feet. On almost any summer day in the Rocky Mountains a scenario similar to the following can happen.

The day began with a pleasant morning temperature of 70° F (20° C). Two friends began a long day hike (15 miles) to a lake for lunch and were to return before dark. Their backpacks contained two sandwiches, two cans of pop, and two light windbreakers. The morning hike went well, and they covered approximately 7.5 miles in 4 hours. Since the morning trek was uphill, the two relatively unfit hikers were working at 70% $\dot{V}o_2$ max. The light lunch consisting of about 400 kcal could not possibly compensate for the 1500 kcal consumed during the hike. Additionally, the morning sun and hard exercise caused a mild dehydration as a result of sweating that was not compensated for by one can of pop. During the lunch break the sky clouded over quickly and the threat of rain loomed.

The two hikers decided to return to the trail head 7.5 miles away. No sooner had they started than a cold, mountain shower began. Windbreakers were soon soaked and ineffective, and even standing under trees could not decrease the growing hypothermia. Dry-bulb temperature had dropped quickly 48° F (9° C). Both hikers were soon quite fatigued because of poor fitness and also a growing hypoglycemia. All factors were contributing to a drop in rectal temperature. Severe shivering and fatigue caused the hikers to stop, losing an important mechanism for heat production. Conversation became irrational, and one hiker decided to go ahead and leave the other, more symptomatic partner behind.

Fortunately, an experienced hiker came along the trail to find the incapacitated hiker barely conscious. A tent was quickly pitched, a fire started, and the symptomatic hiker stripped and placed in a sleeping bag in the tent. The hiking partner, regaining some sense, returned to be placed by the fire. Both were given hot Tang, and after 2 hours of rewarming, they regained body temperature and blood glucose levels and recovered from the previous fatigue. Both hikers eventually walked back to their automobile intact without serious side effects.

The altitude, rain, fatigue, dehydration, and hypoglycemia coupled with a rather moderate temperature resulted in a potentially lethal hypothermia. Fortunately, an experienced backpacker was present to save two inexperienced hikers. The possibility of hypothermia must be anticipated, even in the summer, when enjoying the mountains.

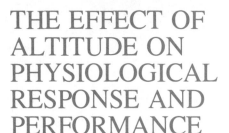

chapter 17

THE EFFECT OF ALTITUDE ON PHYSIOLOGICAL RESPONSE AND PERFORMANCE

MAJOR LEARNING OBJECTIVE

Decreasing barometric pressure with increasing altitude results in decreased partial pressure of oxygen. Altitude acclimatization involves increasing pulmonary ventilation, hemoglobin concentration, and capillary density. Altitude exposure above 1,524 meters (5,000 feet) results in a decrease in aerobic capacity and performance.

APPLICATIONS

Quick ascents to high altitude can result in acute mountain sickness and, perhaps, high altitude pulmonary edema. Exercise can increase symptomatology. Administration of acetazolamide and gradual ascent to high altitude result in reduced symptomatology. There is no known way to reverse the effects of altitude on aerobic mechanisms.

ALTHOUGH our knowledge of the possible deleterious effects of ascending to high altitudes has been recognized for some time, the formal collection of this knowledge has occurred in the relatively recent past. Angello Musso, a well-known Italian physiologist, was one of the first to conduct research in the mountains.[41] In 1894, he and his colleagues made their first expedition to Monte Rosa, altitude 4,600 meters (15,093 feet).

Today, more than 10 million people live at altitudes above 3,658 meters (12,000 feet), mostly in the Andes and Himalayas. The expanding world population makes the possibility of high altitude habitation more likely. Additionally, increased human mobility has resulted in more frequent high altitude recreational sojourns, for example, Mt. McKinley (6,194 meters, 20,320 feet), the tallest mountain in North America, is regularly ascended.

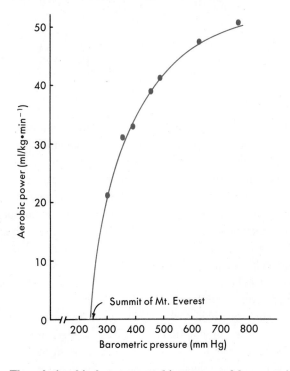

FIG. 17-1 The relationship between aerobic power and barometric pressure. Declining pressure reduces aerobic power. The barometric pressure on the summit of Mt. Everest, thought to be 250 mm Hg., would result in an aerobic power prediction of 5 ml/kg · min^{-1}. (Reprinted by permission of the publisher from Adaptation to extreme altitudes, by West, J.B. In Horvath, S.M., and Yousef, M.K., editors: Environmental physiology: aging, heat, and altitude. Copyright © 1981 by Elsevier Science Publishing Co., Inc.)

427

Mt. Everest, on the other hand, the tallest peak in the world at 8,848 meters (29,030 feet), is rarely ascended. In fact, the first successful attempt was not made until the British team reached the summit in 1953. Arguments have been made about the actual altitude of the summit and whether the barometric pressure is 250 or 235 mm Hg. To the laymen, such an argument seems esoteric. But to the climber or the scientist, the 15 mm Hg difference can cause an already dangerously low aerobic power to be reduced by one-half, that is, from 10 to 15 ml/kg · min^{-1}.[68] Figure 17-1 illustrates the decline in aerobic power with decreasing barometric pressure. West[68] predicts this capacity to be 5 ml/kg · min^{-1} for a 70-kilogram climber at 250 mm Hg barometric pressure.

This chapter probes human understanding of the physiological and performance response during exposure to altitude. A review of the material in Chapter 6 is helpful to reacquaint us with the measurements and terminology of pulmonary physiology.

The following should prove helpful when translating feet to metric and torr units.

Feet	Meters	Torr (mm Hg)
0	0	760
5,000	1,524	620
10,000	3,048	523
20,000	6,096	349
30,000	9,144	226

ALTITUDE—THE PROBLEM

The physical strain imposed on the body with increasing altitude is caused by decreasing barometric pressure. In other words, hypoxia is caused by the declining pressure. The problem is not a lack of oxygen, as such, since the percentage of oxygen in environmental air remains at 20.9% to an extremely high altitude. The problem, instead, is a matter of the decreased tension placed on the oxygen molecules with declining pressure. As described in an earlier chapter, oxygen tension (P_{O_2}) can be calculated by multiplying the barometric pressure times the percentage of oxygen in the air. For example, in Laramie, Wyoming at an altitude of 7,200 feet and an average barometric pressure of 580 torr, the atmospheric P_{O_2} is approximately 121 mm Hg. At sea level in San Diego, for example, the average atmospheric P_{O_2} would be 159 mm Hg. Oxygen molecules at high altitude are less concentrated, thus we sometimes speak of the "thinner" air.

The decreased P_{O_2} in the atmospheric air, in turn, decreases alveolar oxygen tension ($P_{A_{O_2}}$). Hence, the hypoxia is caused by the difficulty of loading oxygen into the blood under the low pressure conditions. Figure 17-2 shows the decline in the saturation of arterial blood with oxygen ($S_{a_{O_2}}$) as the altitude is increased. The purpose of this section of the chapter is to describe how the body responds to a hypoxic stimulus, acutely and chronically, both in physiological and performance terms.

The study of hypoxia

Four procedures have been used to study hypoxia. First, hypoxia can be studied naturally by exposing subjects to terrestrial altitudes such as Pike's Peak (4,300 meters, 14,108 feet). When the biological effects of the total altitude environment are under study, this procedure is used. When, however, only the hypoxia, as such, is under study, a hypobaric (low pressure) chamber is the method of choice. In this case, mobility is limited but hypoxia can be closely controlled. A third method has also been used in which the percentage of oxygen inspired by the subject is manipulated. In this way, altitude can be simulated. For instance, if the altitude of Mt. Everest were to be simulated, a gas mixture containing 7% oxygen would be administered to the subject. Figure 17-3 shows the relationship of oxygen percentage to altitude and barometric pressure. Fourth, the effects of altitude have been studied by measuring responses of those people raised or living at higher altitudes.

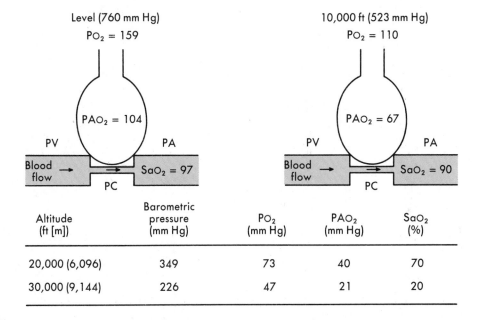

Altitude (ft [m])	Barometric pressure (mm Hg)	PO$_2$ (mm Hg)	PAO$_2$ (mm Hg)	SaO$_2$ (%)
20,000 (6,096)	349	73	40	70
30,000 (9,144)	226	47	21	20

FIG. 17-2 Illustration of the relationship between the partial pressure of atmospheric oxygen (PO$_2$), alveolar oxygen (PAO$_2$), and the percent saturation of arterial blood with oxygen (SaO$_2$) at sea level (760 mm Hg) and at 10,000 feet (523 mm Hg). Blood flow moves through the pulmonary vein (PV), past the alveoli in the pulmonary capillaries (PC), and into the pulmonary artery (PA). The same relationships are also shown for 6,080 and 9,120 meters (20,000 and 30,000 feet). (From Folk, G.E., Jr.: Introduction to environmental physiology, Philadelphia, 1966, Lea & Febiger.)

PHYSIOLOGICAL RESPONSE TO ALTITUDE
Pulmonary ventilation

The first acute response to altitude exposure is an increase in pulmonary ventilation ($\dot{V}E$). This homeostatic response results from the body's need to increase the arterial saturation of oxygen. The resting ventilation does not begin to rise significantly, however, until alveolar oxygen tension (P_{AO_2}) reaches 60 mm Hg (see Figure 17-4). This represents an altitude greater than 3,048 meters (10,000 feet). Increased $\dot{V}E$ is attributed mostly to an increase in tidal volume rather than respiratory rate. Hypoxia stimulates the carotid bodies, causing the elevated $\dot{V}E$.[25] Contrary to popular belief, acute altitude exposure causes the body to become more alkaline. The increase in breathing causes increased CO_2 removal (respiratory alkalosis), which increases blood pH above 7.4. After a period of time, the kidney normalizes the pH by increasing bicarbonate excretion.[17]

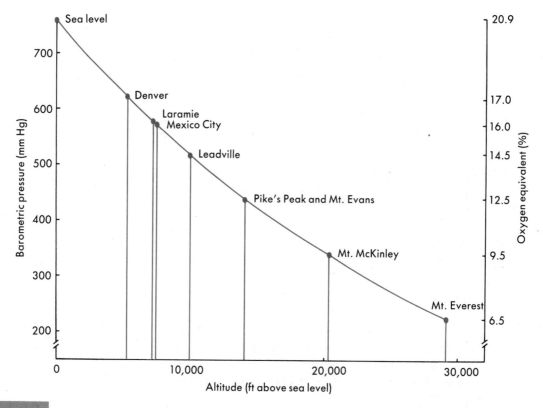

The approximate barometric pressure and the percent oxygen equivalents of various terrestrial altitudes are depicted. (From Consolazio, C.F., Johnson, R.E., and Pecora, L.J.: Physiological measurements of metabolic functions in man, New York, 1963, McGraw-Hill Book Co.)

Most studies have observed an increase of maximal $\dot{V}E$ at moderate altitude.[7,21,27,47] This is true in women[47] as well as men. One exception was a group of college basketball players who resided at 1,000 meters (3,200 feet) and showed no change on short-term exposure to 2,200 meters (7,200 feet).[50] There was an increase in maximal ventilatory equivalent, however, indicating that more ventilation was required for the same oxygen consumption. Parallel increases in noradrenaline and pulmonary ventilation have been observed during exercise at 14% oxygen (3,048 meters, 10,000 feet).[7] Since noradrenaline levels were unchanged during normoxia (20.9% O_2), it is possible that this catecholamine potentiates the exercise ventilatory response at altitude.

Some investigators have observed increases in maximal pulmonary ventilation at high altitude (>4,000 meters) compared to sea level,[6,35] and other investigators have observed no increase.[19,45] In the latter study, no differences were found in a group of women, all experienced climbers and members of the American Women's Himalayan Expedition.[19] This experiment simulated an altitude of 4,100 meters (13,452 feet) and resulted in a decrease in aerobic power similar to that seen in men. Variability may be related to the variability of high altitude symptomatology among subjects, that is, those with more symptoms may be less willing to push themselves to high exercise intensities.

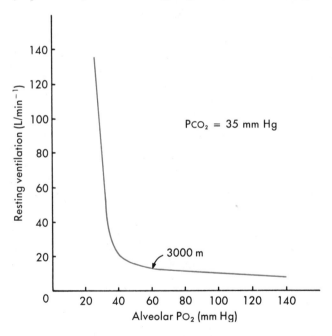

FIG. 17-4 Characterization of the response of resting ventilation as a function of the decline in the alveolar oxygen tension (P_{AO_2}). Note that the curve assumes a P_{CO_2} of 35 mm Hg and that the threshold for increased ventilation occurs at about 3,040 meters (10,000 feet) or 60 mm Hg. (From Scroggin, C.H., Hyers, T.M., Reeves, J.T., and others: High altitude pulmonary edema in the children and young adults of Leadville, Colorado, N. Engl. J. Med. *297*:1269, 1977.)

Oxygen consumption

Absolute submaximal oxygen consumption appears to be unaffected by hypoxia imposed at 4,300 meters (14,108 feet) in men exercising at low to moderate levels.[31] When the working intensity is adjusted to the same percentage of maximal $\dot{V}O_2$ used at sea level, endurance capacity exceeds the sea level performance.[43] Therefore, if exercise is adjusted accordingly, the oxygen delivery system in men seems to function efficiently, and endurance capacity at low to moderate intensities is surprisingly high.

It is clear that aerobic power is seriously affected by hypoxia in both men and women. Decreases in $\dot{V}O_2$ max between -2% and -34% have been recorded at altitudes between 1,524 meters (5,000 feet) and 4,572 meters (15,000 feet).* In fact, a decrease of 3.2% $\dot{V}O_2$ max for each 300-meter (980-foot) increase in elevation above 1,600 meters (5,250 feet) has been estimated[6] (see Figure 17-5).

Although it is indisputable that aerobic power declines with increasing altitude, the varibility in the threshold for significant change may not have been definitively estab-

*References 8, 18, 19, 27, 45, 47.

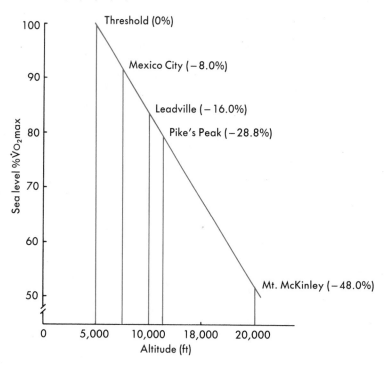

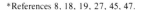

FIG. 17-5   **Buskirk and others[6] plotted the data of several investigations. A regression line predicts the threshold for a decrease in $\dot{V}O_2$ max at 1,600 meters (5,000 feet) and that the decline proceeds at a rate of 3.2% for each additional 300 meters (1,000 feet). For example, aerobic power is predicted to decline by 8.0% at Mexico City (2,280 meters or 7,500 feet) and by 28.8% on Pike's Peak (4,286 meters or 14,100 feet).**

lished. Residence altitude, physical condition, and method of testing may affect the results. A 17.4% $\dot{V}o_2$ max decrease was observed in male runners at 2,300 meters (7,544 feet).[1] A decrease of 10% to 13% $\dot{V}o_2$ max was observed for women at about the same altitude.[47] However, two other studies report declines of 2% and 1% $\dot{V}o_2$ max in swimmers and basketball players, respectively.[20,50] The prediction line discussed (3.2%/500 meters)[6] does not show a standard error, but the plotted points would suggest that the $\dot{V}o_2$ max at 2,300 meters (7,544 feet) could be anywhere between 85% and 100% of sea level values. This variability of response suggests that certain individuals or groups may display characteristics resistant to the hypoxia of moderate altitude. This question should be investigated further.

Cardiac output

Investigations examining cardiac output during submaximal exercise at altitude have produced conflicting results. Some found no change,[55,57] others observed a decrease,[2,66] and others have observed an increase.[65] The data from the third investigation are shown in Figure 17-6 along with the comparable stroke volumes. It can be seen that stroke

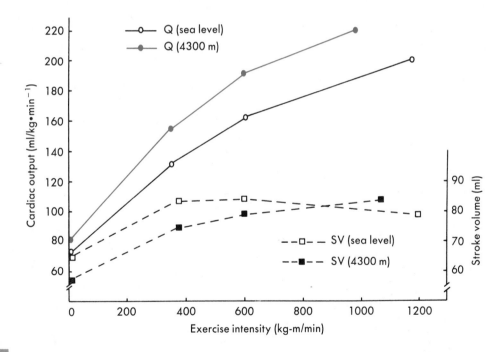

FIG. 17-6   The change in cardiac output ($\dot{Q}$) and stroke volume (SV) with increasing exercise intensity both at sea level (open symbols) and at 4,300 meters (14,108 feet; closed symbols). (From Vogel, J.A., and Hansen, J.E.: Cardiovascular function during exercise at high altitude. In Goddard, R.F., editor: The effect of altitude on physical performance, Chicago, 1966, The Athletic Institute.)

volume values during low exercise intensities at 4,300 meters (14,108 feet) are below sea level values. At the same time, the cardiac outputs are higher. This result was achieved through an overcompensation by the heart rate. Stroke volume is thought to decline at high altitude partly because of a decrease in plasma volume.[46] Failure of the heart rate to overcompensate could cause variable results in the cardiac output response.[42]

The decrease in maximal cardiac output commonly observed at high altitude is a function of a decline in maximal stroke volume and a variable decrease in maximal heart rate.[55,57,66]

Anaerobic response

Although aerobic processes do not appear to be affected when a person performs submaximal exercise at altitude, this is apparently not the case for the glycolytic pathway. For example, one investigator[63] instructed subjects to ride a bicycle ergometer for 20 minutes at a submaximal load (750 kp-m $\cdot$ min^{-1}) while exposed to simulated altitude (4,550 meters, 14,929 feet) in a hypobaric chamber. Significant increases in blood lactic acid concentration were reported. Similar increases have been reported by others.[37] This is not surprising, since lower oxygen tension requires a higher contribution from glycolysis than at sea level.

In contrast, most investigators report a decrease in maximal lactate production at high altitude.[12,18,45] These results, all involving male subjects, indicate a decrease in activity of the glycolytic pathway as well as decreased availability of bicarbonate for lactate buffering. However, an increase in maximal lactate was found in trained women climbers.[19] The majority of data indicate a declining anaerobic power at altitude. Despite these findings, anaerobic performance such as sprinting, discussed in a later section, does not seem to be affected by exposure to hypoxia.

Hemoglobin, hematocrit, and blood glucose

Hemoglobin and hematocrit levels are both increased by acute exposure to altitude, primarily due to dehydration.[25] This would be expected given the need to maximize the oxygen-carrying capacity of the blood.

Blood glucose levels are depressed at high altitude (3,650 meters, 11,976 feet) and the normal rise in free fatty acid levels during exercise is potentiated.[62]

ACCLIMATIZATION TO ALTITUDE

Acclimatization can be both short and long term. Short-term acclimatization is usually characterized by altitude exposure less than a year and perhaps as short a period as 3 to 6 weeks. Long-term acclimatization can include those groups who have lived at altitude from 1 to many years and those who are natives of altitude, perhaps for generations. Those having lived at altitude from 1 to many years can be further differentiated into those who were acclimatized as adults and those who were acclimatized during the developmental growth period. Various acclimatization responses may be expected depending on the characteristics of the group examined, that is, duration and timing of exposure.

Generally, physiological changes associated with acclimatization can be classified into fast response, occurring within a few weeks, and slow response, occurring over many years.[40] A typical fast acclimatization response is the reflex hyperventilation observed almost immediately on high altitude exposure.[40] Additionally, hemoglobin[25] and hematocrit levels have been observed to make an adaptive response (increase) within 3 weeks of exposure to altitude.[65] Slow acclimatization responses involve hypertrophy of tissues and cells and changes in subcellular materials.[40] Examples of slow response adaptations are increased capillary density and pulmonary diffusing capacity,[5] and increased concentration of mitochondria and respiratory chain enzymes.[40] Figure 17-7 provides a summarized illustration of short- and long-term acclimatization to altitude and the advantage they offer, that is, increased oxygen delivery to the tissues.

This section addresses three questions: What are the physiological and performance responses to short-term exposures (up to about 6 weeks)? Do highly trained persons have an advantage relative to the acclimatization process? What differences have been identified between newcomers and altitude natives relative to hypoventilation?

Short-term physiological and performance responses

Since we know that acute changes occur at altitude that can seriously limit our performance, that is, aerobic power, it is reasonable to ask if these changes revert with continued exposure. Many variables do return to, or toward, sea level values. However, we cannot expect a variable such as aerobic power to ever return to its sea level value. Figure 17-8 shows the results of an experiment in which middle-distance runners lived at

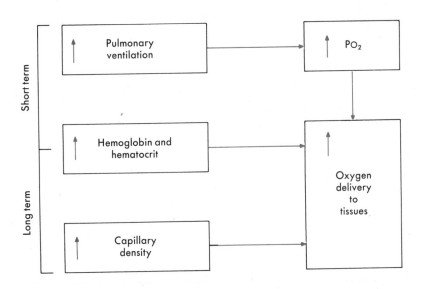

FIG. 17-7   The short-term and long-term acclimatization response to altitude exposure. The biological advantage of this adaptation is improved oxygen delivery to the tissues.

TABLE 17-1 ||||| CHANGES IN ARTERIAL PARTIAL PRESSURE OF OXYGEN
(Pao_2) AND OXYGEN SATURATION (So_2) AT REST AND MAXIMAL
EXERCISE DURING ACUTE ACCLIMATIZATION TO HIGH ALTITUDE
(4,300 meters, 14,108 feet)

	Resting response		Maximal exercise response	
	Pao_2 (mm Hg)	So_2 (%)	Pao_2 (mm Hg)	So_2 (%)
Sea level	93	95	106	96
First week	44	82	45	79
Third week	53	86	55	82

From Vogel, J.A., and Hansen, J.E.: Cardiovascular function during exercise at high altitude. In
Goddard, R.F., editor: The effect of altitude on physical performance, Chicago, 1966, The Athletic
Institute.

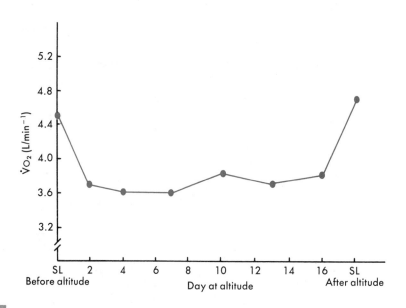

FIG. 17-8   The response of $\dot{V}o_2$ max with 17 days exposure to 3,000 meters (10,135 feet) compared
with before and after altitude values. $\dot{V}o_2$ max is still significantly depressed after 17 days.
(From Dill, D.B., and Adams, W.C.: Maximal oxygen uptake at sea level and at 3,090 m
altitude in high school champion runners, J. Appl. Physiol. *30:*854, 1971.)

an altitude of 3,090 meters (10,138 feet) for 17 days.[18] $\dot{V}O_2$ max made a small return toward sea level values but was still significantly depressed. A partial explanation for this failure to return to sea level values appears in Table 17-1. Although PaO_2 and % SO_2 return toward sea level values after 3 weeks at 4,300 meters (14,108 feet), the change is minimal.[65] Incidentally, cardiac output does return close to sea level values after 3 weeks because of an increase in heart rate at rest and during light exercise and an increase in stroke volume during moderate and heavy exercise.[65] The continued depression of $\dot{V}O_2$ max with exposure indicates that the heart and circulation do not limit the response.

Anaerobic capacity does not appear to return to normal after acclimatization either. Lactic acid measured following an exhaustive bicycle ride after 4 days at 2,300 meters (7,544 feet) was 44% of the sea level norm.[12] After 22 days, the value was further depressed to 51%. Decreased glycolytic activity, therefore, is not positively affected by a 3-week stay at altitude.

Submaximal exercise at altitude represents an entirely different picture. Eight subjects were exercised at the same exercise intensity (75% $\dot{V}O_2$ max) at sea level and following 2 and 12 days at 4,300 meters (14,108 feet).[43] Endurance time increased significantly between sea level and 12 days (62 vs 100 minutes) and between 2 and 12 days (69 vs 100 minutes). These data suggest that the oxygen transport system is not impaired during light and moderate exercise at high altitude. Only when the aerobic system is maximally stimulated does an impairment appear.

Training and acclimatization

Since training promotes circulation and tissue changes related to tissue oxidation, it has been hypothesized that athletes, or highly conditioned people, have an advantage at altitude. This phenomenon was investigated by comparing two groups of newcomers to altitude (4,000 meters, 13,120 feet), one conditioned and the other not, with a group of native (altitude-dwelling) Peruvian Indians.[38] The $\dot{V}O_2$ max of the conditioned newcomers was similar to that of natives at 4,000 meters (13,120 feet) and the $\dot{V}O_2$ max of the nonconditioned newcomers was lowest. In fact, time to exhaustion was higher in the conditioned newcomers compared to natives. However, $\dot{V}_E$ max was highest in the two newcomer groups and the natives showed a hypoventilation response to exercise. The authors concluded that the oxygen transport system of the conditioned newcomers was similar to that of the natives.

A classical study was conducted in which high school track athletes residing in Leadville, Colorado (3,100 meters, 10,171 feet) were compared with a similar group residing in Lexington, Kentucky (sea level).[28] Both groups competed and were tested at both locations. $\dot{V}O_2$ max was equivalent at sea level between groups, and both decreased by 25% at 3,100 meters (10,171 feet). The Leadville group did not show the relative hypoventilation observed in Peruvian natives. The Lexington group won all track events at both altitudes, that is, they were simply faster. The authors concluded that the "handicap of hypoxia at medium altitude is not imposed selectively." In other words, the best athlete will always win at altitude as well as at sea level. But these authors concluded that sea level athletes have an oxygen transport system similar to the acclimatized altitude athlete.

An additional related question can also be asked. Does it make a difference when a person is acclimatized to altitude from birth, migrating during the developmental period, or as an adult? $\dot{V}_{O_2}$ max was compared among three Peruvian groups with these characteristics and a group of lowland residents from the United States visiting at 3,400 meters (11,152 feet).[26] All groups were untrained. There was no significant differences between those born at altitude and those acclimatized during the developmental period. The $\dot{V}_{O_2}$ max of both the Peruvian sea level residents acclimatized to altitude as adults and the U.S. lowlanders was significantly lower than for those born at altitude. This relationship is illustrated in Figure 17-9. Apparently, the most successful adaptations occur when migration to altitude occurs during the developmental period.

THE ADVANTAGE OF ALTITUDE TRAINING

Runners, over the past 10 years, have been interested in training under altitude conditions. They have observed the successful career of Frank Shorter during the 1970s

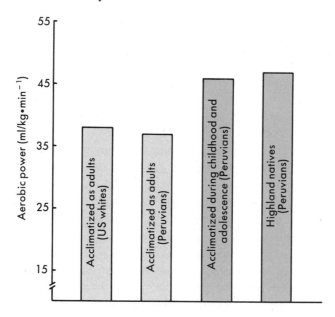

FIG. 17-9   Comparison of aerobic power in two groups acclimatized to 3,400 meters (11,152 feet) as adults (U.S. whites and Peruvians), a group acclimatized during childhood (Peruvians), and a group of highland natives (Peruvians). The group acclimatized during the developmental period made adaptations similar to highland natives. (From Frisancho, A.R.: Human adaptation: a functional interpretation, St. Louis, 1979, The C.V. Mosby Co.)

and associated this success with his residence in Boulder, Colorado. There is some logic, however, in their interest in altitude training. First, altitude acclimatization increases hemoglobin and hematocrit values, which could be expected to improve oxygen-carrying capacity on return to sea level. In reality, the early changes (acute acclimatization) in these variables are the result of hemoconcentration of blood due to decreased plasma volume. Such a change would not improve oxygen-carrying capacity or performance.[13] Second, if sea level training pace can be maintained at altitude, an additional cardiovascular benefit may be realized because of the greater stimulus offered by hypoxia. The converse of this point is also true. Slowing the pace at altitude will provide the same cardiovascular stimulus as at sea level with less joint discomfort.[13]

A related question asks whether an advantage can be achieved in altitude performances by altitude training. This question generated considerable interest when the Olympics were held in Mexico City (2,280 meters, 7,500 feet) in 1968. Both questions, altitude training effects on sea level performance and altitude performance, are addressed in this section.

Sea level performance

Most studies do not support a potentiating effect of training at altitude on sea level performance.[4,6,31,44] Six high school middle-distance runners were taken to 3,090 meters (10,135 feet) and administered six maximal treadmill runs over 17 days.[18] The subjects were tested for sea level $\dot{V}O_2$ max before and after the altitude exposure. Postaltitude $\dot{V}O_2$ max was increased 4.2% above the prealtitude value. It was not clear, however, whether this advantage was a reflection of the hypoxic exposure, the repeated treadmill training, or a combination. Therefore, the experiment was repeated under more controlled conditions.[1] This time 12 middle-distance runners were divided into two groups matched for age, $\dot{V}O_2$ max, and 2-mile run time. One group trained at 2,300 meters (7,544 feet) at 75% of sea level $\dot{V}O_2$ max for 3 weeks and the other group trained at the same intensity at sea level. After 3 weeks, the groups exchanged places and carried out the same training regimen. Using this protocol, training at sea level, without hypoxia, could be directly compared to the combined stimulus of training and hypoxia. Two-mile runs timed initially after altitude exposure were 7.2% slower compared to sea level. The same variable recorded at sea level following the sojourn to altitude was not significantly different from the prealtitude result. Aerobic power was reduced by 17.4% at 2,300 meters (7,544 feet). Figure 17-10 compares $\dot{V}O_2$ max values at the two locations in both groups. For conditioned athletes, training plus hypoxia had no added advantage to training alone.

Altitude performance

The Mexico City Olympic Games in 1968 stimulated considerable interest in the physiological effects of competing at 2,280 meters (7,500 feet) and whether prior altitude training was required. In fact, the U.S. Olympic Track and Field team trained in Alamosa, Colorado at an altitude similar to that of Mexico City. Was this procedure warranted and effective? Nine Swedish Olympic athletes were exposed to the equivalent barometric pressure of Mexico City (580 torr) in a hypobaric chamber.[56] As would be expected, the aerobic power was significantly reduced. Thus, it was hypothesized that all events requiring a high degree of aerobic involvement would be depressed in Mexico City. Another group of American investigators studied performance at an altitude equivalent to Mexico City and found that all events requiring a duration of more than 2 minutes were depressed by 5% to 6%.[21] It was inferred that events requiring less time, and a higher anaerobic component, would not be affected by the altitude.

An improvement in $\dot{V}O_2$ max of 2.6% was observed after 20 days at altitude.[1] Certainly, most athletes would not have the luxury of spending such a long time at altitude and, even then, the 2.6% improvement would most likely be of little practical benefit. Another investigation is instructive on this point.[35] Athletes trained at sea level showed the same physiological and performance decrements at 3,100 meters (10,168 feet) as demonstrated by natives of that altitude. The best athletes won the track events irrespective of their acclimatization.

The psychological factors involved in competing at altitude cannot be discounted, however. A similar altitude race, accompanied with entirely different symptomatology, might be expected to turn out quite differently. A basketball coach who commonly brings his team to Laramie, Wyoming (2,200 meters, 7,200 feet) solves this problem by telling his players that the altitude will not matter because they are playing inside.

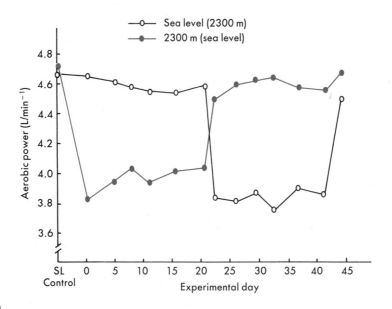

| FIG. 17-10 | Aerobic power measurements in two groups of runners simultaneously training either at sea level or at altitude (2,300 meters or 7,544 feet). The groups demonstrated similar responses at each site, and the hypoxia was not found to potentiate the exercise response. (From Adams, W.C., Bernguer, E.M., Dill, D.B., and others: Effects of equivalent sea-level and altitude training on $\dot{V}O_2$ max and running performance, J. Appl. Physiol. *39:*262, 1975.) |

One problem related to performance at altitude, which has not been directly studied, is the effect of altitude on games, like basketball, which are combined aerobic/anaerobic sports. It is known that more lactic acid is produced during submaximal aerobic activity at altitude.[63] Oxygen debt discrepancies in these games may be more of a problem than we commonly realize. Results of studying a basketball team who travelled to play at an altitude of 2,200 meters (7,200 feet) from a residence altitude of 1,000 meters (3,280 feet) showed no decline in aerobic power.[50] The team did not show an extremely high aerobic power even at 1,000 meters, but they were highly conditioned. It is possible that athletes with well-trained cardiorespiratory systems do not suffer compromises so easily at altitude. Again, basketball is not a sport with a very high aerobic component, like distance running. It could be that the component for these athletes that is compromised at altitude is anaerobic. This topic deserves more research attention.

The Mexico City Olympic results are instructive in that world records were broken in 29% of the sprint events. Such an advance is about average for Olympic competitions. Events lasting longer than 1 minute were depressed by 3%, and those lasting longer than 4 minutes were depressed by 8%. Long-term acclimatization may have been a factor, since the first five runners in the 10,000 meter run were either born or acclimatized to altitude for many years.[10] This finding, however, does not support altitude training for the habitual lowlander nor is it definitive evidence of the advantage of long-term acclimatization.

HIGH ALTITUDE SICKNESS

Recreation at high altitude is not without its hazards. The two clinical entities most common at high altitude are acute mountain sickness (AMS) and high altitude pulmonary edema (HAPE).

Acute mountain sickness

AMS has been observed at an altitude as low as 1,500 meters (4,920 feet) and is observed to some extent in virtually everyone above 5,000 meters (16,400 feet).[25] Symptoms are at their maximum during the first 24 to 48 hours and gradually decline and disappear in 6 or 8 days. Above 6,000 meters (19,680 feet) the symptoms may never disappear.[40] Symptoms include anorexia, headache, nausea, lassitude, insomnia, and fatigue. The symptoms may be less apparent in females[67] and are potentiated by physical activity and the consumption of alcohol.[25] Those persons symptomatic at 3,658 meters (11,998 feet) showed elevated catecholamine levels not seen in asymptomatic persons.[34]

The exact cause of AMS is not known, but it seems to be linked to the hypoxia-induced shift of water from the extracellular compartment to the cells. This shift causes cerebral edema and an increased intracranial pressure[30,53] that is probably related to AMS headache and, perhaps, other symptoms. Treatment includes rest and removal from altitude in the most severe cases. The administration of acetazolamide has been effective in preventing the most severe effects of AMS. Acetazolamide is a carbonic anhydrase inhibitor that leads to an increase in tissue P_{CO_2} and increased $\dot{V}_E$ and Pa_{O_2}.[40] Increasing the Pa_{O_2} removes a major effect of the hypoxia. Another successful method for reducing

\multicolumn{2}{c}{Description of high altitude pulmonary edema (HAPE)}	
Variable	Description
Altitude of occurrence	Usually above 2,736 meters, (9,000 feet)
Time of onset	Within 6 to 36 hours
Symptomatology	
Early	Dry cough, dyspnea, weakness on effort, pain or pressure in substernal area, and occasionally, anorexia, nausea, and vomiting
Late	Noisy respiration with wheezing and bubbling rales, coma in severe cases, tachycardia, and decreased blood pressure
Treatment	Removal from altitude is essential, followed by bed rest and oxygen administration

From Hultgren, H.N.: High altitude altitude pulmonary edema. In Goddard, R.F., editor: The effects of altitude on physical performance, Chicago, 1966, The Athletic Institute.

symptomatology is staging.[25] For example, symptoms at Pike's Peak can be reduced in sea level residents by making an intermediate stop in Denver (1,605 meters, 5,280 feet) for a few days before ascending further.

High altitude pulmonary edema

HAPE is a far more serious and even life-threatening mountain illness. The following box describes the various aspects of this illness.[36] It is imperative that a person showing signs of HAPE be moved as soon as possible to a lower altitude.

TRAINING FOR MOUNTAIN CLIMBING

Every mountaineer has a personal method to prepare for an expedition. Virtually no research has been conducted that indicates the best methods for preparing the body for the rigors of altitude, cold, and heavy physical activity incurred in mountain climbing. However, the following suggestions should be helpful, particularly for the novice climber.[51]

1. Begin training at least 2 months before a climb.
2. Have a complete physical examination, including an exercise electrocardiogram.
3. The training program should stress aerobic power first, and muscular strength, endurance, and flexibility second. Aerobic power can be increased by running, hiking with a pack, cycling, cross-country skiing with a pack, etc.
4. Since mountain climbing involves all the major muscle groups, weight training should involve the arms, shoulders, lower trunk, and legs. Emphasize the antagonists as well as the prime movers and all types of pressing movements.

5. Concentrate on aerobic training 4 days per week and strength training on 2 alternate days.

6. Specificity is important. Use backpacking on foot and skis and actual climbing as much as possible.

SUMMARY

More than 10 million people live at altitudes above 3,658 meters, (12, 000 feet), mostly in the Andes and Himalayas. Opportunities for recreational use of high altitude environments are increasing.

The physical strain imposed on the body with increasing altitude is caused by the decreasing barometric pressure. As the barometric pressure decreases, the oxygen tension declines, making it more difficult to saturate the arterial blood. This decrease in oxygen supply is called hypoxia. On exposure to hypoxia, an increase in resting pulmonary ventilation ($\dot{V}_E$) is observed, usually at altitudes greater than 3,040 meters (10,000 feet). This response leads to an increased CO_2 removal that causes the body fluids to become more alkaline. Maximal $\dot{V}_E$ is increased at moderate altitude in both men and women. Increased exercise ventilation may be related to increased noradrenaline levels. High altitude may or may not stimulate higher maximal ventilation. This may be a result of the subject's inability to demonstrate physiological capacity because of the adverse effects of high altitude symptoms.

Submaximal oxygen consumption in men is unaffected by high altitude (4,100 meters, 13,448 feet) when the exercise intensity at altitude is adjusted to the same relative intensity used at sea level. However, significantly different oxygen consumptions are observed between normoxia and hypoxia (4,100 meters, 13,448 feet) in women. Aerobic power is significantly depressed by hypoxia in both sexes. It is estimated that aerobic power is reduced by 3.2% for each 300 meters (1,000 feet) above 1,600 meters (5,000 feet). Although it is indisputable that moderate and high altitude exposures limit maximal oxygen consumption, the threshold for the production of the effect may be variable.

It is unclear whether submaximal exercise cardiac output changes with altitude. However, maximal cardiac output definitely is decreased. Submaximal lactate production increases at altitude, and most studies indicate a decline in maximal lactate levels.

Acclimatization to altitude occurs initially over the first few weeks (fast response) and also over many years, perhaps generations (slow response). Increased capillary density, pulmonary diffusing capacity, concentration of mitochondria, and respiratory chain enzyme levels have been observed with long-term acclimatization. Hemoglobin concentration and pulmonary ventilation increases are examples of fast-response acclimatization.

Runners exposed to 17 days at 3,090 meters (10,135 feet), showed a small return of $\dot{V}_{O_2}$ max toward sea level values, but these values still remained significantly depressed. Cardiac output values do return to sea level values after 3 weeks at 4,300 meters (14,108 feet). The continued depression of $\dot{V}_{O_2}$ max must, therefore, be related to tissue level changes.

Depressed maximal lactate values do not normalize after 22 days at 2,300 meters

(7,544 feet); in fact, they are depressed by 51%. Submaximal endurance time appears to be improved by 12 days' exposure to altitude. Only at maximal levels of exercise are performance impairments observed.

The oxygen transport system of conditioned altitude newcomers is similar to natives. Athletes from Lexington, Kentucky (sea level) won all the track events against native athletes from Leadville, Colorado (3,100 meters, 10,168 feet) at Leadville. Of course, they won the same events in Lexington. The best athlete wins at altitude even though aerobic performance times are depressed.

The most successful adaptations to altitude are when migrations occur during the developmental period. Natives of high altitude and lowlanders chronically exposed to altitude both hypoventilate during high altitude exercise when compared to newcomers. High altitude natives depend on increased oxygen-carrying capacity of the blood and pulmonary diffusing capacity to maintain oxygen transport.

It does not appear that hypoxia plus training potentiates the effects caused by training alone. Performances at moderate altitude lasting longer than 2 minutes are significantly reduced. Anaerobic performances are essentially unaffected.

Acute mountain sickness (AMS) is observed in people at an altitude as low as 1,500 meters (4,920 feet) and in virtually everyone above 5,000 meters (16,400 feet). Symptoms are at their maximum after 24 or 48 hours and disappear in 6 to 8 days. The symptoms include anorexia, headache, nausea, lassitude, insomnia, and fatigue. The administration of acetazolamide and the use of staging (gradual ascent) reduce the symptoms.

High altitude pulmonary edema (HAPE) is far more serious. Symptomatology is marked by noisy respiration, wheezing, bubbling rales, and coma in severe cases. Removal from altitude is mandatory, and a quick reversal is usually noted.

KEY TERMS

acute hypoxic exposure hypoxia experienced over a period of minutes to several weeks.

AMS acute mountain sickness.

chronic hypoxic exposure hypoxia experienced over a period of months to a lifetime.

HAPE high altitude pulmonary edema.

high altitude altitudes above 3,048 meters, (10,000 feet). The likelihood of both AMS and performance decrements is high.

hypoxia low oxygen content.

low altitude any altitude below 1524 meters, (5,000 feet). The likelihood of AMS and performance decrements is low.

moderate altitude any altitude between 1524 and 3048 meters (5,000 and 10,000 feet). Probable performance decrements and variable occurrence of AMS occur here. Usually the cabin pressure of jet aircraft is kept between 5,000 to 8,000 feet.

torr barometric pressure measured in millimeters of mercury (mm Hg).

REVIEW QUESTIONS

1. How is tissue hypoxia caused at altitude?

2. Explain the mechanism by which the blood becomes alkaline at altitude.

3. Discuss the relationship between increase in altitude and loss of aerobic power. Is there an absolute threshold for loss of aerobic power in all people? Explain.

4. What is the explanation for increased maximal lactate production at altitude?

5. Discuss fast and slow acclimatization to altitude.

6. Knowing what you do about physiological and performance limitations at altitude, how can it be said that the best athletes will always win at altitude?

7. What are the theoretical arguments that support the advantages of altitude training? What does the research support?

8. List the most typical symptoms of AMS. What can be done to modify these symptoms?

REFERENCES

1. Adams, W.C., Bernauer, E.M., Dill, D.B., and others: Effects of equivalent sea-level and altitude training on $\dot{V}O_2$ max and running performance, J. Appl. Physiol. **39:**262, 1975.

2. Alexander, J.K., Hartley, L.H., Modelski, M., and others: Reduction of stroke volume during exercise in man following ascent to 3,100 meter altitude, J. Appl. Physiol. **23:**849, 1967.

3. Astrand, P.O., and Rodahl, K.: Textbook of work physiology, ed. 2, New York, 1977, McGraw-Hill Book Co.

4. Balke, B.: Variation in altitude and its effect on exercise performance. In Falls, H.B., editor: Exercise physiology, New York, 1969, Academic Press, Inc.

5. Buskirk, E.R.: Work capacity of high altitude natives. In Baker, P.T., editor: The biology of high altitude peoples, Cambridge, 1978, Cambridge University Press.

6. Buskirk, E.R., Kollias, J., Picon-Reatigue, E., and others: Physiology and performance of track athletes at various altitudes in the United States and Peru. In Goddard, R.F., editor: The effects of altitude on physical performance, Chicago, 1966, The Athletic Institute.

7. Clancy, L.J., Critchley, J.A.J.H., Leitch, A.G., and others: Arterial catecholamines in hypoxic exercise in man, Clin. Sci. Molec. Med. **49:**503, 1975.

8. Consolazio, C.F.: Submaximal and maximal performance at high altitude. In Goddard, R.F., editor: The effects of altitude on physical performance, Chicago, 1966, The Athletic Institute.

9. Consolazio, C.F., Johnson, R.E., and Pecora, L.J.: Physiological measurements of metabolic functions in man, New York, 1963, McGraw-Hill Book Co.

10. Craig, A.B., Jr.: Olympic 1968: a post mortem, Med. Sci. Sports **1:**177, 1969.

11. Cunningham, W.L., Becker, E.J., and Kreuzer, F.: Catecholamines in plasma and urine at high altitudes, J. Appl. Physiol. **20:**607, 1965.

12. Cunningham, D.A., and Magel, J.R.: The effect of moderate altitude on post-exercise blood lactate, Int. Z. Angew. Physiol. **29:**94, 1970.

13. Daniels, J.T.: Training where the air is rare, Runn. World p. 50, June, 1980.

14. Daniels, J.T., and Chosy, J.J.: Epinephrine and norepinephrine excretion during running training at sea level and altitude, Med. Sci. Sports **4:**219, 1972.

15. Davies, C.T.M., and Few, J.D.: Effect of hypoxia on the adrenocortical response to exercise in man, J. Endocrinol. **71:**157, 1976.

16. Dempsey, J.A., Reddan, W.G., Birnbaum, M.L., and others: Effects of acute through life-long hypoxic exposure on exercise pulmonary gas exchange, Respir. Physiol. **13:**62, 1971.

17. Dill, D.B.: Physiological adjustments to altitude changes, JAMA **205**(11):123, 1968.

18. Dill, D.B., and Adams, W.C.: Maximal oxygen uptake at sea level and at 3,090 m altitude in high school champion runners, J. Appl. Physiol. **30:**854, 1971.

19. Drinkwater, B.L., Folinsbee, L.J., Bedi, J.F., and others: Response of women mountaineers to maximal exercise during hypoxia, Aviat. Space Environ. Med. **50:**657, 1979.

20. Faulkner, J.A.: Training for maximal performance at altitude. In Goddard, R.F., editor: The effects of altitude on physical performance, Chicago, 1966, The Athletic Institute.

21. Faulkner, J.A., Daniels, J.T., and Balke, B.: Effects of training at moderate altitude on physical performance capacity, J. Appl. Physiol. **23:**85, 1967.

22. Faulkner, J.A., Kollias, J., Favour, C.B., and others: Maximal aerobic capacity and running performance at altitude, J. Appl. Physiol. **24:**685, 1968.

23. Folk, G.E., Jr.: Introduction to environment physiology, Philadelphia, 1966, Lea & Febiger.

24. Forster, H.V., Dempsey, J.A., Birnbaum, M.L., and others: Comparison of ventilatory responses to hypoxic and hypercapnic stimuli in altitude-sojourning lowlanders, lowlanders residing at altitude and native altitude residents, Fed. Proc. **28:**1274, 1969.

25. Frisancho, A.R.: Human adaptation: a functional interpretation, St. Louis, 1979, The C.V. Mosby Co.

26. Frisancho, A.R., Martinez, C., Velasquez, T., and others: Influence of developmental adaptation on aerobic capacity at high altitude, J. Appl. Physiol. **34:**176, 1973.

27. Grover, R.F., and Reeves, J.T.: Exercise performance of athletes at sea level and 3100 meters altitude, Med. Thorac. **23:**129, 1966.

28. Grover, R.F., Reeves, J.T., Gorver, E.B., and others: Muscular exercise in young men native to 3100 m altitude, J. Appl. Physiol. **22:**555, 1967.

29. Guyton, A.C.: Physiology of the human body, ed. 6, Philadelphia, 1984, Saunders College Publishing.

30. Hackett, P.H., Rennie, D., and Levine, H.D.: The incidence and importance of prophylaxis of acute mountain sickness, Lancet **2:**1149, 1976.

31. Hansen, J.E., Vogel, J.A., Stelter, G.P., and others: Oxygen uptake in man during exhaustive work at sea level and high altitude, J. Appl. Physiol. **23:**511, 1967.

32. Harris, C.W., Shields, J.L., and Hannon, J.P.: Electrocardiographic and radiographic heart changes in women at high altitude, Am. J. Cardiol. **18:**847, 1966.

33. Heath, D., and Williams, D.R.: Man at high altitude: the pathophysiology of acclimatization and adaptation, Edinburgh, 1977, Churchill Livingstone.

34. Hoon, R.S., Sharma, S.C., Balasubramanian, V., and others: Urinary catecholamine excretion on acute induction to high altitude, J. Appl. Physiol. **41:**631, 1976.

35. Horstman, D.H., Weiskopf, R., and Robinson, S.: The nature of perception of effort at sea level and high altitude, Med. Sci. Sports **11:**150, 1979.

36. Hultgren, H.N.: High altitude pulmonary edema. In Goddard, R.F., editor: The effects of altitude on physical performance, Chicago, 1966, The Athletic Institute.

37. Klausen, K., Dill, D.B., and Horvath, S.M.: Exercise at ambient and high oxygen pressure at high altitude and at sea level, J. Appl. Physiol. **29:**456, 1970.

38. Kollias, J., Buskirk, E.R., Akers, R.F., and others: Work capacity of long-time residents and newcomers to altitude, J. Appl. Physiol. **24:**792, 1968.

39. Laciga, P., and Koller, E.A.: Respiratory, circulatory and ECG changes during acute exposure to high altitude, J. Appl. Physiol. **41:**159, 1976.

40. Lahiri, S.: Physiological responses and adaptations to high altitude. In Robertshaw, D., editor: Environmental physiology II, Baltimore, 1977, University Park Press.

41. Luft, U.C.: Famous fallacies in altitude physiology. In Horvath, S.M., and Yousef, M.K., editors: Environmental physiology: aging, heat and altitude, New York, 1981, Elsevier/North Holland, Inc.

42. MacDougall, J.D., Redden, W.G., Dempsey, J.A., and others: Acute alterations in stroke volume during exercise at 3,100 m altitude, J. Hum. Ergol. **5:**103, 1976.

43. Maher, J.T., Jones, L.G., and Hartley, L.H.: Effects of high-altitude exposure on submaximal endurance capacity of men, J. Appl. Physiol. **37:**895, 1974.

44. Maher, J.T., Jones, L.G., Hartley, L.H., and others: Aldosterone dynamics during graded exercise at sea level and high altitude, J. Appl. Physiol. **39:**18, 1975.

45. Maresh, C.M.: Influence of moderate altitude residents (2200 meters) on the acute mountain sickness and exercise response during early hypobaric hypoxia (4270 meters), Laramie, Wyoming, 1981, University of Wyoming Doctoral dissertation.

46. Merino, C.F.: Studies on blood formation and destruction in polythemia of high altitude, Blood **5:**1, 1950.

47. Miles, D.S., Wagner, J.A., Horvath, S.M., and others: Absolute and relative work capacity in women at 758, 586 and 523 Torr barometric pressure, Aviat. Space Environ. Med. **51:**439, 1980.

48. Montcloa, F., Donayre, J., Sobrevilla, L.A., and others: Endocrine studies at high altitude. II. Adrenal cortical function in sea level natives exposed to high altitudes (4300 meters) for two weeks, J. Clin. Endocrinol. **25:**1640, 1965.

49. Nair, C.S., Gopinathan, P.M., and Shankar, J.: Cardio-pulmonary responses to exercise during acclimatization to altitude and cold, Indian J. Med. Res. **66:**498, 1977.

50. Noble, B.J., and Maresh, C.M.: Acute exposure of college baskeball players to moderate altitude: selected physiological responses. Res. Q. **50:**668, 1979.

51. O'Shea, J.P.: An exercise prescription for mountain climbing, Physic. Sportsmed. **4:**38, 1976.

52. Pace, N., Groswold, R.L., and Grunbaum, B.W.: Increase in urinary norepinephrine excretion during 14 days sojourn at 3800 meters elevation, Fed. Proc. **23:**521, 1964.

53. Peterson, E.W., Bornstein, M.B., and Jasper, H.H.: Cerebrospinal fluid pressure under conditions existing at high altitudes, Arch. Neurol. Psychol. **52:**400, 1944.

54. Politte, L.L., Almond, C.H., and Logue, J.T.: Dynamic electrocardiography with strenuous exertion at high altitudes, Am. Heart J. **75:**570, 1968.

55. Pugh, L.G.C.E.: Cardiac output in muscular exercise at 5,800 meters (19,000 ft.), J. Appl. Physiol. **19:**441, 1964.

56. Saltin, B.: Aerobic and anaerobic work capacity at an altitude of 2,250 meters. In Goddard, R.F., editor: The effects of altitude on physical performance, Chicago, 1966, The Athletic Institute.

57. Saltin, B., Grover, R.F., Blomqvist, C.G., and others: Maximal oxygen uptake and cardiac output after two weeks at 4,300 meters, J. Appl. Physiol. **25:**400, 1968.

58. Sanders, J.S., and Martt, J.M.: Dynamic electrocardiography at high altitude, Arch. Intern. Med. **118:**132, 1966.

59. Schoene, R.B.: Control of ventilation in climbers to extreme altitude, J. Appl. Physiol. **53:**886, 1982.

60. Scoggin, C.H., Hyers, T.M., Reeves, J.T., and others: High altitude pulmonary edema in the children and young adults of Leadville, Colorado, N. Engl. J. Med. **297:**1269, 1977.

61. Squires, R.W., and Buskirk, E.R.: Aerobic capacity during acute exposure to simulated altitude, 914 to 2286 meters, Med. Sci. Sports Exerc. **14:**36, 1982.

62. Stock, M.J., Chapman, C., Stirling, J.L., and others: Effect of exercise, altitude and food on blood hormone and metabolite levels, J. Appl. Physiol. **45:**350, 1978.

63. Sutton, J.R.: Effect of acute hypoxia on the hormonal response to exercise, J. Appl. Physiol. **42:**587, 1977.

64. Timiras, P.S., Krum, A.A., and Pace, N.: Body and organ weights of rats during acclimatization to an altitude of 12,470 feet, Am. J. Physiol. **191:**598, 1957.

65. Vogel, J.A., and Hansen, J.E.: Cardiovascular function during exercise at high altitude. In Goddard, R.F., editor: The effect of altitude on physical performance, Chicago, 1966, The Athletic Institute.

66. Vogel, J.A., Hartley, L.H., Cruz, J.C., and others: Cardiac output during exercise in sea level residents at sea level and high altitude, J. Appl. Physiol. **36:**169, 1974.

67. Ward, M.: Mountain medicine: a clinical study of cold and high altitude, New York, 1975, Van Nostrand Reinhold Co.

68. West, J.B.: Adaptation to extreme altitudes. In Horvath, S.M., and Yousef, M.K., editors: Environmental physiology: aging, heat and altitude, New York, 1981, Elsevier/North Holland, Inc.

69. West, J.B.: Human physiology at extreme altitudes on Mount Everest, Science **223:**784, 1984.

SUGGESTED READINGS

Folk, G.E., Jr.: Introduction to environmental physiology, Philaelphia, 1966, Lea & Febiger.

Frisancho, A.R.: Human adaptation: a functional interpretation, St. Louis, 1979, The C.V. Mosby Co.

Goddard, R.F.: The effects of altitude on physical performance, Chicago, 1966, The Athletic Institute.

Horvath, S.M., and Yousef, M.K.: Environmental physiology: aging, heat and altitude, New York, 1981, Elsevier/North Holland, Inc.

CASE STUDY 1

In June 1977, Carl Maresh, then a doctoral student at the University of Wyoming, and I joined a scientific team from the University of Wisconsin (approximately sea level) on Mt. Evans (4,286 meters, 14,100 feet). The Wisconsin team drove directly from Madison to base camp at approximately 3,040 meters (10,000 feet). They remained there for about 48 hours before moving up to a small shelter-laboratory on the summit. The base camp stop was used to collect some initial data and as an opportunity to *stage* the ascent.

Carl and I arrived from Laramie (2,200 meters, 7,200 feet) on the evening before the move to the summit. We stayed on the summit for the subsequent 48 hours. The staging procedure may have ameliorated the symptoms of acute mountain sickness in the lowlanders but the symptoms were present. Most everyone had headaches, in varying degrees of severity, some were nauseated, and most were anorexic and spent considerable time tucked away in sleeping bags.

During the evening I observed, for the first time, Cheyne-Stokes respiration (named after two nineteenth century physicians, John Cheyne of Scotland and William Stokes of Ireland, who identified this cyclic respiratory phenomenon). This type of respiration, often observed during exposure to hypoxia, is characterized by rhythmical variations in respiratory intensity. Respiration decreases in intensity until total cessation occurs for 5 to 40 seconds. This phase is followed by a gradual increase in intensity, again reaching a point at which the individual sounds dyspneic. Then the pattern repeats itself. Lying awake at night in the shelter on Mt. Evans was reminiscent of a hospital pulmonary ward. A physician, accompanying the team, monitored everyone for signs of pulmonary edema, which did not occur. In fact, no serious medical problems were noted, but at times it seemed a sure bet that one or more of our shelter mates would not take a next breath. They always did.

In contrast to the Wisconsin group, Carl and I were more or less free of altitude symptoms. We did show signs of Cheyne-Stokes respiration, but no other symptomatology was present. In fact, we both continued training at this altitude, since we were preparing for a marathon run in a few weeks.

This exercise experience was interesting because of the grossly increased pulmonary ventilation, which caused us to reduce pace considerably. Our appetites were excellent but we did have trouble sleeping. We didn't know whether to attribute the sleeping trouble to an altitude effect or the suspense created by the respiratory anomalies of our companions. Our relatively symptom-free condition was probably not a function of our physical fitness, since several of the lowlanders were training somewhat strenuously before their arrival in Colorado.

Continued.

Most likely, our advantage was caused by our acclimatization to 2,200 meters (7,200 feet). The exact mechanism of this response has not been investigated extensively. However, Carl, stimulated by the contrast in symptomatology, made this topic the focus of his doctoral dissertation.[45] Seven lowland natives, who resided in Lincoln, Nebraska, were compared with nine moderate altitude natives, residing in Laramie. Comparisons were made at home altitude and in a hypobaric chamber at a simulated altitude of 4,270 meters (14,006 feet). Symptoms, as in the example, were less pronounced in the Laramie residents. Although both groups had decreased aerobic power, the value was reduced by only 15% in the Laramie subjects compared to a 34% decrease in the Lincoln subjects. Experimental data predicted a decrease of 29%.[6] The results of Carl's research indicated that reduced symptomatology over the first 48 hours of exposure may be related to both hormonal and cardiorespiratory differences between the groups at 4,270 meters (14,006 feet).

CASE STUDY 2

The University of Wyoming Mt. McKinley Team was training for a June assault of this 6,177-meter (20,320-foot) peak during the winter months of 1978. Most members were running and cross-country skiing with packs in preparation for the rigors of the Muldrow Glacier route. This is not a highly technical route, but the exertion and windchill exposure in addition to the altitude can be intense. The team, some of whom were lowlanders, met at Estes Park, Colorado (2,280 meters, 7,500 feet) in February. We stayed there over night before the day hike that would bring us within a half day of a winter attempt on Long's Peak (4,334 meters, 14,255 feet). In addition to the Long's Peak attempt, the trip was used to test camping equipment and as an opportunity to practice crampon and ice ax work.

Two of the team members were college students residing at a relatively low altitude level in Idaho and were not highly conditioned. With backpacks loaded for the 3-day trip, the first day's hike began at a trail head at approximately

2,736 meters (9,000 feet). Our destination was base camp, an area at 3,344 meters (11,000 feet), 5 miles away. Before long, the dry trail turned to snow and the trail was steadily uphill. Headaches were common, and the lowlanders were very fatigued. Although it was obvious that these young men were slowing down, the extent of their symptoms was not immediately obvious. After reaching the base camp area, tents were pitched and stoves were lit. It was now late in the afternoon. Only brief stops had been made to rest, and no systematic fluid intake was encouraged. A moderately heavy snow was falling, and the temperature was $-20°$ F ($-29°$ C). After pitching my tent, I noticed the lowlanders standing with their gloves off, staring at an unfolded tent on the ground. They had lost their ability to concentrate on the fairly simple task that confronted them. Mental capacity on Mt. McKinley can be reduced by as much as 50%. Lassitude saps the will, which poses a danger for everyone in the party. Frostbite is not uncommon among persons experiencing altitude, cold, and heavy exertion for the first time. Fortunately, the gloveless climbers were spared this danger by their companions' pushing and cajoling. Rewarming, rest, food, and fluids resulted in a quick recovery.

The next day brought increased symptomatology in almost every member of the party. The symptoms were most likely accentuated by the hard ice ax practice and the attempt at the summit. A number of the expedition behaviors exhibited during this experience were questionable and speak well for climbing groups to practice together under simulated conditions as much as possible. This group learned the following during its trial:

1. The climb should be staged, especially for lowlanders, but others can benefit as well. Strenuous exercise during acute exposure can potentiate AMS.
2. Physical condition is very important for the preparation of climbers. It may not eliminate AMS, but its serious effects can be moderated.
3. Fluid intake must be attended to constantly. Thirst is not an adequate gauge. Dehydration increases the risk of frostbite.
4. Faster, more experienced climbers must be continuously aware of the condition of slower, less experienced companions. Early signs of AMS can be detected and closely followed.

The two Idaho climbers returned home to intensify their training program. In July 1978, they both reached the summit of Mt. McKinley without serious mishap.

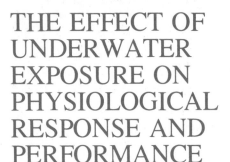

chapter 18

THE EFFECT OF UNDERWATER EXPOSURE ON PHYSIOLOGICAL RESPONSE AND PERFORMANCE

MAJOR LEARNING OBJECTIVE

Divers are subject to extremely high barometric pressures. They experience a decreased heart rate, and oxygen consumption increases as a function of increasing pressure during submaximal exercise.

APPLICATIONS

Diving is a potentially dangerous activity. Hyperventilation before snorkel dives can cause blackout. The duration of scuba dives should be related to diving depth and type of breathing mixture.

■ Hyperventilation is contraindicated before snorkeling. Oxygen breathing during scuba diving can increase diving duration, but mixtures greater than 60% can cause oxygen toxicity.

INCREASED barometric pressure experienced during a descent into deep water is a less common occurrence than decreased barometric pressure (altitude exploration). Man's persistence in exploring the limits of his environment will probably be displayed in seeking the ocean floor. The deepest penetration of the ocean by mechanical means was by Jacques Piccard in 1960 when his submarine *Trieste* reached 35,800 feet below sea level.[30] The probable skin diving limit is around 350 feet; however, an unofficial record is claimed at 728 feet.[30]

This chapter introduces the student to the physiological problems of underwater activity and discusses the implications for underwater sport.

UNDERWATER PROBLEMS

The problem of hyperbarism is also the cause—increased barometric pressure. The sport that makes hyperbarism of concern to exercise physiologists is underwater diving: snorkeling and scuba. Unlike the environmental strains already discussed (heat, cold, and altitude), it is not physiologically possible for humans to acclimatize to the strain of increased barometric pressure. Some mammals, like most diving seals, can descend to depths up to 800 feet with few problems,[9] whereas humans have a limited capacity to exist underwater unless surrounded by an artificial environment, like a submarine. Part of a human's problem in an underwater, high-pressure environment is the limited capacity to store oxygen. Table 18-1 indicates the areas and extent of oxygen storage in the human body. Approximately 2,240 ml can be stored in the lung, blood, muscle, and tissue water.[17] With a resting metabolic rate of 250 ml · min^{-1}, the maximal theoretical limit of breath holding is 9 minutes. Since conscious humans cannot tolerate the full depletion of

TABLE 18-1 ||||| THEORETICAL STORAGE OF OXYGEN IN THE HUMAN BODY

Area	Storage units	Oxygen storage (ml)
Lungs	4.5 L, 16% O_2	800
Blood	5 L, 20 ml O_2/100 ml	1000
Muscle	16 kg, 1.5 ml O_2/100 g	240
Tissue water	40 L, 5 ml/L	200
		TOTAL: 2240 ml

From Scholander, P.F., Hammel, H.T., LeMessurier, H., and others: Circulatory adjustment in pearl divers, J. Appl. Physiol. **17**:184, 1962.

TABLE 18-2 ‖‖‖‖ CHANGES IN ALVEOLAR PARTIAL PRESSURE OXYGEN (P_{AO_2}), NITROGEN (P_{AN_2}) AND CARBON DIOXIDE (P_{ACO_2}) AT 1 (sea level), 2 (33 feet), AND 3 (100 feet) ATMOSPHERES*

	P_{AO_2}	P_{AN_2}	P_{ACO_2}	
Sea level (760 mm Hg)	101	672	40	1 atmosphere
33 feet (1520 mm Hg)	260	1173	40	2 atmospheres
100 feet (3040 mm Hg)	578	2375	40	3 atmospheres

*Oxygen and nitrogen tension varies directly with increasing pressure; carbon dioxide tension is unaffected.

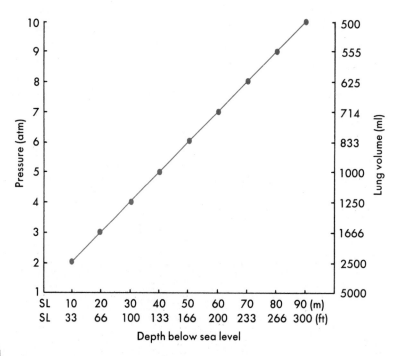

FIG. 18-1 The relationship between increasing depth below sea level and increasing pressure (atmospheres) and the effect on lung volume. As pressure doubles, lung volumes are decreased by half.

oxygen stores, maximal diving time is about 2 minutes. Increased carbon dioxide tension (Pco_2) levels stimulate the need for renewed breathing long before the stores are depleted. Breath holding is further limited when one engages in exercise at the same time.

Barometric pressure at sea level (760 mm Hg) is referred to as 1 atmosphere. Each 33 feet, or 10 meters, of submersion results in the addition of another 760 mm Hg—another atmosphere. Figure 18-1 illustrates the relationship of increasing depth below sea level and increasing pressure (atmospheres) as well as the effect of increasing pressure on lung volume. Since it is compressible, the body and its internal structures are compressed as they are subjected to increasing external pressures. As the pressure doubles, for example, between 2 and 4 atmospheres, the lung volume is halved (2,500 to 1,250 ml). The decreasing lung volume represents another stress of increasing pressure above 760 mm Hg.

Another effect of hyperbarism is the increased diffusion of respiratory gases from the lung into the blood and the increased amount of dissolved gases in the body fluids, especially nitrogen (N_2). Table 18-2 demonstrates the change in the alveolar tension of oxygen, nitrogen, and carbon dioxide during descent from sea level to 33 feet (1 atmosphere) and then to 100 feet (3 atmospheres). Oxygen and nitrogen tensions vary directly with atmospheric pressure, but carbon dioxide tension varies with the release of CO_2 from the blood into the alveoli. Depth does not alter CO_2 release. At 1 atmosphere about 1 L of N_2 is dissolved in the body fluids; at 2 atmospheres 2 L is dissolved and so forth. The deeper the dive, the more N_2 is dissolved. This in itself is not a problem but can be if a very fast ascent is attempted, causing the bends, which is discussed later.

Practical summary. The physiological problem of underwater exploration is directly related to the increased barometric pressure experienced in this environment; there is an inability to store oxygen and a decreased lung volume. Parodoxically, increased oxygen tension results in increased oxygen diffusion into the blood.

UNDERWATER PHYSIOLOGY

Recently, open-sea dives of up to 1,100 feet have been made with use of helium-oxygen gas mixtures.[19] Such diving possibilities have great commercial implications, but they also have scientific challenges, since we know very little about the physiological responses to this strain. A dive of this magnitude represents an atmospheric pressure of greater than 33 atmospheres (25,080 mm Hg).

Seals that are monitored during deep dives show bradycardia, normal blood pressure, and vasoconstriction in the periphery and nonvital organs.[16] Even active muscles have a reduced blood flow, resulting in a highly anaerobic response, with high levels of lactate accumulation. Humans, like seals, show a diving bradycardia[18]; however, some evidence indicates that their exercise response may be more aerobic, with reduced submaximal lactate production.[13,20]

Hypobaric chambers are currently available that can accommodate humans in both resting and exercise conditions, either dry or immersed in water. Some investigations have been conducted in chambers that can alter the barometric pressure but with no possibility of immersion. Pressure and immersion, both experienced by the diver, are separate and unique stimuli.

Immersion at rest is known to increase cardiac output.[8] Placing only the face in cold water produces a bradycardia and an increase in blood pressure.[11] Increased pressure alone causes increased intrapulmonary air turbulance,[14] changes in alveolar-arterial oxygen gradients,[23] increased work of breathing,[22] and decreased ventilation with CO_2 retention.[7] The experiments most applicable to sport diving involve both pressure and immersion stimuli.

Exercise experiments

Some experiments have examined submaximal exercise responses. For example, a group of subjects exercised on a bicycle ergometer at 50, 100, 150, and 200 watts in a hyperbaric chamber.[21] They were tested throughout a range of pressures from 1.45 to 6.76 atmospheres, representing depths from 15 to 190 feet, with and without water immersion. Oxygen consumption ($\dot{V}_{O_2}$) increased linearly with depth in both wet and dry conditions. Respiratory rate and heart rate increased linearly with $\dot{V}_{O_2}$ in both conditions. Immersion alone caused an increase in tidal volume but not increasing depth. Submaximal pulmonary ventilation ($\dot{V}_E$) was depressed as a linear function of pressure. This experiment, like others,[13,20] found an increase in submaximal $\dot{V}_{O_2}$ and a reduction in exercise lactate level. Apparently, the increase in oxygen tension (P_{O_2}) with increased depth results in a more aerobic exercise response. It could be that lactate is more effectively buffered, but there is no direct evidence of such a response. Some have suggested that the increased work of breathing may inflate the $\dot{V}_{O_2}$, but results of one investigation found that when the inspiratory resistance was increased threefold, there was no change in the $\dot{V}_{O_2}$–exercise intensity relationship.[4]

Another experiment studied six men living in a hyperbaric chamber at 49.5 atmospheres (over 1600 feet).[19] The divers' ventilatory function was depressed, and they were rapidly exhausted at moderate levels of exercise from severe dyspnea. However, $\dot{V}_{O_2}$ and heart rate were within normal ranges, indicating that the cause of the exhaustion was probably not circulatory (at 150 and 300 kg-m $\cdot$ min^{-1}: 1.80 and 1.92[1]; 130 and 137 b $\cdot$ min^{-1}, respectively). Dyspnea does not limit submaximal exercise up to 6.76 atmospheres or until the $\dot{V}_{O_2}$ surpassed 2.5 L $\cdot$ min^{-1} or the $\dot{V}_E$ increased above 50 L $\cdot$ min^{-1}.[21]

The physiological response to submaximal exercise with increasing atmospheric pressure is distinguished by an increase in $\dot{V}_{O_2}$, a depression of $\dot{V}_E$ and, at great depths with moderate exercise, exhaustion caused by extreme dyspnea. At 6.76 atmospheres, there is no problem maintaining exercise when the $\dot{V}_{O_2}$ level does not exceed 2.5 L $\cdot$ min^{-1} and the $\dot{V}_E$ is less than 50 L $\cdot$ min^{-1}.

Maximal exercise has also been examined as a function of increasing pressure. For example, $\dot{V}_{O_2}$ max was studied in divers at 1.0, 1.4, 3.0, and 6.0 atmospheres.[12] Values were higher at 1.4 compared to 1.0 and declined at 3.0 and 6.0, but at 6.0 $\dot{V}_{O_2}$ max still exceeded the value obtained at 1.0. Apparently the increased P_{O_2} at 1.4 aided $\dot{V}_{O_2}$ max, but the increased pressure beyond this depth prevented further increases. Two other studies[1,6] showed no differences in $\dot{V}O_2$ max between 1 and 6 atmospheres. Still another investigation,[24] seeking to build on the knowledge of the aforementioned studies, examined $\dot{V}O_2$ max at 1, 4, 7, and 10 atmospheres. Graded exercise to exhaustion on a bicycle ergometer was administered in a hyperbaric chamber. At pressures beyond 4 atmospheres, exercise was terminated by "choking dyspnea" (Figure 18-2). The authors concluded that aerobic power was limited by airway compression, which limited expiration and caused a persistent cough. This work agrees with others who found maximal exercise was limited by dyspnea at 6.76 atmospheres.[21] It was suggested that dyspnea may be due to higher $\dot{V}O_2$ with increasing pressure, increased gas density, CO_2 retention, or a relative decrease in the expiratory reserve volume. At 4.34 atmospheres physical working capacity was decreased between 25% and 33%, again because of severe dyspnea.[5]

A similarity in response between divers and patients with obstructive lung disease, especially bronchospasm in asthmatics, has been noted.[15] Asthmatics display hyperinflation of the lungs, dyspnea in the absence of CO_2 retention, and impaired expiratory flow rates. Hyperbarism could be useful experimental model for studying in the physiological mechanisms involved with obstructive lung disease.

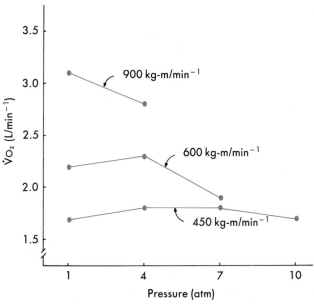

FIG. 18-2   The $\dot{V}O_2$ response during exhaustive tests at 450, 600, and 900 kp-m · min^{-1} while exposed to pressures of 1, 4, 7, and 10 atmospheres. At pressures above 4 atmospheres, exercise is terminated because of severe dyspnea. (From Wood, L.D.H., and Bryan, A.C.: Mechanical limitations of exercise ventilation at increased ambient pressures. In Lambertsen, C.J., editor: Underwater physiology: proceedings of the Fourth Symposium on Underwater Physiology, New York, 1971, Academic Press, Inc.)

Practical summary. During submaximal exercise with increased barometric pressure, $\dot{V}O_2$, respiratory rate, and heart rate are increased, and lactate accumulation is decreased. Fatigue during submaximal exercise with deep underwater exposure and during maximal exercise at most underwater depths is caused by dyspnea.

SPORT APPLICATIONS

The two most common physical activities conducted under hyperbaric conditions are snorkeling and scuba diving. In the former, swimmers use a mask and mouthpiece with an extended breathing tube. To explore shallow underwater areas, a breath is taken and held while the swimmer submerges. About 600 ml of oxygen is available for breath holding after maximal inhalation.[2] Normal breath-holding time is between 30 and 60 seconds. Hypoxia, caused by decreased P_{O_2}, makes the diver come to the surface for a new breath. Underwater time can be extended by hyperventilation before the dive because CO_2 is eliminated. This practice is discouraged because of the increased incidence of blackout.[3] Presumably blackout occurs because reduced CO_2 lowers breathing drive, which in turn decreases brain oxygenation. Skin divers have speculated about the possibility of using a longer tube to allow breathing while more deeply under the surface. However, this would be impossible, since inspiration is not possible at a depth of 2 feet below the surface without a breathing apparatus.[10]

Scuba diving allows breathing below the surface and thus extended diving times. Inspiratory gas must be at a pressure close to the hydrostatic force outside of the chest for inspiration to occur. Scuba equipment allows the delivery of compressed air under pressure. A regulator adjusts the gas pressure to that of the surrounding environment so the diver can inspire. In an open-circuit scuba system, the expiration is released into the water. This rids the body of CO_2 but also gives up the O_2 not utilized by the body. In another scuba system, the closed-circuit apparatus, unused O_2 is redirected back into the body,

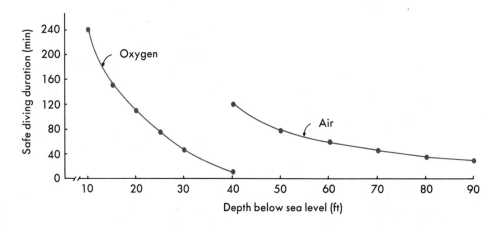

FIG. 18-3   **Safe diving durations as a function of diving depth below sea level using both compressed air and oxygen in scuba tanks.**

and CO_2 is eliminated by sending expired air through a CO_2 absorbent. Air tanks have a capacity of 1,000 to 2,000 L with an approximate diving duration of 30 to 60 minutes. Figure 18-3 shows the relationship of diving depth to diving duration when one breathes air or oxygen from a single 70 cubic foot tank. Oxygen can extend the dive duration.

HAZARDS OF SPORT DIVING

The squeeze

"The squeeze," or high chest pressure, is the chest symptom perceived when the scuba diver holds his breath while descending. Without inspiration, which equalizes the intrapulmonary pressure with atmospheric pressure, the chest would be crushed at a depth of 100 feet.[9]

The bends

The best-known form of decompression sickness (dysbarism) is the bends. At sea level the nitrogen (N_2) in the body tissues is in equilibrium with the atmospheric pressure. As atmospheric pressure increases, more N_2 is forced into the tissues to maintain this equilibrium. N_2 entry into the tissues is a slow process, as is its exit. When the diver ascends slowly, the N_2 has time to diffuse out of the tissues into the blood and eventually out of the lung. However, with a fast ascent the N_2 cannot be removed fast enough, and bubbles form in the tissue fluids.[2] The symptoms caused by these bubbles are referred to as the bends. Bubbles can collect in the small blood vessels causing decreased blood flow, or in the muscles and joints causing pain. Paralysis can occur if the bubbles interfere with the central nervous system. Treatment involves recompression, which decreases the bubble size, and 100% O_2 administration, which increases the rate of bubble elimination.[10] The rate of ascent of the diver should depend on the depth of the dive and the dive duration. If possible, the ascent should not exceed 60 feet/min. For some diving depths and durations, ascending faster than 60 feet/min necessitates decompression.

The chokes

"The chokes" is another form of dysbarism produced by the formation of N_2 bubbles in the venous blood. The bubbles are carried to, and become lodged in, the pulmonary capillaries, causing severe dyspnea.[10] Treatment is the same as with the bends.

Nitrogen narcosis

Another nitrogen-related problem, which should not be confused with the bends, is nitrogen narcosis, also called "rapture of the deep."[9] It involves a different mechanism. When air is breathed at pressures above 3 atmospheres, the inspired nitrogen has an intoxicating effect on the central nervous system. Euphoria and an inability to concentrate set in much as in alcoholic intoxication. At 10 atmospheres the diver can be rendered completely helpless.[2] The breathing of helium-oxygen mixtures can extend the depth and duration of a dive by eliminating nitrogen narcosis, but it does not eliminate the bends, so a slow ascent is still necessary.[10]

Oxygen poisoning

Breathing hyperoxic mixtures below 60% O_2 does not produce harmful effects. However, breathing oxygen mixtures that create alveolar oxygen tensions greater than seven times normal for extended periods, such as 100% O_2, causes abnormal responses. Symptoms include muscle twitching, abnormal breathing, unconsciousness, and convulsions. This entity is called oxygen poisoning and is caused by increased oxygen saturation of hemoglobin in the venous blood. Carbon dioxide transport is disturbed, leading to CO_2 retention and a lowering of pH. Breathing high-oxygen mixtures while diving can be lethal.

Air embolism

Air emboli can be formed by breath holding during a diving ascent. The diver must exhale while ascending. If the breath is held, the air in the lungs expands during ascent, which can cause the lung to rupture. (This condition does not occur in snorkeling, in which the diver descends from and returns to the surface with the breath held.) Air from the lungs enters the pulmonary vein through the rupture and is carried to the heart or cerebral circulation, causing dizziness, blurred vision, or unconsciousness. Although air embolism is not a form of dysbarism, it is treated by decompression to reduce the size of the emboli.[10] If the air exits through the rupture and collects between the chest wall and the lung, a pneumothorax is said to occur. It is sometimes necessary for this air to be removed surgically with a syringe.

Underwater sports are exciting but potentially dangerous. Every attempt should be made to anticipate possible problems and prepare for them.

Practical summary. Snorkeling dives are limited by the decreasing oxygen tension produced by breath holding. Scuba gear facilitates extended diving times but air mixtures can lead to such hazards as oxygen poisoning and nitrogen narcosis. Air embolism can occur when divers do not exhale on ascent.

SUMMARY

Hyperbarism is increased barometric pressure. Unlike altitude, heat, and cold, it is impossible to acclimatize to high pressure. Maximal underwater diving time without breathing support is about 30 to 60 seconds. At that time, P_{CO_2} increases to such a level that a new breath at the surface is required.

Pressure at sea level is approximately 760 mm Hg. Each 33 feet of descent from sea level increases the barometric pressure 1 atmosphere (another 760 mm Hg). Increasing pressure decreases lung volume. Oxygen and nitrogen tensions vary directly with depth, and carbon dioxide level is unaffected by increasing pressure.

Humans exposed to deep dives show bradycardia, as do other diving mammals. Water immersion increases cardiac output, whereas hyperbarism causes intrapulmonary air turbulence, changes in alveolar-arterial oxygen gradients, increased work of breathing, and decreased ventilation with CO_2 retention.

Oxygen consumption during submaximal exercise increases linearly with increasing pressure. Ventilation decreases linearly with pressure. The lactate response to hyperbarism appears to be depressed, which indicates that metabolism is more aerobic. At pressures up to 6.76 atmospheres and $\dot{V}o_2$ and $\dot{V}E$ levels less than 2.5 and 50 L $\cdot$ min^{-1}, respectively, submaximal exercise is tolerated quite well.

Maximal oxygen consumption increases between 1.0 and 1.4 atmospheres, then declines at 3.0 and 6.0 atmospheres but still exceeds the 1.0 response. Values for $\dot{V}o_2$ max at 7.0 and 10.0 atmospheres are depressed because exercise is usually terminated by severe dyspnea. Physical working capacity at 43.4 atmospheres is reduced between 25% and 33%.

Snorkeling, shallow-water diving with a mask and breathing tube, is limited by the swimmer's ability to hold his breath. Usually snorkeling dives last between 30 and 60 seconds, limited by the accumulation of CO_2, which stimulates breathing. Hyperventilation before breath-holding dives is not encouraged because of the high incidence of blackout.

Scuba equipment enables the diver to overcome the human inability to inspire below a depth of about 2 feet. A regulator connected to a compressed air tank adjusts air pressure to that of the environment, allowing inspiration.

The squeeze is high chest pressure experienced when holding the breath instead of inhaling during descent. The bends, a form of decompression sickness (dysbarism), is caused by the diver ascending too quickly. Nitrogen that has diffused into the tissues during exposure to high pressure bubbles out of solution and lodges in small capillaries, joints, and possibly the central nervous system. The resulting pain and paralysis is treated by recompression, which reduces the size of the nitrogen bubbles. The chokes occur when the bubbles lodge in the pulmonary capillaries, resulting in severe dyspnea.

Nitrogen narcosis, "rapture of the deep," is an intoxication caused by breathing air at air pressures greater than 3 atmospheres. Oxygen poisoning is caused by breathing mixtures containing more than 60% O_2. Symptoms include muscle twitching, abnormal breathing, unconsciousness, and convulsions. Breathing helium-oxygen mixtures eliminates nitrogen narcosis but not the bends.

Air emboli are released into the bloodstream or chest cavity from lung ruptures caused by the failure of the scuba diver to exhale while ascending. This condition can be treated with decompression.

KEY TERMS

atmosphere 1 atmosphere is the pressure associated with sea level (760 mm Hg). Two atmospheres is experienced at 10 meters (33 feet) below sea level and is equivalent to the weight of a column of water 10 meters high plus the barometric pressure (1,520 mm Hg).

decompression literally, "to free from pressure"; in underwater physiology, to return the body to sea-level pressure after exposure to deep underwater pressure.

dysbarism decompression sickness, such as the bends, resulting from too rapid decompression.

dyspnea difficult or labored breathing.

embolism obstruction of a blood vessel—in underwater physiology, usually by an air bubble.

hyperbarism increased barometric pressure.

hyperventilation increased air in the lungs above normal. Can lead to respiratory alkalosis due to washing out of carbon dioxide from the blood.

hypoxia low oxygen content.

narcosis unconsciousness.

P partial pressure (tension) of a gas.

scuba self-contained underwater breathing apparatus.

W watts, a unit of power.

REVIEW QUESTIONS

1. Describe hyperbarism in terms of atmospheres.

2. Describe the basis of the pulmonary problem encountered with increasing barometric pressure.

3. How do seals adapt to deep dives?

4. Describe the human physiological and performance response to submaximal exercise underwater. Explain the possible reasons for the lactate response.

5. What is the basis of fatigue during underwater exercise?

6. What is the primary hazard of snorkeling?

7. Contrast diving time associated with the breathing of air and oxygen. What hazard could be associated with oxygen breathing?

8. What is the difference between the bends and nitrogen narcosis?

REFERENCES

1. Anthonisen, N.R., Utz, G., Kryger, M.H., and others: Exercise tolerance at 4 and 6 ata, Undersea Biomed. Res. **3**:95, 1976.

2. Astrand, P.O., and Rodahl, K.: Textbook of work physiology, ed. 2, New York, 1977, McGraw-Hill Book Co.

3. Craig, A.B., Jr.: Causes of loss of consciousness during underwater swimming, J. Appl. Physiol. **16**:583, 1961.

4. Dressendorfer, R.H., Wade, C., and Bernauer, E.: Combined effects of breathing resistance on aerobic work tolerance, J. Appl. Physiol. **42**(3):444, 1977.

5. Dwyer, J., Saltzman, H.A., and O'Bryan, R.: Maximal physical-work capacity of man at 43.4 ata, Undersea Biomed. Res. **4**(4):359, 1977.

6. Fagraeus, L.: Maximal work performance at raised air and helium-oxygen pressures, Acta Physiol. Scand. **91**:545, 1974.

7. Fagraeus, L., Hesser, C.M., and Linnarsson, D.: Cardiorespiratory responses to graded exercise at increased ambient air pressure, Acta Physiol. Scand. **91**:259, 1974.

8. Farhi, L.E., and Linnarsson, D.: Cardiopulmonary readjustments during graded immersion in water at 35° C, Respir. Physiol. **39:**35, 1977.

9. Folk, G.E., Jr.: Introduction to environmental physiology, Philadelphia, 1966, Lea & Febiger.

10. Lambertsen, C.J.: Effects of excessive pressures of oxygen, nitrogen, carbon dioxide, and carbon monoxide: implications in aerospace, undersea, and industrial environments. In Mountcastle, V.B., editor: Medical physiology, ed. 14, St. Louis, 1980, The C.V. Mosby Co.

11. LeBlanc, J.: Man in the cold, Springfield, Ill., 1975, Charles C Thomas, Publisher.

12. Linnarsson, D., and Fagraeus, L.: Maximal work performance in hyperbaric air. In Lambertsen, C.J., editor: Underwater physiology V: proceedings of the Fifth Symposium on Underwater Physiology, Bethesda, Md., 1976, Federation of American Societies for Experimental Biology.

13. Linnarsson, D., Karlsson, J., Fagraeus, L., and others: Muscle metabolites and oxygen deficit with exercise in hypoxia and hyperoxia, J. Appl. Physiol. **36**(4):399, 1974.

14. Murphy, T., Clark, W., Buckingham, I.P.B., and others: Respiratory gas exchange in exercise during helium-oxygen breathing, J. Appl. Physiol. **26:**303, 1969.

15. Permutt, S.: Physiological changes in the acute asthmatic attack. In Austen, K.F., and Lichenstein, L.M., editors: Asthma, New York, 1973, Academic Press, Inc.

16. Schmidt-Nielsen, K.: Animal physiology: adaptation and environment, London, 1975, Cambridge University Press.

17. Scholander, P.F.: Experimental investigations on the respiratory function in diving mammals and birds, Hvalradets Skrifter **22:**1, 1940.

18. Scholander, P.F., Hammel, H.T., LeMessurier, H., and others: Circulatory adjustment in pearl divers, J. Appl. Physiol. **17:**184, 1962.

19. Spaur, W.H., Raymond, L.W., Knott, M.M., and others: Dyspnea in divers at 49.5 ata: mechanical, not chemical in origin, Undersea Biomed. Res. **4**(2):183, 1977.

20. Taunton, J.E., Banister, E.W., Patric, T.R., and others: Physical work capacity in hyperbaric environments and conditions of hyperoxia, J. Appl. Physiol. **28**(4):421, 1970.

21. Thalmann, E.D., Sponholtz, D.K., and Lundgren, C.E.G.: Effects of immersion and static lung loading on submerged exercise at depth, Undersea Biomed. Res. **6**(3):259, 1979.

22. Wood, L.D.H., and Bryan, A.C.: Effect of increased ambient pressure on flow-volume curve of the lung, J. Appl. Physiol. **27:**4, 1969.

23. Wood, L.D.H., and Bryan, A.C.: Mechanical limitations of exercise ventilation at increased ambient pressures. In Lambertsen, C.J., editor: Underwater physiology: proceedings of the Fourth Symposium on Underwater Physiology, New York, 1971, Academic Press, Inc.

24. Wood, L.D.H., and Bryan, A.C.: Exercise ventilatory mechanics at increased ambient pressure, J. Appl. Physiol. **44**(2):231, 1978.

SUGGESTED READING

Lambertsen, C.J.: Underwater physiology: proceedings of the Fourth Symposium on Underwater Physiology, New York, 1971, Academic Press, Inc.

CASE STUDY 1

During the 1960s the U.S. Navy intensified its interest in underwater experimentation. This intensification was stimulated by the greater reliance by the Navy on nuclear submarines and the potential need for underwater rescue. In addition, scientists were interested in human ability to live and work in a deep-sea environment. A series of Sea Lab experiments were undertaken. In Sea Lab II, a submarine-like chamber was lowered to the ocean floor and Navy volunteers spent extended periods (days) living in the chamber. Each day experimental sojourns were planned outside the chamber. The internal pressure of the chamber was equalized to the outside so that the volunteers, in scuba gear, could easily leave the chamber through a port open to the sea. Breathing in the chamber was made possible by a helium-oxygen mixture provided by the mother ship above. The helium mixture caused "Donald Duck" speech, adding comic relief to the serious experiments.

However, this was not the only surprise the subjects provided for the surface-bound experimenters. As a daily ritual, when leaving or returning to the chamber, volunteers were asked to apply maximal force to a torque wrench connected to the side of the chamber. The results were monitored above. The purpose of this small experiment was to follow projected strength loss over the duration of the stay on the ocean floor. Instead of decreased force, however, scientists on the mother ship began to notice gradual increases. After a couple of days, broadcasts from above began to inquire about the fitness status of the volunteers. "Are you feeling any changes in strength, endurance, etc.?" "No, no, we feel just fine. In fact, we feel unusually fit." As the days passed by, strength continued to increase. The scientists above were beginning to dream of future publications, in which long, scholarly conversations speculated on causes. At the experiment's end, with the volunteers being decompressed in a hyperbaric chamber on the deck of the ship, the experimenters began a process of debriefing. Questions about the strength experiments, initially answered with seriousness, finally ended in convulsive laughter and much knee slapping. Puzzled experimenters could not understand why their serious inquiries were met with such disrespect. Finally, the hoax was revealed: working in pairs while conducting the out-of-chamber activities, the subjects decided to work together when it was time for each to take a turn. Each day they would apply a little extra force. The truth ended all fantasies of unique publications and speculation on causes. The playfulness of the human animal is not always compatible with scientific experimentation; on the other hand, it speaks well for human survival instincts under adverse conditions.

Other experiments were far more successful. In fact, human adaptability to underwater life is quite remarkable.

CASE STUDY 2

Hyperbaric oxygenation has been used for treatment of several disorders involving general or local hypoxia. For example, pulmonary edema usually results in decreased arterial oxygenation. Placing a patient in a hyperbaric chamber while breathing oxygen (or given pressurized oxygen) can improve arterial oxygenation. In effect, this procedure increases inspired P_{O_2}, which increases the gradient between the lungs and pulmonary capillaries. Thus more oxygen can be loaded in the arterial blood. Another example is the patient in shock, who suffers from decreased tissue blood flow.

Alveolar oxygen tension increases in proportion to the increase in barometric pressure. For instance, the following calculations illustrate the effect of administering oxygen under pressure on total inspired oxygen tension:

Sea level P_{AO_2} = 1 atmosphere $\times$ 80% O_2 $\times$ 760 mm Hg = 608 mm Hg

Chamber P_{AO_2} = 2 atmospheres $\times$ 80% O_2 $\times$ 760 mm Hg = 1216 mm Hg

With a doubling of inspired oxygen tension, alveolar oxygen tension also doubles. Therefore, the alveolar/capillary gradient is increased.

The major disadvantage of this form of therapy is the possibility of oxygen toxicity. Toxicity develops very rapidly with higher barometric pressures. Therapy usually involves the use of lower barometric pressure and intermittent use of oxygen so that possible toxicity is prevented.

PART FIVE

SPECIAL CONSIDERATIONS

chapter 19

GROWTH AND AGING RELATED TO PERFORMANCE

MAJOR LEARNING OBJECTIVE

Physiological age is a more appropriate measure of growth toward maturity than chronological age. Aging is marked by a decrease in adaptability, but the decrease is more marked in a sedentary population.

APPLICATIONS

Competition is usually based on chronological age, which matches children of vastly different physical maturity. Growth of the skeleton (physiological age) may be an effective means of equalizing competition. Individualized prescriptions for exercise can be applied with small variations to people of all ages.

T**HE** process of growing to maturity has been defined as an increasing ability to adapt.[51] One goal of physical education and sport is to provide activities that promote this adaptation. To accomplish this goal, teachers and coaches should be aware of the physiological consequences of the maturation process. Such knowledge may prevent injury and perhaps supplement natural growth. The first objective of this chapter is to review human biological growth by discussing general growth characteristics, changes in physiological function that are related to exercise and sport performance, and the implications of growth for teaching and coaching.

Extensive changes in attitude have occurred over the last 25 years regarding sport participation during the growing years. This is especially true for the preadolescent years. At one time, physical education did not support preadolescent sport participation. Our culture, however, has demanded earlier participation in sport. Today, most communities offer opportunities for children to play baseball, for example, as early as 6 to 8 years of age. Moreover, most junior high and middle schools offer competitive sports programs during the period of significant pubertal growth. High schools and colleges continue this trend with sport participation when at least some athletes have not completed growth. Many ask whether such activity is physiologically desirable. This chapter addresses this question.

If growth involves increasing adaptability, aging has been defined as a decreasing ability to adapt.[51] Most people reading this book will not have a primary interest in aging by virtue of either their own age or their occupational motivation. The demand for expertise in exercise for aging populations, however, is growing as the population of older persons grows. Sport and physical activity in American culture have most often been associated with youth. Today, we can see a quiet but persistent proliferation of sport competition for seniors and a general interest in movement as an intervention tool to prevent or help in the rehabilitation for disorders common to the aging population. As with children, we can ask whether such participation is safe and capable of promoting physiological function. It might even be asked if exercise can retard the aging process.

EXERCISE AND GROWTH
General characteristics of growth

Perhaps the best way to appreciate the general sequence of growth is to examine the change in stature with increasing chronological age. Figure 19-1 shows this relationship. These data were recorded cross-sectionally (samples of children from each age group) in two separate investigations: St. Louis, Missouri, in 1892-1894[43] and Saginaw, Michigan, in 1963-1964.[35] A linear increase in stature can be seen from age 8 through 17. Also, an increase in stature has taken place over the 71-year period. This *secular trend* is manifested in body weight as well as height, and children reach puberty earlier than in previous generations.[31]

Another way to examine growth data is by the change in growth per year. Figure 19-1 shows the absolute height of children for each age. Such a display does not reveal any change in the rate of the growth process. In contrast, Figure 19-2 displays the same type of data in terms of change per year. It can be seen that both sexes show an acceleration in stature during the period between 12 and 15 years. Thereafter growth decelerates until final maturity. The increase is known as the *adolescent growth spurt* accompanying the onset of puberty.[56] This growth spurt occurs earlier in girls, between 10.5 and 13 years. In boys, it occurs between 12.5 to 15 years.[56] Before puberty, the sexes are roughly the same size. During the period between 10.5 to 13 years, girls tend to be taller. Although the spurt in boys lags about 2 years behind, it attains a greater peak, which to a large extent accounts for the final sex difference in stature.

The adolescent growth spurt in height generally parallels organ growth. Some differences are notable; for example, brain growth is well ahead of the general growth curves. In contrast, heart diameter follows the same pattern as height. This indicates that heart growth is synchronous with general growth, which has implications for participation in

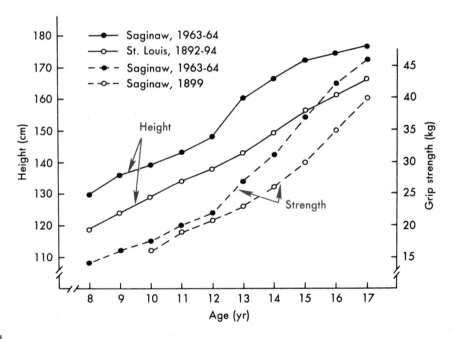

FIG. 19-1   **The relationship of height and grip strength to chronological age. The height data were recorded in Saginaw, Michigan, in 1963-1964 (Montpetit and others[35]) and in St. Louis, Missouri, in 1892-1894 (Porter[43]). The grip strength data were recorded in Saginaw, Michigan, in 1899 and in 1963-1964 (Montpetit and others[35]). Both height and grip strength show a secular trend (increase) from the 1890s to 1963-1964.**

aerobic activities. Figure 19-3 presents the results of an experiment in which heart volume was compared in young competitive swimmers during prepubertal, pubertal, and post-pubertal years.[59] Heart volume corrected for body size (ml · kg^{-1}) was significantly greater during the postpubertal compared to the prepubertal period. During puberty no significant change is noted even though an increase was recorded for boys.

It could be asked what importance these data have for aerobic performance. From a physiological point of view, no difference was observed in aerobic power over the three pubertal periods, when this variable is expressed as a function of body size. Thus, capacity for aerobic exercise is not limited by chronological age or growth stage. In fact, the heart volume data indicate that the training may have a beneficial effect, since the heart is larger than would be expected from body growth alone. This increase is not considered harmful, but performance decisions concerning child athletes should be based on the gestalt of many factors, for example, psychological factors. Teachers and coaches should be cautioned that a child should not be viewed as a small adult.[44] However, from a

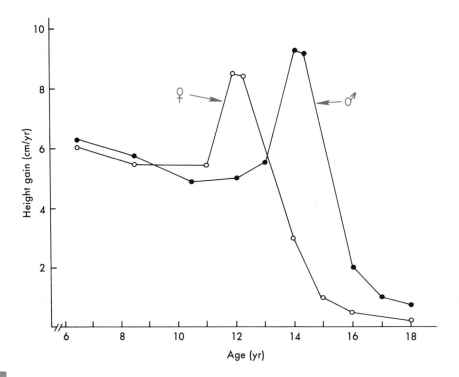

FIG. 19-2   The adolescent growth spurt in boys and girls. Height has been expressed as a rate of change (cm/yr). The growth spurt occurs earlier in girls, on the average at 12 years, than boys, average at 14 years, with the growth peak higher in boys. (Adapted from Tanner, J.M.: Education and physical growth, London, 1967, University of London Press, Ltd.)

strict physiological view, it does not seem that the body is adversely affected by exercise.

Additional physiological variables should also be considered. Figure 19-1 shows the change in grip strength with increasing chronological age. Grip strength increases roughly parallel to the increase in body stature. After age 12, a secular trend is noted, that is, the 1963-1964 data show an increase compared to the data collected in 1899 in the same community. As would be expected, strength increases as the body grows. After puberty, boys tend to become stronger, in absolute terms, than girls.[56] This increase, to a great degree, is related to differences in body size between the sexes. Males do tend to have greater muscle mass from birth, and girls have more fat tissue from birth. These differences are accentuated at puberty as a result of the increase in production of testosterone and estrogen, respectively.[44]

Along with increases in aerobic power during the growing years, other variables are

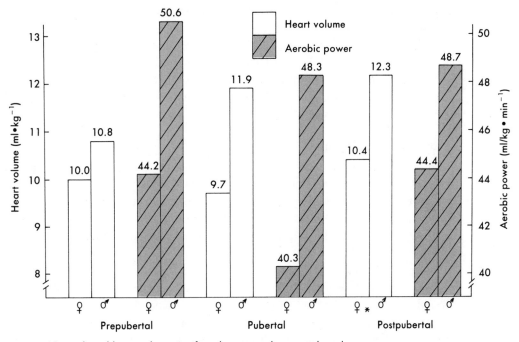

*Postpubertal heart volume significantly greater than prepubertal

FIG. 19-3   A comparison of heart volume and aerobic power in boys and girls classified as prepubertal, pubertal, and postpubertal. No significant differences in aerobic power were noted between groups. Heart volume, corrected for body weight, is significantly higher in both boys and girls in postpubertal compared to prepubertal groups. (Adapted from Wirth, A., Trager, E., Scheele, K., and others: Cardiopulmonary adjustment and metabolic response to maximal and submaximal physical exercise of boys and girls at different stages of maturity, Eur. J. Appl. Physiol. *39:*229, 1978.)

known to increase. Between 10 and 18 years, when aerobic power increases by about 55%, pulmonary ventilation, pulmonary diffusing capacity, and cardiac output increase proportionally—49%, 45%, and 50%, respectively.[60] During this same period, red blood cell and hemoglobin concentrations increase by about 20% in boys.[56] Girls experience less increase, and after age 12, a sex difference can be observed, with boys having larger concentrations. Again, body size differences begin to be apparent at about age 12.

Physiological age

Up to this point the figures presented have been related to chronological age. It is known that children proceed toward and reach puberty at vastly different rates. Thus, two children of the same chronological age can be greatly different in physiological maturity. A measure of the degree to which maturity has been obtained is referred to as *physiological age* (also developmental age). Usually, physiological age is evaluated by progress in the growth of the skeleton. X-rays of bone epiphyses (growth centers), particularly the wrist bones, reveal the progress of the bone toward complete development.[56] It is possible for a female child, for example, to be 14 years old chronologically, but only 10 years old physiologically. At a time when most girls would have reached puberty, such a girl would be significantly behind. Performance expectations would be quite different for a 10 year old compared to a 14 year old. Implications of these individual differences are discussed later.

Aerobic activity and growth

Are prepubescent children biologically handicapped when performing endurance activities? One study examined the response of prepubescent boys to 60 minutes of continuous activity.[30] Heart rate during exercise was found to be lower than adults, with insignificant increases in lactate production. Moreover, the aerobic power of 10-year-old ice hockey players (56.6 ml $\cdot$ kg/min^{-1})[9] was similar to that of adult ice hockey players (55.3 ml $\cdot$ kg/min^{-1}).[15]

Several studies have examined the aerobic power changes of young athletes in training. $\dot{V}O_2$ max was measured in 20 male middle-distance runners over a period of 6 years (all subjects ranged in age from 10 to 18 years).[10] Data supported the view that changes in aerobic power merely paralleled shifts in body size brought on by growth. Similar results were observed in both male and female swimmers (8 to 18 years of age).[59] Exercise blood glucose levels and free fatty acid concentrations were likewise not different between prepubescent and postpubescent swimmers. One study did observe increases in aerobic power, corrected for body weight, in older postpubescent competitive swimmers.[7] The authors attributed the increase to the very heavy training loads placed on the swimmers (3,000 to 5,000 yards per day, September to May, and 8,000 to 12,000 yards per day, June to August) compared to those in other investigations.

The question remains whether children who train during the growth years show improvements beyond changes attributable to growth alone. Young competitive swimmers (9 to 11 years old) were found to increase $\dot{V}O_2$ max by 15% over a 7-month period compared to a 5% increase for nonswimmers.[58] This was a significant difference. A similar result was observed in young cross-country runners (8 to 11 years old).[33] These runners used more fat during submaximal exercise compared to nonrunners. It appears that exercise training supplements the growth changes. There is no evidence, however, that these changes represent "permanent" adaptations that provide an advantage over those who do not train until after puberty. No evidence is yet available that shows preadolescent training to be physiologically harmful.

Implications for teaching and coaching

It does not appear that, from a physiological point of view, childhood exercise and sport are contraindicated after 8 years of age. Few data are available for ages younger than this, and certainly much more can be learned about the age period 8 to 18 years. One area that deserves particular attention is the effect of hard preadolescent training on various orthopedic variables, for example, joint stress and subsequent adult disorders. One study examined the throwing arms of 162 baseball players between 9 and 14 years old. Various skeletal abnormalities were observed in 76 of 80 pitchers. Similar findings were observed in only 7 of 47 other players.[1] A reasonable rule would be to ban those pitches that place undue strain on joints, like curve balls, until skeletal age is more advanced. However, with prudent practice as the key, exercise and sport programs during the elementary years would seem very appropriate, in fact, beneficial.

The junior high and middle school years are interesting and controversial. These years place children in the middle of the adolescent growth spurt. Physiological handicaps, as such, are not indicated, but vast individual differences in physiological age make competition based on chronological age unrealistic. Matching a 14 year old who is advanced in maturity, perhaps with a skeletal age of 18 years, against a child with a retarded physiological growth is less than equal pairing. Competitive groupings would be much more equitable if the critical variable was advancement toward maturity rather than chronological age. Team sports for boys during this period favor those who are more physiologically mature. An interesting paradox exists for girls' sports. Girls who are successful in sports like track and field have been found to initiate menarche (menstruation), an important pubertal point of measure, later than average (13.58 vs 12.33 years).[32] Apparently these sports tend to favor those with prepubertal sex characteristics, for example, less fat. Other studies have not confirmed this hypothesis. It is not known whether delayed menarche is a function of early sport training or just a characteristic of those who succeed in these sports. A sports-induced mechanism would have to show alterations in hormonal release with chronic training.

Swimmers, in contrast, have been found to be advanced in their maturity.[8] Several hypotheses are possible to explain the findings of advanced menarche. For instance, swimming may just attract athletes who are genetically predisposed to early development. The additional fat percentage characteristic of girls after puberty may serve as a flotation advantage. Thus, it is important for teachers and coaches to remember that capacities may not be the same for two persons of the same chronological age. This has implications for team selection and class groupings. Physiological age may be an important criterion. Such information also mitigates the use of rigid norms for children in this age group.

Classical investigations were conducted by Hale[19] in 1956 and Krogman[27] in 1959. They recorded the physiological ages of boys participating in the Little League Baseball World Series. The boys were found to be skeletally more mature than average for their chronological age group. In addition, the more mature boys tended to play the most critical positions. For example, the most advanced players were the pitchers.

High school sport is subject to the same growth implications as other age groups. Many basketball players, for example, do not complete growth until after the high school years. Exercise and sport are certainly not contraindicated, but growth differences should be appreciated and perhaps incorporated into competitive rules.

EXERCISE AND AGING

The life span of man (that is, the maximal limits of life) has not changed "in the last hundred millenia."[21] However, life expectancy has increased. For example, in 1900 life expectancy at birth was 49 years and in 1980 it was 73 years.[21] The limits of human life (that is, life span) seem to be relatively fixed. There is no firm evidence of humans living beyond 110 to 113 years.[24] Recent increases in life expectancy are mainly a result of improvements in medical science. It has been estimated that life span would only be increased by 11.8 years with the elimination of heart disease and by another 2.5 years if cancer were eliminated.[21] There is no evidence that humans could improve on the outer aging limits of the species mentioned. The relevant question for exercise science is whether exercise can reduce the effects of aging, enabling increased performance possibilities and, perhaps, certain health benefits. The effect of exercise on the aging process has not been well studied.[22] Although some evidence suggests long-term health benefits and retardation of aging as a result of exercise, it lacks sufficient definitude. This section of the chapter reviews some of the research dealing with aging populations.

General characteristics of aging

As indicated previously, aging can be characterized as decreased ability to adapt to the environment.[51] This decrease is related to continual cell death.[49] Cardiac output,[50] nerve conduction velocity,[51] bone tissue,[17] and muscle mass[51] decrease while blood pressure and peripheral resistance[51] increase. Lung function also declines, largely a result of a decrease in elastic recoil force and resistance to deformation of the chest wall.[45] For example, there is a decline in maximal voluntary ventilation, forced expiratory volume in 1 second, and vital capacity.[45] These and other factors contribute to a general loss of ability to perform physical exercise and to recover from its effects.[51]

Changes in muscle tissue and force

Muscle force is known to decline with aging. A 28% decrease between ages 25 and 74 years has been noted.[46] This decrease may be related to changes in muscle mass. A decrease in creatinine excretion (33%), related to protein breakdown, was observed between ages 20 and 90 years.[57] The decrease in animal muscle mass[61] is related to both fiber number and fiber diameter.[20] Fitts found the greatest decrease in FT fibers, resulting in an apparent increase in ST fibers from 43% (20 to 29 years) to 55% (60 to 65 years).[28] Both FG and FOG fibers declined.[29] As muscle mass declines, so does the volume of mitochondria.[38] One author[14] observed significant decrements in SDH enzymes in mammalian skeletal muscle with increasing age, but other authors[38] could not find enzymatic changes in humans up to 70 years of age.

Changes in bone tissue

Bone density loss averages 0.75% to 1.0% per year after age 30 to 35 years in women and 50 to 55 years in men.[53] Aging results in an increased probability of bone fracture.[53] The decline in bone density is related to calcium deficiency,[6] which may be caused by decreased calcium levels in the diet or decreased calcium absorption, retention, or use.[53]

Changes in aerobic power

Humans reach their peak in functional capacity at about age 30. Although differences can be expected between individuals and among organs, the average loss of functional

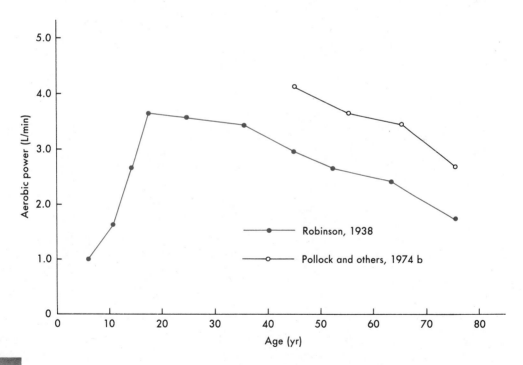

FIG. 19-4   The change in aerobic power with age in males. The Robinson[47] data show a peak at 17.4 years, a relative plateau until age 30, and a linear decline thereafter. Data from the Pollock and others[40] experiment show an upward displacement of the aging line in a group of highly trained older men. The rate of decline is approximately equal, however.

capacity is 0.75% to 1.0% per year.[51] The classic experiment of Robinson[47] in 1938 established the basic relationship of aerobic power to age (Figure 19-4). Ninety-three subjects between ages 6 and 91 years were given a maximal exercise test. Aerobic power, expressed in liters per minute, rose until 17.4 years, plateaued at about 30, and declined thereafter. Similar data were reported in subjects between 30 and 80 years,[4] amounting to a decline of 40% in aerobic power over this period. A 38% decrease in aerobic power for women was found between ages 23 and 70.3 years (Figure 19-5).[39] These subjects were tested before and after a sedentary hiatus of approximately 6 years to confirm the cross-sectional trend with longitudinal data.

A major question related to these findings is whether aerobic mechanisms, as such, decline or whether the change is related to a decrease in muscle mass. When data on aging were corrected for loss in muscle mass, no change in aerobic power was found.[4] Although mitochondrial volume decreases, no decrease can be seen in mitochondria per sarcomere.[18] Moreover, no change in calf muscle blood flow was observed between men age 74

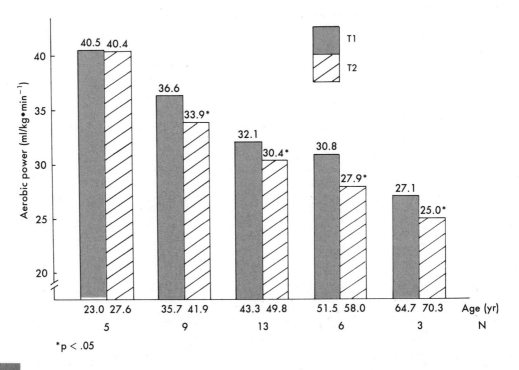

*p < .05

FIG. 19-5   The change in aerobic power with age in females. Subjects were tested twice approximately 6 years apart. On both occasions, aerobic power showed a steady decline. All groups significantly decreased in aerobic power at the second testing, with the exception of the youngest group (23.0 to 27.6 years). (Adapted from Plowman, S.A., Drinkwater, B.L., and Horvath, S.M.: Age and aerobic power in women: a longitudinal study, J. Gerontol. *34*:512, 1979.)

years and those age 25 years.[46] It was concluded that "the muscle cells of the 65-70 year old men are still capable of maintaining as great a metabolic flow as those of young men."[3] In an absolute sense, however, performance declines in parallel with the decrease in muscle mass. Also, performance changes may be related to changes in central circulation.

Cardiac output decreases 0.8% per year in the average sedentary individual.[26] Data have implicated decreases in both maximal stroke volume and heart rate in the cardiac output decrement.[18] Exercise blood pressure increases with age, increasing cardiac effort (heart rate × systolic blood pressure), as a result of increases in arterial peripheral resistance.[13] Heart rate does not appear to be affected at the higher work intensities. Figure 19-6 shows comparative data of a group of young boys ($\overline{X}$ age = 16.7 years) and

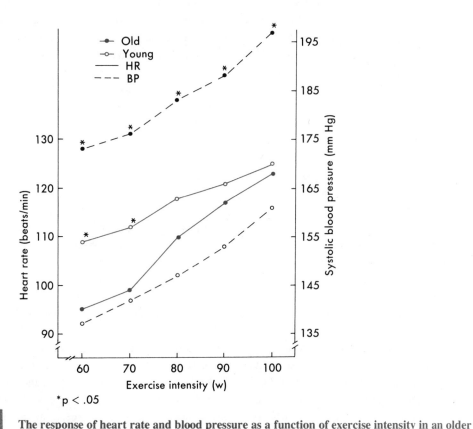

*p < .05

FIG. 19-6 The response of heart rate and blood pressure as a function of exercise intensity in an older group ($\overline{X}$ age = 69.2 years) and a younger group ($\overline{X}$ age = 16.7 years). Blood pressure is significantly higher in the older group at all intensities. Heart rate was significantly different between groups only at the lower intensities. (Adapted from DeVries, H.A., and Adams, G.M.: Comparison of exercise responses in old and young men: I. The cardiac effort/total body effort relationship, J. Gerontol. *27*:344, 1972.)

a group of older men ($\overline{X}$ age = 69.2 years). Blood pressure was significantly higher in the older group at all exercise intensities. Heart rate was significantly higher only at 60 and 70 W. After age 60, left ventricular ejection fraction is significantly lower than in younger subjects.[42]

Training middle-aged and older individuals

Whether the effects of aging can be retarded by exercise interventions has not been extensively studied. Particularly lacking are longitudinal studies of matched groups who exercise compared with those who do not. To date, this question has mainly been examined through the use of cross-sectional sampling. Readers are referred back to Figure 17-4 to see such a comparison. The data of Robinson[47] are plotted along with those of Pollock and others,[40] in which case aerobic power was determined in a group of 25 men between the ages of 40 and 75 years. These men were all highly trained and age group champions. It can be seen that the highly trained group (open circles) remains well above the normal aging line (closed circles). The aging rate appears to be about the same, even though the peak adult value was undoubtedly higher. Certainly the capacity for exercise is higher in the trained group, but the evidence does not support an alteration in the aging process. In a similar comparison, $\dot{V}O_2$ max of former track athletes, 25 to 43 years old, was measured after discontinuance of their careers.[48] The former athletes, untrained at the time, decreased from 71.4 to 41.8 ml $\cdot$ kg/min^{-1} (40%). A control group decreased from 50.6 to 36.5 ml $\cdot$ kg/min^{-1} (28%) over the same period. The average age at the second test was 56.6 years. The two groups were more alike during middle age than during youth. These data combined with those of Pollock and others[40] may suggest an advantage to training, but the suggestion is relatively weak. Such data may merely reflect a hereditary difference.[40]

Several studies have examined the trainability of older persons. Training of those over age 60 did not produce bradycardia at rest.[5] Bradycardia was observed in a somewhat younger middle-aged (49 to 65 years) group.[41] When exercising at a constant submaximal intensity, posttraining heart rate in older men[5] and women[2] is lower, with little change in $\dot{V}O_2$ max.[5,54]

Experiments indicate that relative changes (%) in the strength of older subjects are comparable to those expected in young subjects.[36,37] These changes seem to be attributed to different factors, however. In the young, strength after 2 weeks of training is not accompanied by much hypertrophy of muscle (Figure 19-7). The change has been associated with alterations in neural factors. Thereafter, with continued training, the contribution of hypertrophy increases to account for about 90% of the change at 8 weeks. On the other hand, the contribution of hypertrophy in older subjects never exceeds approximately 35%, with neural factors always making the greatest contribution. Strength changes in the elderly apparently affect the nervous system primarily.

Exercise has been studied to determine its effect on bone mineral content. When older runners (50 to 59 years) were compared to nonexercising control subjects, bone mineral content of the femur and humerus was 20% higher.[52] Women are particularly susceptible to osteoporosis (decreased bone density) and risk of fracture. Studies have shown that bone density can be improved in women who remain physically active.

A group of middle-aged (43-year-old) males was studied to determine the effect of training on anaerobic threshold.[11] After 9 weeks, the previously sedentary subjects increased anaerobic threshold from 49.40% $\dot{V}O_2$ max to 57%. The anaerobic enzymes, creatine phosphokinase and lactate dehydrogenase, increased, and submaximal lactate levels decreased after 8 weeks of training in a group of older men (56 to 70 years).[55]

Aerobic power increased with endurance training in previously sedentary males by 10%,[34] 11%,[55] 12%,[25] 18%,[41] and 24%.[25] Maximal cardiac output improved significantly from 19.4 to 21.4 L/min after 15 weeks of training at 80% $\dot{V}O_2$ max.[34] Moreover, resting

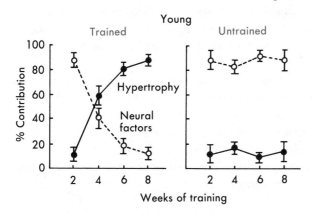

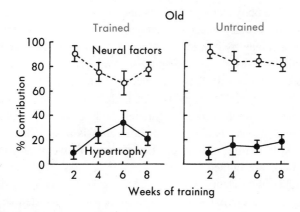

FIG. 19-7 Contributions of hypertrophy and neural factors to strength gain in young and old subjects. Unlike the case in the young group, hypertrophy makes a relatively small contribution to changes in strength. (From Moritani, T., and deVries, H.A.: Neural factors versus hypertrophy in the time course of muscle strength gain, Am. J. Phys. Med. *58:*115, 1979; and Moritani, T., and deVries, H.A.: Potential for gross muscle hypertrophy in older men, J. Gerontol. *35:*672, 1980.)

muscle glycogen (vastus lateralis) and aerobic enzyme (maleate dehydrogenase and succinate dehydrogenase) levels increased following 8 weeks of endurance training.[55] Both anaerobic and aerobic pathways have shown evidence of improvement with training during middle age.

Training changes in a younger group (36.8 years) were compared with changes in an older group (52.9 years) before and after a 4-month physical fitness program.[23] No significant differences were observed in $\dot{V}o_2$ max, total lipids, cholesterol, triglycerides, or blood glucose levels.

The question has been asked whether long-term training (6 to 10 years) changes depend on previous activity level.[25] Two previously sedentary middle-aged (45 to 55 years) groups improved aerobic power by an average of 18% after 6 or 7 years. However, a group of previously active or semiactive men improved by only 1%. The latter group was absolutely higher before and after training but had apparently reached genetic, environmental, and aging limits for change.

Still another investigation studied the trainability of older men ($\overline{X}$ age = 69.5 years; range = 51 to 87 years).[12] All trained 3 times per week. The most significant findings occurred in the oxygen transport system, although pulmonary and strength changes were also observed. With proper precautions, because of the higher probability of heart disease, older subjects not only respond to exercise with a favorable attitude, they can achieve significant physiological gains as well. The question of alteration of the aging process remains, requiring additional investigation.

SUMMARY

The process of growing to maturity has been defined as an increasing ability to adapt. From birth to physical maturity, body stature increases linearly. American children have exhibited a secular trend in this century, meaning that height and weight have increased above previous generations and puberty is reached earlier. When growth data are plotted as a rate of change (cm/yr), an adolescent growth spurt, increased acceleration in growth at the onset of adolescence, is observed. This spurt occurs earlier in girls (10.5 to 13 years) than in boys (12.5 to 15 years). The boys' peak is higher, accounting for the final sex difference in stature. Organ growth generally parallels body growth. For example, heart growth parallels general stature. No significant difference is observed in aerobic power, corrected for body size, before, during, or after puberty. This indicates that the capacity for aerobic exercise is not limited by age.

Strength increases parallel body stature increases. After puberty, boys are stronger than girls, prompted by larger muscle mass resulting from increased testosterone secretion. Between ages 10 and 18 years, pulmonary ventilation, pulmonary diffusing capacity, and cardiac output increase proportionately.

Physiological age distinguishes progress toward final maturity. This variable can be measured by skeletal x-rays and displays wide individual differences.

Young athletes adapt well to endurance training. Most studies support significant relationships between aerobic power changes and body size changes. Several studies have found that with very heavy training increases occur greater than could be expected from body size changes alone.

Competition during the elementary years can be beneficial; however, little is known physiologically about children under 8 years and the potential adult consequences of competition at this age. More attention should be paid to physiological age for equalizing competition and class groupings during the junior high and middle school years. Boys successful in sport during this period tend to be advanced physiologically, and girls successful in track and gymnastics tend to be late to mature. Female swimmers are advanced in maturity, perhaps because of the advantage of postpubertal body fat.

Aging is defined as a decrease in the ability to adapt to the environment. Cardiac output, pulmonary function, nerve conduction velocity, bone tissue, and muscle mass decline with age, and blood pressure and peripheral resistance increase.

Accompanying a decrease in muscle mass is a decrease in the ability to apply force, that is, strength. This decrease is related to diminished fiber number and diameter, with the greatest decrease found in FT fibers. Bone tissue is lost at a rate of 0.75% to 1.0% per year after age 30 to 35 years in women and 50 to 55 years in men.

Aerobic power (L/min) rises during growth to a peak at about 17.4 years, where it essentially plateaus until age 30 and declines thereafter. Functional capacity decreases by about 0.75% to 1.0% after age 30. This decrease seems to run parallel to the decline in muscle mass. Cardiac output and left ventricular ejection fraction are lower in older subjects as well. Blood pressure is higher.

Highly trained middle-aged runners have an aerobic power higher than their sedentary counterparts, but no good evidence shows that the aging curve has been any more than displaced upward. This results in greater performance capacity but aging proceeds at the same rate.

Middle-aged and older individuals appear to be quite trainable from a physiological point of view. Submaximal heart rate is reduced by training. There is little change in $\dot{V}o_2$ max. Strength changes (%) are comparable with younger subjects. These changes are not accompanied by large increases in hypertrophy typical of younger trainees. Bone mineral content, anaerobic threshold, and aerobic power increase with training.

KEY TERMS

adolescence transition period between childhood and adult development.

adolescent growth spurt rapid acceleration in stature at the onset of puberty.

aging decreasing ability to adapt.

chronological age age from birth.

growth increasing ability to adapt.

life expectancy probable age of death.

life span maximal attainable age.

menarche onset of menstruation.

osteoporosis decrease in bone density often associated with aging.

physiological age (also **developmental age**) age based on maturation of the body, usually the skeleton, according to established norms.

puberty attainment of sexual maturity.
pubescent arriving at puberty.

REVIEW QUESTIONS

1. What explanation can you provide for the secular increase in body stature from the 1890s to the 1960s?

2. Explain the relationship between heart volume and aerobic power from childhood (prepuberty) through adolescence (postpuberty). What can we deduce from these data relative to childhood competition in endurance activities?

3. Define physiological age and contrast it with chronological age. How might this concept be used to equalize childhood and adolescent competition?

4. Discuss the relationship between sports performance and age at menarche. What hypotheses may explain this phenomenon?

5. What muscle components decrease when muscle mass declines with aging?

6. Explain the physiological factors that account for the decline in aerobic capacity with aging. Is it possible that the rate of decline may be decreased with increased physical activity?

7. Discuss the rationale associated with the trainability of aging exercisers.

REFERENCES

1. Adams, J.E.: Injury to the throwing arm. A study of traumatic changes in the elbow joints of boy baseball players, Calif. Med. **102:**127, 1965.

2. Adams, G.M., and deVries, H.A.: Physiological effects of an exercise training regimen upon women aged 52 to 79, J. Gerontol. **28:**50, 1973.

3. Asmussen, E.: Aging and exercise. In Horvath, S.M., and Yousef, M.K., editors: Environmental physiology: aging, heat and altitude, New York, 1981, Elsevier/North Holland.

4. Asmussen, E., Fruensgaard, K., and Norgaard, S.: A follow-up longitudinal study of selected physiologic functions in former physical education students—after forty years, J. Am. Geriatr. Soc. **23:**442, 1975.

5. Barry, A.J., Daly, J.W., Pruett, E.D.R., and others: The effects of physical conditioning on older individuals. I. Work capacity, circulatory-respiratory function, and electrocardiogram, J. Gerontol. **21:**182, 1966.

6. Bell, G.H., Cuthbertson, D., and Orr, J.: The strength and size of bone in relation to calcium intake, J. Physiol. **100:**299, 1941.

7. Bell, G.H., and Ribisl, P.M.: Maximal oxygen uptake during swimming of young competitive swimmers 9 to 17 years of age, Res. Q. **50:**574, 1979.

8. Bugyi, B., and Kausz, I.: Radiographic determination of the skeletal age of the young swimmers, J. Sports Med. Phys. Fitness **10:**269, 1970.

9. Cunningham, D.A., Telford, P., and Swart, G.T.: The cardiopulmonary capacities of young hockey players: age 10, Med. Sci. Sports **8:**23, 1976.

10. Daniels, J., Oldridge, N., Nagle, F., and others: Differences and changes in $\dot{V}O_2$ among young runners 10 to 18 years of age, Med. Sci. Sports **10:**200, 1978.

11. Davis, J.A., Frank, M.H., Whipp, B.J., and others: Anaerobic threshold alterations caused by endurance training in middle-aged men, J. Appl. Physiol.: Respir. Environ. Exerc. Physiol. **46:**1039, 1979.

12. deVries, H.A.: Physiological effects of an exercise training regimen upon men aged 52 to 88, J. Gerontol. **25:**325, 1970.

13. deVries, H.A., and Adams, G.M.: Comparison of exercise responses in old and young men: I. The cardiac effort/total body effort relationship, J. Gerontol. **27:**344, 1972.

14. Ermini, M.: Aging changes in mammalian skeletal muscle, Gerontology **22:**301, 1976.

15. Ferguson, R.J., Marcotte, G.G., and Montpetit, R.R.: A maximal oxygen uptake test during ice skating, Med. Sci. Sports **1:**207, 1969.

16. Fitts, R.H.: Aging and skeletal muscle. In Smith, E.L., and Serfass, R.C., editors: Exercise and aging: the scientific basis, Hillside, N.J., 1981, Enslow Publishers.

17. Garn, S.W., Rohmann, C.G., and Wagner, B.: Bone loss as a general phenomenon in man, Fed. Proc. **26:**1729, 1967.

18. Grimby, G., Nilsson, N.J., and Saltin, B.: Cardiac output during submaximal and maximal exercise in active middle-aged athletes, J. Appl. Physiol. **21:**1150, 1966.

19. Hale, C.J.: Physiological maturity of little league baseball players, Res. Q. **27:**276, 1956.

20. Hanzlikova, V., and Gutmann, E.: Ultrastructural changes in senile muscle, Adv. Exp. Med. Biol. **53:**421, 1975.

21. Hayflick, L.: Origins of aging. In Horvath, S.M., and Yousef, M.K., editors: Environmental physiology: aging, heat and altitude, New York, 1981, Elsevier/North Holland.

22. Holloszy, J.O.: Exercise, health and aging: a need for more information, Med. Sci. Sports Exerc. **15:**1, 1983.

23. Ismail, A.H., and Montgomery, D.L.: The effect of a four-month physical fitness program on a young and an old group matched for physical fitness, Eur. J. Appl. Physiol. **40:**137, 1979.

24. Johnson, R.E.: Some reflections on ageism. In Horvath, S.M., and Yousef, M.K., editors: Environmental physiology: aging, heat and altitude, New York, 1981, Elsevier/North Holland.

25. Kasch, F.W.: The effects of exercise on the aging process, Physic. Sportsmed. **4:**64, 1976.

26. Katori, R.Y.O.: Normal cardiac output in relation to age and body size, Tohuku J. Exp. Med. **128:**377, 1979.

27. Krogman, W.M.: Maturation age of 55 boys in the little league world series, 1957, Res. Q. **30:**54, 1959.

28. Larsson, L., and Karlsson, J.: Isometric and dynamic endurance as a function of age and skeletal muscle characteristics, Acta Physiol. Scand. **104:**129, 1978.

29. Larsson, L., Sjodin, B., and Karlsson, J.: Histochemical and biochemical changes in human skeletal muscle with age in sedentary males, age 22-65 years, Acta Physiol. Scand. **103:**31, 1978.

30. Macek, M., Vavra, J., and Novosadova, J.: Prolonged exercise in prepubertal boys, Eur. J. Appl. Physiol. **35:**291, 1976.

31. Malina, R.M.: Secular changes in growth, maturation, and physical performance. In Hutton, R.S., editor: Exercise and sport sciences reviews, Philadelphia, 1979, The Franklin Institute Press.

32. Malina, R.M., Harper, A.B., Avent, H.H., and others: Age at menarche in athletes and non athletes, Med. Sci. Sports **5:**11, 1973.

33. Mayers, N., and Gutin, B.: Physiological characteristics of elite prepubertal cross-country runners, Med. Sci. Sports **11:**172, 1979.

34. Miyashita, M., Haga, S., and Mizuta, T.: Training and detraining effects on aerobic power in middle-aged and older men, J. Sports Med. Phys. Fitness **18:**131, 1978.

35. Montpetit, R.R., Montoye, H.J., and Leading, L.: Grip strength of school children, Saginaw, Michigan: 1899 and 1964, Res. Q. **38:**231, 1967.

36. Moritani, T., and deVries, H.A.: Neural factors versus hypertrophy in the time course of muscle strength gain, Am. J. Phys. Med. **58:**115, 1979.

37. Moritani, T., and deVries, H.A.: Potential for gross muscle hypertrophy in older men, J. Gerontol. **35:**672, 1980.

38. Orlander, J., Kiessling, K.H., Larson, L., and others: Skeletal muscle metabolism and ultrastructure in relation to age in sedentary men, Acta Physiol. Scand. **104:**249, 1978.

39. Plowman, S.A., Drinkwater, B.L., and Horvath, S.M.: Age and aerobic power in women: a longitudinal study, J. Gerontol. **34:**512, 1979.

40. Pollock, M.L., Miller, H.S., and Wilmore, J.: Physiological characteristics of champion American track athletes 40 to 75 years of age, J. Gerontol. **29:**645, 1974.

41. Pollock, M.L., Dawson, G.A., Miller, H.S., and others: Physiologic responses of men 49 to 65 years of age to endurance training, J. Am. Geriatr. Soc. **24:**97, 1976.

42. Port, S., Cobb, F.R., Coleman, R.E., and others: Effect of age on the response of the left ventricular ejection fraction to exercise, N. Engl. J. Med. **303:**1133, 1980.

43. Porter, W.T.: The growth of St. Louis children, Trans. Acad. Sci. St. Louis **6:**263, 1894.

44. Rarick, G.L., and Seefeldt, V.: Characteristics of the young athlete. In Thomas, J.R., editor: Youth sports guide for coaches and parents, Washington, D.C., 1977, The Manufacturers Life Insurance Co. and National Association for Sport and Physical Education.

45. Reddan, W.G.: Respiratory system and aging. In Smith, E.L., and Serfass, R.C., editors: Exercise and aging: the scientific basis, Hillside, N.J., 1981, Enslow Publishers.

46. Richardson, D., and Schewchuk, R.: Comparison of calf muscle blood flow responses to rhythmic exercise between mean age 25- and 74-year-old men, Proc. Soc. Exp. Biol. Med. **164:**550, 1980.

47. Robinson, S.: Experimental studies of physical fitness in relation to age, Arbeitsphysiologie **10:**251, 1938.

48. Robinson, S., Dill, D.B., Robinson, R.D., and others: Physiological aging of champion runners, J. Appl. Physiol. **41:**46, 1976.

49. Shock, N.W.: Metabolism and age, J. Chronic Dis. **2:**687, 1955.

50. Shock, N.W.: The physiology of aging, Sci. Am. **206:**100, 1962.

51. Smith, E.L.: Age: the interaction of nature and nurture. In Smith, E.L., and Serfass, R.C., editors: Exercise and aging: the scientific basis, Hillside, N.J., 1981, Enslow Publishers.

52. Smith, E.L.: Bone changes in the exercising older adult. In Smith, E.L., and Serfass, R.C., editors: Exercise and aging: the scientific basis, Hillside, N.J., 1981, Enslow Publishers.

53. Smith E.L., Sempos, C.T., and Purvis, R.W.: Bone mass and strength decline with age. In Smith, E.L., and Serfass, R.C., editors: Exercise and aging, the scientific basis, Hillside, N.J., 1981, Enslow Publishers.

54. Stamford, B.A.: Physiological effects of training upon institutionalized geriatric men, J. Gerontol. **28**:441, 1973.

55. Suominen, H., Heikkinen, E., Liesen, H., and others: Effects of 8 weeks' endurance training on skeletal muscle metabolism in 56–70-year-old sedentary men, Eur. J. Appl. Physiol. **37**:173, 1977.

56. Tanner, J.M.: Education and physical growth, London, 1967, University of London Press, Ltd.

57. Tzankoff, S.P., and Norris, A.H.: Effect of muscle mass decrease on age-related BMR, J. Appl. Physiol.: Respir. Environ. Exerc. Physiol. **43**:1001, 1977.

58. Vaccaro, P., and Clarke, D.H.: Cardiorespiratory alterations in 9 to 11 year old children following a season of competitive swimming, Med. Sci. Sports **10**:204, 1978.

59. Wirth, A., Trager, E., Scheele, K., and others: Cardiopulmonary adjustment and metabolic response to maximal and submaximal physical exercise of boys and girls at different stages of maturity, Eur. J. Appl. Physiol. **39**:229, 1978.

60. Yamaji, K., and Miyashita, M.: Oxygen transport system during exhaustive exercise in Japanese boys, Eur. J. Appl. Physiol. **36**:93, 1977.

61. Yiengst, M.J., Barrows, C.H., and Shock, N.W.: Age changes in the chemical composition of muscle and liver in the rat, J. Gerontol. **14**:400, 1959.

SUGGESTED READINGS

Brewer, V., Meyer, B.M., Keele, M.S., and others: Role of exercise in prevention of involutional bone loss, Med. Sci. Sports Exerc. **15**:445, 1983.

Hale, C.J.: Physiological maturity of little league baseball players, Res. Q. **27**:276, 1956.

Hensley, L.D., East, W.B., and Stillwell, J.L.: Body fatness and motor performance during preadolescence, Res. Q. Exerc. Sport **53**:133, 1982.

Holloszy, J.O.: Exercise, health and aging: a need for more information, Med. Sci. Sports Exerc. **15**:1, 1983.

Horvath, S.M., and Yousef, M.K.: Environmental physiology: aging, heat and altitude, New York, 1981, Elsevier/North Holland.

Oyster, N., Morton, M., and Linnell, S.: Physical activity and osteoporosis in post-menopausal women, Med. Sci. Sports Exerc. **16**:44, 1984.

Rarick, G.L., and Seefeldt, V.: Characteristics of the young athlete. In Thomas, J.R., editor: Youth sports guide for coaches and parents, Washington, D.C., 1977, The Manufacturers Life Insurance Co. and National Association for Sport and Physical Education.

Robinson, S.: Experimental studies of physical fitness in relation to age, Arbeitsphysiologie **10**:251, 1938.

Shephard, R.J., and Sidney, K.H.: Exercise and aging. In Hutton, R.S., editor: Exercise and sport sciences reviews, Philadelphia, 1979, The Franklin Institute Press.

Shock, N.W.: The physiology of aging, Sci. Am. **206**:100, 1962.

Smith, E.L., and Serfass, R.C.: Exercise and aging: the scientific basis, Hillside, N.J., 1981, Enslow Publishers.

Spirduso, W.W.: Exercise and the aging brain, Res. Q. Exerc. Sport **54**:208, 1983.

Tanner, J.M.: Education and physical growth, London, 1967, University of London Press, Ltd.

CASE STUDY 1

When I was in junior high school, the sports program at each grade level was separated into two divisions called "lightweights" and "heavyweights." I was classified a lightweight for 3 years. Presumably those administering the program were concerned with equalizing competition. They probably weren't concerned with anything as esoteric as physiological age but simply felt that the little guys shouldn't be subjected to the battering from larger classmates of the same chronological age. At any rate, it meant that two teams played where ordinarily there would be one. I appreciated the system, although it was not without some social consequences. Some highly skilled "heavyweights" with little playing time looked longingly at the "shrimps" who got to play and often expressed their vehemence verbally, at the very least. Lightweights weren't always satisfied either. The heavyweight team was often the more socially esteemed. Of course, the tables could be turned. The physiologically advanced 13-year-old seventh grader sometimes played with older ninth graders. Such a person was often a ship without a port on both sides.

Social implications aside, the benefits of basing competition on some measure of physiological age are many. (Body weight, by the way, is probably not the best criterion.) More players can take advantage of competitive sport. Safety afforded to bone epiphyses by decreasing the likelihood of mismatched body size should be obvious. Since performance in sport often is heavily loaded on the side of body size, playing time becomes more a matter of execution than pure size. (This discussion may sound as though there is an assumption of value in competition for junior high and middle school youngsters. On the contrary, no value judgment is intended, only the realistic view that sports competition exists, so it should be dealt with as intelligently as possible.)

A very narrow view can be taken of child growth knowledge. For example, growth data have been used to select ballet students, since larger bodies classically have not been as aesthetically acceptable.[56] The U.S. Air Force Academy at one time had a rigid height limitation based on cockpit size, with obvious basketball implications.

Growth logic can be applied to the selection of elite age-group teams. Given equal exposure to practice, the more physiologically advanced child usually performs better, especially in games like football and basketball. A coach could make a team selection based on physiological age. No coach would do such a thing without having knowledge of skill.

How could growth knowledge be used to aid team selection or class grouping? First, it would be necessary to use some measure of physiological age. The most valid measure would be by determination of bone development by x-ray of the wrist bones. Groupings could then be based on age toward maturity, not on chronological age. The most valid educational use would involve the establishment of several groups or teams, not just one elite team. (The most successful procedure would incorporate skill, mental, and psychological data as well.)

A second technique, less technical to administer, would involve determination of the progress of development of secondary sex characteristics. Growth of breasts, genitalia, and pubic hair is used to identify developmental stage.[56] The stages could be incorporated with other measures for selection and placement. Although the social impact of such a system could be touchy, in the hands of a competent professional such a system would provide tremendous educational benefits.

Some argue against such procedures as a form of postnatal "genetic engineering," that is, manipulating human characteristics for controlling environmental conditions. It would be quite correct to argue against control for purposes of elite selection. On the other hand, control for the purposes of achieving educational goals is another question. That is already done when we arbitrarily break groups down based on chronological age. Physiological age may be a better criterion.

CASE STUDY 2

STUDENT: Do you mean to tell me that my 55-year-old sedentary father should start running?

PROFESSOR: Not should, but could.

STUDENT: You mean my rusty, old father could indeed start running?

PROFESSOR: Well, no, not start running, but with time and motivation, it's certainly possible. If he hasn't been exercising for a number of years, a more prudent beginning would be easy walking. And I wouldn't start that until after he had been cleared with a stress test.

STUDENT: You mean putting the old boy on the treadmill. He might croak. He hasn't pushed himself away from the TV set in 30 years.

PROFESSOR: Well, it's his decision, but certainly a stress test is essential. You know that the treadmill can be adjusted so that most everyone can exercise.

STUDENT: Yes, I remember. But, assuming that he's cleared for exercise, how does he begin?

PROFESSOR: There's no evidence that the principles that apply to younger people can't be applied to middle-aged exercisers as well. The application of the exercise stimulus may be more gradual, but not quantitatively different. It's certainly essential to remember the effect of lowered maximal values on the strain of performance.

STUDENT: What do you mean?

PROFESSOR: You're aware of the decline in aerobic power with age. Because of this decline any absolute physical load represents a larger relative load, percentagewise, in an older individual than in the young. There is no apparent change in submaximal exercise $\dot{V}o_2$ with aging. For example, a given physical load may result in a $\dot{V}o_2$ of 1.5 L/min in a group of 25 year olds as well as in a group of 50 year olds. If aerobic power decreases by 1% per year after age 30, the relative physiological strain on a group of 50 year olds would, on the average, be 20% higher.

STUDENT: However, that shouldn't affect the exercise prescription if it's described in relative terms.

PROFESSOR: Right! Depending on how long the older person has been sedentary, you may wish to cut back on the percentage until initial musculoskeletal and cardiovascular adjustments are made, but that speaks to the application of the principles, not the principles themselves.

STUDENT: Well, maybe the old boy should try it after all.

PROFESSOR: If *he* wants to!

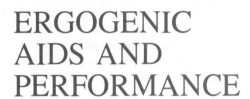

chapter 20

ERGOGENIC AIDS AND PERFORMANCE

MAJOR LEARNING OBJECTIVE
Athletic "doping" is a widely used practice.
Research with supplements is difficult because
special research protocols are required and
because it is sometimes impossible to study
athletes using drug dosages in life situations.

APPLICATIONS
The use of illegal substances may be more of an
educational problem than a physiological
problem. Emphasis on winning by our culture
counteracts any reasonable attempt by scientists
to provide objective truth. If winning were not
so important, drugs would not seem so
important.

BOTH scientific and lay journals in the 1980s are full of reports of drug use, especially anabolic steroids, to aid sport performance. Drug use in sport is not a recent phenomenon. The first reported death from drug usage in sport occurred in the 1890s.[13] It is not difficult to believe that drugs have been used to gain performance benefits for many, many years. When competition is taken seriously, performers will look for substances or methods to provide them with an edge. The question for us is neither a legal or a moral one, the importance of these areas notwithstanding. In exercise physiology we need to concern ourselves with questions like: Do real physiological and performance effects occur? Are there pathological side effects that contraindicate use?

Our discussion should begin with some basic definitions. First, the topic of aiding performance is often categorized under the term *ergogenic aids*. The term is a combination of the word *ergo,* meaning work, and *genic,* meaning producing. Therefore, the term literally refers to aids to the production of work. Ergogenic aids have been defined as ''substances and phenomena that are work-producing aids, and these aids are thought to enhance performance above levels anticipated under normal conditions.''[49]

International competition organizations use the term *doping* to identify ergogenic practices that are illegal. The International Olympic Committee (IOC) has specifically defined doping. The main components of the definition are as follows[64]:

1. Doping involves taking a foreign substance into the body, or
2. ''Physiological substances taken in abnormal quantities,'' or
3. ''Taken by an abnormal route of entry.''
4. Taking a foreign substance for the purpose of gaining a performance advantage in an ''artificial and unfair manner.''
5. Also, any medical intervention that ''boosts the athlete's performance'' is thought to be doping.

Interpretation of the IOC definition is often problematic. For example, would megadoses of vitamin C be considered doping? Certainly, vitamin C is not a foreign substance, nor is it normally taken by an abnormal route of entry. On the other hand, it is a substance required in physiological processes. Would vitamin C administration in large doses be considered artificial or unfair? Although the letter of the definition is not always clear, certainly the spirit is, that is, the IOC wants to prohibit those practices that might provide an unfair advantage.

Experimental concerns

The field of exercise physiology and other disciplines related to sports medicine are charged with the professional responsibility to determine whether substances provide an advantage. Experimentation in this area is full of difficulties. Most doping techniques have both objective and subjective effects. Therefore, it is necessary to determine whether a substance changes a physiological process in a beneficial way or merely alters the athlete's psychological state positively. Highly sophisticated experiments must be designed to discover the truth. When any substance is administered during experimentation, a *placebo* (a substance appearing like but not having the effect of the authentic substance) must be administered to a comparative group or the same group at a different time. This technique enables the researcher to assess the subjective effect of receiving a substance, albeit inert. Another important element of these experiments is the *control* group. Quite often experiments involve the chronic administration of a substance at the same time that training is taking place. To control for the effect of the training alone, one group might train without taking either the substance or a placebo.

Other experimental problems make the study of ergogenic aids difficult. Experiments with animals provide a relatively pure approach to the determination of physiological effects. However, substance use and abuse usually involves much more than just the physiological effect, which makes animal studies less than realistic. Experiments are often conducted using therapeutic dosages, and actual use by athletes involves much greater quantities. The conclusions of many experiments are suspect as a result of the failure to use *double blind* techniques, that is, techniques in which neither the researcher nor the subject know the contents of the substance provided. If either person knows the true contents, there is the possibility of unconscious suggestions by the investigator or increased motivation by the subject to perform better. All difficulties aside, sophisticated experimentation is needed with a variety of substances used by athletes.

The purpose of this chapter is to review the evidence regarding the performance-enhancing characteristics of a variety of substances. Specifically, this review is limited to *stimulants* (amphetamines, caffeine, and nicotine), *depressants* (morphine and alcohol), *cardiovascular enhancers* (blood doping, beta blockers, and hyperoxia), *steroids, vitamins,* and, *minerals.*

STIMULANTS

Amphetamines

Amphetamines (β-phenylisopropylamine) were first synthesized in 1927. Because they act as a central nervous system stimulant, reducing the sense of fatigue, amphetamines have become widely used. In 1970, 65 different amphetamines, or substances producing approximately the same effect, were being produced by 40 companies.[20] Amphetamines are known on the street as "bennies," "speed," and "uppers." In addition to their fatigue-reducing qualities, they are also used as appetite suppressants.

Fatigue-reduction possibilities make amphetamines attractive for athletes seeking endurance performance advantages. In addition, amphetamines may have other effects that are related to athletic performance. For example, increased cardiac output, oxygen uptake, muscle and liver glycogenolysis, vasoconstriction of peripheral blood vessels, and vasodilation in skeletal muscle and the respiratory vessels may all be affected by the use of amphetamines.

Increases in isometric strength have been observed following the administration of amphetamines.[34] Another study found increases in knee extension strength but not in elbow flexion strength.[11] This same experiment found no change in leg power with these drugs. There does not seem to be a logical reason why amphetamines would selectively affect one muscle group and not another.

The results of animal studies that have examined the effect of amphetamines on endurance are contradictory. No significant change in swimming endurance could be found in rats treated with four drug doses (4, 8, 12, or 16 mg/kg body weight) at four different times of administration before the swim (36, 60, 90, or 120 minutes).[14] However, another study found increased endurance performance with low doses of amphetamines but not with high doses.[25] Still another study, which administered amphetamines to mice over a period of 6 weeks, found a 70% longer exhaustive swim time than in comparable untreated animals.[23]

Human studies have also been contradictory. For instance, significant increases in work performance were found during the latter stages of a cycling, strength, and endurance test.[8] This test does have a short-term endurance component, but it is highly anaerobic as well. Interestingly, an increase in peak lactate production has been observed with amphetamine administration.[11] This may explain the results in the cycling, strength, and endurance test.[8] On the other hand, no differences could be found between amphetamine and placebo treatments in six trained subjects who rode to exhaustion on a bicycle ergometer.[33]

Another study attempted to determine the role of amphetamines during endurance performance in humans.[11] A well-controlled double blind experiment was conducted with six healthy males. The drug treatment used 15 milligrams of amphetamine sulfate per 70 kilograms of body weight 2 hours before the endurance task. Although no change was observed in aerobic power, the subjects rode significantly longer under the drug's influence, and as cited earlier, peak lactate level was significantly higher. Apparently the symptoms of fatigue were masked, with the drug allowing the longer ride. Since we depend on our sensations to safely guide our performance, the use of amphetamines could be dangerous.

Another example of the possibly dangerous consequences of amphetamine use, not to mention psychological dependency, is the drug's effect on peripheral blood vessels. The drug constricts the vessels, thus decreasing their role in the dissipation of body heat. Such an effect could prove life threatening during endurance performances in hot environments.

Practical summary. Amphetamine use may improve the performance of strength tasks. Although somewhat contradictory, it appears likely that the fatigue-masking qualities of the drug may provide performance enhancement during endurance tasks. The possible dangerous side effects of such a practice make such use unwise, especially in hot environments. Animal data are not as convincing as human data concerning the endurance question.

Caffeine

Recent studies indicate that caffeine may improve endurance performance. The proposed physiological effect that enables the improvement is an increase in the oxidation of fat, stimulated by caffeine intake. In 1978, investigators at Ball State University reported results of their work with nine cyclists.[15] Under one condition, subjects rode a bicycle ergometer to exhaustion 1 hour following consumption of 330 milligrams of caffeine (2.5 cups of coffee). In a second condition, subjects rode after consuming 200 milliliters of hot water with 5 milligrams of decaffeinated coffee (placebo condition). The caffeine ride was 19.5% longer than the placebo ride. Ratings of perceived exertion were significantly lower, and fat oxidation was significantly increased with caffeine. The following year, the same group[35] reported similar results. Using a 2-hour isokinetic cycle exercise, the caffeine condition resulted in the production of significantly more work. Fat oxidation was significantly higher during the second hour of the test (these results are shown in Figure 20-1). Carbohydrate level was not different between these conditions, indicating that it was not spared, which the authors originally thought was involved in the mechanism of

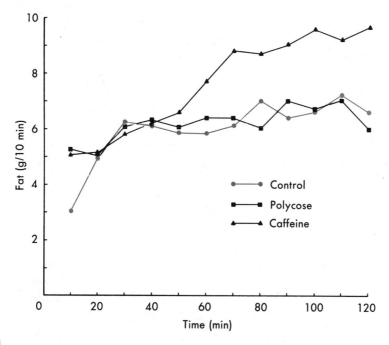

| **FIG. 20-1** | Mean fat use during a 2-hour isokinetic cycling exercise with no additive (control), carbohydrate feeding (polycose), or caffeine supplementation. Fat use during the caffeine trial became significantly higher at 50 to 60 minutes and remained significantly higher during the second hour. No other significant differences were noted. (Adapted from Ivy, J.L., Costill, D.L., Fink, W.J., and others: Influence of caffeine and carbohydrate feedings on endurance performance, Med. Sci. Sports *11:*6, 1979.) |

caffeine action. The beneficial effect of caffeine rests with increased release of free fatty acids. However, benefits are accompanied by increased diuresis, which can be an irritant to the athlete.

In a related study, the effect of caffeine and training was examined in 60 mature rodents.[63] When the caffeine-fed group was compared to the noncaffeine group, both of whom had trained for 9 weeks, the caffeine group reduced body weight and fat cell size by 22% and 25% more than the noncaffeine group. The implication of this study points to possible beneficial body composition effects of chronic use of caffeine during training.

Although more experimentation is necessary, caffeine appears to be beneficial to endurance performance. The possible advantages of caffeine to performance must be evaluated in the final analysis by also considering the possible negative side effects, that is, increased cardiac frequency.

Nicotine

Nicotine is known to stimulate the cardiovascular system at rest. What effect does nicotine have during exercise, and what implications may this potential effect have on performance? Two studies have recently (1980-1981) examined the acute effect of nicotine on the physiological response to submaximal exercise. One measured left ventricular function at rest and during exercise to 85% of age-predicted maximal heart rate in six young male smokers and six nonsmokers.[5] Subjects smoked two cigarettes before exercise and one during the first minute of exercise. Time to 85% maximal heart rate was not different between the groups. Smoking significantly altered several variables at rest compared to the nonsmoking trial: increased heart rate, blood pressure, and ventricular contractility; and decreased end-diastolic volume and pulmonary transit time. The only significant difference during exercise was a decreased pulmonary transit time, that is, blood transit through the pulmonary system. The authors concluded that smoking does not significantly alter cardiac function during submaximal exercise.

In another study, 16 habitual smokers were tested with and without smoking while riding a bicycle ergometer (supine).[9] After smoking, exercise cardiac output, oxygen consumption, and heart rate increased and stroke volume decreased during a 30-minute submaximal ride.

Two rather large epidemiological studies have recently examined the relationship between smoking and endurance variables. Maximal oxygen consumption was determined in 597 males between the ages of 16 to 69 years.[47] When the data were corrected for differences in age, body weight, skinfold fat, and drinking habits, smokers were found to have significantly lower $\dot{V}O_2$ max values. In a similar study, 586 males from the Indiana State Police Force exercised to exhaustion on a treadmill.[45] Smokers had significantly lower exercise durations and maximal heart rates, and significantly higher maximal systolic blood pressure levels. It should be remembered when interpreting these data that smokers usually have an inactive life-style as well, that is, determining specific causation is not always possible.

Practical summary. Smoking definitely provides increased cardiovascular strain at rest, but the effect during submaximal exercise is benign. However, endurance performance appears to be adversely affected by smoking. There is a definite need to pay more attention to the chronic effects of smoking, particularly using prospective designs.[64] To find a group of subjects foolish enough to begin smoking and continue for months and years is fortunately difficult, if not impossible.

DEPRESSANTS

Alcohol

A committee of the American College of Sports Medicine thoroughly examined the literature related to alcohol and developed a position statement. Such a statement was necessary, since alcohol is widely used by athletes, and many people have advocated its use as an ergogenic aid. The major points of the position statement are as follows:

1. The acute ingestion of alcohol can exert a deleterious effect on a wide variety of psychomotor skills, such as reaction time, hand-eye coordination, accuracy, balance, and complex coordination.

2. Acute ingestion of alcohol will not substantially influence metabolic or physiological functions essential to physical performance, such as energy metabolism, maximal oxygen consumption ($\dot{V}O_2$ max), heart rate, stroke volume, cardiac output, muscle blood flow, arteriovenous oxygen difference, or respiratory dynamics. Alcohol consumption may impair body temperature regulation during prolonged exercise in a cold environment.

3. Acute alcohol ingestion will not improve and may decrease strength, power, local muscular endurance, speed, and cardiovascular endurance.

4. Serious and continuing efforts should be made to educate athletes, coaches, health and physical educators, physicians, trainers, the sports media, and the general public regarding the effects of acute alcohol ingestion on human physical performance and on the potential acute and chronic problems of excessive alcohol consumption.

Alcohol may have a beneficial effect used in small quantities, in that it eliminates psychological inhibitions.[64] It should hardly be recommended for this reason in light of the epidemic proportions of alcohol addiction in the United States.

Morphine

The abuse of "hard drugs" is a growing problem in sport, especially on the professional level. Little is known about the effect of these drugs on performance because of obvious legal and moral problems inherent in such experimentation. Morphine has been used with injured players because of the inhibitory effect it has on pain perception. It is banned for this reason. Research with morphine has been conducted in pulmonary physiology. Evidence related to the effect of morphine on exercise ventilatory response is contradictory. One investigation found that morphine significantly depressed ventilatory response at any given level of exercise.[52] A parallel reduction in exercise $\dot{V}_{O_2}$ was also noted. The data of another study did not support this finding in that depressed ventilation was found without a concomitant decrease in $\dot{V}_{O_2}$.[45] These authors made an interesting observation relative to $\dot{V}_{CO_2}$. Under normal conditions, as discussed in an earlier chapter, pulmonary ventilation is directly linked to $\dot{V}_{CO_2}$. Since $\dot{V}_{CO_2}$ did not change under the morphine condition, the link was broken. The protective effect offered by $\dot{V}_{CO_2}$ control of ventilation may have been lost.

CARDIOVASCULAR ENHANCERS
"Blood doping"

"Blood doping" and "blood packing" are slang terms for what might better be called *induced erythrocythemia*. These terms refer to a technique in which blood is withdrawn from an athlete, stored, and reinfused at a later date. The concept is quite rational. That is, if blood volume, red blood cell count, and hemoglobin concentration are positively related to oxygen transport, then increasing these variables may benefit endurance activities. In fact, the result of such a procedure is not unlike that observed with altitude exposure. Following the initial research in this area some concern was expressed that high levels of polycythemia would interfere with circulatory dynamics because of increased frictional properties of blood. To date, however, no known contraindication have been observed.[26]

The first study in this area was reported in 1972 by Ekblom and others.[21] Increases were observed in hemoglobin, $\dot{V}_{O_2}$ max, and physical working capacity following reinfusion. A subsequent study confirmed the significant increase in $\dot{V}_{O_2}$ max.[22] However, no changes were found in cardiac output, stroke volume, and heart rate. The lack of a double blind protocol and a control group in the earlier studies has been criticized.[66] When these experimental procedures were incorporated into an experiment, no increase in treadmill run time or perceived exertion could be found,[67] even though hemoglobin was increased significantly. In contrast, significant increases in $\dot{V}_{O_2}$ max and treadmill run time were reported using these procedures.[10]

One investigation attempted to resolve the conflict in the literature.[67] It was thought that the contradictory findings were the result of the quantity of blood infused and the time between withdrawal and infusion. Positive results had not been observed when less than 800 ml were infused and when the interval between withdrawal and infusion was less than 21 days. The latter factor may not allow hemoglobin to return to prewithdrawal levels. Twelve experienced distance runners ran a race-pace 5 mile treadmill run under control, infusion (RBCs diluted to 920 ml with normal saline solution), and placebo (920 ml normal saline solution) conditions. Runners controlled treadmill speed to simulate race conditions. Only the trial run after the blood infusion was significantly different (29:26 vs 30:17 for the infusion trial after saline injection). Perceived exertion, both central and local, was significantly reduced as well. Hemoglobin and red blood cell count were significantly higher, but hematocrit was not. Treadmill run results of this study are shown in Figure 20-2.

It appears that blood doping can be used to augment performance if appropriate procedures are followed, that is 920 milliliters of diluted RBCs are reinfused 21 days after withdrawal. The extent of its use in competition has been limited, however, in light of revelations following the 1984 Olympics, blood doping may become more popular.

Beta blockers

Beta blockers have been widely used with cardiac patients to reduce heart rate and blood pressure and, therefore, the cardiac symptomatology that arises from increased cardiovascular response. Beta blockers, as the name implies, block beta adrenergic receptors in the heart (selective), or in both the heart and sites in the vascular system, bronchi, and smooth muscle (nonselective). Normally these receptors are responsive to the neurotransmitters acetylcholine and norepinephrine. For example, norepinephrine increases

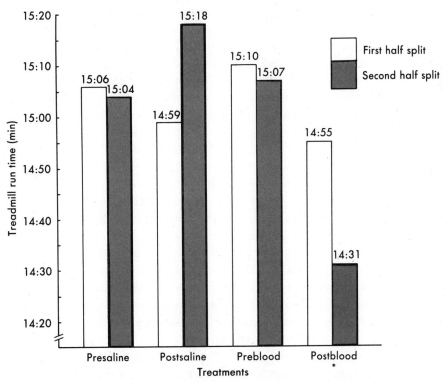

*Total time (first and second half) significantly faster than other three treatments.

FIG. 20-2   Five mile treadmill run times (first and second half splits) during a placebo treatment (before and after saline administration) and a blood infusion treatment (before and after blood administration). (Adapted from Williams, M.H., Lindhjem, M., and Schuster, R.: The effect of blood infusion upon endurance capacity and ratings of perceived exertion, Med. Sci. Sports *10:*113, 1978.)

heart rate. Beta blockers inhibit this influence. Typical examples of beta blockers used in clinical medicine are timolol and propranol.

Many sports combine heavy exercise intensity with motor precision, for example, the biathlon, which combines demanding bouts of cross-country skiing with rifle shooting. High heart rates presumably may interfere with shooting accuracy. Beta blockers have been proposed as an aid to these sports.

The value of beta blockers for performances requiring force, velocity, coordination, and anaerobic metabolism has been examined.[31] Subjects performed with an inert placebo and under the influence of the beta blocker oxprenolol. No significant changes were observed in exercises such as isometric knee extension, vertical jumping, and stair running. Beta blockade did result in significant reductions in total ergometer work in 1 minute, blood lactate level after 1 minute, and maximal heart rate. The beta blocker reduced heart rate, but at the same time it appeared to lower anaerobic capacity.

Nine Finnish Olympic ski jumpers were given oxprenolol or a placebo before four international competitions.[59] No significant difference was observed even though six jumpers had longer jumps with beta blockade. The extreme tachycardia was eliminated, but a high incidence of leg numbness was noted during the blockade trials.

Another effect of beta blockers that may mitigate their use is the probability that cardiac output is decreased in the presence of the heart rate reduction. It does not appear at this time that beta blockade is an effective ergogenic aid.

Oxygen breathing

The addition of higher than normal percentages of oxygen (hyperoxia) to the inspired air has been known for some time to benefit some performances. Despite a lack of evidence that recovery is enhanced with oxygen breathing, many teams provide supplemental oxygen to athletes returning to the bench.[39] Supplemental oxygen during performance provides obvious technical problems.

During endurance activity, performance has been enhanced with oxygen percentages up to 66%[4] and perhaps up to 100%.[69] Studies that used performances lasting less than 2 minutes were unable to show a positive effect from oxygen breathing.[12,44] This is probably a result of the anaerobic nature of performances of this type.

Increased endurance performance capacity is known to occur with oxygen breathing. The mechanism that allows this effect is unclear. It has been suggested that oxygen breathing may increase aerobic power.[62] Other probable factors are reduced work of breathing and a decreased production of lactic acid.

STEROIDS

No other drug has been as controversial or as abused in the past decade as steroids. In sports in which a premium is placed on body size, steroid use is epidemic. Table 20-1 shows estimated steroid usage in various sports for males and females.[57] With all this use, it would be expected that a clear picture of steroid effectiveness would be available; however, such is not the case.

TABLE 20-1 ||||| INCIDENCE OF STEROID USE
AMONG MALE AND FEMALE ATHLETES

Sport	Males* (%)	Females* (%)
Strength/power		
Weightlifting	95+	15
Powerlifting	99+	25
Shotput, discus, javelin	80	20
Football	70	—
Decathlon	60	—
Sprinting	40	1
Endurance		
Running		
Middle distance	10	1
Long distance	10	1
Bicycling long distance	10	—

Adapted from Stone, J.: Steroids, Natl. Strength Condition. Assoc.
J. **5**:13, 1983.
*18 years and older; taken at same point in career.

Steroids used by athletes are synthetic derivatives of testosterone. Testosterone has both anabolic (muscle building) and androgenic (promoting secondary sex characteristics) properties. Males produce testosterone primarily in the testes but also produce small amounts in the adrenal glands. (See an illustration of the pituitary-testes axis in Figure 20-3.) Females produce very small amounts of testosterone in their adrenal glands. About 1% of the total produced is found in its free and active form in the blood. The remainder is bound to protein in the tissues. Free testosterone is converted to 17-ketosteroids, primarily in the liver, and is eventually excreted in the urine.[58]

Synthetically produced steroids attempt to remove the androgenic characteristics, thus leaving only the anabolic factor. Even though prescribed steroids are called *anabolic steroids,* all have retained some androgenic properties.[58]

The two important research questions are as follows: Do anabolic steroids increase muscle hypertrophy and, in turn, is performance improved? Are there side effects to anabolic steroid use, and, if so, do these effects make the benefit/risk ratio too high for recommendation to athletes?

As with all drug research, certain research protocols are necessary to achieve valid results, for example, placebo and double blind designs. Certain additional problems are inherent with research on anabolic steroids:

1. Specificity of subject sample—untrained persons with little or no initial muscle hypertrophy may make unusually large gains with or without steroid use.
2. Drug dosage—therapeutic daily dosages (15 mg) may not be as high as those used by athletes in training (100 to 150 mg).

3. Training dosage—in the practical world steroid use is combined with intense training.

4. Diet and dietary supplementation—athletes engaged in intense resistance training require large caloric intakes and most supplement their diets with protein.

These factors must be considered when planning research protocols so that results are related to actual practice.

Performance effects

Does the administration of anabolic steroids enhance endurance performance? Twenty-one college students were trained with a running program.[38] Subjects were randomly assigned to three groups: steroid (3 mg stanozolol per day), placebo, and control. All groups received a dietary supplement of 90% protein powder. There were no significant differences between groups in mile run time, cable tension strength, skinfold fat, body weight, or $\dot{V}O_2$ max. Thirty-six albino rats were subjected to a similar protocol (drug,

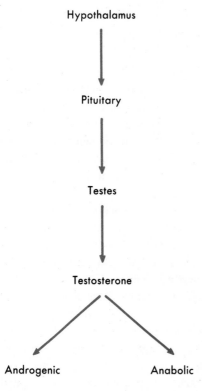

Hypothalamus

Pituitary

Testes

Testosterone

Androgenic   Anabolic

FIG. 20-3   Pituitary-testes axis. Human testosterone has both androgenic (stimulation of secondary sex characteristics) and anabolic (muscle-building) properties. (From Taylor, William N., M.D.: Anabolic steroids and the athlete, Jefferson, N.C., 1982, McFarland & Co., Inc., Publishers. Reprinted by permission of the publisher.)

placebo, and control).[30] Each group was further subdivided into sedentary and exercise (running) treatments. The relative organ weight (per kilogram of body weight) was greater in the exercised animals because of the leaner body composition of the running animals. No significant difference was noted for body weight between drug and placebo groups. Also, hypertrophy of leg muscles was not observed. Another investigation examined the interaction of steroid administration and an exercise program that included both running and progressive resistance training (each 3 days per week).[43] Subjects included six nonathletes and six wrestlers. The experiment was double blind. Both nonathletes and wrestlers gained significantly more weight with dinabol. There was no significant change in $\dot{V}O_2$. It does not appear that steroid administration significantly affects endurance performance or physiological variables related to that performance.

Perhaps the most important performance question is related to muscle hypertrophy and strength development. A few investigations have examined relatively untrained subjects. Although some studies have observed increases in muscle mass and strength,[70] others have not been able to document change.[24,37] One of the negative studies did not use a placebo treatment, and another study found significant changes in muscle size and strength but not when compared to a placebo treatment.[29] It appears that the conclusion that no improvements are possible with untrained subjects may be correct.[58]

Most investigations using trained subjects have found significant improvements in muscle mass and strength.[50,56,61] All studies reported here used comparable experimental controls (double blind and placebo treatments). One investigator studied 16 healthy males who had just completed a beginning weight training class.[61] Subjects were paired on the basis of initial strength tests (bench press and squat) and randomly assigned to an experimental (10 ml dinabol per day) or placebo group. Training consisted of four sets (5 reps) of four exercises at 80% of IRM (repetition maximum). Unlike most studies of trained subjects, no dietary control or protein supplement was provided. Following the 5 weeks of training, the experimental group significantly exceeded the placebo group in bench press, squat, body density, lean body mass, percent of fat, and fat in kilograms.

At least two studies have not found beneficial results.[16,27] As an example, nine competitive lifters were tested under placebo, testosterone, and nandrolone decanoate conditions.[16] In this experiment, not only a synthetically produced anabolic steroid was tested, but testosterone was also examined. A number of measures derived from Cybex (isokinetic) testing were evaluated under each condition. Seven of the variables did not differ among treatments. Both nandrolone and placebo treatments were significantly greater than the testosterone treatment during elbow flexion at 180 degrees/second, that is, showing the power of the placebo. The only difference that favored nandrolone over the placebo was ankle plantar flexion at 30 degrees/second. Perhaps the most interesting finding had to do with subjective reports of the subjects. Reports confirmed feelings of increased strength during the administration of both steroids yet no such finding during the placebo treatment. Apparently, at the very least, steroids provide a feeling of strength. Such a feeling could be powerful enough to entice use regardless of real effects.

Experts from the American College of Sports Medicine have reviewed the steroid literature and developed a ''Position Stand on the Use of Anabolic-Androgenic Steroids in

Sports'' (see box).[2] It was concluded that small increases in strength, important to competition, are exhibited by some, but not all, ''experienced weight trainers.''

Practical summary. It would be easy to find evidence that supports either positive or no performance benefits from anabolic steroids. Final answers to the steroid question require the test of further experimentation.

Side effects

Discussion of side effects is often used to scare athletes from use. Judging by the wide use of anabolic steroids, the perceived benefits counterbalance the possible risks. Virtually no evidence exists relative to the side effects of steroid administration in normal

---

SUMMARY POINTS OF THE AMERICAN COLLEGE OF SPORTS MEDICINE POSITION STAND ON THE USE OF ANABOLIC-ANDROGENIC STEROIDS IN SPORTS

Based on a comprehensive literature survey and a careful analysis of the claims concerning the ergogenic effects and the adverse effects of anabolic-androgenic steroids, it is the position of the American College of Sports Medicine that:

1. Anabolic-androgenic steroids in the presence of an adequate diet can contribute to increases in body weight, often in the lean mass compartment.
2. The gains in muscular strength achieved through high-intensity exercise and proper diet can occur by the increased use of anabolic-androgenic steroids in some individuals.
3. Anabolic-androgenic steroids do not increase aerobic power or capacity for muscular exercise.
4. Anabolic-androgenic steroids have been associated with adverse effects on the liver, cardiovascular system, reproductive system, and psychological status in therapeutic trials and in limited research on athletes. Until further research is completed, the potential hazards of the use of the anabolic-androgenic steroids in athletes must include those found in therapeutic trials.
5. The use of anabolic-androgenic steroids by athletes is contrary to the rules and ethical principles of athletic competition as set forth by many of the sports governing bodies. The American College of Sports Medicine supports these ethical principles and deplores the use of anabolic-androgenic steroids by athletes.

Summary points reprinted with permission of the American College of Sports Medicine. Copyright 1984, American College of Sports Medicine. Contact the American College of Sports Medicine for complete position stand.

subjects. Androgenic side effects have been proposed, since most synthetically produced steroids do not completely remove these characteristics. For instance, the appearance of a spectrum of male secondary sex characteristics can be predicted in females. Since high steroid levels in tissues tell the body that testosterone need not be produced, steroid administration could produce testicular atrophy. These side effects have not been scientifically documented even though they may be correct.

Current knowledge of the side effects of steroids has been derived from patients who receive therapeutic dosages of steroids to correct various pathological conditions. Rather alarming side effects have been reported concerning the clinical use of steroids.[36] Short-term use appears to be benign and reversible with discontinuation of the drug; however, 80% of 69 patients showed alterations in liver function. Long-term use has resulted in the diagnosis of *peliosis hepatis* and *hepatocellular carcinoma*. Both are potentially deadly. Also, patients treated with steroids for aplastic anemia have developed *myeloid leukemia*. Such a result may have occurred without steroid administration.

Another important side effect of steroid administration is the development of mood changes and aggressive behavior.[2] These responses are related to blood testosterone levels that are known to alter brain waves (electroencephalogram). Production of antisocial aggressive behavior may be advantageous when the interaction is limited to a barbell but can be otherwise unpleasant or perhaps dangerous. It has been suggested that this aggressive behavior may explain the positive strength changes observed in some lifters, that is, high motivation to train.

Steroid use is racing ahead in epidemic proportions. Presently, scientists know very little about possible side effects. The performance data are still controversial. While athletic associations are increasing efforts for detection of anabolic steroid use among athletes, the scientific community needs to devote considerable effort to further understanding of this potentially deadly drug.

VITAMINS

The folklore of vitamin supplementation is so pervasive in athletics that there is no doubt of wide acceptance of benefits and consequent employment by athletes. Vitamins are claimed to do everything from curing the common cold to promoting performance. They certainly are essential to our daily nutrition "as regulators of metabolic processes, usually acting as coenzymes."[66] These regulatory functions have caused speculation as to their role in athletic performance.

Fat-soluble vitamins (A, D, E, and K) can be toxic if taken in excess because they are stored in bodily tissues, mainly in the liver. Excessive intake of water-soluble vitamins (C and B complex: thiamin, riboflavin, pyridoxine, folic acid, cyanocobalamin, biotin, and pantothenic acid) is not usually a problem because the excess is removed by the kidney and excreted. However, vitamin C and niacin are known to be toxic in large amounts. There is a tendency among some athletes to consume megadoses of vitamins. In some cases, this practice may be harmless, but in others, vitamin toxicity may result.

Table 20-2 reviews all the vitamins, indicating their major function, toxicity, and a sample of evidence related to performance. Investigators have been unable to find a

TABLE 20-2 |||||| VITAMINS: MAJOR FUNCTION, TOXICITY, AND EVIDENCE FOR AND AGAINST PERFORMANCE ENHANCEMENT

Vitamin	Major function	Toxicity	Evidence of performance enhancement
A	Maintain vision	In excess	Wald and others[60]—no significance in submaximal or maximal exercise over 6-month deficiency period
B₁ (thiamin)	Energy metabolism	Nontoxic	Keys and others[41]—no benefit to physical performance from supplementation
B₂ (riboflavin)	Energy metabolism	Nontoxic	Horwit[32]—not beneficial
Niacin	Energy metabolism	In excess	Hilsendager and Karpovich[31]—insignificant effect on endurance Bergstrom and others[6]—short-term, near maximal, and prolonged submaximal work unchanged
B₆ (pyridoxin)	Amino acid metabolism	Nontoxic	Lawrence and others[42]—no effect on swimming endurance capacity
B₁₂ (cyanocobalamin)	Carbohydrate and fat metabolism	Nontoxic	Montoye and others[48]—no effect on half mile run
Pantothenic acid	Carbohydrate and fat metabolism	Nontoxic	No objective evidence available
Folic acid (folacin)	DNA synthesis	Nontoxic	No objective evidence available
B complex	Energy metabolism	Nontoxic, except niacin	Contradictory Simonson and others[54]—no effect Early and Carlson[19]—less fatigue with supplemented subjects
C (ascorbic acid)	Not completely determined	In excess	Contradictory Spioch and others[55]—significant effect Keren[40]—no beneficial effect
D	Calcification of bones; calcium and phosphate metabolism	In excess	Berven[7]—no effect on physical working capacity of children
E	Antioxidant; prevents oxidation of fatty acids	In excess	Contradictory Cureton[17]—significant effect on run to exhaustion in wrestlers Shephard and others[53]—insignificant effect on college swimmers

From Williams, M.H.: Vitamin, iron and calcium supplementation: effect on human physical performance. In Haskell, W., Scala, J., and Whittam, J., editors: Nutrition and athletic performance, Palo Alto, 1982, Bull Publishing Co.

beneficial effect of extradietary supplementation of vitamins A, B_1, B_2, niacin, B_6, B_{12}, pantothenic acid, folic acid, and D. Evidence is contradictory relative to B complex, C, and E.

It has been argued that vitamins may not be beneficial when dietary intake is adequate, but many athletes are using extremely high exercise intensities with ad lib calories taken from food products containing little or no vitamins. This argument is valid and should stimulate future research. Such research is complicated, since it is difficult to scientifically control experiments in which athletes randomly become vitamin deficient. Most institutions that protect the health and welfare of human subjects would probably not approve of experiments in which athletes are systemically made to be vitamin deficient.

MINERALS

Minerals are "physiological compounds that help regulate such functions as oxygen transport, excitability of muscle and nerve tissue, acid-base balance, and water metabolism."[66] Iron is found in hemoglobin, myoglobin, and the cytochromes, all involved in oxygen transport and aerobic ATP production. Women are more likely to become iron deficient as a result of the loss of iron in the menstrual discharge. One report indicates that 25% of trained field hockey players, 35% of moderately active females, and 8% of sedentary females are iron deficient.[28] The average daily intake of iron is not sufficient to replace loss in females. Women athletes undergoing hard training would probably prevent the possibility of anemia (decreased RBCs) by adding iron to their diets. However, little research is available to evaluate the effect of supplementation. It is still not known whether performance would be improved. Athletes taking iron supplements should be prudent in their intake, since iron cannot be excreted and can accumulate in the liver.

Calcium, an essential ingredient in the skeleton as well as a mandatory component of muscle contraction, nerve transmission, and blood clotting mechanisms, does not become deficient with a balanced diet.[66] Zinc was found to be at low normal levels in long distance runners.[18] This may suggest the need for supplementation; however, no performance decline was noted. Zinc is a trace mineral required for blood cell production, tissue repair, growth, and reproductive function.

SUMMARY

This chapter deals with an examination of whether various supplemental aids alter physiological function or benefit performance, and whether harmful side effects may occur. These aids are most commonly referred to as ergogenic aids, which literally means producing work. Since many ergogenic aids are not endogenous substances and can take the form of drugs, their effects may provide an unfair advantage. The job of the exercise physiologist is to determine whether any advantage at all can be shown. Experimentation is difficult because of the possible subjective effect of supplementation. Control groups, placebo substances, and double blind administration are techniques that aid the investigator in the search for real effects.

Many athletes believe that their performance can be augmented with the use of stimulants. Amphetamines have been administered in the hopes that the athlete may become fatigue resistant. This drug has produced increased strength in some muscle groups but not in others. The fatigue-masking qualities of the drug may provide performance enhancement during endurance tasks. However, this same effect could be fatal, especially in hot environments.

Another stimulant recently recognized as having possible benefits is caffeine. Caffeine appears to be beneficial to endurance performance by recruiting fat for exercise metabolism and sparing carbohydrate.

Although the evidence concerning the cardiovascular effects of nicotine during submaximal exercise is contradictory, maximal performance is definitely inhibited. Lower $\dot{V}O_2$ max values and treadmill exercise durations have been observed in smokers.

Alcohol is classed as a depressant and may remove psychological inhibitions inherent in athletics if used in small quantities. However, alcohol, in any quantity, is not recommended by the American College of Sports Medicine. Morphine, another depressant, is sometimes used in sport to inhibit pain perception. Administration of this drug destroys the link between pulmonary ventilation and $\dot{V}CO_2$, thus eliminating the primary factor in the control of exercise hyperpnea.

"Blood doping," or induced erythrocythemia, has been advocated as a means of increasing hemoglobin, hematocrit, and blood volume and, in turn, improving oxygen transport. It appears that "blood doping" can be used to augment endurance performance if appropriate procedures are followed. Those procedures include withdrawing and reinfusing more than 800 milliliters of blood and allowing at least 21 days for the reconstitution of the subject's blood values.

Beta blockers, drugs that inhibit heart rate and blood pressure, have been proposed as an effective means of reducing the effects of anxiety or previous exercise on motor control tasks. Research indicates that this class of drugs reduces anaerobic capacity and does not benefit ski jumping.

Hyperoxia, increased oxygen percentages in the inspired respiratory air, is known to benefit endurance performance but technical difficulties limit its application. On the other hand, recovery from exercise does not seem to be enhanced by hyperoxia.

No other drug has been as controversial or as misused in the past decade as steroids. Steroids attempt to mimic the anabolic effects (muscle building) of testosterone while minimizing its androgenic effects (promotion of secondary sex characteristics). The evidence concerning the effects of steroids on muscle mass and strength is contradictory in both untrained and trained groups. Well-controlled studies have found both positive gains and no improvement. Side effects of the drug have not been examined in normal subjects. However, when steroids are used for long-term therapeutic intervention, cases of liver carcinoma and leukemia have been observed.

Extradietary supplementation of vitamins A, B_1, B_2, niacin, B_6, B_{12}, pantothenic acid, folic acid, and D have not proven effective for sports performance. Evidence is contradictory relative to B complex, C, and E. Vitamin toxicity is a concern for the fat-soluble vitamins (A, D, E, and K) and vitamin C and niacin (water soluble).

Iron deficiency may be a problem for menstruating women training at high intensities. It is not known whether iron supplementation is beneficial; however, since iron cannot be excreted, it should be taken with caution.

KEY TERMS

anabolic related to protein synthesis, muscle building.

anabolic steroids synthetic derivative of testosterone used by athletes that retains the property of protein synthesis.

androgenic related to the promotion of male secondary sex characteristics.

beta blockers drugs that block beta adrenergic receptors in the heart, resulting in reduced heart rate and blood pressure.

blood doping slang term for induced erythrocythemia.

cardiovascular enhancer ergogenic aids that promote efficient function of the cardiovascular system.

depressants substances that decrease the body's vital functions.

doping slang term for the intake of substances that may provide a performance advantage.

double blind a research technique in which neither the researcher nor the subject knows the contents of the substance provided.

ergogenic aids "substances and phenomena that are work-producing aids, and those aids are thought to enhance performance above levels anticipated under normal conditions."[49]

hyperoxia excess oxygen content.

induced erythrocythemia technique for increasing red blood cells by withdrawing blood, storing it, and reinfusing it in the same person at a later date.

minerals physiological compounds that regulate functions such as oxygen transport, excitability of muscle and nerve tissue, acid-base balance, and water metabolism.

placebo a substance appearing like but not having the effect of the authentic substance.

stimulants substances that enhance the body's vital functions.

vitamins essential elements of daily nutrition that regulate metabolic processes.

REVIEW QUESTIONS

1. Discuss the experimental design problems that complicate the study of ergogenic aids.

2. Discuss the possible dangerous consequences of amphetamine use in the heat. Be sure to include the physiological response that is primarily affected.

3. What is the proposed mechanism by which caffeine might provide a performance benefit? How is this mechanism related to the concept of glycogen sparing?

4. How would you explain to athletes why alcohol abuse may hinder performance?

5. What is the theory underlying the possible beneficial effects of blood doping? What procedures seem to ensure the beneficial effects?

6. Explain the difference between the anabolic and the androgenic properties of steroids. What can be concluded regarding changes in muscle mass resulting from steroid administration? What are the potential side effects?

7. What is the general conclusion regarding the use of vitamin supplementation for athletes? What argument can be made against this conclusion?

8. Does the exercise scientist have an obligation to discuss the possible moral and ethical implications of working with athletes? Why?

REFERENCES

1. American College of Sports Medicine: Position statement on the use of alcohol in sports, Med. Sci. Sports Exerc. **14**:9, 1982.

2. American College of Sports Medicine: Position stand on the use of anabolic-androgenic steroids in sports, Sports Med. Bull. **19**:13, 1984.

3. Avakian, E.V., Horvath, S.M., Michael, E.D., and others: Effect of marihuana on cardiorespiratory responses to submaximal exercise, Clin. Pharmacol. Ther. **26**:777, 1979.

4. Bannister, R.G., and Cunningham, D.J.C.: The effects on the respiration and performance during exercise of adding oxygen to the inspired air, J. Physiol. (Lond.) **125**:118, 1954.

5. Behr, M.J., Leon, K.-H., and Jones, R.H.: Acute effects of cigarette smoking on left ventricular function at rest and exercise, Med. Sci. Sports Exerc. **13**:9, 1981.

6. Bergstrom, J., Hultman, E., Jorfeldt, L., and others: Effect of nicotinic acid on physical working capacity and on metabolism of muscle glycogen in man, J. Appl. Physiol. **26**:170, 1969.

7. Berven, H.: The physical working capacity of healthy children. Seasonal variation and effect of ultraviolet radiation and vitamin D supply, Acta Paediatr. **148**:1, 1963.

8. Borg, G., Edstrom, C.-C., Linderholm, H., and others: Changes in physical performance induced by amphetamine and amobarbital. In Whitlock, F.A., Charalampous, K.D., Lynn, E.J., and others, editors: Amphetamines: medical and psychological studies, New York, 1974, MSS Information Corporation.

9. Brundin, T.: Effects of tobacco smoking on the blood temperature during exercise, Acta Physiol. Scand. **479**:43, 1980.

10. Buick, F.J., Gledhill, N., Froese, A.B., and others: Effect of induced erythrocythemia on aerobic work capacity, J. Appl. Physiol.: Respir. Environ. Exerc. Physiol. **48**:636, 1980.

11. Chandler, J.V., and Blair, S.N.: The effect of amphetamines on selected physiological components related to athletic success, Med. Sci. Sports Exerc. **12**:65, 1980.

12. Christensen, E.H., Krogh, A., and Lindhard, J.: Investigations on heavy muscular work, Q. Bull. Health Organiz. League Nations **3**:388, 1934.

13. Cooper, D.L.: Drugs and the athlete, JAMA **221**:1007, 1972.

14. Cooter, G.R., and Stull, G.A.: The effect of amphetamine on endurance in rats, J. Sports Med. Phys. Fitness **14**:120, 1974.

15. Costill, D.L., Dalsky, G.P., and Fink, W.J.: Effects of caffeine ingestion on metabolism and exercise performance, Med. Sci. Sports **10**:155, 1978.

16. Crist, D.M., Stackpole, P.J., and Peake, G.T.: Effects of androgenic-anabolic steroids on neuromuscular power and body composition, J. Appl. Physiol.: Respir. Environ. Exerc. Physiol. **54**:366, 1983.

17. Cureton, T.K.: Wheat germ oil, the "wonder" fuel, Scholast. Coach **24:**36, 1955.

18. Dressendorfer, R., and Sockolov, R.: Hypozincemia in runners, Physic. Sportsmed. **8:**97, 1980.

19. Early, R., and Carlson, B.: Water soluble vitamin therapy on the delay of fatigue from physical activity in hot climate conditions, Intern. Z. Ange. Physiol. **27:**43, 1969.

20. Edison, G.R.: Amphetamines: a dangerous illusion. In Whitlock, F.A., Charalampous, K.D., Lynn, E.J., and others, editors: Amphetamines: medical and psychological studies, New York, 1974, MSS Information Corporation.

21. Ekblom, B., Goldbarg, A.N., and Gullbring, B.: Response to exercise after blood loss and reinfusion, J. Appl. Physiol. **33:**175, 1972.

22. Ekblom, B., Wilson, G., and Astrand, P.O.: Central circulation during exercise after venesection and reinfusion of red blood cells, J. Appl. Physiol. **40:**379, 1976.

23. Estler, C.-J., and Cabrys, M.C.: Swimming capacity of mice after prolonged treatment with psychostimulants. II. Effect of metamphetamine on swimming performance and availability of metabolic substrates, Psychopharmacology **60:**173, 1979.

24. Fowler, W.M., Gardner, G.W., and Egstrom, G.H.: Effect of an anabolic steroid on physical performance of young men, J. Appl. Physiol. **20:**1038, 1965.

25. Gerald, M.C.: Effects of (+)-amphetamine on the treadmill endurance performance of rats, Neuropharmacology **17:**703, 1978.

26. Gledhill, N.: Blood doping and related issues: a brief review, Med. Sci. Sports Exerc. **14:**183, 1982.

27. Golding, L.A., Freydinjer, J.E., and Fisher, S.S.: Weight, size, and strength—unchanged with steroids, Physic. Sportsmed. **2:**39, 1974.

28. Haymes, E.: The effect of physical activity level on selected hematological variables in adult women. Paper presented at AAHPERD Convention, Houston, Texas, March, 1972.

29. Hervey, G.R., Hutchinson, I., Knibbs, A.V., and others: "Anabolic" effects of methandiaone in men undergoing athletic training, Lancet **7988:**699, 1976.

30. Hickson, R.C., Heusner, W.W., Van Huss, W.D., and others: Effects of dianabol and high-intensity sprint training on body composition of rats, Med. Sci. Sports **8:**191, 1976.

31. Hilsendager, D., and Karpovich, P.: Ergogenic effect of glycine and niacin separately and in combination, Res. Q. **35:**389, 1964.

32. Horwit, M.: Riboflavin. In Goodhart, R., and Shils, M., editors: Modern nutrition in health and disease, Philadelphia, 1980, Lea & Febiger.

33. Hueting, J.E., and Poulus, A.J.: Amphetamine, performance, effort and fatigue, Pflugers Arch. **318:**260, 1970.

34. Ikai, M., and Steinhaus, A.: Some factors modifying the expression of human strength, J. Appl. Physiol. **16:**157, 1961.

35. Ivy, J.L., Costill, D.L., Fink, W.J., and others: Influence of caffeine and carbohydrate feedings on endurance performance, Med. Sci. Sports **11:**6, 1979.

36. Johnson, F.L.: The association of oral androgenic-anabolic steroids and life threatening disease, Med. Sci. Sports **7:**284, 1975.

37. Johnson, L.C., and O'Shea, J.P.: Anabolic steroid: effects on strength development, Science **164:**957, 1969.

38. Johnson, L.C., Roundy, E.S., Allsen, P.E., and others: Effect of anabolic steroid treatment on endurance, Med. Sci. Sports Exerc. **7**:287, 1975.

39. Karpovich, P.V., and Sinning, W.E.: Physiology of muscular activity, Philadelphia, 1971, W.B. Saunders Co.

40. Keren, G.: The effect of high dosage vitamin C intake on aerobic and anaerobic capacity, J. Sports Med. Phys. Fitness **20**:145, 1980.

41. Keys, A., Henschel, A.F., Mickelsen, O., and others: The performance of normal young men on controlled thiamine intake, J. Nutr. **26**:399, 1943.

42. Lawrence, J., Smith, J., Bower, R., and others: The effect of alphatocopherol (vitamin E) and pyridoxine HCl (vitamin B_6) on the swimming endurance of trained swimmers, J. Am. College Health Assoc. **23**:219, 1974.

43. Loughton, S.J., and Ruhling, R.O.: Human strength and endurance responses to anabolic steroid and training, J. Sports Med. Phys. Fitness **17**:285, 1977.

44. Margaria, R., Camporesi, E., Aghemo, P., and others: The effect of O_2 breathing on maximal aerobic power, Pflugers Arch. **336**:225, 1972.

45. Martin, B.J., Zwillich, C.W., and Weil, J.V.: Morphine reduces ventilation without changing metabolic rate in exercise, Med. Sci. Sports Exerc. **12**:285, 1980.

46. McHenry, P.L., Faris, J.V., Jordan, J.W., and others: Comparative study of cardiovascular function and ventricular premature complexes in smokers and non-smokers during maximal treadmill exercise, Cardiology **39**:493, 1977.

47. Montoye, H.J., Gayle, R., and Higgins, M.: Smoking habits, alcohol consumption and maximal oxygen uptake, Med. Sci. Sports Exerc. **12**:316, 1980.

48. Montoye, H.J., Spata, P., Pinckney, V., and others: Effects of vitamin B_{12} supplementation on physical fitness and growth on young boys, J. Appl. Physiol. **7**:589, 1955.

49. Morgan, W.P.: Ergogenic aids and muscular performance, New York, 1972, Academic Press, Inc.

50. O'Shea, J.P.: Biochemical evaluation of effects of stanozolol on adrenal, liver and muscle function in man, Nutr. Rep. Int. **10**:381, 1974.

51. Rusko, H., Kantola, H., Luhtanen, P., and others: Effect of beta-blockade on performances requiring force, velocity, coordination and/or anaerobic metabolism, J. Sports Med. Phys. Fitness **20**:139, 1980.

52. Santiago, T.V., Johnson, J., Riley, D.J., and others: Effects of morphine on ventilatory response to exercise, J. Appl. Physiol.: Respir., Environ. Exerc. Physiol. **47**:112, 1979.

53. Shephard, R., Campbell, R., Pimm, P., and others: Do athletes need vitamin E, Physic. Sportsmed. **2**:57, 1974.

54. Simonson, E., Enzer, N., Baer, A., and others: The influence of vitamin B (complex) surplus on the capacity for muscular and mental work, J. Industr. Hygiene **24**:83, 1942.

55. Spioch, F., Kobza, R., and Mazur, B.: Influence of vitamin C upon certain functional changes and the coefficient of mechanical efficiency in humans during physical effort, Acta Physiol. Pol. **17**:251, 1966.

56. Stamford, B.A., and Moffat, R.: Anabolic steroid: effectiveness as an ergogenic aid to experienced weight trainers, J. Sports Med. Phys. Fitness **14**:191, 1974.

57. Stone, J.: Steroids, Natl. Strength Condition. Assoc. J. **5**:13, 1983.

58. Taylor, W.N.: Anabolic steroids and the athlete, Jefferson, N.C., 1982, McFarland & Co., Inc., Publishers.

59. Videman, T., Sonck, T., and Janne, J.: The effect of beta-blockade in ski jumpers, Med. Sci. Sports **11**:266, 1979.

60. Wald, G., Brouha, L., and Johnson, R.: Experimental human vitamin A deficiency and ability to perform muscular exercise, Am. J. Physiol. **137**:551, 1942.

61. Ward, P.: The effect of an anabolic steroid on strength and lean body mass, Med. Sci. Sports **5**:227, 1973.

62. Welch, H.: Hyperoxia and human performance: a brief review, Med. Sci. Sports Exerc. **14**:253, 1982.

63. Wilcox, A.R.: The effects of caffeine and exercise on body weight, fat-pad weight, and fat-cell size, Med. Sci. Sports Exerc. **14**:317, 1982.

64. Williams, M.H.: Drugs and athletic performance, Springfield, Ill., 1974, Charles C Thomas, Publisher.

65. Williams, M.H.: Nutritional aspects of human physical and athletic performance, Springfield, Ill., 1976, Charles C Thomas, Publisher.

66. Williams, M.H.: Vitamin, iron and calcium supplementation: effect on human physical performance. In Haskell, W., Scala, J., and Whittam, J., editors: Nutrition and athletic performance, Palo Alto, 1982, Bull Publishing Co.

67. Williams, M.H., Lindhjem, M., and Schuster, R.: The effect of blood infusion upon endurance capacity and ratings of perceived exertion, Med. Sci. Sports **10**:113, 1978.

68. Williams, M.H., Wesseldine, S., Somma, T., and others: The effect of induced erythrocythemia upon 5-mile treadmill run time, Med. Sci. Sports Exerc. **13**:169, 1981.

69. Wilson, G.D., and Welch, H.G.: Effects of hyperoxic gas mixtures on exercise tolerance in man, Med. Sci. Sports **7**:48, 1975.

70. Win-May, M., and Mya-tu, M.: The effects of anabolic steroids on physical fitness, J. Sports Med. Phys. Fitness **15**:266, 1975.

SUGGESTED READINGS

Casal, D.C., and Leon, A.S.: Failure of caffeine to affect substrate utilization during prolonged running, Med. Sci. Sports Exerc. **17**:174, 1985.

Gray, M.E., and Titlow, L.W.: The effect of pangamic acid on maximal treadmill performance, Med. Sci. Sports Exerc. **14**:424, 1982.

Hanley, D.F.: Drug use and abuse. In Strauss, R.H., editor: Sports medicine and physiology, Philadelphia, 1979, W.B. Saunders Co.

Kanstrup, I., and Ekblom, B.: Blood volume and hemoglobin concentration as determinants of maximal aerobic power, Med. Sci. Sports Exerc. **16**:256, 1984.

Morgan, W.P.: Ergogenic aids and muscular performance, New York, 1972, Academic Press, Inc.

Powles, A.C.P.: The effect of drugs on the cardiovascular response to exercise, Med. Sci. Sports Exerc. **13**:252, 1981.

Taylor, W.N.: Anabolic steroids and the athlete, Jefferson, N.C., 1982, McFarland & Co., Inc., Publshers.

Whitlock, F.A., Charalampous, K.D., Lynn, E.J., and others: Amphetamines: medical and psychological studies, New York, 1974, MSS Information Corporation.

Wilcox, A.R.: The effects of caffeine and exercise on body weight, fat-pad weight, and fat-cell size, Med. Sci. Sports Exerc. **14:**317, 1982.

Williams, M.H.: Drugs and athletic performance, Springfield, Ill., 1974, Charles C Thomas, Publisher.

Williams, M.H.: Nutritional aspects of human physical and athletic performance, Springfield, Ill., 1976, Charles C Thomas, Publisher.

Williams, M.H.: Vitamin, iron and calcium supplementation: effect on human physical performance. In Haskell, W., Scala, J., and Whittam, J., editors: Nutrition and athletic performance, Palo Alto, 1982, Bull Publishing Co.

CASE STUDY 1

Twenty years ago, I was a member of a research team at the University of Illinois that was studying the effect of vitamin E on performance and various physiological variables. The design and results of that study are not the subject of this case study. The point I wish to make has been made over and over again in medicine: sometimes the contents of a capsule are not as important as what the patients feel they will gain from the capsule. Many "miraculous" cures have taken place with pills containing absolutely nothing of benefit. I'm sure the same is true of many supplements taken by athletes. If the process of receiving perceived aids results in improved performance, or the perception of improved performance, the apparent causal link between supplement and performance will be firmly entrenched.

One of the subjects in that experiment is a case in point. This gentleman was a university professor who asked if he could continue the supplement following termination of the experiment protocol. Without too much thought, or consideration of what treatment group the professor was in, permission was quickly granted. Daily, the professor would appear at the door of the physical fitness lab for his allotment of vitamin E. After this went on for a while, someone asked what professor X was doing. It was explained that he thought he had received such a great physiological change from the supplement that he was sure it was a miracle drug and that he had asked to continue with the vitamin. A group of us discussed the matter and discovered that he had participated in the placebo group that received a capsule filled with fat. Our initial response was to roar with laughter. The more difficult task was to inform him of the actual contents of the capsule. Our solution to that problem and the human subject implications is not as important to the point of this case study. The importance of the matter is in the great power of receiving something you believe will be effective. You can see how many athletes become "hooked" on supplements irrespective of the accumulated evidence.

CASE STUDY 2

PROFESSOR: It looks like you have changed your muscle mass 100% since you were a freshman.

ATHLETE: Well, I have grown quite a bit in the last couple of years.

PROFESSOR: Training hard?

ATHLETE: Well, yes, and I have a little help from my friends.

PROFESSOR: What do you mean by that?

ATHLETE: You know, I have friends at the gym where I train who have everything you need.

PROFESSOR: Pills you mean?

ATHLETE: Sure.

PROFESSOR: Steroids?

ATHLETE: Yes.

PROFESSOR: But you've been lifting fantastic amounts of daily weight. Don't you think that has anything to do with your muscle mass and performance success?

ATHLETE: Of course. I work harder than most anyone in my weight class. I'm not national champion just because of a few steroids.

PROFESSOR: Why do you take them then?

ATHLETE: I'm not sure they work. I know I feel stronger when I take them. I know I've improved. I don't know what to attribute to what. What I do know is that I want to be the Olympic champion. The difference could be a pound or two. I know others are taking steroids. I'm not going to give up my one chance just in case they do work.

PROFESSOR: Haven't you heard about the possible side effects: testicular atrophy, liver carcinoma, leukemia?

ATHLETE: Sure, and it scares me some. But, you know, to be Olympic champion is worth it. If I could be champion I'd gladly die the next day.

Dialogues like this do take place. The answer to such problems does not lie with experimentation, detection methods, and codes of conduct. The answer is embedded within our human desire to achieve at any cost. Until we can make an impact here, our scientific efforts will be explanatory rather than important.

chapter 21

PHYSIOLOGICAL BASIS OF EXERCISE PERCEPTIONS

MAJOR LEARNING OBJECTIVE
Exercise perceptions are useful for providing information about the perceptual intensity of exercise and for predicting physical working capacity.

APPLICATIONS
The Borg scale can be used to evaluate exercise and sport effort. It can be viewed as an aid to coaching and teaching to be used in combination with performance (for example, time) and physiological data (for example, heart rate).

U NTIL the late 1960s, little interest was exhibited in the sensations of physical effort reported during exercise. For the most part, exercise perceptions were thought to be unimportant and/or unable to be measured. However, it seemed obvious to a few investigators that control of exercise intensity depended to a large extent on monitoring these sensations. For example, pain and discomfort while running signal the need to make decisions relative to pace and even whether exercise will be continued. Understanding more about exercise perception is now thought to be an essential element in the scientific attempt to account for human performance.

Recently, a number of investigators have become increasingly concerned with how exercise perceptions are sensed. In other words, they asked what the physiological basis of exercise perceptions is. This chapter brings the reader up to date regarding current knowledge in this area.

PSYCHOPHYSICAL MEASUREMENT

The first experimental step in the study of exercise perceptions required the development of a reliable and valid measurement tool. Many exercise scientists in the 1960s questioned whether varying sensations of work could be quantified.

Fortunately, a rating scale was developed by Gunnar Borg, professor of psychology at the University of Stockholm. Borg, as a psychologist, was interested in relating sensation of effort (output) to easily quantifiable physical stimuli (input). Therefore, the bicycle ergometer was chosen to provide known physical exercise intensities and easily attainable physiological responses, that is, heart rate.[6] An exercise test was constructed in which intensity was periodically increased and exercise perceptions were recorded simultaneously with heart rate. Borg developed a simple rating scale in which recorded perceptions were theoretically matched with physiological response (see Figure 21-1). He termed perceptual responses "ratings of perceived exertion (RPE)." In fact, because the scale values (6 to 20) approximately parallel the heart rate range of a young person (60 to 200 beats per minute), Borg has suggested that heart rate can be predicted from RPE in the following manner: heart rate = RPE × 10.[7]

The scale, which has become known as the Borg or RPE scale, is a simple, easily understood format in which numbers are selected that coincide with the individual's perceptions of how intense the exercise feels. The number 6 on the scale can be viewed as the baseline of sensation for the work being performed, that is, no exertion at all. The top of the scale, 20, would be the most exhausted a person could feel for the exercise being performed, that is, maximal exertion. Each person estimates the intensity level that corresponds to his or her perception of effort at any point in time, or level of exercise, during a particular task.

517

It should be pointed out that many other measurement options are open to investigators interested in measuring RPE. Two of these options are magnitude estimation and effort production.[7] The detailed discussion necessary to explain these psychophysical measurement techniques will not be given here.

RELIABILITY AND VALIDITY OF THE BORG SCALE

Exercise physiologists have been concerned about the reproducibility (reliability) of RPE; that is, can the sensations be duplicated in the same test from one day to the next? Such an experiment was performed using a progressive protocol, work loads presented incrementally from low to high, and a random protocol.[39] Correlation coefficients computed between repeat tests were 0.80 and 0.78 for the progressive and random protocols. Using a modification of the Borg scale, others found reliability coefficients of a higher magnitude, 0.991 and 0.996 for walking and 0.985 and 0.987 for running.[27]

Another question of interest concerns the validity of the Borg scale, that is, do the perceptual ratings really assess the physiological strain imposed by the work? Generally, the Borg scale is thought to be valid to the extent that the scale ratings parallel metabolic measures. Since RPE is linearly related to heart rate in most exercise tasks, the scale is considered to be valid.

6

7   Very, very light

8

9   Very light

10

11   Fairly light

12

13   Somewhat hard

14

15   Hard

16

17   Very hard

18

19   Very, very hard

20

FIG. 21-1   The Borg scale for rating perceived exertion (RPE). The number *6* on the scale is associated with no exertion, and *20* with maximal exertion.

Practical summary. Ratings of perceived exertion measured with the Borg scale are considered reliable and valid estimates of effort for use in practical environments.

GENERAL DESCRIPTION OF EXERCISE PERCEPTIONS
Exercise intensity

As mentioned, the Borg scale was developed to follow the pattern of heart rate during bicycle ergometer exercise. As exercise intensity is incrementally increased, heart rate increases and, in turn, RPE increases (see Figure 21-2). As the data in Figure 21-2 suggest, the Borg heart rate prediction formula (RPE × 10) *generally* describes the linear relationship, however, *specifically* this is not the case. For example, at 900 kpm a subject might perceive the effort to be 9 at a heart rate of 125. The equation predicts heart rate to be 9 × 10 = 90. Studies have found exercise intensity and RPE to be correlated at about the 0.85 level.[7] The lack of a perfect correlation expresses the error in the heart rate prediction.

Practical summary. Most research supports the linear relationship between heart rate and RPE but does not support the use of the formula RPE × 10 = Heart rate.

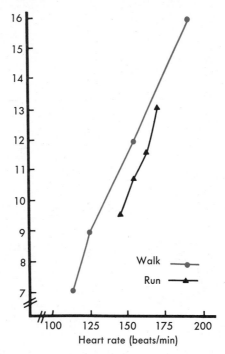

FIG. 21-2   **Exercise perceptions expressed as a function of heart rate. RPE rises linearly with increasing heart rate during walking and running. (From Noble, B.J., Metz, K.F., Pandolf, K.B., and others: Perceived exertion during walking and running, Med. Sci. Sports 5:116, 1973.)**

Walking and running responses

It has been known for some time that the rate of body metabolism (oxygen consumption) is higher while running than while walking at lower velocities,[5] for example, below 5 mph. To bring this speed range into perspective, preferred walking speed in a group of college students has been calculated to be 3.11 mph.[25] For speeds greater than 5 mph, the metabolic cost of walking is higher than that of running. Obviously, from a metabolic point of view, it would be best to walk at less than and run at more than 5 mph. It was suspected that RPE would respond in the same way.

Generally, RPE was found to react in the same way as oxygen consumption (see Figure 21-3). However, the speed at which walking felt more difficult was less than 5 mph, specifically 4.2 mph.[25] For the first time, it became clear that the RPE was partly, but not completely, explained by the metabolic cost of exercise.

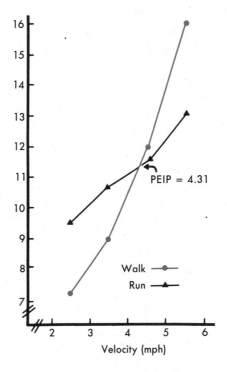

FIG. 21-3   Exercise perceptions during walking and running. Subjects perceive the effort of running to be harder than walking at lower speeds and vice versa at higher speeds. PEIP = Perceived exertion intersection point. (From Noble, B.J., Metz, K.F., Pandolf, K.B., and others: Perceived exertion during walking and running, Med. Sci. Sports 5:116, 1973.)

Comparison in other modes of exercise

RPE was compared in various other modes of exercise as well.[12] In addition to comparing perceptions of equivalent exercise intensities, RPE was compared at equivalent metabolic levels (oxygen consumption or heart rate). Exercise perceptions while bicycling were found to be significantly higher than while running at given submaximal oxygen consumptions. However, since maximal oxygen consumption while bicycling is lower than while running, when comparisons were made at equivalent percentages of $\dot{V}O_2$ max, no differences were observed. In others words, if an individual works at 50% of maximum in each type of exercise, perceptions of exertion will not be significantly different. Therefore, exercise seems to be rated in relation to a task-related maximum.

When swimming and running were compared, no differences were observed in given submaximal oxygen consumptions. Although the authors did not discuss comparisons relative to maximal values, presumably swimming sensations would have been lower at equal percentages of maximal oxygen consumption. Arm exercise comparisons do not appear to conform to the same principle as strictly leg comparisons. This is undoubtedly a result of the much smaller muscle mass in the arms.

Effect of exercise duration on exercise perceptions

Most investigations have examined RPE during relatively short-term work. A few exceptions are notable and provide us with insight into perceptions during long-term exposure. Virtually every study found that perceptions increased over time. RPE was measured during walking and running at speeds from 2.0 to 6.5 mph and over 30 minutes.[35] Not only did RPE increase over time, but as speed increased in separate treatments, so did the rate at which RPE increased. Similar results were observed during a simulated marathon run (2 to 3 hours) on a treadmill.[3] Although pulmonary ventilation and oxygen consumption remained stable, heart rate tended to increase with time.

RPE, heart rate, and performance time were recorded in one runner participating in the Mechanicsburg, Pennsylvania marathon.[26] Measurements were recorded after 8.2, 14.2, 20.2, and 26.2 miles. Heart rate remained stable at 140 beats/min. Conversely, RPE increased from 13 at 8.2 miles to 19 at 26.2 miles. Performance time was quite stable compared to RPE, with incremental times recorded at 47, 51, 46, and 52 minutes, respectively. The fatigue process involved in a long-duration performance necessitates the recruitment of additional motor units to sustain the exercise. This additional recruitment as well as increased core temperature, most likely accounts for the increased heart rate and the RPE as well when speed is held constant on a treadmill. Muscle soreness may also cause increases in the RPE. Therefore, motor unit recruitment, body temperature, and muscle soreness may contribute to increasing RPE during long-duration exercise.

Perceptual responses to recovery from marathon running have also been examined.[30] RPE during race-pace treadmill exercises was significantly elevated 2 to 3 and 6 to 8 days after the marathon. Muscle soreness and stiffness seemed to be related to the increased perceptual ratings following a marathon run.

Influence of physical training on exercise perceptions

Five college men trained 3 days per week for 5 weeks. Following training, the RPE at a heart rate of 150 beats per minute did not change significantly, but the treadmill time to reach 150 increased. Therefore, the heart rate and RPE time curve were shifted to the right with training. Another study involved training eight young males (21 to 32 years) 5 days per week for 8 weeks.[12] Maximal oxygen uptake was improved from 2.90 L/min to 3.35 L/min. RPE was lower for given $\dot{V}_{O_2}$ levels after training, but no differences were evidenced when results were expressed in percent of $\dot{V}_{O_2}$ max, that is, relative to aerobic power. Thus, effort is perceived to be less following training when the metabolic level of the exercise is equivalent. However, since fitness ($\dot{V}_{O_2}$ max) improved with training, comparison at the same metabolic level represents two different percentages of maximum. It appears that, relative to $\dot{V}_{O_2}$ max, RPE remains unchanged with training. More experimentation is required here.

PHYSIOLOGICAL BASIS OF EXERCISE PERCEPTIONS

Perhaps the best way to begin to explain the physiological basis of exercise perceptions is to examine each variable that has been hypothesized to be related to perceptual ratings. In that way we can begin to describe an explanatory model. The complexity of the problem and the rather recent origin of this research indicate that investigators in this area have made only very preliminary progress.

Heart rate

The search for heart rate (HR) as a possible cue to perceptual ratings has used considerable experimental energy. Although the reasonable correlations found between HR and RPE[6] stimulated early research activity, it does not seem reasonable that HR, as such, is sensed as a basis for effort perceptions.

Running and walking were compared to determine whether the pattern of HR change with increased speed was paralleled by similar perceptual changes.[25] Results showed that HR did not seem to explain the perceptual response and that another factor, most likely emanating from local musculature, was primarily responsible. HR was not eliminated as a contributing factor, but certainly the power of its implication was reduced. In another experiment, no significant differences in RPE were found between equal exercise intensities when HR was significantly increased by increased environmental heat.[31] Therefore, HR, as such, was eliminated as the sole parameter affecting exertion ratings and a "complex and yet unresolved integration of several parameters" was said to be involved.

Although HR measures physiological strain and is found to be linearly related to RPE,[24] factors in addition to the HR seem to be involved in setting exercise perceptions.

Ventilation

Respiratory sensations are known to be well perceived.[1] Increases in ventilation during exercise were detected when tidal volume increased by 700 ml.[45] Therefore, it was hypothesized that artifically increasing ventilation, by adding 1.75% and 3.5% CO_2 to the inspired air while subjects ran and cycled, would incrementally increase RPE in proportion to the elevated ventilation. The only significant difference observed in RPE was at 7 mph (the highest speed) on the treadmill when 3.5% CO_2 induced a ventilation increase of approximately 30 L/min. It was suggested that ventilatory cues do not make significant contributions until approximately 70% $\dot{V}O_2$ max (7 mph) is reached. The reason that subjects were unable to detect increases in ventilation at lower levels of work is unclear. Perhaps local muscular discomfort predominates at lower exercise intensities and overpowers the pulmonary cues.

Ventilation shows great potential as a perceptual cue during exercise. Certainly respiratory sensations are consciously perceived. However, during low-level exercise these cues are most likely masked by other, more intense stimuli. It appears that high-level exercise may show ventilation to be a powerful factor in the setting of RPE; however, the experimental work is yet to be accomplished.

Oxygen consumption

Similar to HR, oxygen consumption has been shown to be linearly related to RPE.[24] This observation has led some researchers to speculate that this parameter plays an important role in setting effort perceptions. Two experiments attempted to discover whether exercises that showed a common oxygen consumption level (power output) would result in similar RPE responses.[32,41] Pedal speed and resistance were manipulated while power output was held constant. RPE was observed to be significantly higher at a pedaling rate of 40 rpm compared to 60 and 80 rpm. A distressed cardiorespiratory system could not have caused the higher RPE at 40 rpm. Muscular and joint discomfort associated with high resistance/low repetition (40 rpm) exercise must dominate the perceptual rating.

As was the case with HR, $\dot{V}O_2$ has not been found to be a primary cue in the setting of perceptual intensity. Again, local muscular factors seem to be more important, at least for submaximal exercise on the bicycle ergometer.

Catecholamines

Catecholamine concentration, particularly norepinephrine (NE), has been shown to increase with increasing work load above 50% $\dot{V}O_2$ max.[15] Another study found little change in either NE or epinephrine (E) at 200 and 400 kpm/min; however, both increased, especially NE, at 750 kpm/min.[13] In general, RPE increases linearly with exercise intensity. In this study, at the point where catecholamines rose precipitously, subjects passed the midpoint of the rating scale and began rating exercise as "laborious" rather than "light." Catecholamines may play a role during heavy exercise in setting exercise perceptions.

Blood glucose

To study the possible role of blood glucose level in setting exercise perception, long-distance runners were exposed to 2-hour treadmill runs under placebo and glucose ingestion conditions.[3] Blood glucose level decreased with time, particularly after 1 hour, during the placebo run. RPE was significantly lower during the glucose run. Therefore, glucose depletion was suggested as a factor in exertion ratings during long-duration exercise. The central nervous system, via glucoreceptors, was thought to be involved in the sensing process.

Lactic acid

It is always tempting to implicate the accumulation of lactic acid with increasing perceptual intensity. The research evidence does not always support this hypothesis. However, the data from several studies are in conflict, so that the final chapter is yet to be written. For example, 27 elite distance runners were studied during a submaximal run (12 mph, 0%) on the treadmill.[27] RPE was found to correlate 0.61 with lactate accumulation. These authors, on the basis of this correlation compared to other computed relationships, suggest that lactic acid is the best single predictor of RPE. Other authors have reported similar correlations (between 0.63 and 0.77).[11] On the other hand, a correlation of only 0.15 was reported between these variables with a mixed sample of normal volunteers, rehabilitation patients, and a long-distance competitive cyclist.[18]

Further evidence of confusion regarding the role of lactic acid has been reported.[12,41] One investigation[12] indicates that RPE may be set as a function of lactate concentrations, that is, when lactate was equal in two different modes of exercise, RPE was also equivalent. In the other study,[41] bicycle trials were administered to subjects in which pedal rate and resistance were manipulated so the power output, and therefore oxygen uptake, was equated. RPE was found to be significantly higher during 60 rpm trials compared to 40 and 80 rpm. However, lactate concentration was not significantly different between trials. In summary, the accumulation hypothesis involving lactic acid remains open to question.

EXPLANATORY MODELS

Most scientific papers dealing with RPE offer some statement relative to the contribution of various physiological variables to the setting of perceptual intensity. A few of these papers distinguish themselves by having made some attempt to identify the dimensions of an explanatory model.

The following two factors were proposed to explain the variability in RPE when exercises involving different muscle masses were compared[12]:

> *Local factor* — "the feeling of strain in working muscles"
> *Central factor* — "perceived tachycardia, tachypnea, and even dyspnea"

The local factor is said to predominate in exercise involving small muscle masses. Large muscle group exercise places stress on pulmonary ventilation and circulation in addition to causing local discomfort. This model is the most often quoted explanation of perceptual variability during exercise.

Most research supports the presence of a local factor, but attempts to directly examine the factors involved conclude that these factors are "difficult or probably impossible to quantify."[33] Likewise, most authors support the existence of the central factor. Although most central factors, (HR, $\dot{V}O_2$, $\dot{V}E$, and respiratory rate) have been found to be correlated with RPE, when these factors were tested experimentally they were not found to be primary. However, these factors do undeniably contribute to the overall sense of exertion.

Figure 21-4 depicts a model proposed to further explain the factors related to RPE.[19] This model suggests that the relationships between subjective ratings and specific physiological events during different types of physical work can be more precisely defined and compared using "subordinate" differentiated ratings that are close to the level of the discrete symptoms.[33] That is, ratings of specific body areas should be obtained, not just overall ratings. For example, during bicycle exercise, ratings of *local* discomfort in the legs, *central* discomfort in the chest, as well as *overall* discomfort ratings could be requested.

Several authors have used the concept of *differentiated ratings* in their investigations. Differentiated ratings, simply stated, refer to an attempt to independently specify perceptual intensities arising from local and central cues. Because bicycle and treadmill ergometers are most typically used, local is defined as cues arising from the legs, and

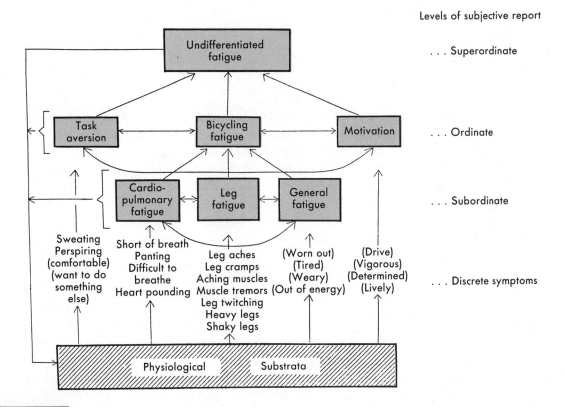

FIG. 21-4 An explanatory model that depicts the interaction of several factors related to the setting of exercise perceptions. This model suggests a direct link between specific physiological events (cues) and the rating of perceived exertion. (From Pandolf, K.B.: Influence of local and central factors in dominating rated perceived exertion during physical work, Percept. Mot. Skills 46:683, 1978.)

central is defined as cardiac and pulmonary sensations. In addition, an overall rating is requested. Therefore, in a graded test protocol, three ratings would be requested at least once during each stage.

It appears that sensory information must pass through several steps so that perceptual ratings can be expressed. Physiological consequences of exercise stimuli range from feedback from muscles and tendons to high breathing rates associated with the accumulation of high amounts of lactic acid. How these responses are mediated by the central nervous system and recognized as symptoms is not entirely clear. Symptoms are most likely filtered through a maze of stored data related to personality, motivation, past experience, health status, cultural patterns, etc. before being translated into perceptual ratings. For example, the intensity of the symptom is tested against whether the symptom had been experienced before and its previous consequences. The result of this integration is the assignment of a rating number or the adjustment of exercise effort to compensate for the sensation. The proposed steps in this process can be summarized as follows:

1. Exercise stimulus
2. Physiological response
3. Sensory response (symptomatology)
4. Reference filter
5. Perceptual intensity rating or physical adjustment

PRACTICAL CONSIDERATIONS

Experimentation with exercise perceptions has largely involved theoretical questions to date. However, several practical implications are evident from the data. These implications have a bearing on the conduct of exercise and sport programs.

One important practical consideration relates to controlling exercise intensity. Hospital-based and commercial exercise programs can often afford to directly monitor certain physiological variables that, when maintained at specified levels, control exercise intensity. Most individually initiated or school/community exercise programs necessitate less elaborate and less expensive techniques of control. Teaching people how to monitor their sensations would be an excellent way to accomplish intensity control under these circumstances. Recent research indicates that cardiac patients who maintain exercise intensities equivalent to a rating of 12 to 14 on the Borg scale stay approximately within the recommended exercise target heart rate (that is, 70% to 90% of heart rate range). Popular running literature urges joggers to "stay in touch" with their bodies, that is, to monitor feelings so that appropriate judgments can be made about adjustment of intensity. The "talk test," which cautions joggers to regulate pace so that talking with a companion is possible, is a practical suggestion that helps to control metabolism at an efficient level. It is known that when exercise is intense enough to produce lactic acid, respiration increases precipitously. Such an intensity will not allow comfortable talk and will bring the jogger closer to fatigue. Another example can be drawn from the research of William P. Morgan at the University of Wisconsin. His work identified two types of cognitive styles in marathon runners.[23] The more successful runners practiced what is called *association*.

These runners are in constant contact with their body functions and attempt to adjust pace based on their perceptions. The less successful marathoners mostly practiced *dissociation,* which diverts the attention from body function to ''more pleasant'' thoughts to relieve boredom and discomfort. Association is thought to be the preferential behavior for the purpose of precise control. Dissociation could be harmful, since it literally means ''losing touch'' with the body.

Preliminary studies indicate that practice with the Borg scale may help individuals evaluate sensations and maintain target intensity levels, for example, heart rate.[28] Asking exercisers to rate various running velocities and providing them with heart rate feedback provides a sense of their prescribed target level. Of course, they must be cautioned that increased environmental heat or altitude will necessitate an adjustment. Also, patients who have ischemic cardiac responses with no chest discomfort have to be especially careful in using this procedure.

Experiences with uphill and downhill running are often prescribed as beneficial for the road runner. Experiments have found that joggers do not fully compensate for increased metabolic rates in uphill running by decreasing their speed.[42] Practice with sensation/heart rate relationships in a number of environmental situations is probably necessary for more exact control of exercise intensity.

Sports coaches and physical education teachers have used the concept of percentage intensity assignments as a means of prescribing intensity and motivation for many years. Athletes are asked to swim or run a lap at 80% intensity and football players are urged to give 110% for their alma mater. Knowledge of how perceptions increase as a function of exercise intensity increases would be helpful to both students/athletes and teachers/coaches. For example, it is assumed that 80% of maximal time for a given distance will result in a perceptual interpretation of 80%. This, in fact, is not always the case. Perceptual intensity, depending on the individual, may be more or less than real time intensity. Students have often been criticized for loafing when they have only interpreted their intensity to be different from what the instructor expected. Neither was in error relative to their own perception, but both were in error relative to the other's perception. Such situations require recognition of the possibility for this confusion and the ability of the teacher/coach to learn more about the student/athlete's perceptions. Discussion and performance feedback would instruct both the student/athlete and the teacher/coach. Track coaches have used this kind of feedback in a more practical form to teach athletes for many years. Recent research with swimming indicates that swimmers consistently swim at intensities higher than requested.

Ratings of exercise perception have become a common component of exercise stress evaluations. Knowledge of how an individual is responding physiologically is absolutely essential, but information about how the subject feels is likewise important. This is particularly true when physiological and psychological responses are out of synchrony. For example, cardiac patients have been observed to rate exercise sensations (ES) in a graded evaluation as 7 (very, very light) for the entire test. Such patients are either hiding their feelings or have rather serious perceptual defects that could result in overexertion. On the other hand, patients wanting remuneration for workmen's compensation or seeking early retirement have been known to rate work above 15 (hard) with heart rates below 100. Most likely such a response, showing a large physiological/psychological discrepency, is indicative of the need for counseling.

SUMMARY

Several physiological variables have been examined to discover possible internal cues for the setting of exercise perceptions. Although both heart rate and $\dot{V}O_2$ increase in a parallel fashion with RPE, neither seems to adequately explain the perceptual rise during exercise of increasing intensity. Pulmonary ventilation, since it is known to be systematically sensed, has been the subject of experimentation. This variable is strongly linked to perception at exercise intensities above 70% $\dot{V}O_2$ max. Below this level the ventilatory cue may be masked by other competing cues. Catecholamines, especially norepinephrine, may also play a role in heavy exercise. When runners receive a supplement of blood glucose during long-duration exercise, their perceptions are lower than after receiving a placebo substance. The central nervous system is implicated in this response. Finally, although several studies have found significant relationships between lactate acid production and exercise perceptions, others have failed to support this anaerobic by-product as a definite cue. Since perceptual ratings provide a gestalt view of how the body senses its exercise experience, perhaps all of these variables share responsibility for sensory input. Exactly how they interact during various types of exercise is yet to be explained. However, the concept of perceived exertion is being used beneficially in many practical environments.

KEY TERMS

Borg scale a psychophysical scale that translates perceptions of exertion into numerical ratings (RPE).

central rating a rating of exertion usually associated with the cardiorespiratory system and generally located in the chest region.

cognitive association a cognitive strategy during exercise in which attention is maintained on body functions.

cognitive dissociation a cognitive strategy during exercise in which attention is directed away from body functions.

differentiated ratings the local and central ratings of perceived exertion.

local rating a rating of exertion sensed at the site of primary muscle contraction, for example, the legs during cycling.

overall rating (undifferentiated rating) a rating of exertion associated with the entire body undifferentiated as to anatomical location or physiological system.

RPE rating of perceived exertion.

REVIEW QUESTIONS

1. Explain how the Borg scale was developed and assess its reliability and validity.

2. Describe the relationship between heart rate and perceived exertion in both general and specific terms.

3. How does the walking and running experiment indicate the presence of a local factor involvement in perceived exertion?

4. Why does perceived exertion continue to rise throughout a marathon run when performance time (minute/mile) may be relatively stable?

5. What role does pulmonary ventilation play in the setting of perceived exertion at both lower and higher exercise intensities?

6. We often think of lactic acid accumulation as being synonymous with muscular fatigue. How is this variable related to perceived exertion?

7. How might the use of differentiated ratings of perceived exertion be valuable in the assessment of progressive physical fatigue?

8. Given what you know about the increase in pulmonary ventilation at the so-called anaerobic threshold and the general response of RPE to endurance exercise, why might the talk test be a useful means of regulating exercise intensity?

REFERENCES

1. Bakers, J.H.C.M., and Tenney, S.M.: The perception of some sensations associated with breathing, Respir. Physiol. **10**:85, 1970.

2. Bar-Or, O., Skinner, J.S., Buskirk, E.R., and others: Physiological and perceptual indicators of physical stress in 41 to 60 year old men who vary in conditioning level and in body fitness, Med. Sci. Sports **4**:96, 1972.

3. Bell, C.W.: Perceptual, biochemical and physiological responses in long term work, an investigation of the influence of glucose ingestion, unpublished doctoral dissertation, University of Pittsburgh, 1975.

4. Bergstrom, R.M., Halttunen, P.K., and Viljanen, A.V.: The voluntary regulation of breathing in man, Acta Physiol. Scand. **84**:428, 1972.

5. Boje, O.: Energy production, pulmonary ventilation and length of steps in well-trained runners working on a treadmill, Acta Physiol. Scand. **7**:362, 1944.

6. Borg, G.: A simple rating scale for use in physical work tests, Kungl Fysiografiska Sallskapets I Lund Forhandlinger, **31**:1962.

7. Borg, G., and Noble, B.J.: Perceived exertion, Exerc. Sport Sci. Rev. **2**:131, 1974.

8. Cafarelli, E., and Noble, B.J.: The effect of inspired CO_2 on subjective estimates of exertion, Ergonomics **79**:581, 1976.

9. Davies, C.T.M., Few, J.D., Foster, K.G., and others: Plasma catecholamine concentration during dynamic exercise involving different muscle groups. Cited in Sargeant, A.J., and Davies, C.T.M.: Perceived exertion during rhythmic exercise involving different muscle masses, J. Hum. Ergol. **2**:3, 1973.

10. Docktor, R., and Sharkey, B.J.: Note on some physiological and subjective reactions to exercise and training, Percept. Mot. Skills **32**:233, 1971.

11. Edwards, R.H.T., Melcher, A., Hesser, C.M., and others: Physiological correlates of perceived exertion in continuous and intermittent exercise with the same average power output, Eur. J. Clin. Invest. **2**:108, 1972.

12. Ekblom, B., and Goldbarg, A.N.: The influence of physical training and other factors on the subjective rating of perceived exertion, Acta Physiol. Scand. **83:**399, 1971.

13. Frankenhaeuser, M., Post, B., Nordheden, B., and others: Physiological and subjective reactions to different physical work loads, Percept. Mot. Skills **28:**343, 1969.

14. Gamberale, F.: Perceived exertion, heart rate, oxygen uptake and blood lactate in different work operations, Ergonomics **15:**545, 1972.

15. Howley, E.T.: The effect of different intensities of exercise on the excretion of epinephrine and norepinephrine, Med. Sci. Sports **8:**219, 1976.

16. Hueting, J.E., and Sarphati, H.R.: Measuring fatigue, J. Appl. Psychol. **50:**535, 1966.

17. Hueting, J.E., and Poulus, A.J.: Amphetamine, performance, effort and fatigue, Proceedings of Netherlands Society for Physiology and Pharmacology, Eleventh Federation Meeting of Medical-Biological Societies, Amsterdam, 1970.

18. Kay, C., and Shephard, R.J.: On muscle strength and the threshold of anaerobic work, Int. Zangew. Physiol. **27:**311, 1969.

19. Kinsman, R.A., and Weiser, P.C.: Subjective symptomatology during work and fatigue. In Simonson, E., and Weiser, P.C., editors: Psychological aspects and physiological correlates of work and fatigue, Springfield, Illinois, 1976, Charles C Thomas, Publisher.

20. Michael, E., and Eckardt, L.: The selection of hard work by trained and non-trained subjects, Med. Sci. Sports **4:**107, 1972.

21. Michael, E., and Hackett, P.: Physiological variables related to the selection of work effort on a treadmill and bicycle, Res. Q. **43:**216, 1972.

22. Morgan, W.P., and Borg, G.: Perception of effort in the prescription of physical activity. In Craig, T., editor: Mental health and emotional aspects of sports, Chicago, 1976, American Medical Association.

23. Morgan, W.P., and Pollock, M.L.: Psychologic characterization of the elite distance runner. Conference on the marathon: physiological, medical epidemiological and psychological studies, New York, 1976, The New York Academy of Sciences.

24. Noble, B.J., and Borg, G.: Perceived exertion during walking and running, Proceedings of the Seventeenth International Congress of Applied Psychology, Liege, Belgium, 1971.

25. Noble, B.J., Metz, K.F., Pandolf, K.B., and others: Perceived exertion during walking and running. II, Med. Sci. Sports **5:**116, 1973.

26. Noble, B.J.: Perceived exertion during a marathon run: a case study, unpublished manuscript, 1976.

27. Noble, B.J., and Norris, R.: Reliability of perceived exertion ratings, unpublished manuscript, 1974.

28. Noble, B.J.: The use of perceived exertion to control exercise intensity, unpublished manuscript, 1972.

29. Noble, B.J.: Physiological basis of perceived exertion: a tentative explanatory model, unpublished manuscript, 1977.

30. Noble, B.J., Maresh, C.M., Allison, T.G., and others: Cardiorespiratory and perceptual recovery from a marathon run, Med. Sci. Sports **3:**239, 1979.

31. Pandolf, K.B., Cafarelli, E., Noble, B.J., and others: Perceptual responses during prolonged work, Percept. Mot. Skills **35:**975, 1972.

32. Pandolf, K.B., and Noble, B.J.: The effect of pedaling speed and resistance changes on perceived exertion for equivalent power outputs on the bicycle ergometer, Med. Sci. Sports **5**:132, 1973.

33. Pandolf, K.B.: Influence of local and central factors in dominating rated perceived exertion during physical work, Percept. Mot. Skills **46**:683, 1978.

34. Pandolf, K.B., Burse, R.L., and Goldman, R.F.: Differentiated ratings of perceived exertion during physical conditioning of older individuals using leg-weight loading, Percept. Mot. Skills **40**:563, 1975.

35. Robertson, R.J.: The effect of exercise duration on the psychophysical and physiological responses to walking and running, unpublished doctoral dissertation, University of Pittsburgh, 1973.

36. Robertson, R.J., Gillespie, R.L., McCarthy, J., and others: Differentiated perceptions of exertion. Part I, Percept. Mot. Skills **49**:683, 1979.

37. Robertson, R.J., Gillespie, R.L., McCarthy, J., and others: Differentiated perceptions of exertion. Part II, Percept. Mot. Skills **49**:691, 1979.

38. Sargeant, A.J., and Davies, C.T.M.: Perceived exertion during rhythmic exercise involving different muscle masses, J. Hum. Ergol. **2**:3, 1973.

39. Skinner, J.S., Hutsler, R., Bergsteinova, V., and others: The validity and reliability of a rating scale of perceived exertion, Med. Sci. Sports **5**:94, 1973.

40. Skinner, J.S., Borg, G.A.V., and Buskirk, E.R.: Physiological and perceptual reactions to exertion of young men differing in activity and body size. In Franks, B.D., editor: Exercise and fitness, Chicago, 1969, The Athletic Institute.

41. Stamford, B.A., and Noble, B.J.: Metabolic cost and perception of effort during bicycle erogmeter work performance, Med. Sci. Sports **6**:226, 1974.

42. Smith, S.L.: Perceived exertion and heart rate control, doctoral dissertation, University of Pittsburgh, 1973.

43. Turner, M.G.: The effects of positive and negative work on differentiated ratings of perceived exertion, masters thesis, University of Wyoming, 1979.

44. Weiser, P.C.: Interrelationships of the motor and metabolic support systems during work and fatigue. In Simonson, E., and Weiser, P.C., editors: Psychological aspects of fatigue, Springfield, Ill., 1974, Charles C Thomas, Publisher.

45. West, D.W.M., Ellis, C.G., and Campbell, E.J.M.: Ability of man to detect increases in his breathing, J. Appl. Physiol. **39**:372, 1975.

SUGGESTED READINGS

Borg, G.A.V.: Psychophysical bases of perceived exertion, Med. Sci. Sports Exerc. **14**:377, 1982.

Borg, G., and Noble, B.J.: Perceived exertion, Exerc. Sport Sci. Rev. **2**:131, 1974.

Mihevic, P.M.: Cardiovascular fitness and the psychophysics of perceived exertion, Res. Q. Exerc. Sport **54**:239, 1983.

Noble, B.J.: Practical application of perceived exertion, Med. Sci. Sports Exerc. **14**:406, 1982.

Noble, B.J., and Allen, J.G.: Perceived exertion in swimming, Swimming Technique **21**:11, 1984.

Noble, B.J., Borg, G.A.V., Jacobs, I., and others: A category—ration perceived exertion scale: relationship and muscle lactates and heart rate, Med. Sci. Sports Exerc. **15**:523, 1983.

Pandolf, K.B.: Influence of local and central factors in dominating rated perceived exertion during physical work, Percept. Mot. Skills **46:**683, 1978.

Reilly, T., and Ball, D.: The net physiological cost of dribbling a soccer ball, Res. Q. Exerc. Sport **55:**267, 1984.

Stephenson, L.A., Kolka, M.A., and Wilkerson, J.E.: Perceived exertion and anaerobic threshold during the menstrual cycle, Med. Sci. Sports Exerc. **14:**218, 1982.

CASE STUDY 1

As a physical education teacher you are often called on to document changes that take place in your students over a period of time. Often physiological tests are time-consuming and require expensive equipment. However, it is possible to predict these changes from perceptual data that we know to be directly related to variables like HR and oxygen consumption.

Let's take as an example a 16-year-old high school girl. You, as the physical education teacher, want to measure perceptual changes that occur over the course of a school year. Simply ask the student to run, step up on a bench, or ride a stationary bicycle at three arbitrarily determined submaximal levels in which the loads and rates can be controlled rather rigorously. Bench stepping (18 inches) is a practical example. The three loads, lasting 2 minutes each, with at least 5 minutes recovery time between loads, can be controlled by having the student step in cadence with a metronome (12, 24, 36 steps/min). During the last 15 seconds of each load, the student is asked to rate her exertion on the Borg scale. The load (ft-lb/min) can be determined by the formula: bench height (ft) × body weight (lb) × stepping rate (steps/min). For example, 1.5 ft × 100 lb × 12 steps/min = 1800 ft-lb/min.

Repeating this test at the end of the year should provide a clear indication of change, if it has occurred, and a new estimate of the student's working capacity. Such a test is relatively quick, reasonably valid, and easy to manage.

CASE STUDY 2

With a very general interpretation, Borg's prediction equation for heart rate (RPE × 10 = HR, for example, 15 [hard] × 10 = 150) is useful. However, because factors other than HR are involved in setting the perception, you cannot expect a perfect prediction. How can we explain the extreme ratings that do not conform to the prediction?

Consider the seventh grade football player who rates his exercise effort as very, very light (7) throughout every exercise intensity of a graded exercise test. To fully evaluate this response, additional data must be recorded. The easiest method of interpretation would be to determine simultaneous HRs. For example, if HRs of 130, 150, and 170 beats per minute were recorded on a bike test using work loads of 300, 600, and 900 kg/min, Borg's formula would predict ratings of 13, 15, and 17. Ratings of 7 at each load would indicate that the perception was certainly not predictive of physiological effort. Not even a high pain threshold could possibly explain this "macho" response. Assuming that instructions were adequately explained and understood, it would be best to look for reasons other than physiological to explain this large perceptual discrepency. Possibly such a player was trying to impress you, the coach, with his ability to give 110% without complaint.

Another extreme sometimes observed is the student who rates effort to be hard (15) or very hard (17) in the presence of evidence that cardiac cost is low, for example, HR = 100 or 120. Again, it is unlikely that a student would be so out of shape or have such a low pain threshold to account for the perceptual response. It would be best to look for an ulterior motive. For instance, some teachers place unfit students in the weight room and will not allow them to engage in regular activities. Weight lifting may be a preferred activity. Of course, many other explanations are possible.

Both extreme responses discussed require additional counseling by the teacher or other specialist.

CASE STUDY 3

A sophomore swimmer races in the 500 yard freestyle in a high school swimming meet. His time is 6:49 with 100 yard splits of 72, 82, 78, 92, and 84 seconds. The coach suggests the swimmer has "gone out" too fast; however, the swimmer indicates that he had a great deal left at the end. Further inquiry reveals that the swimmer thought he was maintaining an even pace. Performance improvement in this swimmer requires knowledge of, and practice in, pacing.

What must the swimmer learn to acquire a sense of pace? First, the swimmer must learn how he feels at various paces of the 100 yard freestyle. Second, he must connect these feelings with the actual time, particularly the predicted race time. Third, he must practice swimming repeat 100s at the correct "feeling" and match this against time.

Let's assume that our swimmer has a maximal 100 yard freestyle time of 65 seconds. Therefore, a predicted race goal of 78 seconds, if maintained over 500 yards, would result in a performance increase of 18 seconds. This pace would be approximately 83% of maximum. Next, the swimmer is asked to swim 100s at 70%, 80%, and 90% of maximum, perceptually determined. With this information the coach can ask the swimmer to repeat certain performances while the swimmer is given periodic time feedback, for example, slow it up a bit or that's just right. The swimmer should be asked to concentrate on his feelings so that times can be repeated using this information.

Although even pacing in a race is theoretically the most efficient procedure, it should be remembered that swimming one 100 is not the same as swimming five back-to-back 100s. A fatigue drop-off is likely. However, the goal of even pacing is not impossible.

Making athletes aware of pacing may improve their performance significantly. It should not be viewed as a substitute for hard training but as a valuable supplement.

GLOSSARY

acclimation physiological change in response to heat stress caused by artificial environments, such as saunas.

acclimatization physiological change in response to heat stress caused by natural environments, such as a visit to a hotter environment.

acute hypoxic exposure hypoxia experienced over a period of minutes to several weeks.

adaptation general term referring to the ability of organisms to adjust to their environments.

adenosine triphosphate (ATP) a high-energy phosphate bond that serves as the immediate source of energy for muscle contraction.

adipose tissue hyperplasia increasing the number of adipocytes.

adipose tissue hypertrophy enlargement of existing adipocytes.

adolescence transition period between childhood and adult development.

adolescent growth spurt rapid acceleration in stature at the onset of puberty.

aerobic literally, ''with oxygen''; refers to one of two metabolic systems that produce ATP for muscle contraction. The other system is anaerobic.

aerobic power the maximal amount of oxygen that can be consumed per minute during maximal exercise.

afferent refers to neurons that carry sensory impulses from the periphery to the spinal cord.

aging decreasing ability to adapt.

all-or-none law the law stating that when either a muscle or a nerve fiber is stimulated above threshold, it will respond maximally.

amino acids the basic chemical building blocks of protein in food.

AMS acute mountain sickness.

anabolic related to protein synthesis, muscle building.

anabolic steroids synthetic derivative of testosterone used by athletes, which retains the property of protein synthesis.

anaerobic literally, ''without oxygen''; refers to one of two metabolic systems that produce ATP for muscle contraction. The other system is aerobic.

anaerobic decay the decline of peak anaerobic power output with repeated maximal contractions over time (usually <60 seconds). This measurement is said to indirectly estimate the capacity of the lactic acid system.

anaerobic power the maximal ability of the anaerobic systems (ATP-PC and lactic acid) to produce energy.

androgenic related to promoting male secondary sex characteristics.

anemia a condition marked by a below normal red blood cell concentration.

association the act of combining.

535

athletic pseudonephritis a transient condition found in athletes following exercise and marked by the increased excretion of protein, cells, and other substances. This condition mimics a kidney disease known as glomerular nephritis.

atmosphere one atmosphere is the pressure associated with sea level (760 mm Hg). Two atmospheres is experienced at 10 meters (33 feet) below sea level and is equivalent to the weight of a column of water 10 meters high plus the barometric pressure (1,520 mm Hg).

A-V oxygen difference the difference in oxygen saturation between arterial and venous blood.

basal metabolic rate the minimal energy expenditure necessary to maintain life.

beta blockers drugs that block beta adrenergic receptors in the heart, resulting in reduced heart rate and blood pressure.

blood doping slang term for induced erythrocythemia.

blood pressure the pressure measured in the vascular system that is associated with cardiac contraction (systolic) and relaxation (diastolic).

body composition division of the body into two principal tissue components—fat and lean.

body core central portion of the body. The temperature of the core (98.6° F [37° C]) is measured in the rectum, esophagus, or tympanum.

body shell casing of the body, the skin, which is the interface between the body and the environment at which heat dissipation takes place.

Bohr effect the shift of the oxyhemoglobin dissociation curve to the right as a function of increased P_{CO_2} and lower pH.

Borg scale a psychophysical scale that translates perceptions of exertion into numerical ratings (RPE).

bradycardia a condition in which the heart rate is lower than normal.

calorimetry a means of determining caloric values by measurement of heat produced, either through direct combustion of food samples or through measurement of changes in temperature brought about by the metabolism of food.

cardiac catheterization a technique that measures heart function in which a catheter is passed through a vein into the heart.

cardiac output the amount of blood pumped from the heart each minute.

cardiovascular enhancer ergogenic aids that promote efficient function of the cardiovascular system.

central rating a rating of exertion usually associated with the cardiorespiratory system and generally located in the chest region.

chronic hypoxic exposure hypoxia experienced over a period of months to a lifetime.

chronological age age from birth.

clo measurement unit used to evaluate the heat transfer value of clothing.

cognitive association a cognitive strategy during exercise in which attention is maintained on body functions.

cognitive dissociation a cognitive strategy during exercise in which attention is directed away from body functions.

cold tolerance the ability of the body to adapt its physiological processes to protect against cold temperatures.

cold zone homoiothermy maintained by thermogenesis (increasing metabolic rate above normal).

concentric contraction force created by shortening of muscle, as in the up portion of a push-up; sometimes referred to as positive exercise.

conduction movement of heat from one tissue to another, caused by physical contact with a temperaure gradient (high to low).

contraction since this term usually implies change in length of muscle, generally shortening, and we know that other length changes are possible (lengthening), contraction should be defined as the "attempt to shorten."

convection movement of heat from the body by circulation of air or water across its surface.

cool zone heat conservation is necessary but increased heat production by increasing metabolic rate is not required.

cutaneous vasoconstriction the process by which skin blood vessels are compressed to reduce blood flow and, therefore, loss of body heat.

decompression literally, ''to free from pressure''; in underwater physiology, to return the body to sea-level pressure after exposure to deep underwater pressure.

dehydration excessive water loss.

densiometry measurement of body density for the purpose of determining body fat and lean proportions.

depressants substances that decrease the body's vital functions.

differentiated ratings the local and central ratings of perceived exertion.

dissociation the act of separating.

doping slang term for the intake of substances that may provide a performance advantage.

double blind a research technique in which neither the researcher nor the subject know the contents of the substance provided.

dynamic exercise exercise marked by a change in joint angle, sometimes referred to as isotonic exercise.

dysbarism decompression sickness, such as the bends, resulting from too rapid decompression.

dyspnea difficult or labored breathing.

eccentric contraction force created by lengthening of muscle, as in the down portion of a push-up; sometimes referred to as negative exercise.

echocardiography a technique that measures heart function in which sound waves are reflected from heart structures.

efferent refers to neurons that carry motor impulses from the spinal cord to an effector organ in the periphery, that is, skeletal muscle.

electrocardiography a technique that measures electrical changes during the cardiac cycle.

electrolytes ions, primarily sodium, potassium, and chloride, that play an important role in water balance.

embolism obstruction of a blood vessel—in underwater physiology, usually by an air bubble.

epinephrine a hormone secreted by the adrenal medulla that stimulates ATP production by its action on fat and muscle cells.

ergogenic aids substances and phenomena that are work-producing aids; these aids are thought to enhance performance above levels anticipated under normal conditions.

euhydration normal hydration ($\pm 1\%$ to 2%).

evaporation transfer of water to water vapor, with a resulting decrease in temperature of the object previously holding the water.

excess postexercise oxygen consumption (EPOC) oxygen consumption greater than resting values recorded during the recovery period following exercise.

exercise proteinuria excess protein in the urine following exercise.

fatty acids one of the basic chemical building blocks of fat in food. Fatty acids are used as a fuel for aerobic metabolism.

fiber the cylindrical cell, ranging in length from 2 to 50 mm, which makes up skeletal muscle.

fiber type muscle fibers are characterized (typed) according to their contractile speed (fast or slow) or metabolic capacities (oxidative or glycolytic).

glomerular filtration rate (GFR) the rate at which blood entering the kidney is filtered through the glomerulus.

glucagon a hormone secreted by the pancreas that stimulates ATP production by its action on fat cells and the liver.

glucose a monosaccharide carbohydrate used as a fuel for aerobic and anaerobic metabolism.

glycogen the storage form of glucose.

glycogen depletion the removal of carbohydrates from storage in muscle tissue or liver resulting from long-duration, high-intensity exercise.

glycogen repletion the process of restoring carbohydrates in muscle tissue or liver following long-duration, high-intensity exercise.

glycolysis the anaerobic process by which glycogen is broken down to lactic acid to produce ATP for muscular contraction.

glycolytic enzymes substances that cause or accelerate the process of anaerobic glycolysis, for example, phosphofructokinase.

growth increasing ability to adapt.

HAPE high altitude pulmonary edema.

heart rate the number of times the heart beats each minute.

heat strain response of the body to the heat stress.

heat stress temperature stimulus acting on the body.

hematocrit the percentage of red blood cells in blood.

hemoglobin complex iron-protein molecule important in the transport of oxygen and carbon dioxide in blood.

high altitude altitudes above 3,048 meters (10,000 feet). The likelihood of both AMS and performance decrements is high.

high-density lipoprotein (HDL) a lipoprotein fraction of total cholesterol responsible for breaking down cholesterol; also thought to protect against coronary artery disease.

hyperbarism increased barometric pressure.

hypercapnia excess carbon dioxide content in the blood.

hyperoxia excess oxygen content.

hyperplasia change in tissue cross section caused by growth of new fibers.

hyperpnea increase in depth and rate of breathing as with exercise.

hypertrophy the increased cross-sectional dimension of the muscle fiber.

hyperventilation increased air in the lungs above normal. Can lead to respiratory alkalosis due to washing out of carbon dioxide from the blood.

hypocapnia low carbon dioxide content in the blood.

hypoventilation decreased air in the lungs below normal. Can lead to respiratory acidosis due to retention of carbon dioxide in the blood.

hypoxia low oxygen content.

induced erythrocythemia technique for increasing red blood cells by withdrawing blood, storing it, and reinfusing it in the same person at a later date.

insulin a hormone secreted by the pancreas that promotes the uptake of blood glucose and amino acid by the cells. This hormone also inhibits the effects of epinephrine and glucagon.

isocapnia normal carbon dioxide content.

isokinetic contraction dynamic contraction in which the speed of movement is constant throughout a range of movement.

isokinetic exercise exercise in which the angular velocity of muscle contraction is held constant.

isometric contraction muscular force resulting in no change in muscle length or movement of the skeleton.

isometric exercise exercise in which tension is produced without changing the joint angle, also referred to as static exercise.

kilocalorie (kcal) the unit of measure used to describe both energy intake and energy expenditure.

Krebs cycle also known as the tricarboxylic acid cycle; describes the mechanism by which carbohydrate, fat, and protein are degraded to carbon dioxide, hydrogen ions, and electrons. The electrons are subsequently transported to oxygen, forming water and energy (ATP).

lactic acid an end product of anaerobic glycolysis.

left ventricular hypertrophy increasing the cross section of the heart's left ventricle.

life expectancy probable age of death.

life span maximal attainable age.

local rating a rating of exertion sensed at the site of primary muscle contraction, for example, the legs during cycling.

low altitude any altitude below 1,524 meters (5,000 feet). The likelihood of AMS and performance decrements is low.

low-density lipoprotein (LDL) a lipoprotein fraction of total cholesterol responsible for transporting triglycerides in the blood.

maximal exercise exercise that continues to exhaustion or until maximal physiological values are attained.

menarche onset of menstruation.

MET one MET is equivalent to resting metabolic rate. Thus, 5 MET would refer to a metabolic rate that is five times that of rest.

metabolic rate the rate at which the body produces energy and, therefore, heat. This variable is used as a measure of the degree to which the body adapts to the cold.

metabolism the chemical changes within the body that provide energy and maintain life.

minerals physiological compounds that regulate functions such as oxygen transport, excitability of muscle and nerve tissue, acid-base balance, and water metabolism.

minimal weight the lowest safe weight for athletic competition, usually associated with wrestling.

moderate altitude any altitude between 1,524 and 3,048 meters (5,000 and 10,000 feet). Probable performance decrements and variable occurrence of AMS occur here. Usually the cabin pressure of jet aircraft is kept between 5,000 and 8,000 feet.

motor unit a single motor neuron (efferent) and all the muscle fibers that it innervates.

narcosis unconsciousness.

neuromuscular junction the anatomical site at which the neuron's axon terminates in muscle tissue. Also called the motor endplate.

neuron the basic anatomical unit of the nervous system. It consists of a cell body, dendrites, and an axon.

obesity fat accumulation greater than 15% above normal.

onset of blood lactate accumulation (OBLA) the point at which lactic acid concentration begins to increase in the blood.

osmolality a measure of the number of particles contained in a solution.

osteoporosis decrease in bone density often associated with aging.

overall rating (undifferentiataed rating) a rating of exertion associated with the entire body undifferentiated as to anatomical location or physiological system.

oxygen consumption the amount of oxygen that the body consumes each minute.

oxygen debt a term that has been used to explain the excess postexercise oxygen consumption.

oxyhemoglobin chemical combination of oxygen with hemoglobin.

P partial pressure (tension) of a gas.

peak anaerobic power output an indirect measurement of the ATP-PC system in which the highest production of power ($kg\text{-}m \cdot sec^{-1}$) is recorded during maximal exercise over a short period of time (<10 seconds).

percentage of maximal oxygen consumption (%$\dot{V}o_2$ max) a measurement unit used to express the intensity of physiological effort. For example, exercising at 50% $\dot{V}o_2$ max would demonstrate an exercise intensity one-half of one's maximal ability to consume oxygen.

phosphocreatine a substance found in limited quantities in muscle cells that when broken down anaerobically provides inorganic phosphate necessary to reconstitute ATP.

phosphorylation the process by which inorganic phosphate is provided so that adenosine triphosphate can be reconstituted from adenosine diphosphate.

physiological age (also **developmental age**) age based on maturation of the body, usually the skeleton, according to established norms.

placebo a substance appearing like but not having the effect of the authentic substance.

plasma clearance the extent to which the kidney excretes unwanted substances.

power performance of work with time as a consideration ($P = W \times T^{-1}$). Power is measured in watts.

proprioception the peripheral control process by which feedback is provided concerning position, length, and tension in muscles, tendons, or joints.

puberty attainment of sexual maturity.

pubescent arriving at puberty.

radiation movement of heat from one object to another without direct physical contact and in proportion to the temperature difference between the objects (high to low temperature).

reabsorption the process by which the kidney returns usable substances to the blood.

reflex arc an anatomical unit that conducts impulses via an afferent neuron through the spinal cord and directly into an efferent neuron, producing an involuntary response in an effector organ.

renal blood flow (RBF) the rate at which blood enters the kidney (glomerulus) through the afferent arteriole.

respiratory enzymes substances that cause or accelerate the process of aerobic energy production, for example, succinate dehydrogenase.

respiratory exchange ratio (R) the ratio of carbon dioxide produced and oxygen consumed used as a measure of nutrient use.

RPE rating of perceived exertion.

sarcomere the basic contractile unit in the muscle fiber.

scuba self-contained underwater breathing apparatus.

shivering involuntary muscle contraction by which the body can increase its metabolic rate and adjust to cold temperatures.

skinfold measurement determination of fat-pad thickness at various anatomical sites for the purpose of predicting total body fat percentage.

sliding filament hypothesis the proposition that explains how protein filaments within the sarcomere move to cause muscle fiber contraction.

somatotype determination of body structure by identifying the relative contributions of three components: endomorph (flesh), mesomorph (muscle), and ectomorph (linearity).

specific dynamic action an increase in metabolic rate associated with the digestion of food.

spot reduction the theory that exercise over a specific anatomical area (spot) will result in exclusive fat reduction in that area.

stimulants substances that enhance the body's vital functions.

stroke volume the amount of blood pumped from the heart with each beat.

submaximal exercise exercise at an intensity below that observed for maximal exercise.

synapse an anatomical unit that serves as the connective link between neurons.

thermogenesis production of heat by physiological processes.

torque production of angular force, for example, in an isokinetic test.

torr barometric pressure measured in millimeters of mercury (mm Hg).

total anaerobic power output synonymous with anaerobic power output, reflecting the actions of both the ATP-PC and the lactic acid systems, specifically associated with the total production of power over a 30-second period (Wingate test).

ventricular mass the size of the left ventricular walls, which may increase (hypertrophy) with certain types of training.

ventricular volume the size of the left ventricular cavity, which may increase (hypertrophy) with certain types of training.

vitamins essential elements of daily nutrition that regulate metabolic processes.

volume stress the stimulus for the increase in cardiac stroke volume, thought to be a result of training that exposes the heart to high levels of blood exchange.

$\dot{V}o_2$ **max** maximal oxygen consumption or aerobic power.

W watts, a unit of power.

work when muscular contraction results in shortening (concentric) of muscle, the resulting body movement is considered work ($W = f \times d$). Work is also performed when muscles lengthen (eccentric), in which case, muscles are said to be worked on. Since work does not involve time, which is usually the case in sport and exercise, and can be accomplished when no movement occurs ($d = 0$), such as with isometric force, "exercise" is the preferred term to use as an encompassing term for force created by muscular contraction within the context of sport and exercise.

zone of intolerable cold maintenance of homoiothermy is impossible (core temperature falls).

zone of thermal comfort narrow thermal zone in which homoiothermy is maintained.

INDEX

Page numbers with *t* designate a table appears on the page.